Perspectives in Basic and Applied Toxicology

Perspectives in Basic and Applied Toxicology

Edited by

BRYAN BALLANTYNE
MD, DSc, PhD, MFOM, FAACT, FRCPath, FIBiol, DATS
Director of Applied Toxicology, Union Carbide Corporation, USA
Adjunct Professor of Toxicology and Pharmacology
University of West Virginia, USA

WRIGHT
London Boston Durban Singapore Sydney Toronto Wellington

John Wright
is an imprint of Butterworth Scientific

First published 1988

British Library Cataloguing in Publication Data

Perspectives in basic and applied toxicology.
1. Toxicology
I. Ballantyne, Bryan
615.9 RA1211

ISBN 0-7236-0837-7

Photoset by
Mathematical Composition Setters Ltd, 7 Ivy Street, Salisbury, Wiltshire
Printed and bound by
Butler & Tanner, Frome, Somerset

Preface

This book is a collection of essays on various aspects of toxicology for which there is a need for review, or which are not given sufficient attention in textbooks and monographs on toxicology. An objective in many of these contributions is to relate fundamental knowledge of toxicology, gained in the laboratory, to its application in assessing relevance of that information to the causation of adverse health effects, predicting hazardous situations, defining protective and precautionary measures, and the recognition and management of intoxication in humans. It is hoped that this volume will be informative and of use to undergraduate and graduate toxicologists, pharmacologists, physicians, industrial hygienists, and other health professionals.

The past decade has seen very marked changes in the scope and practice of toxicology, as well as in attitudes towards the interpretation, implications, and applications of toxicological knowledge. Some of these changes are scientifically, ethically and professionally desirable, others are not.

Toxicology conducted for safety evaluation purposes must be one of the most regulated areas of contemporary science. Quality control and good laboratory practice should be central to any investigational procedure. Thus it is abhorrent that the need for regulated toxicology was highlighted by individuals within certain contract and consulting laboratories who falsified reports, and even inserted non-existent data. National and international regulations governing the toxicology testing requirements for materials used in particular applications are now beginning to develop some scientific rationalization, but this is still at an early stage. All too often the regulations tabulate a 'shopping list of requirements', irrespective of all the factors that need to be taken into account during hazard evaluation. In many instances the methodology to be applied is specified, sometimes in fine detail. This has led to an attitude with some organizations of undertaking toxicology testing procedures merely to 'satisfy the regulations', rather than undertaking investigations appropriate to assessing toxicity, evaluating hazard, and allowing the development of protective and precautionary measures. Clearly this attitude is conducive to malpractices, inappropriate testing, excessive use of *in vivo* procedures, and may result in documentation which will not allow a reasonable assessment of 'in-use' hazards. Thus, the currently less than satisfactory system may result in testing that is carried out 'according to the regulatory cookbook', producing studies which may not be totally appropriate for evaluating potential adverse health effects because of an absence of basic and applied scientific rationalization in their design. The development of a toxicology testing programme for any given material requires an in-depth consideration of a multiplicity of factors, which may be unique to that material or its intended use. In no way can a handbook of specified test requirements and specific protocols substitute for a careful and scientifically reasoned approach to toxicology testing. There is a clear need to maintain scientific integrity, to analyse the reasons for conducting a series of studies, and be continually aware of the ethical and moral aspects of conducting health-related studies. An integrated approach to satisfy all these factors emphasizes the need for a greater degree of cooperation and informed discussion between government, academia, and industry and their trade organization representatives. Europe has perhaps the lead in this respect, and certainly has much to teach the United States in terms of reasoned and reasonable approaches in the area of mandated toxicology testing.

An unfortunate trend, seen at its worst both in industry and government, is the manner in which toxicology and occupational medicine are organized. It is not unusual that health-related groups are directed by 'managers' lacking not only formal education and training in any of the health sciences, but also with little or no appreciation of biology and variability in biological systems. It is frequently reasoned that by having such a lay overview of professional activities, 'the various factors can be viewed in their widest perspective'! It may also be reasoned that such a structure allows the representation of 'best interest', to the partial exclusion of professional guidance. The ramifications of lay control of professional activity and expression argues for independence of recommendations in matters such as, for example, classification and permissible exposures. It is unfortunate that, even within central government, political and financial gains may override serious health concerns. Perhaps one of the most recent repulsive examples of this was the attempted prevention, by US White House personnel, of testimony by the US Surgeon General to a congressional hearing concerned with the banning of advertising relating to the smoking of cigarettes. It is well appreciated that the Office of Management and Budget has played a major and determining lead in weakening the Government's role in protecting the workplace, and the public in general, from environmental hazardous xenobiotics (*Lancet*, January 4, 1986, p. 33; February 8, 1986, pp. 325–326). Indeed, as this Preface is being written there has been a Presidential veto of a clean water bill, which he described rather curiously as being 'loaded with waste'! For someone who professes the sanctity of life by public exhibitions of abhorrence at abortion, there is a curious paradox in the same individual permitting increased likelihoods for developmentally toxic materials to harm the embryo and foetus as a consequence of allowing (policy directing) measures which allow decreased standards of public health.

An issue closely related to that of the lay control of professional activity is a trend that, irrespective of qualifications and experience, anyone can indulge in health hazard evaluation, including the interpretation and extrapolation of toxicology information. In an editorial entitled 'Everybody wants to be a Toxicologist' (*J. Toxicol., Cut. Ocular Toxicol.* **3**, 1 (1984)), Dr Edward M. Jackson has drawn attention to the desire of chemists, engineers and even lawyers to be toxicologists, and the potential consequences of this attitude. An appreciation of what constitutes an adverse health effect demands an in-depth knowledge of variability, and what constitutes normality, in biological systems. A sound knowledge of biology is an essential prerequisite to any training course in toxicology, and equally important is that the professional toxicologist maintain competence in the biological sciences.

An important feature of the past decade in toxicology has been the enhanced effort to develop and validate methods for the prediction, or confirmation, of adverse health effects based on *in vitro* approaches. This has been partly due to the activity of animal welfare groups, and in part to a continual recognition on the part of toxicologists of the need for such tests on scientific, ethical and economic grounds. Although many of these approaches hold considerable promise as routine screening procedures to assess the potential for adverse biological effects, at present many of the methods require that there be *in vivo* studies to confirm the results when a positive test is obtained, and to get a more precise definition of usable dose-response relationships. It is unfortunate, however, that a few groups are modifying methods in a manner which may give a less stringent assessment of toxicity (i.e. potential to harm), and hence a greater probability for product safety clearance. In some instances dose is decreased, using a supposed justification that the method gives a response more representative of the sensitivity of the human. In the long-term this can only have adverse product safety repercussions. Also disturbing in the area of developing tests for assessing potential human adverse health effects is the practice of patenting scientific methodology.

The results of toxicology studies, and their interpretation, may have far reaching implications for health-related issues in the workplace, home and general environment. These applied aspects of toxicology are frequently overshadowed by political, commercial, regulatory and technological issues and pressures. These factors may well lead to scientifically and ethically unsatisfactory conclusions and controls if the basic health issues are not reiterated and an impartial stance taken by the toxicologist. There are many examples which indicate that there is no utopia with respect to protection of mankind against xenobiotics, and it is thus of prime importance that the toxicologist and his professional colleagues should be sure of the ethical and moral foundations of their work and its implications, and that they should give impartial opinion in a professional manner. Unfortunately, and perhaps not unexpectedly, there is evidence that some toxicologists have too great a dependence on formal bureaucratic lines of authority and reporting. For example, Dr Daniel A. Bronstein evaluated responses from Society of Toxicology members, having a US mailing address, who replied to a questionnaire concerning potential ethical problems in the practice of toxicology (*Fund. Appl. Toxicol.* 7, 525 (1986)). One of his major conclusions from this restricted survey was that (some) toxicologists may not qualify as members of a 'learned profession', defined on the basis of independence of judgement. In a pathetically inadequate, and at times silly, response from the Ethics Committee of the Society of Toxicology (*Fund. Appl. Toxicol.* 7, 531 (1986)) they conclude with the amazing statement that, 'The use of an ethics questionnaire to arrive at Professor Bronstein's conclusions may be within the bounds of situational ethics but, certainly, is extraordinary in the eyes of one trained in the scientific method'!

There is no doubt that a small proportion of the toxicology community is ethically and morally deficient, and deliberately biased in their interpretations and extrapolation of toxicological information; the proportion is probably about the same as that for any other professional community. For the remaining majority, there is a constant need to examine social and moral values in the context of their work. Clearly there must be a sensible balance between the desirable and what is possible and acceptable with respect to protection of the community from xenobiotic-induced adverse health effects, but there should be a constant vigilance to avoid the inadequate.

Toxicity is concerned with defining the potential to develop adverse health effects, their nature, incidence, mechanism of production and reversibility. The implications with respect to human health are clear, as is the need to ensure that toxicology information is made available to the scientific and medical communities. It is my clear conviction that all information relating to human health should be accessible in a readily available form, and with all the information that is necessary to allow the reader to reach his own conclusions on the adequacy of the study design and conduct in terms of the objectives of the investigation, and to formulate his own conclusions. It is unfortunate that publication of information may be inhibited by considerations of security, commercial secrecy, and in a few cases an amoral desire not to inform of potential adverse health effects for certain products or processes. With respect to the US industrial situation, the likelihood for significant adverse health effects being overlooked or ignored has been markedly reduced by the substantial risk reporting requirement of Section 8(e) of the Toxic Substance Control Act. Ultimately there is nothing to be gained, and in most cases much to loose, from suppressing information which has a bearing on the causation of adverse human health effects, their recognition and management. Here perhaps more than with many other branches of knowledge, is the guidance of Albert Einstein appropriate: 'The right to search for truth implies also a duty. One must not conceal any part of what one has recognized as true.'

One objective of this deliberately provocative and irate Preface is to encourage those with responsibility for the training of toxicologists to instill a greater concern about ethical and moral issues as fundamental to the practice of toxicology as a profession with wide-ranging social implications.

I wish to thank Ms Jacquie Cochran for conscientiously typing much of the manuscript for this book to be a standard format, and with the most professional of style and manner. It has been a pleasure to work with Mr Roy Baker of John Wright and to experience his guidance, tact and kindness. Finally, I wish to thank my wife, Yvonne B. Ballantyne, for her never failing patience and support during the preparation of this book, and for the unenviable task of proofreading the manuscript.

Bryan Ballantyne
Charleston, West Virginia, USA
February, 1987

Contributors

Mohamed B. Abou-Donia PhD
Laboratory of Neurotoxicology, Department of Pharmacology, Duke University Medical Center, Durham, North Carolina 27710, USA

Bryan Ballantyne MD, DSc, PhD, MFOM, FAACT, FRCPath, FIBiol, DATS
Applied Toxicology Department, Union Carbide Corporation, Danbury, Connecticut 06817, USA

Clark D. Carrington PhD
Laboratory of Neurotoxicology, Department of Pharmacology, Duke University Medical Center, Durham, North Carolina 27710, USA

David B. Doman MD
Connecticut Belair Medical Park, Wheaton, Maryland, and School of Medicine, George Washington University, Washington DC, USA

Paul Grasso DSc, MD, FRCPath, DCP, DTM&H
Robens Institute, University of Surrey, Guildford, Surrey GU2 5XM, UK

Yigal Greener PhD
Sterling-Winthrop Research Institute, Columbia Turnpike, Rensselaer, New York 12144 USA

Peggie J. Guzzie MS, PhD
Bushy Run Research Center, RD 4, Mellon Road, Export, Pennsylvania 15632, USA

Ernest S. Harpur BSc, PhD, MPS
Department of Pharmaceutical Sciences, Aston University, Aston Triangle, Birmingham B4 7ET, UK

George H. Lambert MD, PhD
Division of Neonatology, Department of Pediatrics, Michael Reese Hospital and Medical Center, Chicago, Illinois 60616, USA

Daniel M. Lapadula PhD
Laboratory of Neurotoxicology, Department of Pharmacology, Duke University Medical Center, Durham, North Carolina 27710, USA

A. Philip Leber PhD, DABT
Barberton Technical Center, PPG Industries Inc., Barberton, Ohio 44203, USA

Timothy C. Marrs MD, MSc, FRCPath, MIBiol, DipRCPath (Tox)
Section of Pathology and Clinical Toxicology, Medical Division, Chemical Defence Establishment, Porton Down, Wiltshire SP4 OJQ, UK

Arthur G. Ramage BSc, MPhil, PhD
Academic Department of Pharmacology, School of Medicine, Royal Free Hospital (University of London), London NW3 2PF, UK

Ronald S. Slesinski PhD, DABT
Bushy Run Research Center, RD 4, Mellon Road, Export, Pennsylvania 15632, USA

John A. Thomas PhD, DATS
Department of Pharmacology and Toxicology, School of Medicine, Northwestern University, Chicago, Illinois 60601, USA

Rochelle W. Tyl PhD, DABT
Bushy Run Research Center, RD 4, Mellon Road, Export, Pennsylvania 15632, USA

Tipton R. Tyler PhD, DABT
Applied Toxicology Department, Union Carbide Corporation, Danbury, Connecticut 06817, USA

H. Michael D. Utidjian MB BS, MFOM, DIH
Central Medical Department, American Cyanamid Company, Wayne, New Jersey 07470, USA

Contents

Chapter 1

Biochemical Methods for Assessment of Neurotoxicity

Mohamed B. Abou-Donia, Daniel M. Lapadula and Clark D. Carrington

INTRODUCTION

Neural tissues are composed of neurones that can be divided into two separate functional entities, the cell body and the axon. Synthesis of macromolecules, metabolic processes, and maintenance of cellular homeostasis are carried out in the cell body. Propagation of electrical impulses and transportation of nutrients and cellular components from the cell body to the terminal are carried out through the axon. Information is transferred from one cell to another via release of neurotransmitters across the synapse. Neurotoxic agents may exert their neurotoxicity on any one or more of these neural sites.

Until recently, the most reliable procedure for assessing the neurotoxic effects of chemicals was the correlation of clinical observation and the results of histopathological examinations. Although exposure to some neurotoxicants may produce severe neurologic dysfunction, it may not evoke a detectable tissue lesion. Non-specific neuropathologic lesions result when a neurotoxicant produces a severe vascular disturbance to the nervous system. In contrast, specific lesions are produced when a neurotoxic agent interferes with particular structures and functions of the neuron.

There are a few biochemical methods that have been standardized for neurotoxicity testing. Although there is sparse literature on the use of biochemical methods in detecting neurotoxic effects, nevertheless the available information could serve as a basis for the development of such methods. The use of biochemical tests to study neurotoxicity does not replace neuropathological examination. It can, however, supplement the microscopic examination of neural tissues. Biochemical tests have the following advantages: (1) most of them are technically simple; (2) they can be performed on a large number of test animals; (3) they may be presented in quantitative form that can be statistically analysed; (4) their results may be correlated with the dose and the time course of the clinical condition; and (5) some of the biochemical tests may be carried out with biopsied nerves or blood from humans. This review is a survey of biochemical methods that may be performed to test for neurotoxicity, and these methods are classified into three areas: (1) biochemical markers; (2) metabolic processes of the nervous system; and (3) biochemical correlates of neuropathological lesions.

BIOCHEMICAL MARKERS

Biochemical tests used to screen for neurotoxicity usually include markers for specific functions of the nervous system. These may involve the measurement of RNA, DNA or protein levels, or subcellular enzyme activities. These tests may be used for both characterizing or identifying toxic effects and defining their mechanisms of action.

Nervous tissues are heterogeneous cellularly, morphologically, physiologically and biochemically. Because the neurochemistry of various regions of the brain is different, whole brain analysis is not usually the most useful method for studying brain functions in normal or in intoxicated subjects. There are three approaches to the processing of neural tissues for biochemical testing: (1) separation of the tissue into its anatomical regions, (2) isolation of specific cell types, or (3) preparation of subcellular fractions by centrifugation. In many cases, one or more of these approaches may be utilized.

Anatomical Regions

The brain may be separated into the following anatomical regions: cerebellum, thalamus, hypothalamus, striatum, hippocampus, etc. (Glowinski and Iverson, 1966). It is essential to separate brain tissue by its anatomic sections since these vary considerably in their physiological and biochemical functions. Also, specific diseases and neurotoxicants affect only specific areas in the nervous tissue. Thus, while lead affects GABA (γ-aminobutyric acid) levels in cerebellum (Silbergeld et al., 1980), acrylamide produces changes in striatal dopamine receptors (Bondy et al., 1981). Furthermore, there is a selectivity in the distribution of neurotoxicants in various parts of nervous tissues, e.g. chlordecone (Fujimore et al., 1982), manganese (Bonilla et al., 1982), *O*-4-bromo-2,5-dichlorophenyl *O*-methyl phenylphosphonothioate (leptophos; Abou-Donia, 1976, 1979a, 1980), *O*-ethyl *O*-4-nitrophenyl phenylphosphonothioate (EPN; Abou-Donia, et al. 1983a,b,c,d), and tri-*o*-cresyl phosphate (TOCP: Nomeir and Abou-Donia, 1984, 1985). Knowledge of the anatomical localization of neurotoxicants may give some insight into their molecular target site interactions (Abou-Donia, 1983a; Abou-Donia and Nomeir, 1985).

Cellular Classification

Based on function and embryonic origin, neural tissue cells are classified into two groups, neurones and glia. These cell types not only vary in their functions, but may also vary in their sensitivity to the neurotoxic action of neurotoxic chemicals. Neuronal and glial cell populations may be isolated from whole brain or specific brain areas by forcing the tissues through fine sieves (Rose and Sinha, 1970). Cellular dissociation may be facilitated by the use of proteolytic enzymes. The neuronal fraction consists mainly of perikarya cut off from their dendrites. The neuronal perikarya-enriched fraction is then separated from the smaller glial cells (also containing some synaptosomes) by centrifugation. These enriched fractions may be used to test the sensitivity of neuronal and glial cells to the neurotoxic agent.

Subcellular Fractions

Subcellular fractions may be isolated using differential centrifugation techniques (Gray and Whittaker, 1962; Rose and Sinha, 1970). Subcellular fractions are isolated (*Fig* 1.1) by homogenization of brain tissue in isotonic (0·32 M) sucrose followed by centrifugation at 1000 × g for 60 minutes to sediment nuclei, cellular debris, and myelin fragments (P_1 fraction). The supernatant from the P_1 fraction is centrifuged at 17000 × g for 60 minutes to sediment the P_2 fraction which consists of mitochondria , myelin, nerve endings and lysosomes. Centrifugation of the S_2 supernatant at 100 000 × g for 60 minutes sediments the microsomal fraction.

The P_2 fraction may be fractionated further into three major morphological

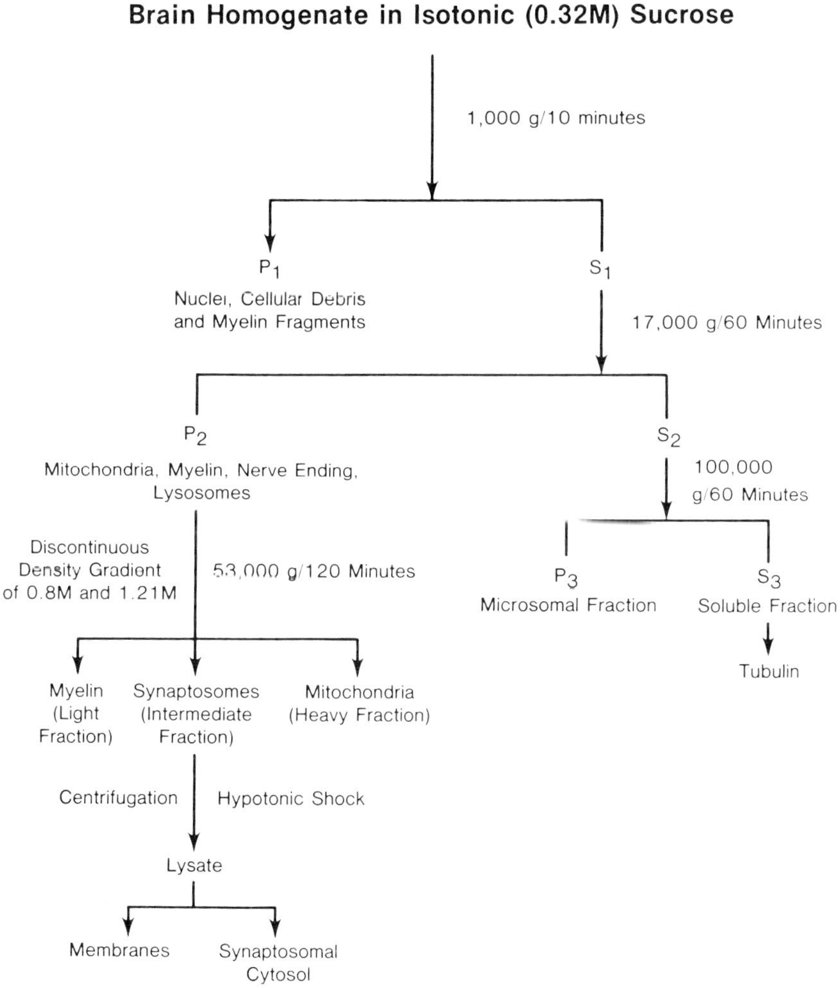

Fig. 1.1 Preparation of brain subcellular fractions.

fractions by centrifuging in a discontinuous density gradient of 0·8 M and 1·2 M sucrose at 53 000 × g for 120 minutes. The myelin fraction is present in the lightest fractions while the heaviest is composed of mitochondria. The intermediate density fraction is composed of synaptosomes which consist of presynaptic terminal enlargements that escape disintegration. Osmotic lysis disrupts synaptosomes and allows the isolation of synaptosomal membrane and the soluble fraction by centrifugation. It is possible to regard synaptosomes as miniature, non-nucleated neurones. They are labile structures and contain intraterminal mitochondria. The degree of subcellular fraction enrichment may be assessed by assaying various subcellular biochemical markers (*Table* 1.1).

Table 1.1. Biochemical markers of brain subcellular fraction.

Fraction	*Subcellular component*	*Marker*	*Reference*
P_1	Nuclei	DNA	Steele and Busch, 1963
	Nuclear membrane	RNA polymerase	Roeder and Rutter, 1969
P_2	Mitochondria:	Cardiolipin	Eichberg et al., 1964
	Inner membrane	D-3-hydroxybutyrate NAD^+ oxidoreduction	Fitzgerald et al., 1974
		Fumarase (L-malate hydrolase, EC4.2.1.2)	Whittaker and Barker, 1972
		Malate hydrolase and other enzymes of tricarboxylic acid cycle and electron transport chain	Whittaker, 1959
	Outer membrane	Monoamine oxidase	Schnaitman et al., 1967
	Lysosomes	Acid hydrolase	Koening et al., 1964
		β-Glucuronidase	Fishman and Bernfeld, 1955
		β-Glucosidase	Robins et al., 1968
		β-Galactosidase	Robins et al., 1968
		N-arylamidase	Boer, 1974
	Myelin	2′,3′-cyclic nucleotide-3′-phosphohydrolase	Konat and Clausen, 1977
		Cerebrosides	Eichberg et al., 1964
	Synaptosome	Acetylcholine	Gray and Whittaker, 1962
	Synaptosome cytoplasm	Choline acetyltransferase	Whittaker et al., 1964
		Glycolytic enzymes (except hexokinases)	Gray and Whittaker, 1962
		Potassium	Mangan and Whittaker, 1966
	Neuronal cells	Guanyl cyclase	Gorids et al., 1974
		Tyrosine hydroxylase	Kuczenski and Mandell, 1972
	Oligodendroglial cells	Glyceride galactosyl transferase	Radin et al., 1972
		Butyrylcholinesterase	Koelle, 1954
P_3	Microsomes	Acetylcholinesterase	Whittaker, 1965
		NADPH: cytochrome C oxidoreductase	Miller and Dawson, 1972
		D-Glucose-6-phosphate phosphohydrolase	Poduslo, 1975
S_3	Soluble	L-Lactate:NAD oxidoreductase, EC1.1.1.27	Kornberg, 1955
		Glycolytic enzymes (except hexokinases)	Gray and Whittaker, 1962
		Potassium	Mangan and Whittaker, 1966

Specific Subcellular Markers

Macromolecules

DNA may be used as an index for cellular proliferation and cell number in nervous tissues. DNA can be used to estimate cell size by relating it to tissue weight and RNA or protein content. An example is the evaluation of the effect of lead exposure during early development, where there was a reduction in brain weight and a decrease in total brain proteins, without a change in number of brain cells (Krigman and Hogan, 1974).

Early action of toxic agents may be manifested as a disturbance of the DNA-repair enzyme system. Chemicals may interact with the DNA molecule either by directly binding to the nucleic acid moiety or to its associated chromosomal proteins. Such changes in DNA molecules usually interfere with its functions, and these may be used for studying neurotoxic diseases. In order to detect cellular proliferation in peripheral neuropathy induced by acrylamide, the uptake of tritiated thymidine into Schwann cell DNA was determined using autoradiography (Bradley and Asbury, 1970). Methyl mercury reduced [^{3}H] uridine incorporation into spinal cord ganglion neurones (Carmichael and Cavanagh, 1976). DNA analysis may also be used as an indicator of photoreceptor degeneration since loss of the photoreceptor corresponds to loss of retinal DNA. This method has been used to investigate retinal degeneration resulting from drugs and light deprivation (Dewar et al., 1975, 1977a), and in a study of the toxic effects of phenothiazine on the retina (Dewar et al., 1978).

RNA and proteins in nervous tissues are macromolecules that may be changed as the result of exposure to neurotoxic chemicals. A simple technique to study RNA and protein synthesis is to use radiolabelled precursors, determining their rate of incorporation into macromolecules *in vitro* or *in vivo* (Dunn, 1975). For example, mercury was reported to inhibit amino acid transport across the blood–brain barrier (Partridge, 1976) and similar results were obtained with lead (Lorenzo and Gerwitz, 1977). Also exposure to acrylamide (Schotman et al., 1978) methyl mercury (Verity et al., 1977), and carbon disulphide (Savolainen and Jarvisalo, 1977) produced changes in brain protein synthesis.

Lipids

Complex lipids (phospholipids, cerebrosides, sulphatides, and gangliosides), glycolipids and glycoproteins have essential functions in the neural tissue (Zuber, 1978). They are major constituents of the plasma membrane, ion channels, neurotransmitter receptors and myelin. Complex lipids comprise neuronal membrane.

The effects of several neurotoxic agents on lipids have been studied. Neonatal exposure to lead decreased the total brain content of phospholipids, galactolipids, plasmalogens and cholesterol (Van Gelder, 1978). In old rats, chronic treatment with lead acetate resulted in accumulation of N-acetylneuraminic acid in the hypothalamus and in the midbrain reticular formation (Merkurieva et al., 1980). Hydrogen sulphide and sulphur dioxide reduced total lipids and/or phospholipids in brain (Haider et al., 1980). An early effect of carbon disulphide toxicity was the accumulation of N-acetylneuraminic acid in the olfactory bulb of rabbits (Merkurieva et al.,1978).

Recently, the effect of neurotoxicants on lipid peroxidation has been studied. In this process, oxygen reacts directly with lipids resulting in the formation of free radicals and semi-stable peroxides. The harmful effect results from the reactivity of these free radicals with membranes and subcellular organelles. Thallium, nickel, cobalt (Hassan and Ali, 1981), hydrogen sulphide and sulphur dioxide (Haider et al., 1980) have all been found to increase lipid peroxidation. The organophosphorous insecticide metosystox (*O*-dimethy-*S*-2-ethylsuphenyl ethylthiophosphate) decreased total lipids, phospholipids, cholesterol, esterified fatty acids and gangliosides (Islam et al., 1983).

Neurotransmitters

Synaptic transmission is carried out by neurotransmitters. The synthesis, storage, release, interaction with postsynaptic membrane receptors, re-uptake, and/or degradation of the neurotransmitter may be affected by neurotoxicants, thus disturbing the nervous system. The major transmitters and their marker enzymes are listed in *Table* 1.2. Furthermore, some peptides have been identified as chemical messengers (Burgen et al., 1980).

Many neurotoxic agents have been shown to alter the turnover rate and consequently the metabolic half-life of the neurotransmitter (Costa, 1970). Changes in brain catecholamine concentration have been implicated in the neurotoxicity of carbon disulphide since it increased dopamine and decreased norepinephrine concentrations by inhibiting dopamine β-hydroxylase (McKenna and Destefano, 1975). Also, manganese inhibited dopamine formation by inhibiting tyrosine hydroxylase in the striatum (Bonilla, 1980). Organophosphorous insecticides exert their acute effect by inhibiting acetylcholinesterase that leads to the accumulation of acetylcholine at acetylcholine receptors in the central and peripheral nervous systems (Abou-Donia, 1985).

Specific high-affinity Na^+-dependent uptake transport systems are responsible for concentrating neurotransmitters and their precursors in nerve endings (Iverson, 1971). Lead (Silbergeld and Goldberg, 1975), the chlorinated hydrocarbon chlordecone (Chang-Tsui and Ho, 1979) and erythrosin B (Lafferman and Silbergeld, 1979) have all been shown to interfere with neurotransmitter uptake processes.

Influx of Ca^{++} upon depolarization of the nerve endings triggers the release of neurotransmitters from synaptic endings (Cotman et al., 1976). Lead (Bondy et al., 1979) and manganese (Kirpekar et al., 1970) have all been reported to interfere with calcium-dependent neurotransmitter release.

Released neurotransmitters bind to specific receptors of the postsynaptic membrane. This binding has the following characteristics: it is reversible, stereospecific, non-enzymatic, and attains equilibrium with low dissociation constants (Yamamura et al., 1981). Studies on receptor binding are carried out using radiolabelled agonists or antagonists of a given neurotransmitter in order to determine binding kinetics and receptor density after the removal of excess ligand by filtration or centrifugation (Damstra and Bondy, 1980). Recent studies have shown that the following neurotoxic chemicals affect putative neurotransmitter receptors: acrylamide (Bondy et al., 1981), 3,4,3′,4′-tetrachloribiphenyl (Agrawal et al., 1981, 1982), chlordecone (Seth et al., 1981), lead and mercury

Table 1.2 Receptors and their endogenous ligands, agonists and antagonists.

Receptor	*Endogenous ligand*	*Agonist*	*Antagonist*
Adenosine	Adenosine	Cyclohexyladenosine	Diethyl-8-phenylxanthine
Adrenergic:	Epinephrine Norepinephrine		
α-Adrenergic		Clonidine	α-Ergocryptine
β-Adrenergic		Isoproterenol	L-propranolol
Cholinergic:	Acetylcholine		Atropine
Muscarinic		Carbachol oxotremorine-M	Quinuclidinyl benzilate
Nicotinic		Nicotine	α-Bungarotoxin D-tubocurarine
Dopamine:	Dihydroxyphenyl ethylamine		
DA_1		Apomorphine	Haloperidol
DA_2		Propylnorapomorphine	Domperidone
Excitatory	L-Asparate	N-methyl-D-asparate	
Amino acid	L-Glutamate		
GABA:	γ-Aminobutyric acid	Piperidine-4-sufonic acid	
Barbiturate			
Benzodiazepine		Diazepam	Methyl-β-carboline-carboxylic acid
Picrotoxinin			Picrotoxinin
Glycine	Glycine		Strychnine
Histamine:	Histamine		
H_1			Doxepin, mainserin
H_2			Pyrilamine, tiotidine
Opiate:	Enkephalin- (5-L-Leucine) Enkephalin- (5-L-methionine) Endorphin	Enkephalin (2-D-alanine-5-L-methionine) Dihydromorphine	Naloxone
μ		Morphine	
κ		Ethylketocyclazocinene	
σ		SKF-10,047	
ε		Enkephalinamide	

(Bondy and Agrawal, 1980), cadmium (Hedlund et al., 1979), *O,O*-diisopropyl-phosphorofluoridate (DFP) and tri-*o*-cresyl phosphate (Ali et al., 1984).

Ion channels regulate many neuronal functions. While the Na^+ channel polarizes membranes, the K^+ channel depolarizes them. The Na^+/K^+ ATPase pump is required for maintaining the appropriate Na^+ and K^+ concentrations. The Na^+ channel is inactivated by several naturally occurring toxins which are used as probes to study this channel (Hille, 1976). These toxins are tetrodotoxin and saxitoxin (Agnew et al., 1978), batrachotoxin and veratridine (Albuquerque and Daly, 1976), and peptide toxins such as scorpion toxin (Catterall, 1977). Recently a scorpion toxin was shown to have K^+ channel affinity (Carbone et al., 1982).

Na^+/K^+-adenosine triphosphatase (ATPase) is comprised of two polypeptide chains; the smaller is a glycoprotein and the larger binds adenosine triphosphate (ATP) internally and ouabain externally (Carilli et al., 1982). Chlordecone was reported to inhibit Na^+/K^+-ATPase and to decrease ouabain binding to synaptosomes in mice (Desaiah et al., 1980).

Ca^{2+} entry through a Ca^{2+}-selective channel triggers neurotransmitter release from the nerve terminal. This Ca^{2+}-selective channel is regulated by depolarization, neurotransmitters and hormones (Reichardt and Kelly, 1983). Nerve endings contain several Ca^{2+}-calmodulin-dependent protein kinases and a Ca^{2+}-phospholipid activated kinase, each with their own specific substrates. Calmodulin and other Ca^{2+} binding proteins bind to cytoplasmic Ca^{2+}, resulting directly or indirectly in the activation of other enzymes through their Ca^{2+} dependent kinase. It is believed that neurotransmitter vesicle release is regulated via the phosphorylation state of the phosphoprotein synapsin I, which is present in nerve terminals, and is associated with synaptic vesicles (Dolphin and Greengard, 1981).

Few studies have been reported on the effect of neurotoxicants on calcium channels. Manganese was shown to block neurotransmitter release (Kirpekar et al., 1970), and some other heavy metals were shown to interfere with calcium-mediated neurotransmitter release (Bondy et al., 1979).

Protein Phosphorylation

Cyclic nucleotides often regulate nerve terminal functions. When agonists bind to receptors on the nerve membrane, the binding can result in the activation of second messenger systems initiated by cyclic AMP, cyclic GMP and Ca^{2+} with subsequent changes in protein kinases and protein phosphorylation. It is believed that following phosphorylation, conformational changes may occur in membrane proteins, which result in a change in the ion permeabilities of the membrane. Thus, the effect of neurotoxic agents on the nervous system may be examined by measuring adenylate cyclase activity, cyclic nucleotide levels and the extent of protein phosphorylation.

Although protein phosphorylation has been recognized as a dynamic regulatory process for post-translational modification in the nervous system for many years, the role of this function in neurotoxic responses has only recently been investigated (Abou-Donia et al., 1984). While endogenous protein phosphorylation is known to be involved in the interaction of proteins, the precise response of specific proteins will vary depending upon the type of toxicant being investigated. Endogeneous protein phosphorylation involves the donation of a terminal phosphate group from ATP to either serine, tyrosine or threonine. The regulation of phosphorylation is usually under the control of a specific protein kinase for a particular protein or group of proteins. Many of the kinases are controlled by second messengers (cAMP, Ca^{++}, phorbol esters, cGMP) which can either stimulate or inhibit the kinase, frequently by the interaction with a regulatory subunit or protein such as calmodulin. The important role protein phosphorylation plays in the regulation of responses of the nervous system becomes obvious when one considers the wide number of proteins known to be phosphorylated. This list includes neurofilaments, microtubule accessory protein-2 (MAP-2), tubulin, protein I (a neurone-specific protein), tyrosine hydroxylase and dopamine β-hydroxylase. Recent studies in this field have focused on identification of proteins which are altered in response to neurotoxicants. It has been shown that triethyltin (TET) results in a specific decrease in myelin and the phosphorylation of myelin basic protein (O'Callaghan et al., 1983), and that tubulin phosphorylation is increased 21 days after tri-*o*-cresyl phosphate (TOCP) intoxication (Abou-Donia et al., 1984; Patton et al., 1983, 1985). However, it must be emphasized that alterations in endogenous protein phosphorylation *in vitro* may not accurately reflect those occurring *in vivo*.

The diverse number of proteins which are phosphorylated makes it difficult to predict which proteins, if any, will be altered in response to a specific neurotoxicant. An effect on protein phosphorylation may be a side effect, or a primary or secondary cause of the lesion produced. This is much more difficult to discern, since many toxicants need to be metabolized prior to exerting their effects (Abou-Donia, 1983a; Abou-Donia and Nomeir, 1985). For example, although TOCP and 2,5-hexanedione (2,5-HD) both produce lesions which result in a Wallerian-type degeneration, their effects on protein phosphorylation are different. TOCP enhances Ca^{++} stimulated phosphorylation of α and β tubulin while treatment with 2,5-HD results in a decrease in the phosphorylation of these same proteins (Patton, Lapadula and Abou-Donia, unpublished observation).

Endogenous protein phosphorylation is known to result from the interplay of at least three different proteins: protein kinase, protein phosphatase, and a substrate protein (which may be the same as the kinase, if it is phosphorylated). If an effect on protein phosphorylation is observed, it can not be assumed that the effect is only on the protein kinase. O'Callaghan et al. (1983) have demonstrated that in a triethytin-induced neuropathy, it is most likely that the amount of substrate protein (myelin basic protein) is reduced, resulting in a diminished phosphorylation of that protein. In TOCP treated animals, the activity of a protein kinase is apparently altered. This conclusion is supported by the results that TOCP treatment neither altered phosphatase activity, nor the amount of protein, and that TOCP enhanced the phosphorylation of a wide variety of substrate proteins (Abou-Donia et al., 1984; Patton et al., 1983, 1985).

Membrane-Bound Enzymes

ACETYLCHOLINESTERASE (AChE)

This enzyme, also known as specific or true cholinesterase (EC 3.1.1.7), is found in neurones at the neuromuscular junction and in some tissues (Abou-Donia, 1985). AChE hydrolyzes acetylcholine (ACh), which is released as the result of cholinergic stimulation. This enzyme is present on the postsynaptic membrane, and on the plasma membrane of the entire cholinergic neurone. Inhibition of AChE enhances transmission at all cholinergic synapses. However, since this enzyme is present in excess at cholinergic synapses, it is necessary to inhibit 60 to 90% of the enzyme before the onset of cholinergic dysfunction.

Two active sites are recognized in the AChE-active centre: an anionic site and an esteratic site. The nitrogen atom and methyl groups of the choline moiety of ACh interact with the anionic site, while the carbonyl carbon atom of the acetyl moiety of ACh binds to the esteratic site (Koelle, 1963). Organophosphorous compounds only attack the esteratic site by forming a phosphoric acid ester with enzyme. The phosphorylated enzyme formed by some inhibitors is hydrolyzed very slowly, or, with other compounds, the phosphorylation reaction is virtually irreversible. This irreversibility may result from 'ageing', a process that involves the loss of one of the alkyl groups on the phosphorylated enzyme, resulting in the negatively charged monoalkoxyphosphorylated enzyme (Koelle, 1963). Inhibition of AChE results in the accumulation of endogenous ACh in nerve tissue and effector organs. This leads to the development of signs and symptoms that mimic the muscarinic, nicotinic, and central nervous system action of ACh.

NEUROTOXIC ESTERASE

Neurotoxic esterase or neuropathy target enzyme (NTE) is the putative target for organophosphorous compound-induced delayed neurotoxicity (OPIDN) Johnson, 1969, 1982). Some organophosphorous compounds with anti-esterase activity are also capable of producing OPIDN in humans and sensitive animal species (farm animals, dogs, cats and chickens; Smith et al., 1930; Abou-Donia, 1981, 1985). There is a delay period of 6 to 14 days before onset of ataxia and paralysis. Neural lesions are seen as Wallerian-type degeneration of axons and myelin of the central and peripheral nervous systems. This effect was first observed in humans exposed to tri-*o*-cresyl phosphate (TOCP; Smith et al., 1930). Several organophosphorous pesticides produce OPIDN (Abou-Donia, 1981).

NTE is a membrane bound protein (Richardson et al., 1979) with a molecular weight of 155 000 to 178 000 daltons (Williams and Johnson, 1981; Williams, 1983; Carrington and Abou-Donia, 1985a). The target size of NTE from hen brain was determined by radiation inactivation to be 105 000 (Carrington et al., 1985). NTE is transported in the sciatic nerve of hens at a fast axonal transport rate of about 150 mm/day (Carrington and Abou-Donia, 1985b). Recently, two NTE isozymes (NTE_A and NTE_B) have been reported (Chemnitius et al., 1983). NTE has been identified as being responsible for the phenylvalerate-hydrolyzing activity in hen brain that is susceptible to inhibition only by delayed neurotoxic compounds such as mipafox (Johnson, 1977, 1982). To produce OPIDN, NTE must not only be inhibited, but also has to undergo ageing. Although NTE is a good marker enzyme for screening organophosphorous compounds for the potential to produce delayed neurotoxicity, it may not be relevant to the molecular mechanisms of OPIDN (Abou-Donia, 1981). NTE has not been isolated, and its biochemical and physiological functions are not known. Moreover, in young chicks and in rats treated with delayed neurotoxic organophosphorous esters, NTE is present, becomes inhibited, and ages without subsequent development of OPIDN (Abou-Donia, 1981, 1985).

METABOLIC PROCESSES OF THE NERVOUS SYSTEM

Energy Metabolism

Large amounts of energy are required in order for nervous tissue, and brain in particular, to maintain the transport of ions and proteins essential for its function and to sustain its highly active biosynthetic processes. Thus, glucose availability and maintenance of the enzymes essential for energy production are critical to neuronal function. Recent studies have shown that some neurotoxic chemicals affect glucose metabolism and energy production both in the central and peripheral nervous systems. Examples of this group are: methyl mercury (Bull and Lutkenhoff, 1975), lead (Bull et al., 1979), hexachlorophene (Cammer and Moore, 1972), and organotin compounds (Lock, 1976). Also, glycolytic enzymes were shown to be inhibited by alcohol (Merkurieva et al., 1980) and carbon disulphide (Sabri et al., 1979). An *n*-hexane metabolite, 2,5-hexanedione, was shown to inhibit some glycolytic enzymes such as the sulphydryl enzymes glyceraldehyde-3-phosphate dehydrogenase (Sabri et al., 1979; Graham and Abou-Donia, 1980) phosphofructokinase (Sabri et al., 1979), and enolase (Howland et al., 1980). Enolase was also shown to be inhibited by acrylamide (Howland et al., 1980). Heavy metals inhibit energy metabolism by inhibiting some glycolytic and tricarboxylic acid cycle enzymes (Simpson, 1964). Likewise, carbon monoxide and carbon disulphide disrupt energy metabolism by inhibiting the cytochrome system and oxidative phosphorylation (Hopkins, 1972).

The regional rate of brain glucose consumption depends upon the relative metabolic activity of the brain areas. This metabolic activity may be determined by the uptake of [^{14}C]-2-deoxyglucose (2-DG) and its subsequent phosphorylation by hexokinase to 2-deoxyglucose-6-phosphate (2-DG-P; Sokoloff et al., 1977). The 2-DG-P trapped in various regions of the brain may be taken as an index of glucose use and neuronal activity.

Axonal Transport

Introduction

Studies of axoplasmic transport for different neurotoxicological problems have recently increased in the literature. Many neurotoxicants have both direct and indirect effects on axonal transport. One of the problems facing neurotoxicology is investigating whether alterations in transport are the cause of a neurological problem, or a result of the treatment. Detection of axonal transport defects are difficult with further complications occurring in the determination of which of the many rates of transport are being affected (Ochs, 1982). The different rates of transport which could be affected are fast anterograde (approximately 200 to 500 mm day^{-1}), retrograde, and slow anterograde. To complicate matters even further, slow anterograde transport can be subdivided into at least two components, slow component A (SC_a, 0·5–1 mm/day) and slow component B (SC_b, 2–15 mm/day; Tytell et al., 1981). Although more than six rates of slow transport have been reported, we will deal with only the two major classifications of slow transport. Procedures for studying axonal transport vary widely from laboratory to laboratory. In general, there are two possible problems which a toxic insult can induce. The first is an alteration in either all the rates of transport or only in one specific rate of transport. The second is an alteration in the quality of proteins transported; in other words, the transport rate of a specific protein is altered, and in this case, the overall rate of transport may not be affected.

Axonal Transport in Toxic Neuropathies

$\beta\beta'$-IMINODIPROPRIONITRILE (IDPN)

IDPN primarily induces a neuropathy in which there is an accumulation of neurofilaments in the proximal portion of the axon (Chou and Hartmann, 1964, 1965). Griffin et al. (1978) found that in rats SC_a was selectivity stopped by IDPN treatment. SC_b was also inhibited, but not to the same degree. Since neurofilaments and microtubules make up the majority of SC_a, SDS-PAGE (sodium dodecyl sulphate-polyacrylamide gel electrophoresis) revealed that SC_a was virtually stopped, with the neurofilament triplet proteins (70K, 160K and 210K) being the most affected. Other rates of transport were not affected by this treatment.

ORGANOPHOSPHOROUS COMPOUNDS

Several organophosphorous compounds which produce organophosphorous ester-induced delayed neurotoxicity (OPIDN; Abou-Donia, 1981) have been investigated for an effect on axonal transport with conflicting results. In this neuropathy, there is a delay of 6 to 14 days before the onset of a Wallerian-type degeneration. There is a proliferation of smooth endoplasmic reticulum early on in the neuropathy, but its relationship to any alteration in axonal transport is unknown. The first reported alteration of transport by delayed neuropathic organophosphorous compounds was demonstrated in the rat optic system by Reichert and Abou-Donia (1980) after local application of the neurotoxicant. More recently an inhibition of the slow component of axonal transport has been reported in hen sciatic nerve (Padilla et al., 1983). However, further work is needed to elucidate a direct role of alterations in axonal transport in the production of this neuropathy.

ACRYLAMIDE

Morphologically, acrylamide neuropathy is characterized by an accumulation of neurofilaments in the axonal terminal (Prineas, 1969). Rasool and Bradley (1978) found a 75% decrease in tubulin binding of colchicine in animals having a clinical neuropathy. In general, there is an alteration in the rate of slow transport, and a minimal, if any, change in the rate of fast transport. However, Sidenius and Jakobsen (1983) found that although the rate is not altered, there is a significant reduction in the fractional amount of label in the sciatic nerve. When consided with the work by Souyri et al. (1981), there is an implication that axoplasmic filamentous swellings may quantitatively reduce the amount of fast transported material in the axon terminal. Jakobsen and Sidenius (1983) also found that retrograde axonal transport was reduced in a dose-dependent manner. They suggested that the retention of protein in the distal axons is accounted for by the accumulation of filaments. The filaments block the retrograde flow of proteins leading to an accumulation of SER in the terminal region of the axon.

ALIPHATIC HEXACARBONS

This class of compounds also produces a distal axonopathy with the primary morphological feature being an accumulation of neurofilaments in the distal part of the axon. Fast axonal transport has been found to be impaired (Mendell et al., 1977), probably due to the accumulation of the neurofilaments (Griffin et al., 1982). Any alterations in axonal transport are most likely secondary to some direct effect of the neurotoxic meabolite 2,5-hexanedione.

CARBON DISULPHIDE

Prolonged exposure leads to a neuropathy that is also characterized by an increase in neurofilaments. Free thiol groups on neurofilaments may be involved in the binding to CS_2 (Mäkinen et al., 1977).

MUSCLE SPINDLE INHIBITORS

Colchicine, vincristine and vinblastine are examples of neurotoxicants which are known to interact with microtubules and inhibit axonal transport. Under numerous circumstances, these compounds have been shown to interrupt fast transport (Kreutzberg, 1969; Paulson and McClure, 1974, 1975) presumably by the disruption of the microtubular network.

Cytoskeletal Proteins

Cytoskeletal elements (microtubules, intermediate filaments and microfilaments) which make up the backbone structure of cells are particularly important to neurones. Due to the extreme length of some neurones (axons of up to 1 meter) these stable proteins are important for the normal functioning of the neurone. Microtubules are primarily made up of tubulin (α and β subunits) and microtubule accessory proteins (MAP). These tubules are approximately 24 nM in diameter. Intermediate filaments in the neurone are known as neurofilaments, which are approximately 10 nM in diameter. Neurofilaments are made up of at least three distinct proteins designated by their molecular weights as being in the range of 65–70 K (70 K the most common designation), 140–170 K (160 K), and 190–220 K (210 K). Microtubules and neurofilaments appear to be linked to one another by cross-bridge structures. Microfilaments are composed of actin complexes and generate contractile units in non-muscle cells. All three filaments have been postulated to have a role in axonal transport. These three classes of filament networks share some common properties. These properties include: (1) the ability to form linear protein polymers; (2) they consist of a backbone protein and various accessory proteins; (3) the cytoskeleton is isolatable by treatment with detergents, eg. Triton X-100, which removes membrane and other cellular elements.

Since neurofilaments as well as their glial cell (astrocytes) counterpart, glial fibrillary acidic protein (GFAP), are found only in nervous tissue, these proteins become valuable markers for neurotoxicity. GFAP in particular is known to increase in response to traumatic or toxic injury (O'Callaghan and Miller, 1983; O'Callaghan et al., 1983) through the extensive proliferation of astrocytes. This protein is therefore a marker for assessing the response of the nervous system to a toxic insult which results in astrocytic proliferation.

Neurofilaments as well as microtubular proteins are known to be profoundly influenced by various toxic chemicals, and are probably the primary sites of action of many toxicants. These compounds include IDPN, acrylamide, aliphatic hexacarbons, organophosphorous compounds, carbon disulphide (see sections on axonal transport and protein phosphorylation on pages 8 and 11). Recently we have been able to demonstrate a direct *in vivo* crosslinking of neurofilaments in rats that were treated with 2,5-hexanedione (*Fig.* 1.2). Polyacrylamide gel electrophoresis of cytoskeletal proteins from treated rats revealed several protein bands which were not present in control animals. Through the use of monoclonal antibodies to the neurofilament triplet proteins, crosslinking of the 70 K and 160 K neurofilament proteins was demonstrated using the method of Towbin et al. (1979). Incubation of the nitrocellulose with primary antibody was followed by a second antibody, and finally with I^{125} Protein A and exposed to X-ray film. Only those protein bands originally derived from the neurofilament proteins are

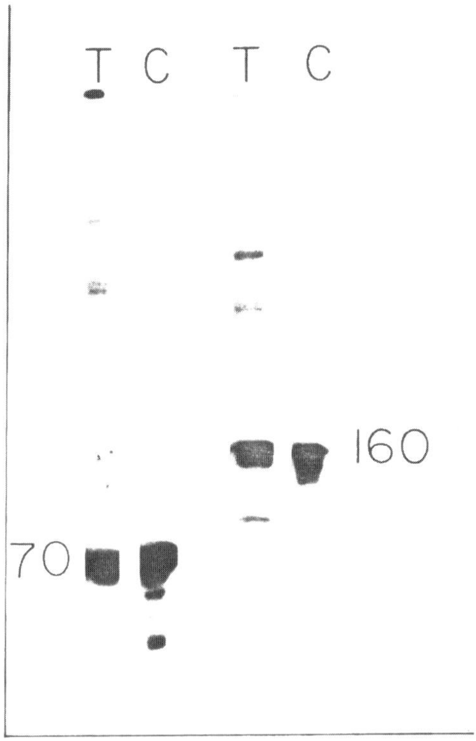

Fig. 1.2 Immunoblots to the 70 K or 160 K neurofilament proteins from control (C) or 2,5-hexanedione-treated (T) rats. Immunoblots were prepared by blotting proteins from SDS-polyacrylamide gels to nitrocellulose paper. The paper was incubated with primary antibody (anti-70 K or 160 K antibody) followed by a second antibody (rabbit anti-mouse IgG), and finally by ^{125}I-Protein A. The nitrocellulose was exposed to X-ray film for 24 hours. High molecular weight immunoreactive products to both the 70 K and 160 K neurofilament antibodies are seen in 2,5-hexanedione-treated animals. There is also a diminished amount of immunoreative breakdown product in both the 70 K and 160 K immunoblot of 2,5-hexanedione-treated animals.

detected on the film. Numerous high molecular weight bands, as well as material that did not enter the stacking gel, have been shown to be neurofilamental in origin. Another significant finding shown by immunoblots was the decreased amount of immunoreactive breakdown products, which was most evident in the 70 K neurofilament protein of spinal cords from 2,5-hexanedione treated rats.

BIOCHEMICAL CORRELATES OF NEUROPATHOLOGICAL CHANGES

Changes During Wallerian Degeneration

Wallerian degeneration describes the changes that take place in the distal part of an axon that has been cut or crushed. These changes are classified into histopathological and biochemical aspects.

Histopathological Changes

These changes include the following stages in order of succession:

a. Primary degeneration of axon followed by a secondary degeneration of myelin in the order: axon swelling; axon disintegration; loss of normal myelin structures with swelling; tumefaction; and breakdown of myelin sheaths.
b. Cellular proliferation and removal of myelin lipids as follows: degradation of myelin fragments; proliferation of Schwann cell and infiltration by macrophages (phagocytosis); inflammatory cellular lesions that are reactive to the parenchymatous lesions; gradual disappearance and catabolism of phagocytized material.
c. Fibrosis.

Biochemical Changes

These changes result from the liberation of the normal biochemical constituents of axon and myelin (protein, phospholipids, glycolipids and cholesterol—*Fig.* 1.3). Normally myelin may stain red with certain blue dyes such as toluidine blue and cresyl violet. It also stains blue with luxol fast blue. Two final breakdown products, triglycerides and cholesterol esters, are easily identified by their black colour when stained with sudan black, and their red colour when stained with Scharlach R, sudan IV, or oil red O.

In Wallerian degeneration, there is an increase in wet weight and in levels of DNA, RNA, phosphorous, amino acids, carbohydrates and proteins, including collagen (*Table* 1.3). In contrast, there is a decrease in the amounts of lipids and other chemicals such as adenosine triphosphate, thiamine and creatine. Also, cholesterol esters appear. Most of these changes are associated with stage *b*, except for the decrease in acetylcholine and the increase in collagen which are associated with stages *a* and *c* respectively.

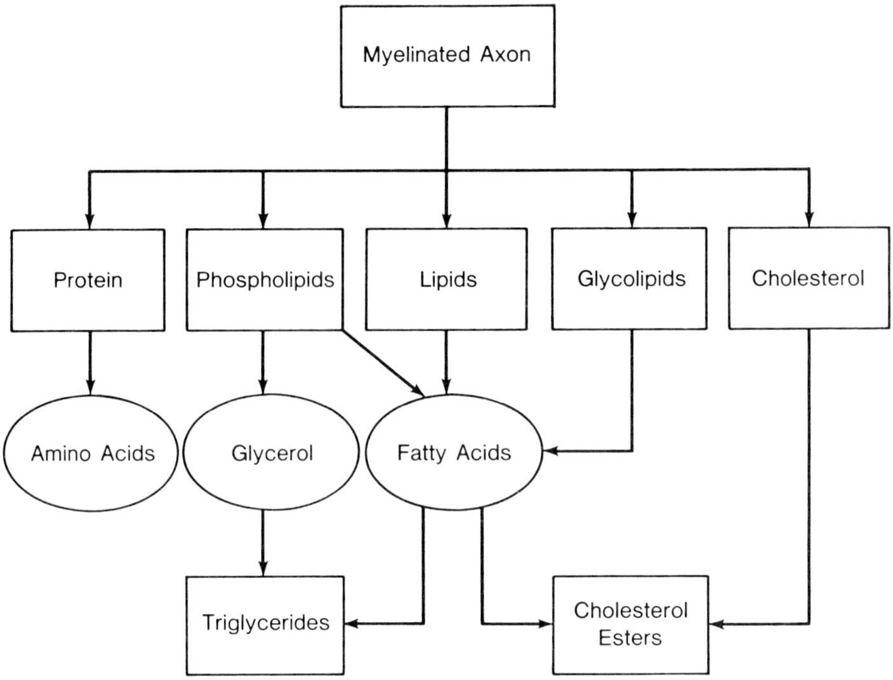

Fig. 1.3 Biochemical changes in the Wallerian degeneration of myelinated axons.

Table 1.3. Chemical changes in peripheral nerves during Wallerian degeneration.

Chemical	*Change*[a]	References
Net weight	+	Webster, 1973
DNA	+	McCaman and Robins, 1959
RNA	+	Oderfeld-Nowak and Niemierko, 1969
Protein[b]	+	McCaman and Robins, 1959
Amino acids[c]	+	Porcellati and Thompson, 1957
Carbohydrates[d]	+	Stewart et al, 1965
Phosphorus[e]	+	McCaman and Robins, 1959
Lipids[f]	–	McCaman and Robins, 1959; Domonkos and Heiner, 1968
Others:		
Adenosine triphosphate	–	Stewart et al., 1965; Greengard et al., 1954
Acetylcholine	–	Brown ad Feldberg, 1936
Nicotine adenine nucleotide	–	Greengard et al., 1954
Thiamine	–	Mucal and Wyss, 1944
Creatine	–	Stewart et al., 1965

[a] Abbreviations: (+) increase, (–) decrease.
[b] Including collagen.
[c] The following amino acids were increased: asparate, glutamate, glutamine, alanine, taurine, serine, glycine, valine, leucine and threonine.
[d] The following carbohydrates were increased: glycogen, glucose, fructose, glucose-6-phosphate and lactate.
[e] Phosphorus includes inorganic and soluble P and organic acid-soluble phosphorus.
[f] The following lipids were decreased: cephalins, lecithins, sphingomyelins, phosphorus-free sphingolipids, ethanolamine, phosphoglycerides, phosphatidylcholine, phosphatidylserine, fatty aldehydes, fatty acids and cholesterol. Also total lipid phosphorus was decreased.

Biochemical Correlates of Neurotoxicants Inducing Wallerian-Type Degeneration

Many neurotoxic agents produce Wallerian-type degeneration (Cavanagh, 1964, 1973; Spencer and Schaumberg, 1981; Abou-Donia, 1979b, 1981, 1985), e.g. organophosphorous compounds, acrylamide, and *n*-hexane and some of its metabolites. Although these neurotoxicants cause Wallerian-type degeneration of the axon and myelin, they exhibit distinct patterns of morphology and distribution of the neuropathologic lesions (Abou-Donia, 1983b; Abou-Donia et al., 1985). Since all of these neuropathies are characterized by Wallerian-type degeneration, it might be possible to use biochemical correlates of Wallerian degeneration (*Table* 1.3) as indices for these neurotoxicities (Dewar and Mofett, 1979).

Many published studies pertaining to biochemical correlates of neurotoxicity have been reviewed. The following parameters, which may account for the variability of the published results, should be considered in assessing these data: (*a*) the purity of chemical used; (*b*) dosage, frequency, and duration of administration; (*c*) route of administration; (*d*) criteria used for neurotoxicity; (*e*) species of test animal; and (*f*) animal age.

Effect on Protein

PROTEIN CONTENT

Neither the concentration of amino acids nor their patterns in spinal cord protein was significantly different in DFP-treated cats from untreated controls (Porcellati, 1966a). On the other hand, DFP and TOCP treatments produced a 60 to 80% increase in the amounts of free serine, threonine, and glutamine in hen peripheral nerve (Montanini and Porcellati, 1964). The increase in free amino acids reached its peak at the sixteenth day for TOCP-treated hens, and at the thirteenth day for control hens.

PROTEIN SYNTHESIS

In the cat, DFP produced a temporary increase in the incorporation of [^{14}C]leucine and [^{14}C]lysine into the protein of the spinal nerves and spinal ganglia after one week, followed by a significant decrease in protein synthesis (Porcellati, 1966a). Similarly, DFP depressed the incorporation rate of [^{14}C]leucine and [^{14}C]lysine into spinal cord proteolipid protein (Porcellati, 1965). On the contrary, in the rat, a species less sensitive to OPIDN, an increase in protein turnover occurred two days after the administration of the non-delayed neurotoxic organophosphorous compound (2-diethoxyphosphinylthioethyl-dimethylamine acid oxalate; Clouet and Waelsch, 1963).

PROTEIN DEGRADATION

DFP and TOCP caused an increase of the neutral proteinase activity in the hen spinal cord and peripheral nerve (Porcellati et al., 1961). Onset of the increase occurred after one week, and reached its peak on the sixteenth to twentieth day after the administration. By the sixth day, there was an increase in the free amino acid concentration in the peripheral nerve. In contrast, tetraethylpyrophosphate, a compound that does not produce OPIDN, did not produce changes similar to those of DFP and TOCP (Porcellati, 1961). Following DFP administration in cats, neutral proteinase activity also increased in the spinal ganglia, spinal nerve and spinal cord. It is noteworthy that a number of organophosphorous compounds inhibited neutral proteinase enzymes *in vitro* when added to normal nervous tissues of hen (Clouet and Waelsch, 1963).

Effect on Lipids

LIPID CONTENT

In neural tissues of hens treated with organophosphorous compounds capable of causing delayed neurotoxicity (i.e. TOCP, DFP, mipafox), no change was detected in the following lipid constituents: total lipid phosphorous , acid-soluble phosphorus, and total phospholipid (Webster, 1954; Porcellati and Mastrantonio, 1964; Joel et al., 1967). An increase in peripheral nerve cholesterol esters reported in TOCP-treated hens (Berry and Cevallos, 1966) was not confirmed in hen brain, spinal cord and peripheral nerves following TOCP (Williams et al., 1966) or mipafox (Joel et al., 1967) administration. Lipids that were increased in neural tissues after treatment with TOCP (Berry and Cevallos, 1966) or DFP (Porcellati and Mastrantonio, 1964) are: phosphatidyl choline, mono- and diglycerides, phosphoryl ethanolamine, phosphoryl choline, and glycerophosphate in hens and phosphoryl choline in the sciatic nerve of DFP-treated rats (Nelson and Barnum, 1960). Only cerebrosides and triglycerides were decreased in peripheral nerve of TOCP-treated hens (Berry and Cevallos, 1966). Glycerylphosphorylethanolamine and glycerylphosphorylcholine were increased 70% in the hen peripheral nerves 13 days after TOCP treatment (Montanini and Porcellati, 1964).

LIPID SYNTHESIS

Studies on the effects of TOCP, DFP and mipafox on the incorporation of radiolabelled precursors have been carried out mostly in the hen, with fewer studies in the cat, rat and mouse. No change was found in the incorporation of [^{32}P]phosphate into acid-soluble phosphorus in the peripheral nerves and spinal cord of TOCP-treated hens (Webster, 1954). On the other hand, the initial decrease in incorporation of [^{14}C]acetate into lipids of peripheral nerves of hens treated with DFP was not observed at fifteenth and seventeenth day (Austin, 1957). A decrease in [^{14}C]acetate into peripheral nerve lipids was also reported after treating hens with mipafox (Majno and Karnovsky, 1961).

Although treatment of hens with TOCP produced no change in the incorporation of [^{32}P]phosphate into total phospholipid of peripheral nerve and spinal cord (Webster, 1954), there was a decrease in the incorporation of [^{32} P]phosphate into specific phospholipids in the peripheral nerves of hens treated with DFP and TOCP (Porcellati and Mustrantonio, 1964). This study also showed an increase in [^{32}P]phosphate incorporation into phosphorylcholine and phosphoryl ethanolamine. Also, the synthesis of phosphatidyl serine in the peripheral nerve was not affected by DFP or TOCP treatment of hens (Porcellati and Mastrantonio, 1964). DFP or TOCP partially inhibited the incorporation of [^{3} H]inositol into polyphosphoinositides of the hen peripheral nerve (Porcellati, 1967b).

LIPID DEGRADATION

Delayed neurotoxic organophosphorus compounds do not affect phospholiphases or lipases *in vitro* (Adams, 1965). The concentration of total phospholipids remains unchanged in the peripheral nerves of hens treated with delayed neurotoxic compounds for at least thirty days (Porcellati and Mastrantonio, 1964; Berry and Cevallos, 1966; Joel et al., 1967). On the other hand, the lysolecithin content in peripheral nerve was decreased (Berry and Cevallos. 1966). Also, a moderate increase in phospholid breakdown has been reported (Porcellati and Mastrantonio, 1964). This was accompanied by a moderate increase in the phosphoryl choline and phosphoryl ethanolamine phosphohydrolase activities (Porcellati, 1966b), indicating accelerated degradative processes.

FATTY ACID METABOLISM

Conflicting results have been obtained on the effect of delayed neurotoxic organophosphorous compounds on fatty acid compositions of neural tissues from treated animals. TOCP treatment changed the free fatty acid composition, showing a decrease of 16 : 0 and 16 : 1, and an increase of 18 : 1 and 18 : 2 (Berry and Cevallos, 1966) On the contrary, mipafox treatment did not affect the polyunsaturated fatty acid patterns of brain, spinal cord and peripheral nerve (Joel et al., 1967). Minor changes were noted in the amounts of tetranoic and pentanoic acids, which might have resulted from the starvation that characterized treated animals in later stages of intoxication.

Comparison Between Lipid and Protein Changes that Occur During Wallerian Degeneration and Chemically Induced Wallerian-Type Degeneration

In contrast to Wallerian degeneration, delayed neurotoxic organophosphorous compounds result in stability of the spinal cord and peripheral nerve lipid concentration. In Wallerian degeneration there are decreases in the amounts of phospholipids, in total cholesterol and cerebrosides. Cholesterol esters are detected and there are alterations in the fatty acid pattern (Johnson et al., 1949, 1950; McCaman, 1962; Miani, 1962; Berry et al., 1965). Furthermore, lysophosphatides of peripheral nerve increase during Wallerian degeneration (Berry et al., 1965; Domonkos and Heiner, 1968), but decrease following TOCP administration (Berry and Cevallos, 1966). These discrepancies might be related to the delay period before onset of histopathologic lesions in OPIDN. This explanation is supported by the finding that detectable phospholipid degradation takes place in the hen peripheral nerve only after 6 to 14 days following TOCP poisoning (Montanini and Porcellati, 1964). In Wallerian degeneration, there is an increase in the incorporation rates of various radiolabelled precursors in the peripheral nerve lipids, both *in vivo* and *in vitro* (Majno and Karnovsky, 1958). In contrast, these biochemical changes do not occur during OPIDN (Majno and Karnovsky, 1961; Porcellati, 1966b, 1967a). Also, a greater rate of labelling of lipid *in vitro* takes place only in later stages of the delayed metabolic process (Majno and

Karnovsky, 1961). Moreover, no change occurs in the enzymes involved in phospholipid biosynthesis (Porcellati, 1967a).

On the other hand, similar findings were obtained with the incorporation of [^{14}C]acetate in the sciatic nerve of mipafox-treated animals, and in transected sciatic nerve and spinal cord (Majno and Karnovsky, 1961; Karnovsky and Majno, 1961). In the rat, incorporation of [^{14}C]acetate is diminished in the proximal parts of the sciatic nerve (where no histopathologic lesion is seen), and enhanced in the degenerated branches (Majno and Karnovsky, 1961). Likewise in the hen, incorporation of [^{14}C]acetate is depressed in early stages of intoxication, and is increased in the later stages (Karnovsky and Majno, 1961).

The major change in lipid metabolism that occurs during the early stages of OPIDN and which does not take place during Wallerian degeneration (after transection) is the decreased rate of [^{32}P]phosphate incorporation into phospholipid in the peripheral nerve (Porcellati, 1967a).

On the other hand, the time course of changes of acidic and neutral proteinase activities is similar in both OPIDN and Wallerian degeneration (Porcellati, 1966a). The possible involvement of lysosomal enzymes in both processes has been proposed (Porcellati, 1966a). Similarly, incorporation of amino acids into nerve protein and proteolipid protein is increased during nerve degeneration in OPIDN and Wallerian degeneration (Porcellati, 1966a). Finally, there is a comparable decreased rate of protein synthesis, both in spinal ganglia at the early stages of DFP poisoning, and in peripheral nerve during nerve degeneration after administration with diptheria toxin, that produces segmental demyelination (Matheson and Cavanagh, 1967).

Hydrolases

The hydrolytic enzymes such as acid phosphatase, β-glucuronidase and β-galactosidase are lysosomal enzymes (DeDuve et al., 1955). Increases in these enzyme activities in peripheral nerves may be used as markers for Wallerian degeneration. These changes have been found to be transient (Hollinger and Rossiter, 1952; Hollinger et al., 1952). The changes are associated with an increase in the number of Schwann cells and endoneural cells (mostly fibroblasts and macrophages), and do not precede the degeneration of axons and myelin. Thus, these changes seem to reflect the cellular proliferation characteristic of stage *b* of Wallerian degeneration.

The changes in hydrolases in animals treated with neurotoxic agents have been investigated histologically and biochemically. TOCP treatment caused an increase in acid phosphatase activity of sciatic nerve and neuroglia of hens (Glees, 1967). Leptophos, an organophosphorous insecticide capable of causing OPIDN (Abou-Donia et al., 1974; Abou-Donia and Preissig, 1976a,b), produced a dose- (Abou-Donia, 1978a) and a time- (Abou-Donia, 1978b) dependent increase in hen plasma acid phosphatase activity. Also, acrylamide produced an increase in the activities of β-glucuronidase and β-galactosidase in rat tibial nerve (Kaplan and Murphy, 1972; Dewar et al., 1977b).

Methyl mercury chloride affects sensory ganglion cells and produces axonal degeneration in the sensory fibres of peripheral nerve (Cavanagh and Chen, 1971; Jacobs et al., 1975). Methyl mercury does not produce Wallerian-type degeneration, but causes contemporaneous degeneration along the whole fibre. Rats treated with this neurotoxicant showed dose-dependent increases in the β-glucuronidase and β-galactosidase activities in the distal end of the posterior tibial nerve.

The increase in lysosomal hydrolase activity perhaps represents proliferation of Schwann cells and macrophages. The determination of these enzyme activities seems to offer an easy method for detecting chemically-induced degeneration of the peripheral nervous system. Also, assays of these enzymes in the plasma of treated animals have been proposed as an early warning index to detect over exposure to this type of neurotoxic chemical.

Another enzyme, 2′, 3′-cyclic nucleotide 3′-phosphohydrolase, a myelin marker, has been used as a marker for organophosphorous compounds that produce delayed neurotoxicity. Thus, DEF (S,S,S-*tri*-n-butyl phosphorotrithionate) produced an increase in the enzyme activity in brains of treated hens which was dose-dependent and corresponded with the development of OPIDN (Abou-Donia et al., 1986). This enzyme was used to study the effects of triethyltin on myelination in developing brain (Konal and Clausen, 1977).

Central nervous system degeneration related to microglial and astrocytic hypertrophy has also been studied by measuring β-glucuronidase activity in the brain. Thus, the copper chelating agent cuprizone, which produces encephalopathy in mice, produced a several-fold increase in brain β-glucuronidase activity (Bowen et al., 1974).

Miscellaneous

Effect of other neurotoxicants on proteins

Methyl mercury reduced the incorporation of [^{14}C]leucine into brain protein (Farris and Smith, 1975) and inhibited protein synthesis in cerebral cortical slices of rats (Yoshino et al., 1966). In contrast, methyl mercury increased protein synthesis in brains of treated rats (Brubaker et al., 1973). Isoniazid (Holtz and Palm, 1964; Cavanagh, 1967) and desoxypyridoxine (Vilter et al., 1953) produced a deficiency in pyridoxal phosphate which interfered with critical neural functions.

Effect on Vitamins

Alcohol produces thiamine deficiency which interferes with neural energy metabolism (Fennelly et al., 1964). TOCP antagonized the absorption of vitamin E from the gastrointestinal tract (Myers and Mulder, 1953).

SUMMARY

Biochemical tests can play a major role in detecting, predicting, and screening for neurotoxicity. These tests, however, do not replace *in vivo* experiments in animals, but rather they compliment neurotoxicity studies in model animal systems. Many neurotoxic chemicals need biochemical activation and undergo biochemical detoxification. The active neurotoxic agent attacks a specific neurotoxicity target in the nervous system. These processes are limited by repair mechanisms. Also, in many instances, animals exposed to neurotoxic chemicals may suffer anorexia and become malnourished. The hen is particularly sensitive to the starvation and poor nutrition states (Majno and Karnovsky, 1961; Porcellati and Mastrantonio, 1964). Proper controls including restricted and force fed animals should be carried out for most of the *in vivo* experiments using biochemical tests. All of these factors are strain-and species-dependent, and thus the response to a test neurotoxicant can be expected to be a function of strain, species and, sometimes, age. Care must therefore be taken in analysing and assessing the results of studies which determine biochemical correlates to neurotoxicity.

ACKNOWLEDGEMENTS

The secretarial work of Mrs Mary Greene is appreciated. This review was supported in part by NIOSH Grants No. OHO2003 and OHO0823, and NIEHS Grant No. ES 02717.

REFERENCES

Abou-Donia M. B. (1976) Pharmacokinetics of a neurotoxic oral dose of leptophos in hens. *Arch. Toxicol.* **36**, 103–110.

Abou-Donia M. B. (1978a) The role of acid phosphatase in delayed neurotoxicity induced by leptophos in hens *Biochem. Pharmacol.* **27**, 2055–2058.

Abou-Donia M. B. (1978b) Increased acid phosphatase activity in hens following an oral dose of leptophos. *Toxicol. Lett.* **2**, 199–203.

Abou-Donia M. B. (1979a) Pharmacokinetics and metabolism of a topically-applied dose of *O*-4-bromo-2,5-dichlorophenyl *O*-methyl phenylphosphonothioate in hens. *Toxicol. Appl. Pharmacol.* **51**, 311–328.

Abou-Donia M. B. (1979b) Delayed neurotoxicity of phenylphosphonothioate esters. *Science* **205**, 713–715.

Abou-Donia M. B. (1980) Metabolism and pharmacokinetics of a single oral dose of *O*-4-bromo-2,5-dichlorophenyl *O*-methyl phenylphosphonothioate (leptophos) in hens. *Toxicol. Appl. Pharmacol.* **55**, 131–145.

Abou-Donia M. B. (1981) Organophosphorous ester-induced delayed neurotoxicity. *Annu. Rev. Pharmacol. Toxicol.* **21**, 511–548.

Abou-Donia M. B. (1983a) Toxicokinetics and metabolism of delayed neurotoxic organophosphorus esters. *Neurotoxicology* **4**, 113–130.

Abou-Donia M. B. (1983b) Interaction between neurotoxicities induced by organophosphorus and long chain hexacarbon compounds. *Neurotoxicology* **4**, 117–136.

Abou-Donia M. B. (1985) Biochemical toxicology of organophosphorus compounds In; Blum K. and Manzo L. K. (eds) *Neurotoxicology*, 423–444. New York; Marcel Dekker, Inc.

Abou-Donia M. B., Abdel-Kader H. M. and Abou-Donia S. A. (1983a) Tissue distribution, elimination, and metabolism of *O*-ethyl *O*-nitrophenyl phenylphosphonothioate in hens following daily dermal doses. *J. Am. Coll. Toxicol.* **2**, 391–404.

Abou-Donia M. B., Abdo K. M., Timmons P. R. et al., (1985a) Brain acetylcholinesterase, acid phosphatase, and 2′,3′-cyclic nucleotide-3′-phosphohydrolase and plasma butyrylcholinesterase activities in hens treated with a single dermal neurotoxic dose of *S,S,S*-tri-*n*-butyl phosphorotrithioate. *Toxicol. Appl. Pharmacol.* *82*, 461–473.

Abou-Donia M. B., Hernandez Y. M., Ahmed N. S. et al (1983b) Distribution and metabolism of *O*-ethyl *O*-4-nitrophenyl phenylphosphonothiate after a single oral dose in one-week old chicks. *Arch. Toxicol.* **54**, 83–96.

Abou-Donia M. B., Kinnes C. G., Abdo K. M. et al (1983c) Physiologic disposition and metabolism of *O*-ethyl *O*-4-nitrophenyl phenylphosphonothioate in male cats following a single dermal administration *Drug Metab. Dispo.* **11**, 31–36.

Abou-Donia M. B., Lapadula D. M., Campbell G. et al (1985). The joint neurotoxic action of inhaled methyl butyl ketone vapor and dermally applied *O*-ethyl *O*-4-nitrophenyl phenylphosphonate in hens: potentiating effect. *Toxicol. Appl. Pharmacol.* **79**, 69–82.

Abou-Donia M. B. and Nomeir A. A. (1985) The role of pharmacokinetics and metabolism in species sensitivity to neurotoxic agents. *Fund. Appl. Toxicol.* *6*, 190–207.

Abou-Donia M. B., Othman M. A., Shawer M. F. et al., (1974) Neurotoxic effect of leptophos. *Experientia* **30**, 63–64.

Abou-Donia M. B. and Pressig S. H. (1976a) Delayed neurotoxicity of leptophos: toxic effects on nervous system of hens. *Toxicol. Appl. Pharmacol.* **35**, 269–282.

Abou-Donia M. B. and Pressig S. H. (1976b) Delayed neurotoxicity of continuous low-dose oral administration of leptophos to hens. *Toxicol. Appl. Pharmacol.* **38**, 595–608.

Abou-Donia M. B., Patton S. E. and Lapadula D. M. (1984) Possible role of endogeneous protein phosphorylation in organophosphorous compound-induced delayed neurotoxicity. In: Narahasi T. (ed.) *Cellular and Molecular Neurotoxicity*, 265–283. New York: Raven Press.

Abou-Donia M. B., Reichert B. L. and Ashry M. A. (1983d) The absorption, distribution, excretion and metabolism of a single oral dose of *O*-ethyl *O*-4-nitrophenyl phenylphosphonothioate in hens. *Toxicol. Appl. Pharmacol.* **70**, 18–28.

Adams C. W. M. (1965). *Neurohistochemistry*. Amsterdam: Elsevier.

Agnew W. S., Levinson S. R., Brabson J. S. et al (1978) Purification of the tetrodotoxin-binding component associated with the voltage-sensitive sodium channel from *Electrophorus electricus* electroplax membranes. *Proc. Natl Acad. Sci.*, **75**, 2606–2610.

Agrawal D. K., Misra D., Agarwal S. et al., (1982) Influence of sex hormones on parathion toxicity in rats: antiacetylcholinesterase activity of parathion and paraoxon in plasma, erythrocytes, and brain. *J. Toxicol. Environ. Health* **9**, 451–459.

Agrawal D. K., Squibb R. E. and Bondy S.C. (1981) The effects of acrylamide treatment upon the dopamine receptor. *Toxicol. Appl. Pharmacol.* **58**, 89–99.

Albuquerque E. X. and Daly J. W. (1976). In Cuatracasas P. (ed.) *The Specificity of Animals, Bacterial and Plant Toxins*, 297–338. London: Chapman and Hall.

Ali S. F., Abou-Donia M. B. and Bondy S. C. (1984) Modulation of avian muscarinic high affinity binding sites by a neurotoxic organophosphate. *Neurochem. Pathol.* **2**, 267–275.

Austin L. (1957). Lipid biosynthesis and chemically induced paralysis in the chicken. *Br. J. Pharmacol.* **12**, 356–360

Berry J. F. and Cevallos W. H. (1966) Lipid class and fatty acid composition of peripheral nerve from normal and organophosphorus-poisoned chickens. *J. Neurochem.* **13**, 117–124.

Berry J. F., Cevallos W. H. and Wade R. R. (1965) Lipid class and fatty acid composition of intact peripheral nerve and during Wallerian degeneration. *J. Am. Oil Chem. Soc.* **42**, 492–500.

Boer G. J. (1974) A microassay for arylamidase activity. *Anal. Biochem.* **59**, 410–411.

Bondy S. C. and Agrawal A.K. (1980) The inhibition of cerebral high affinity receptor sites by lead and mercury compounds. *Arch. Toxicol.* **46**, 249–256.

Bondy S. C., Harrington M. L., Anderson C. L. et al (1979) Low concentration of an organic lead compound alters transport and release of putative neurotransmitters. *Toxicol. Lett.* **3**, 35–41.

Bondy S. C., Tilson H. A. and Agrawal A. K. (1981) Neurotransmitter receptors in brains of acrylamide-treated rats. II. Effects of extended exposure to acrylamide. *Pharmacol. Biochem. Behav.* **14**, 533–537.

Bonilla E. (1980) L-tyrosine hydroxylase activity in the rat brain after chronic oral administration of manganese chloride. *Neurobehav. Toxicol. Teratol.* **2**, 37–41.

Bonilla E., Salazar E., Villasmil J. J. et al. (1982) The regional distribution of manganese in the normal human brain. *Neurochem. Res.* **7**, 221–27.

Brown G. L. and Feldberg W. (1936) The acetylcholine metabolism of a sympathetic ganglion. *J. Physiol.* **88**, 265–283.

Bowen D. M. Flack R. H. A., Martin R. O. et al., (1974) Biochemical studies on degenerative neurological disorders. 1: Acute experimental encephalitis. *J. Neurochem.* **22**, 1099–1107.

Bradley W. G. and Asbury A. K. (1970) Radioautographic studies of Schwann cell behaviour. 1 : Acrylamide neuropathy in the mouse. *J. Neuropath. Exp. Neurol.* **29**, 500–506.

Brubaker P. E., Klein R., Herman S. P. et al., (1973) DNA, RNA and protein synthesis in brain, liver and kidneys of asymptomatic methyl mercury treated rats. *Exp. Mol. Path.*, **18**, 263–280.

Bull R. J. and Lutkenhoff S. D. (1975) Changes in the metabolic responses of brain tissue to stimulation, *in vitro*, produced by *in vivo* administration of methyl mercury. *Neuropharmacol.* **14**, 351–359.

Bull R. J., Lutkenhoff S. D., McCarty G. E. et al (1979) Delays in the postnatal increase of cerebral cytochrome concentrations in lead exposed rats. *Neuropharmacol.* **18**, 83–92.
Burgen A. S. V., Kosterlitz H. W. and Iversen L. L. (1980) *Neuroactive Peptides*. London: Royal Society.
Cammer W. and Moore C. L. (1972) The effect of hexachlorophene on the respiration of brain and liver mitochondria. *Biochem. Biophys. Res. Comm.* **46**, 1887–1894.
Carbone E., Wanke E., Prestipino G. et al (1982) Selective blockage of voltage-dependent K^+ channels by a novel scorpion toxin. *Nature.* **206**, 90–91.
Carilli C. T., Farley R. A., Perlman D. M., et al (1982) The active site structure of Na^+- and K^+-stimulated ATPase. *J. Biol. Chem.* **257**, 5601–5606.
Carmichael N. and Cavanagh J. B. (1976) Autoradiographic localisation of ^3H-uridine in spinal ganglion neurones of the rat and the effects of methyl mercury poisoning. *Acta. Neuropath. Berl.* **34**, 137–148.
Carrington D. C. and Abou-Donia M. B. (1985a) Characterization of [^{3}H]di-isopropylphosphoroflouridate-binding proteins in hen brain. Rates of phosphorylation and sensitivity to neurotoxic and non-neurotoxic organophosphorous compounds. *Biochem. J.* **228**, 537–544.
Carrington D. C. and Abou-Donia M. B. (1985b) Axoplasmic transport and turnaround of neurotoxic esterase in hen sciatic nerve. *J. Neurochem.* **44**, 616–621.
Carrington D. C., Fluke D. J. and Abou-Donia M. B. (1985) Target size of neurotoxic esterase and acetylcholinesterase as determined by radiation inactivation. *Biochem. J.* **231**, 789–792.
Catterall W. A. (1977) Activation of the action potential Na^+ ionophore by neurotoxins. *J. Biol. Chem.* **252**, 8669–8676.
Cavanagh J. B. (1964) Peripheral nerve changes in orthocresyl phosphate poisoning in the cat. *J. Path. Bact.* **87**, 365–383.
Cavanagh J. B. (1967) On the pattern of change in peripheral nerves produced by isoniazid intoxication in rats. *J. Neurol. Neurosurg. Psychiatr.* **30**, 26–33.
Cavanagh J. B. (1973) Peripheral neuropathy caused by chemical agents. *CRC Crit. Rev. Toxicol.* **2**, 365–417.
Cavanagh J. B. and Chen F. C. K. (1971) The effects of methylmercury dicyandiamide on the peripheral nerves and spinal cord of rats. *Acta Neuropath. Berl.* **19**, 208–215.
Chang-Tsue Y. H. and Ho I. K. (1979) Effects of kepone (chlordecone) on synaptosomal gamma-aminobutyric acid uptake in the mouse. *Neurotoxicology* **1**, 357–361.
Chemnitius J. M., Haselmeyer K. H. and Zech R. (1983) Neurotoxic esterase: Identification of two isoenzymes in hen brains. *Arch. Toxicol.* **53**, 235–244.
Chou S. M. and Hartmann H. A. (1964) Axonal lesions and waltzing syndrome after IDPN administration in rats. *Acta Neuropath.* **3**, 428–450.
Chou S. M. and Hartmann H. A. (1965) Electron microscopy of focal neuroaxonal lesions produced by β,β'-iminodiproprionitrile (IDPN) in rats. *Acta Neuropath*, **4**, 590–603.
Clouet D. H. and Waelsch H. (1963) Amino acid and protein metabolism of the brain. IX. The effect of an organophosphorus inhibitor on the incorporation of ^{14}C-lysine into the proteins of rat brain. *J. Neurochem.* **10**, 51–63.
Costa E. (1970) Simple neuronal models to estimate turnover rate of noradrenergic transmitters *in vivo*. In: Costa E. and Giobocini E. (ed.) *Advances in Biochemical Psychopharmacology. II. Biochemistry of Simple Neuronal Models.* New York: Raven Press.
Cotman C. W., Haycock J. W. and White W. F. (1976) Stimulus secretion coupling processes in brain: analysis of noradrenaline and gamma-aminobutyric acid release. *Am. J. Physiol.* **254**, 475–505.
Damstra T. and Bondy S. C. (1980) The current status and future of biochemical assays for neurotoxicity. In Spencer P. S. and Shaumburg H. H. (ed.) 820–833. *Experimental and Clinical Neurotoxicology*. Baltimore, Maryland, and London: Williams and Wilkins.
DeDuve C., Pressman B. C., Gianetto R., Wattiaux R. and Appelmans F. (1955) Tissue fractionation studies and intracellular distribution patterns of enzyme in the rat liver tissue. *Biochem. J.* **60**, 604–617.
Desaiah D., Gilliland T., Ho I. K. and Mehendale H. M. (1980) Inhibition of mouse brain synaptosomal ATPases and ouabain binding by chlordecone. *Toxicol. Lett.* **6**, 275–285.
Dewar A. J., Barron G. and Reading H. W. (1977a) The effect of anti-inflammatory drugs on retinal dystrophy in the rat. *Toxicol. Appl. Pharmacol.* **42**, 65–74.
Dewar A. J., Barron G. and Yates C. M. (1975) The effect of light deprivation on the progress of retinal degeneration in two strains of dystrophic rat. *Exp. Eye Res.* **21**, 507–514.

Dewar A. J. and Moffett B. J. (1979) Biochemical methods for detecting neurotoxicity. A short review. *Pharmacol. Ther.* **5**, 545–562.

Dewar A. J. Moffett B. J. and Sitton M. F. (1977b) Lysosomal enzyme changes in peripheral neuropathy. *Proc. Int. Soc. Neurochem.* **6**, 626.

Dewar A. J. Yates C. M., Barron G. et al. (1978) The effect of chronic chlorpromazine administration on the albino rat retina. *Toxicol. Appl. Pharmacol.* **43**, 501–506.

Dolphin A. C. and Greengard P. (1981) Neurotransmitter- and neuromodulator-independent alterations in phosphorylation of protein I in slice of rat facial nucleus. *J. Neurosci.* **1**, 192–203.

Domonkos J. and Heiner L. (1968) On the possibility of lysophosphatide formation during Wallerian degeneration. *J. Neurochem.* **15**, 93–98.

Dunn A. J. (1975) Intercerebral injections inhibit amino acid incorporation into brain protein. *Brain Res.* **99**, 405–409.

Eichberg J., Whittaker V. P. and Dawson R. M. C. (1964) The distribution of lipids in subcellular particles of guinea-pig brain. *Biochem. J.* **92**, 91–100.

Farris F. F. and Smith J. C. (1975) *In vivo* incorporation of ^{14}C leucine into brain protein of methylmercury treated rats. *Bull. Environ. Contam. Toxicol.* **13**, (4), 451–455.

Fennelly J., Frank C., Baker H. et al (1964) Peripheral neuropathy of the alcoholic. 1: Aetiological role of aneurin and other B-complex vitamins. *Br. Med. J.* **2**, 1290–1292.

Fishman W. H. and Bernfeld P. (1955) Glucuronidases. In: Colowick S. P. and Kaplan N. O. (ed.) *Methods in Enzymology. Vol. 1*, 262–269. New York: Academic Press.

Fitzgerald G. G., Kaufman E. E., Sokoloff L. et al (1974) D(-)-β-hydroxybutyrate dehydrogenase activity in closed cell lines of glial and neuronal origin. *J. Neurochem.* **22**, 1163–1166.

Fujimori K., Benet H., Mehendale H. M. et al (1982) Comparison of brain discrete area distribution of chlordecone and mirex in the mouse. *Neurotoxicology* **3**, 125–130.

Glees P. (1967). A morphology and neurological analysis of neurotoxicity illustrated by tri-cresyl phosphate intoxication in the chick. In: Davey D. G. (ed.) *Neurotoxicity of Drugs, Proceedings of the European Society for the Study of Drug Toxicity. Vol. 8.* Amsterdam: Excerpta Medica.

Glowinski J. and Iverson L. L. (1966) Regional studies of catecholamines in the rat brain. I. The disposition of ^{3}H-norephinephrine, ^{3}H-dopamine, and ^{3}H-DOPA in various regions of the brain. *J. Neurochem.* **13**, 655–699.

Goridis C., Massarelli R., Sensenbrenner M. et al (1974) Guanyl cyclase in chick embryo brain cell cultures: evidence of neuronal localization. *J. Neurochem.* **23**, 135–139.

Graham D. G. and Abou-Donia M. B. (1980) Studies on the molecular pathogenesis of hexane neuropathy. I. Evaluation of the inhibition of glyceraldehyde-3-phosphate dehydrogenase by 2,5-hexanedione. *J. Toxicol. Environ. Health* **6**, 621–631.

Gray E. G. and Whittaker V. P. (1962) The isolation of nerve endings from brain: and electron microscopic study of cell fragments derived by homogenization and centrifugation. *J. Anat.* (London) **96**, 79–87.

Greengard P., Brink F. and Colowick S. P. (1954) Some relationships between action potential oxygen consumption and coenzyme content in degenerating peripheral axons. *J. Cell. Comp. Physiol.* **44**, 395–420.

Griffin J. W., Fahnstock R. G. and Price D. L. (1982) Fast axonal transport through focal regions of cytoskeletal segregation produced by chemical neurotoxins. *Neurology* **32**, A214.

Griffin J. W., Hoffman P. N., Clark A. W. et al (1978) Slow axonal transport of neurofilament proteins: Impairment by β,β'-iminodiproprionitrile administration. *Science* **202**, 633–635.

Haider S. S., Hassan M. and Islam F. (1980) Effect of air pollutant hydrogen sulfide on the levels of total lipids, phospholipids, and cholesterol in different regions of guinea-pig brain. *Ind. J. Exper. Biol.* **18**, 418–420.

Hassan M. and Ali S. F. (1981) Effects of thallium, nickel, and colbalt administration on the lipid peroxidation in different regions of the rat brain. *Toxicol. Appl. Pharmacol.* **57**, 8–13.

Hedlund B., Gamara M. and Bartfai I. (1979) Inhibition of striatal muscarinic receptors *in vivo* by cadmium. *Brain Res.* **168**, 216–218.

Hille B. (1976) Gating in sodium channels of nerve. *Ann. Rev. Physiol.* **38**, 139–152.

Hollinger D. M. and Rossiter R. J. (1952) Chemical studies of peripheral nerve during Wallerian degeneration. 5: β-glucuronidase. *Biochem. J.* **52**, 659–663.

Hollinger D. M., Rossiter R. J. and Upmalis H. (1952) Chemical studies of peripheral nerve during Wallerian degeneration. 4: Phosphatases. *Biochem. J.* **52**, 652–659.

Holtz P. and Palm D. (1964) Pharmacological aspects of vitamin B. *Pharmacol. Rev.* **16**, 113–178.

Hopkins A. (1972) Toxic neuropathy due to industrial agents. In: Dyck P. J. (ed.) *Peripheral Neuropathy. Vol. II*, Part H, Ch. 60, 1207–1226 Saunders.

Howland R. D., Vyas I. L., Lowndes H. E. and Argentieri T. M. (1980) The etiology of toxic peripheral neuropathies: *in vitro* effects of acrylamide and 2,5-hexanedione on brain enolase and other glycolytic enzymes. *Brain Res.* **202**, 131–142.

Islam F., Tayyaba K. and Hassan M. (1983) Organophosphate metasystox-induced increment of lipase activity and lipid peroxidation in cerebral hemisphere: diminution of lipids in discrete areas of the brain. *Acta Pharmacol. Toxicol.* **53**, 121–124.

Iverson L. L. (1971) Role of transmitter uptake mechanisms in synaptic neurotransmission. *Br. J. Pharmacol.* **44**, 571–591.

Jacobs J. M., Carmichael N. and Cavanagh J.B. (1975) Ultrastructural changes in the dorsal root and trigeminal ganglia of rats poisoned with methylmercury. *Neuropath. Appl. Neurobiol.* **1**, 321–337.

Jakobsen J. and Sidenius P. (1983) Early and dose-dependent decrease of retrograde axonal transport in acrylamide-intoxicated rats. *J. Neurochem.* **40**, 447–454.

Joel C. D., Moser H. W., Majno G. et al (1967) Effects of bio-(monoisopropylamino)fluorophosphine oxide (mipafox) and of starvation on the lipids in the nervous system of the hen. *J. Neurochem.* **14**, 479–488.

Johnson A. C., McNabb A. R. and Rossiter R. J. (1949) Chemical studies of peripheral nerve during Wallerian degeneration. I. Lipids. *Biochem. J.* **45**, 500–508.

Johnson A. C., McNabb A. R. and Rossiter R. J. (1950) Chemistry of Wallerian degeneration. A review of recent studies. *Arch. Neurol. Psychiatr.* **64**, 105–121.

Johnson M. K. (1969) The delayed neurotoxic effect of some organophosphorus compounds. Identification of the phosphorylation site as an esterase. *Biochem. J.* **114**, 711–717.

Johnson M. K. (1977). Improved assay of neurotoxic esterase for screening organophosphates for delayed neurotoxicity potential. *Arch. Toxicol.* **31**, 113–115.

Johnson M. K. (1982) The target for initiation of delayed neurotoxicity by organophosphorus esters. Biochemical studies and toxicological applications. *Rev. Biochem. Toxicol.* **4**, 141–202.

Kaplan M. I. and Murphy S. D. (1972) Effect of acrylamide on rotarod performance and sciatic nerve β-glucuronidase activity of rats. *Toxicol. Appl. Pharmacol.* **22**, 259–268.

Karnovsky M. L. and Majno G. (1961) In: Folch-Pi J. (ed.) Chemical Pathology of the Nervous System, 261–266 London: Pergamon.

Kirpekar S. M., Dixon W. and Pratt J. C. (1970) Inhibitory effect of manganese on norepinephrine release from the splenic nerves of cat. *J. Pharmacol. Exper. Ther.* **174**, 72–76.

Koelle G. B. (1954) The histochemical localization of cholinesterases in the central nervous system of the rat. *J. Comp. Neurol.* **100**, 211–236.

Koelle G. B. (1963) Cholinesterase and anticholinesterase agents. In *Handbuch der Expermentellen Pharmakologie. Vol. 15*, 187–298. Berlin: Springer-Verlag.

Koenig H., Gaines D., McDonald T. et al., (1964) Studies of brain lysosomes. I. subcellular distribution of five acid hydrolases, succinate dehydrogenase and gangliosides in rat brain. *J. Neurochem.* **11**, 729–743.

Konat G. and Clausen J. (1977) Triethyl lead-induced intoxication as an experimental model of hypomyelination. *Proc. Int. Soc. Neurochem.* **6**, 215.

Kornberg A. (1955) Lactic dehydrogenase of muscle. In: Colowick S. P. and Kaplan N. O. (ed.) *Methods of Enzymology. Vol. 1*, 441–443. New York: Academic Press.

Kreutzberg G. (1969) Neuronal dynamics and axonal flow IV. Blockage of intraaxonal enzyme transport by colchicine. *Proc. Natl Acad. Sci.* (USA) **62**, 722–728.

Krigman M. R. and Hogan E. L. (1974) Effect of lead intoxication on the postnatal growth of the rat nervous system. *Environ. Health Perspect.* **7**, 187–199.

Kuczenski R. T. and Mandell A. J. (1972) Regulatory properties of soluble and particulate rat brain tyrosine hydroxylase. *J. Biol. Chem.* **247**, 3114–3116.

Lafferman S. A. and Silbergeld E. K. (1979) Erythrosin B inhibition of neurotransmitter accumulation by rat brain homogenate. *Science* **206**, 363–365.

Lock E. A. (1976) Increase in cerebral fluids in rats after treatment with hexachlorophene or triethyltin. *Biochem. Pharmacol.* **25**, 1455–1458.

Lorenzo A. V. and Gerwitz M. (1977) Inhibition of ^{14}C-tryptophane transport into brain of lead-exposed neonatal rabbits. *Brain Res.* **132**, 386–392.

McCaman R. E. (1962) In: Korey S. R. Pope A. and Robins E. (ed.) *Ultrastructure and Metabolism of the Nervous System*, 169–181. Baltimore, Maryland: Williams and Wilkins.

McCaman R. E. and Robins E. (1959) Quantitative biochemical studies of Wallerian degeneration in the peripheral and central nervous systems. I: chemical constituents. *J. Neurochem.* **5**, 18–31.
McKenna M. J. and Destefano V. (1975) A proposed mechanism of action of carbon disulfide on dopamine-β-hydroxylase. *Toxicol. Appl. Pharmacol.* **33**, 137.
Majno G. and Karnovsky M. L. (1958) A biochemical and morphological study of myelination and demyelination. II. Lipogenesis *in vitro* by cat nerve following transection. *J. Exper. Med.* **108**, 197–214.
Majno G. and Karnovsky M. L. (1961) A biochemical and morphological study of myelination and demyelination. III. Effect of an organophosphorus compound (mipafox) on the biosynthesis of lipids by nervous tissue of rats and hens. *J. Neurochem.* **8**, 1–16.
Mäkinen A., Savolainen H., Lehtonen E. et al. (1977) Reduced sulfhydryl groups of rat neurons, glial cells and neurofilaments. *Res. Commun. Chem. Pathol. Pharmacol.* **16**, 577–580.
Mangan J. L. and Whittaker V. P. (1966) The distribution of free amino acids in subcellular fractions of guinea-pig brain. *Biochem. J.* **98**, 128–137.
Matheson D. F. and Cavanagh J. B. (1967) Protein synthesis in peripheral nerve and susceptibility to diptheric neuropathy. *Nature* **214**, 721–722.
Mendell J. R., Zarife S., Saida K. et al., D. (1977) Alterations of fast axoplasmic transport in experimental methyl *n*-butylketone neuropathy. *Brain Res.* **133**, 107–118.
Merkurieva R. V., Bushinskaia L. J., Aulika B. V. et al., (1978) The activity of lysosomal and cytoplasmic enzymes under the experimental influence of carbon bisulfide. *Vopr. Med. Khim.* **2**, 151–156.
Merkurieva R. V., Kotov A. V., Silov V. G. et al., (1980) *Experimental study of Biochemical and Physiological Mechanisms of Cerebral Activity Influenced by Alcohol*, 93–94. Nauka: Minsk Publishing House.
Miani N. (1962) The relationship between axon and Schwann cell phospholipid metabolism of degenerating and regenerating peroneal-tibial nerves of the rabbit *in vitro*. *J. Neurochem* **9**, 525–536.
Miller E. K. and Dawson R. M. C. (1972) Can mitochondria and synaptosomes of guinea-pig brain synthesize phospholipids? *Biochem. J.* **126**, 805–807.
Montanini I. and Porcellati G. (1964) Protein metabolism of peripheral nerves during demyelination by organophosphorous compounds. *Ital. J. Biochem.* **13**, 230–239.
Mucalt A. V. and Wyss F. (1944) Uber den Aneuringehalt des peripheren Nerven wahrend der Degeneration. *Helv. Physiol. Pharmacol. Acta.* **2**, 445–448.
Myers D. K. and Mulder H. E. W. (1953) Effect of tri-*ortho*-cresyl phosphate on the absorption of tocopherol. *Nature* (London) **172**, 773.
Nelson W. L. and Barnum C. P. (1960) The effect of diisopropylphosphorofluoridate (DFP) on mouse brain phosphorus metabolism. *J. Neurochem.* **6**, 43–49.
Nomeir A. A. and Abou-Donia M. B. (1984) Disposition of tri-*o*-cresyl phosphate (TOCP) and its metabolites in various tissues of the male cat following a single dermal application of [^{14}C]TOCP. *Drug Metab. Dispos.* **12**, 705–711.
Nomeir A. A. and Abou-Donia M. B. (1985) Studies on the metabolism of the neurotoxic tri-*o*-cresyl phosphate. Distribution, excretion, and metabolism in male cats after a single dermal application. *Toxicology* **38**, 15–33.
O'Callaghan J. P. and Miller D. B. (1983) Nervous-system specific proteins as biochemical indicators of neurotoxicity. *Trends Pharmacol. Sci.* **4**, 388–390.
O'Callaghan J. P., Miller D. B. and Reito L. W. (1983) Acute postnatal exposure to triethyltin in the rat: effects on specific protein composition of subcellular fractions from developing and adult brain. *J. Pharmacol. Exper. Ther.* **224**, 466–472.
Ochs J. (1982) *Axonal Transport and Its Relation to Other Nerve Functions*. New York: Wiley.
Oderfeld-Nowak B. and Niemierko S. (1969) Synthesis of nucleic acids in the Schwann cells as the early cellular response to nerve injury. *J. Neurochem.* **16**, 235–248.
Padilla S. S., Lapadula D. M., Reiter L. W. et al., (1983) Alteration of slow axonal transport in hens treated with tri-*o*-cresyl phosphate (TOCP). *Fed. Proc. Fed. Am. Soc. Exper. Biol.* **42**, 870.
Partridge W. M. (1976) Inorganic mercury: selective effects on blood–brain barrier transport systems. *J. Neurochem.* **27**, 333–335.
Patton S. E., Lapadula D. M., O'Callaghan J. P. et al., (1985). Changes in *in vivo* brain and spinal cord protein phosphorylation after a single oral administration of tri-*o*-cresyl phosphate to hens. *J. Neurochem.* **45**, 1567–1577.

Patton S. E., O'Callaghan J. P., Miller D. B. et al., (1983) Effect of oral administration of tri-*o*-cresyl phosphate on *in vitro* phosphorylation of membrane and cytosolic proteins from chicken brain. *J. Neurochem.* **41**, 897–901.

Paulson J. C. and McClure W. O. (1974) Microtubules and axoplasmic transport. *Brain Res.* **73**, 333–337.

Paulson J. C. and McClure W. O. (1975) Inhibition of axoplasmic transport by colchicine, podophyllotoxin and vinblastine: an effect on microtubules. *Ann. NY Acad. Sci.* **253**, 517–527.

Poduslo S. E. (1975) The isolation and characterization of a plasma membrane and a myelin fraction derived from oligodendroglia of calf brain. *J. Neurochem.* **24**, 647–654.

Porcellati G. (1961) Proteinase activity of nervous tissues during experimental demyelination. *Proc. VIIth Intern. Congr. Neurol.* 815–822.

Porcellati G. (1965) Il metabolismo proteico nella degenerazione e rigenerazione del tessuto nervoso periferico. *Farmaco* **20**, 586–605.

Porcellati G. (1966a) In: Peeters H. (ed.) *Protides of the Biological Fluids, Vol. 13*, 115–126. Amsterdam: Elsevier.

Porcellati G. (1966b) In: Cazzullo C. L. (ed.) *Convegno Internazionale di Studi sulla Sclerosi Multipla*, 195–206. Gallarate: La Tipografica Varese.

Porcellati G. (1967a) The effect of organophosphorous compounds on nerve phospholipid metabolism. *Prog. Biochem. Pharmacol.* **3**, 49–58.

Porcellati G. (1967b) Organofosforici demielinizzanti e lipogenesi del nervo periferico. *Acta Neurol. (Napole)* **22**, 168–172.

Porcellati G. and Mastrantonio M. A. (1964) Phospholipid metabolism of peripheral nerves during myelination by organophosphorus compounds. *Ital. J. Biochem.* **13**, 332–352.

Porcellati G., Millo A. and Manocchio I. (1961) Protinase activity of nervous tissues in organophosphorus compound poisoning. *J. Neurochem.* **7**, 317–320.

Porcellati G. and Thompson R. H. S. (1957) The effect of nerve section on the free amino acids of nervous tissue. *J. Neurochem.* **1**, 316–325.

Prineas J. (1969) The pathogenesis of dying back polyneuropathies: part II. An ultrastructural study of experimental acrylamide intoxication in the cat. *J. Neuropathol. Exper. Neurol.* **28**, 598–621.

Radin N. S., Brenkert A., Arora R. C. et al., (1972) Glial and neuronal localization of cerebroside-metabolizing enzymes. *Brain Res.* **39**, 163–166.

Rasool C. G. and Bradley W. G. (1978) Axonal transport in acrylamide neuropathy. In Canal N. and Pozza G. (ed.) *Peripheral Neuropathies*, 159–165. Amsterdam: Elsevier/North Holland.

Reichardt L. F. and Kelly R. B. (1983) A molecular description of nerve terminal function. *Ann. Rev. Biochem.* **52**, 871–926.

Reichert B. L. and Abou-Donia M. B. (1980) Inhibition of fast axoplasmic transport by delayed neurotoxic organophosphorus esters: a possible mode of action. *Mol. pharmacol.* **17**, 56–60.

Richardson R. J., Davis C. S. and Johnson M. K. (1979) Subcellular distribution of marker enzymes and of neurotoxic esterase in adult hen brain. *J. Neurochem.* **32**, 607–615.

Robins E., Hirsch H. E. and Emmons S. S. (1968) Glycosidases in the nervous system. I. Assay, some properties, and distribution of β-galactosidase, β-glucuronidase, and β-glucosidase. *J. Biol. Chem.* **243**, 4246–4249.

Roeder R. G. and Rutter W. J. (1969) Multiple forms of DNA-dependent RNA polymerase in eukaryotic organisms. *Nature* **224**, 234–236.

Rose S. P. R. and Sinha A. K. (1970) Separation of neuronal and neuropil cell fractions: A modified procedure. *Life Sci.* **9**, 907–912.

Sabri M. I., Moore C. L. and Spencer P. S. (1979) Studies on the biochemical basis of distal axonopathies. Inhibition of glycolysis produced by neurotoxic hexacarbon compounds. *J. Neurochem.* **32**, 683–690,

Savolainen H. and Jarvisalo J. (1977) Effects of CS_2 intoxication on protein metabolism in rat brain. *Chem. Biol. Interact.* **17**, 51–59.

Schnaitman C., Erwin V. G. and Greenswalt J. W. (1967) The submitochondrial localization of monoamine oxidase. An enzymatic marker for the outer membrane of rat liver mitochondria. *J. Cell Biol.* **32**, 719–720.

Schotman P., Gipon L., Jennekens F. G. I. et al., (1978) Polyneuropathies and CNS protein metabolism. III. Changes in protein synthesis induced by acrylamide intoxication. *J. Neuropathol. Exper. Neurol.* **37**, 820–837.

Seth P. K., Agrawal A. K. and Bondy S. C. (1981) Biochemical changes in the brain consequent to

dietary exposure of developing and mature rats to chlordecone (kepone). *Toxicol. Appl. Pharmacol.* **26**, 262–267.
Sidenius P. and Jakobsen J. (1983) Anterograde axonal transport in rats during intoxication with acrylamide. *J. Neurochem.* **40**, 697–704.
Silbergeld E. K. and Goldberg A. M. (1975) Pharmacological and neurochemical investigations of lead-induced hyperactivity. *Neuropharmacol.* **14**, 431–444.
Silbergeld E. K., Hruska R. E. Miller L. P. et al., (1980) Effects of lead *in vivo* and *in vitro* on GABAergic neurochemistry. *J. Neurochem.* **34**, 1711–1718.
Simpson J. (1964) Biology and disease of the peripheral nerves. *Br. Med. J.* **2**, 709–714.
Smith M. I., Elvove E., Valer P. J., et al., (1930) Pharmacological and chemical studies of the cause of so-called ginger paralysis. *US Public Health Rep.* **45**, 1073–1716.
Sokoloff L., Reivich M., Kennedy C. et al., (1977) The ^{14}C-deoxyglucose method for the measurement of local cerebral glucose utilization: theory, procedure and normal values in the conscious and anaesthetized albino rat. *J. Neurochem.* **28**, 897–916.
Souyri F., Chretien M. and Droz B. (1981) 'Acrylamide-induced' neuropathy and impairment of axonal transport of proteins. I. Multifocal retention of fast transported proteins at the periphery of axons as revealed by light microscope radiography. *Brain Res.* **205**, 1–13.
Spencer P. S. and Schaumburg H. H. (1980) *Experimental and Clinical Neurotoxicology* 929. Baltimore, Maryland: Williams and Wilkins.
Steele W. J. and Busch H. (1963) Studies on acidic nuclear proteins of the Walker tumor and liver. *Cancer Res.* **23**, 1153–1157.
Stewart M. A., Passonneau J. V. and Lowry O. H. (1965) Substrate changes in peripheral nerve during ischaemia and Wallerian degeneration. *J. Neurochem.* **12**, 719–727.
Towbin H., Staehelin T. and Gordon J. (1979) Electrophoretic transfer of proteins from polyacrylamide gels to nitrocellulose sheets: procedure and some applications. *Pro. Natl. Acad, Sci.* (USA) **76**, 4350–4354.
Tytell M., Black M. M., Garner J. A. et al., (1981) Axonal transport: Each major rate component reflects the movement of distinct macromolecular complexes. *Science* **214**, 179–181.
Van Gelder G. A. (1978) Lead and the nervous system. In: Oehme F. W. (ed.) *Toxicity of Heavy Metals in the Environment. Part I*, 101–121. Basel and New York: Dekker.
Verity M. A., Brown W. J., Cheung M. et al., (1977) Methyl mercury inhibition of synaptosomes and brain slice protein synthesis: *in vivo* and *in vitro* studies. *J. Neurochem.* **29**, 673–679.
Vilter R. W. Mueller J. F., Glazer H. et al., (1953) The effect of vitamin B deficiency induced by desoxypyridozine in human beings. *J. Lab. Clin. Med.* **42**, 335–357.
Webster G. R. (1954) The distribution and metabolism of phosphorus compounds in normal and demyelinating nervous tissue of the chicken. *Biochem. J.* **57**, 153–158.
Webster G. R. (1973) Phospholipase A activities in normal and sectioned rat sciatic nerve. *J. Neurochem.* **21**, 873–876.
Whittaker V. P. (1959) The isolation and characterization of acetylcholine-containing particles from brain. *Biochem J.* **72**, 694–706.
Whittaker V. P. (1965) The application of subcellular fractionation techniques to the study of the brain function. *Prog. Biophys. Mol. Biol.* **15**, 39–96.
Whittaker V. P. (1966) Some properties of synaptic membranes isolated from the central nervous system. *Ann. NY Acad. Sci.* **137**, 982–998.
Whittaker V. P. and Barker L. A. (1972) The subcellular fractionation of brain tissue with special reference to the preparation of synaptosomes and their component organelles. In: Fried R. (ed.) *Methods of Neurochemistry. Vol. 2*, 1–5. New York: Dekker.
Whittaker V. P., Michaelson I. A. and Kirkland R. J. A. (1964) The separation of synaptic vesicles from nerve-ending particles (synaptosomes). *Biochem. J.* **90**, 293–303.
Williams C. H., Johnson N. J. and Casterline J. L. (1966) Cholesterol content of spinal cord and sciatic nerve of hens after organo-phosphate and carbamate administration. *J. Neurochem.* **13**, 471–474.
Williams D. G. (1983) Intramolecular group transfer is a characteristic of neurotoxic esterase and is independent of the tissue source of the enzyme. *Biochem. J.* **209**, 817–829.
Williams D. G. and Johnson M. K. (1981) Gel electrophoretic identification of hen brain neurotoxic esterase, labelled with tritiated diisopropylphosphoroflouridate. *Biochem. J.* **199**, 323–333.
Yamamura H. I., Enna S. J. and Kuhar M. J. (1981) *Neurotransmitter Receptor Binding*. New York: Raven Press.

Yoshino Y., Mozei T. and Nakao K. (1966) Biochemical changes in the brain in rats poisoned with an alkylmercury compound with special reference to the inhibition of protein synthesis in brain cortex slices. *J. Neurochem.* **13**, 1223–1230.

Zuber V. L. (1978) Intensity of metabolism of various fractions of cerebral phospholipids under hyperphenylalaninemia. *Vopr. Med. Khim.* **2**, 163–166.

Chapter 2

Chemical Excitants of Cutaneous Pain

A. G. Ramage

INTRODUCTION

Pain is generally acknowledged to be primarily a signal that body tissue is undergoing damaging stimulation. This chapter will be concerned with pain caused by the application of chemicals to the intact skin, which cause pain without, at least initially, damaging the skin. These substances will be termed chemical irritants. There are also many substances that cause pain when applied to the broken skin or injected into the skin, e.g. K^+, histamine and bradykinin. Chemical irritants, e.g. capsaicin, have been used clinically as counter-irritants, because as well as causing pain they provoke an inflammatory response and so relieve more deeply seated muscle pain. Recently chemical irritants, e.g. ω-chloracetophenone (CN; tear gas), have been used by the police and armed services as riot-control agents. To understand how such chemicals cause pain a knowledge of the types of sensory nerves which innervate the skin is required.

Somatosensory Receptors

The skin contains many types of nerve endings which transmit information to the central nervous system about touch, temperature and pain. A controversy exists about whether pain is a distinct modality, or a combination of modalities (e.g. touch and temperature) interpreted as pain when diverse somatosensory receptors are being stimulated. The weight of evidence is now overwhelming in favour of the specificity hypothesis (see Burgess and Perl, 1973; Iggo, 1974).

Sensory or afferent cutaneous nerve bundles contain two distinct morphological types of nerve fibres: myelinated having a fast conduction velocity and unmyelinated having a slow conduction velocity. The myelinated fibres vary in diameter. The large diameter fibres are termed 'A alpha' (11–6 μm) and the smaller 'A delta' (6–11 μm), while the even smaller (1·5–0·3 μm) unmyelinated fibres are termed 'C-fibres'. However, sensory nerve fibres from muscle are divided into Type I, II, III and IV. This nomenclature is sometimes applied also to cutaneous afferents. Therefore, A alpha becomes synonymous with group II, A delta with group III and C-fibre with group IV.

The A alpha fibres are concerned with conveying information on touch, pressure and vibration, and can be divided by their response to constant pressure into slowly, rapidly, and fast adapting fibres respectively. The nerve endings are enscapsulated to form specialized receptors which have been identified in the skin as Ruffini ends and Meissner and Pacinian corpuscles. The small myelinated (A delta) and C-fibres are primarily responsible for transmitting information on pain and temperature. As pain is a perception and an adequate stimulus is difficult to define, pain receptors are called nociceptors, i.e. somatosensory receptors, which respond to stimuli that threaten damage to the skin. No morphologically distinct end organs have been detected in association with either A delta or C nociceptor afferents, and they are presumed to terminate in apparently unspecialized free nerve endings. A network of non-myelinated fibres in the hairy skin of man with 'penicillate' endings, which are located close to the corioepidermal junction with axon twigs occasionally penetrating the epidermis, have been suggested to be involved in nociception (Cauna, 1973).

Additionally there exists a group of A delta and C-fibres which respond to low threshold mechanical stimulation. There appears to be a fairly large amount of these C-fibre receptors in the cat and very few in monkeys, but none have yet been identified in man.

Nociceptors

Nociceptors can be divided into two groups, mechanical and thermal (Iggo, 1974). The mechanical ones are associated with A delta or C-fibres. The A delta fibres are thought to be responsible for first or fast pain sensation described as pin pricking. The function of a high threshold C-mechanoreceptor is uncertain, again due to the paucity of such receptors in man.

Thermal nociceptors are known to be related to both C and A delta fibres. The A delta fibres have been identified only fairly recently in primates. However, the C-thermal nociceptors, which are also termed C-polymodal nociceptors (Bessou

Table 2.1. Summary of skin sensation and associated types of afferent nerve fibres.

	Afferent fibres[a]		
Sensation	*A alpha*	*A delta*	*C*
Touch Pressure Vibration	+ + +	+	+ (cat only?)
Thermoreceptor (warm + cold)	−	+	+ + +
Nociceptors: Mechanical	−	+ + + (fast pain) (pin pricking)	+
Thermal (polymodal nociceptor)	−	+ (primates only?)	+ + + (slow pain) (burning)

[a] (+) Indicates the relative importance of a particular sensation with a type of nerve fibre.
(−) Indicates the absence of a sensation with a type of nerve fibre.

and Perl, 1969), have been extensively studied. They are characterized by their high threshold to mechanical and thermal stimulation and they respond to weak acid applied to the skin. Following an initial stimulation of one of these receptors, there may be an enhancement of their response to a second stimulation and a lowering of their thresholds to either mechanical or thermal stimuli. This corresponds to hyperalgesia. C-polymodal nociceptor afferents constitute 80 to 90% of the C-fibre population. Activation of these sensory receptors in man is associated with a 'burning/itching' pain. This correlates well with the observation that stimulation of only afferent C-fibres in man causes a burning pain sensation. The existence of A delta 'polymodal nociceptors' or thermal nociceptors explains the observation that first pain can be produced in man by noxious heat (Lewis and Pochin, 1937). For a more detailed review see Price and Dubner (1977). Table 2.1 shows a simplified classification of the types of somatosensory receptors found in the skin.

CHEMICAL IRRITANTS AND INFLAMMATION

The main chemical irritants which will be discussed are capsaicin (CAP) and the structurally related substance *n*-nonanoylvanillylamine (VAN), as well as dibenzoxazepine (CR), ω-chloracetophenone (CN) and *o*-chlorobenzylidene malononitrile (CS), all of which cause burning pain sensations when applied to human skin (Janscó, 1960; Ballantyne et al., 1973). The structures of these compounds are shown in *Fig.* 2.1. Of these chemical irritants, capsaicin has received the most attention (Buck and Burks, 1986). The first description of the effects of capsaicin was made in 1878 by Högyes, who reported that an alcoholic extract of paprika caused a burning pain sensation when applied to the skin, and concluded that capsaicin acts mainly on sensory nerves. Further interest in the action of capsaicin occurred when Janscó (1960) observed that its parenteral application together with related acyl amides abolishes the sensation of chemical

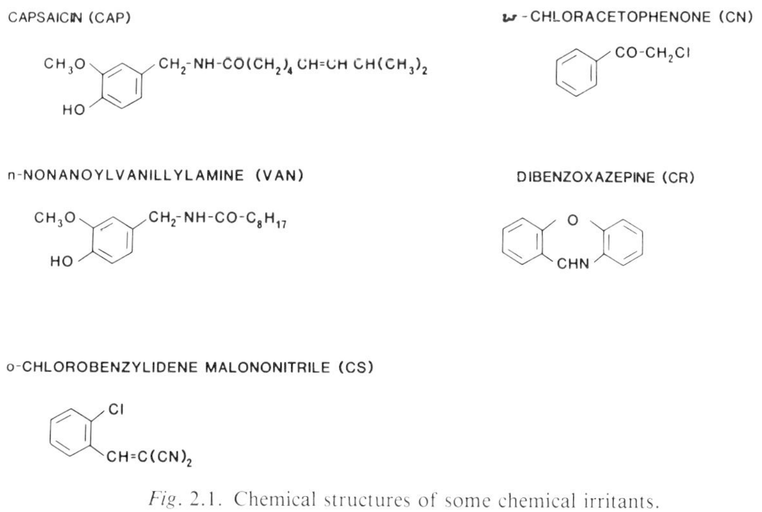

Fig. 2.1. Chemical structures of some chemical irritants.

'pain' stimuli, but leaves a response to mechanical stimuli intact. More recently the observation that capsaicin pretreatment causes substance P depletion in the spinal cord (Gasporovic et al., 1964; Jessel et al., 1978) emphasized the importance of capsaicin as a 'tool' to elucidate mechanisms involved in 'pain' pathways in the peripheral and central nervous system.

Observations at the beginning of this century on the effect of mustard oil on the conjunctiva of the cat and rabbit suggested the involvement of sensory nerves in inflammation. Bruce (1913) showed that when the right eye of the cat or rabbit was anaesthetised, mustard oil applied to both eyes caused severe chemosis in the unanaesthetized eye only. Furthermore, when mustard oil was applied just after transection of the trigeminal nerve, when the sensory nerve endings were still present, severe chemosis developed, but if the sensory nerves were allowed to degenerate, the response to mustard oil was abolished. From such experiments, Bruce concluded that vasodilatation caused by the irritation was the result of an axon reflex.

This observation was substantiated by Breslauer (1919), who found that mustard oil failed to produce reactive hyperemia (i.e. local vasodilatation) in human skin from which sensory nerves had degenerated. Lewis and Grant (1924), in their analysis of the triple response in man, found that severe mechanical or thermal stimulation caused a red central area surrounded by a bright red flare to that patch of the skin. This flare failed to develop if the nerves to the skin had degenerated. They also concluded that the flare was due to an axon reflex.

These observations together with that of Bayliss (1901), that vasodilatation occurs when afferent nerves are stimulated antidromically, led to the suggestion that afferent nerves can release a substance which causes vasodilatation. This substance is at present believed to be substance P (Lembeck, 1983). Janscó reported that capsaicin desensitization blocked the release of this substance, for no antidromic vasodilatation was observed. Further, he demonstrated that chemical irritants can be divided into two classes: those compounds whose inflammatory responses are blocked by capsaicin or sensory denervation and compounds such as dextrose to which the inflammatory response was not blocked (Janscó, 1960; Janscó et al., 1967; 1968). The observation that the inflammatory reaction to mustard oil, xylene and ω-chloracetophenone is not completely abolished was explained by suggesting that these compounds have both classes of action. However, although the inflammatory response to other groups of compounds such as 48/80, thuryl nicotinate, and histamine was unaffected by denervation, the flare was absent. He therefore concluded that capsaicin blocks irritants which act by stimulation of the 'pain' nerve endings to cause an inflammatory response, while the other class act by the release of vasoactive substances from most other cells.

CHEMICAL IRRITANTS AND SOMATOSENSORY RECEPTORS

Pórszász and Janscó (1959) were the first to try and identify which type of somatosensory receptors were involved in capsaicin's ability to block the response to 'painful' chemical injury. They recorded electrical nerve activity from small fibres of the saphenous nerve of the rat. Application of capsaicin to the paws caused the production of low amplitude spikes (action potentials) in the electrical recording, but not the high amplitude spikes associated with touch. It was suggested that these small action potentials were related to 'pain' fibres. Szolcsányi (1977), after intra-arterial injection of capsaicin, observed a considerable reduction of one of the small elevations, which are associated with unmyelinated fibres, of the compound action potential of the saphenous nerve in the cat. Whereas the A alpha and A delta elevations were the same. Foster and Ramage (1981), recording from eight different types of sensory receptors in the cat skin, showed that topical application of capsaicin and the capsaicin derivative *n*-nonanoylvanillylamine only excited C-polymodal nociceptors (*Figs*. 2.2 and 2.3) and warm thermoreceptors. Furthermore, topical application of capsaicin to the rat hindlimb was also found to excite C-polymodal nociceptors and warm thermoreceptors (Kenins, 1982). The selectivity of capsaicin to C-polymodal nociceptors explains why animals pretreated with capsaicin still respond to touch and mechanical pain (Janscó, 1960). Furthermore, taken together with the observations that capsaicin blocks antidromic vasodilatation and that C-fibres must be activated before antidromatic vasodilatation occurs (Hinsey and Gasser, 1930), the latter effect is probably mediated by pain receptors rather than temperature receptors (Celander and Folkow, 1953), and indicates that C-

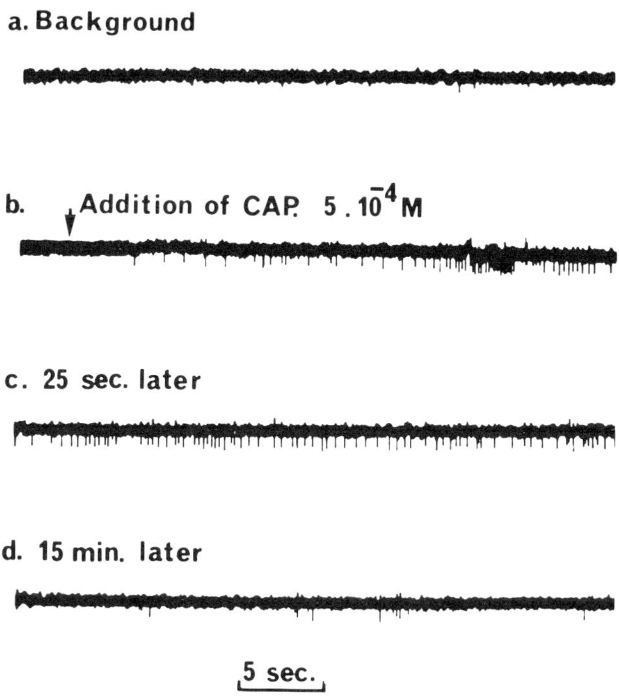

Fig. 2.2. Electrical activity recorded from a fine filament of the saphenous nerve of the cat containing a C-polymodal nociceptor (conduction velocity 0·55 m/sec): *a*. background activity before experimental interventions; *b*. activity on application of capsaicin (CAP 5×10^{-4} M) to the cutaneous receptive area; *c*. activity 25 seconds later; *d*. the return of background activity 15 minutes after application of capsaicin.

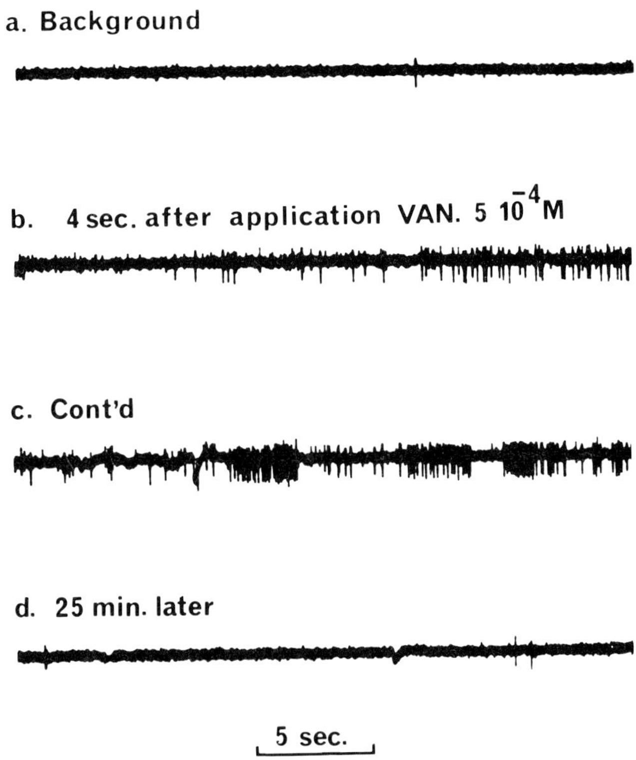

Fig. 2.3. Electrical activity recorded from a fine filament of the saphenous nerve of the cat containing a C-polymodal nociceptor (conduction velocity 0·7 m/sec): *a.* background activity before experimental interventions; *b.* activity recorded 4 seconds after application of *n*-nonanoylvanillylamine (VAN 5×10^{-4} M) to the cutaneous receptive field; *c.* is continuous with *b*; *d.* the return to background activity 25 minutes later. (From Foster and Ramage, 1981.)

polymodal nociceptors are probably the somatosensory receptors involved in the axon reflex, i.e. antidromic vasodilatation.

An examination of the effect of other chemical irritants not structurally related to capsaicin on somatosensory receptors was also carried out by Foster and Ramage (1981). Table 2.2 shows the effect of these agents on the eight types of somatosensory receptors that were isolated. These agents also show selectivity for C-polymodal nociceptors and, where tested, to warm thermoreceptors. However, the ability of chemical irritants to excite warm thermoreceptors could be related to their ability to cause an increase in skin temperature due to vasodilatation. All agents caused a bout of irregular activity when applied to the receptor area of C-polymodal nociceptors (*Fig.* 2.3). A similar pattern has been observed in human polymodal nociceptors to application of a nettle leaf or acetic acid (Van Hees and Gybels, 1972; Torebjörk, 1974; Torebjork and Hallin, 1974). Such activity in these receptors was associated with 'burning/itching' pain. This sensation was also obtained when chemical irritants were applied to human skin. Furthermore, in the cat studies all chemical irritants showed self-tachyphylaxis

Table 2.2. Summary of the selective effects of irritants on somatosensory receptors.[a].

Unit type	*Cond. vel.* (*m*/sec)	*CR*	*VAN*	*CN*	*CS*	*CAP*
A-mechanoreceptors:						
Low threshold	30–50					
Rapidly adapting		0/6	0/7	0/3	—	0/1
Slowly adapting		0/16	0/17	0/6	0/4	0/4
A-delta mechanoreceptors (nociceptors)	4–35	0/5	0/3	0/2	0/2	0/2
C-mechanoreceptors:						
Low threshold	0.8–1.4	0/7	0/6	0/1	—	0/3
Polymodal	0.3–1.2	13/13	9/9	4/4	2/2	3/3
Very high threshold	0.5–1	0/4	0/4	0/1	—	0/1
Thermoreceptors:						
Warm	0.7,0.9	2/2	—	—	—	1/1
Cold	—	0/1	—	—	—	—

[a] The numerator of each fraction represents the number of units which responded, and the denominator the number of units tested.

Cond. vel. = conduction velocity;— = not determined; CR = dibenzoxazepine; VAN = *n*-nonanoylvanillylamine; CN = ω-chloracetophenone; CS = *o*-chlorobenzylidene malononitrile; CAP = capsaicin. (After Foster and Ramage, 1981.)

and, although the data is incomplete, the evidence suggests that chemical irritants also show cross-tachyphylaxis. If this is so, it might be inferred that these irritants have the same mode of action or act on the same pharmacological receptor. Sensory units which did respond to chemical irritants were also sensitive to heat, suggesting that there may be a common process involved in the ability of sensory receptors to detect heat and to be stimulated by chemical irritants. Within this context, it was reported (Foster and Ramage, 1981) that the initial testing of three C-polymodal nociceptors to noxious heat (50°C) abolished the expected response to chemical irritants, and also the response of warm thermoreceptors to warmth after excitation by chemical irritants was abolished. However, the gross response of C-polymodal nociceptors to mechanical deformation was not altered by chemical irritants except by *n*-nonanoylvanillylamine, which did show a tendency to reduced mechanical responsiveness of C-polymodal nociceptors, particularly at high concentrations. Interpretation of these observations must be speculative, since these observations are the results of only one laboratory and that, also, noxious heat will initiate the inflammatory reaction and may thereby alter the access of the irritant to its site of action.

If the basis of the selectivity of chemical irritants is chemical, the conclusion drawn from quantitative studies of pain production by a series of structurally related acyl amides applied to the rat eye, that capsaicin was a structurally specific drug having several critical moieties for the binding to a receptor molecule, is most interesting. Such properties would make these chemical irritants valuable tools in pain studies (Szolcsanyi and Janscó-Gábor, 1975). However, the basis of this selectivity might be due to a distributional basis, in that the nerve endings of polymodal receptors and warm thermoreceptors are superficially located within the skin surface, while the other types of receptors are deeper, and would therefore receive a smaller amount of the irritant than the more superficial receptors. Furthermore, the fact that A alpha somatosensory receptors are encapsulated may be a barrier preventing the chemical irritants from affecting them. Finally, another possible basis for this selectivity may be due to the combination of fibre size with other unknown properties which underlies the differential sensitivity of nerve fibres to local anaesthetics, i.e. the ability to block 'pain' fibres before touch fibres.

However, close-arterial injection of chemical irritants also excites A delta and C high threshold mechanoceptors (nociceptors) as well as C-polymodal nociceptors (Ramage, 1977). In these experiments, substances which cause pain when applied to broken skin or injected into the skin were also given close-arterially. Bradykinin and 5-hydroxytryptamine were found to consistently excite C-polymodal nociceptors but not A delta mechanical nociceptors, which were excited by KC1. The effect of close-arterial injections of capsaicin and other alogenic substances to one of these high threshold A delta nociceptors is shown in *Fig*. 2.4. This A delta nociceptor only responded to KCl and capsaicin, and both drugs reversibly blocked the response to mechanical stimulation. These results suggest that chemical irritants will excite other sensory receptors, and that such excitation is dependent on accessibility. The following observations support such a view. Exposure of the isolated rabbit vagus nerve, which is mostly composed of C-fibres, to dibenzoxazepine and *n*-nonanoylvanillylamine caused a reversible reduction in the electrical evoked compound action potentials of between 20 to 40% (Ramage, 1977), and that capsaicin has been shown to depolarize the rat vagus nerve and reduce the electrically evoked compound action potentials of A and C-fibres (see Foster and Ramage, 1981) support such a conclusion. These results indicate also that there does not seem to be a discrete pharmacological receptor as in the case for many neurotransmitters, but a special ability of these

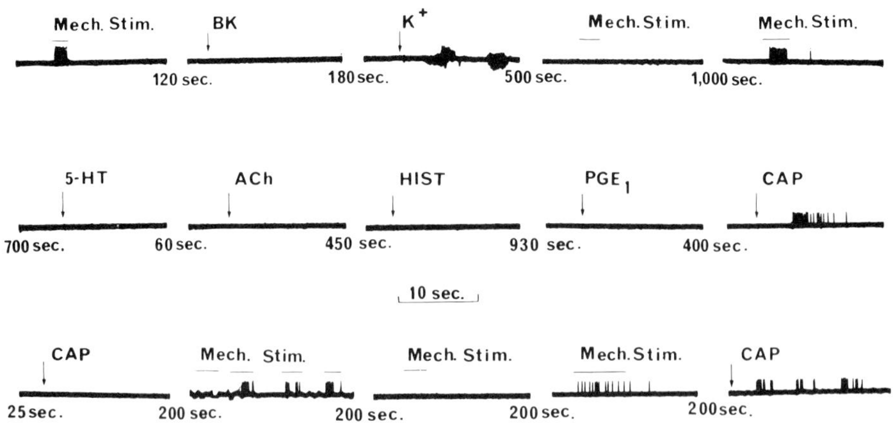

Fig. 2.4. Electrical activity recorded from a fine filament of the saphenous nerve of the cat containing an A delta mechanical nociceptor (conduction velocity 10 m/sec). The time between each section of the record is indicated and the record runs from top left to bottom right. Close intra-arterial injection of the following have been given: bradykinin (BK 30 μg), potassium chloride (K^+ 5 mg), 5-hydroxytryptamine (5-HT 60 μg), acetylcholine (ACh 30 μg), histamine (HIST 60 μg), prostaglandin E_1 (PGE_1 30 μg) and capsaicin (CAP 9 μg). Mechanical stimulation (Mech. stim.) is indicated by a line above the recording.

chemical irritants to alter, in some manner, the properties of the nerve membrane. More recently the effect of capsaicin on myelinated fibres of the frog sciatic nerve has shown that capsaicin does not affect the early part and the slow K^+ conductance, but suppresses the second part of the fast K^+ channels (Dubois, 1982). However, frogs do not respond to capsaicin. Topical application of capsaicin to the rat saphenous nerve only blocks conduction in C-polymodal nociceptors, but not in C cold receptors and myelinated fibres (Petsche et al., 1983). Therefore, more studies on mammalian axons are required to elucidate the mechanism by which capsaicin and other chemical irritants cause their action on nerve membranes.

Capsaicin application renders man and other animals insensitive to further noxious chemical stimuli, and this insensitivity can last for some time. Attempts have been made to relate this insensitivity to morphological changes. Repeated application of 1% capsaicin to the cornea of the rat resulted in ultra-structural changes being restricted to partly or completely naked nerve endings. These ultra-structural changes were mitochondrial swelling and a reduction in the number of microvesicles in the nerve terminal (Szolcsányi et al., 1975). If capsaicin pretreatment is carried out in neonatal rats, it causes a life-long insensitivity to chemical irritants. The insensitivity is accompanied by a destruction of the small neurones, but not the large neurones in dorsal root ganglia (Janscó et al., 1977). The question arises, is this loss of small neurones associated exclusively with C-fibres or are small myelinated (A delta) fibres also affected? Further examination of the saphenous nerve has also shown that there is a 60 to 70% loss of C-fibres, and a 10% reduction in small myelinated fibres (Janscó et al., 1980). This degeneration is also associated with the loss of the following peptides: substance P, somatostatin, vasoactive intestinal polypeptide, and cholecystokinin (Janscó et al., 1981). Furthermore, this degeneration can only be caused in rats up to 14 days of age. The destruction of cell bodies of primary sensory peptidergic neurones has been shown to be due to capsaicin interference with the action of nerve growth factor (NGF) since the latter can also partially antagonize the effect of capsaicin (Otten et al., 1983). However, further studies are also required with the other structurally unrelated chemical irritants to investigate whether they also possess such an action.

Recently, Weston (1982) has indicated differences between *n*-nonanoylvanillylamine and the other chemical irritants using blister base experiments in humans. The repeated application of potassium chloride, bradykinin and all chemical irritants to the blister base causes self-tachyphylaxis. The repeated application of *n*-nonanoylvanillylamine produced non-specific desensitization to all other chemical irritants and to KCl. Only repeated application of KCl rendered blister bases insensitive to *n*-nonanoylvanillylamine. Cross-tachyphylaxis occurred between *o*-chlorobenzylidene malononitrile and dibenzoxazepine, and after repeated application of bradykinin, the response to all chemical irritants was reduced. As expected, capsaicin showed similarities to *n*-nonanoylvanillylamine.

It is therefore evident that the mechanism of action of these chemical irritants in causing pain is not yet fully understood. Though they selectively excite C-afferents, this may be due to the ability to these agents to gain access to the nerve membrane, since C-afferents are supposed to have 'free' nerve endings. Until a good model of these 'free' nerve endings has been discovered, the action of the chemical irritants will not be fully understood as 'single' fibre recordings from small diameter afferent is extremely difficult.

REFERENCES

Ballantyne B., Beswick F. W. and Price-Thomas D. (1973) The presentation and management of individuals contaminated with solutions of dibenzoxazepine (CR). *Med. Sci. Law* **13**, 265–268.

Bayliss W. M. (1901) On the origin from the spinal cord of the vaso-dilator fibres of the hind-limb, and on the nature of these fibres. *J. Physiol.* **26**, 173–209.

Bessou P. and Perl E. R. (1969) Responses of cutaneous sensory units with unmyelinated fibres to noxious stimuli. *J. Neurophysiol.* **32**, 1025–1043.

Breslauer F. (1919) Die Pathogenese der trophischen Gewebsschaden nach der Nervenverletzuny. *Dtsch. Z. Chirurgie* **150**, 50–81.

Bruce A. N. (1913) Vaso-dilator axon-reflexes. *Quart. J. Exp. Physiol.* **6**, 334–354.

Buck S. H. and Burks T. F. (1986) The neuropharmacology of capcaisin: review of some recent observations. *Pharmac. Rev.* **38**, 179–226.

Burgess P. R. and Perl E. R. (1973) Cutaneous mechanoreceptors and nociceptors. In: Iggo. A. (ed.) *Handbook of Sensory Physiology. Vol. 2. Somatosensory Systems*, 30–78. Berlin: Springer-Verlag.

Celander O. and Folkow B. (1953) The nature and the distribution of afferent fibres provided with axon reflex arrangement. *Acta Physiol. Scand.* **29**, 359–370.

Cauna N. (1973) The free penicillate nerve endings of the human hairy skin. *J. Anat.* **115**, 277–288.

Dubois J. M. (1982) Capsaicin blocks one class of K^+ channels in the frog node of Ranvier. *Brain Res.* **245**, 327–375.

Foster R. W. and Ramage A. G. (1981) The action of some chemical irritants on somatosensory receptors of the cat. *J. Neuropharmacol* **20**, 191–198.

Gasparovic J., Hadzovic S., Hakovic S. et al. (1964) Contribution to the theory that substance P has a transmitter role in sensitive pathways. *Med. Exp.* **10**, 303–306.

Hees J. Van and Gybels J. M. (1972) Pain related to single afferent C fibres from human skin. *Brain Res.* **48**, 397–400.

Hinsey J. C. and Gasser H. S. (1930) The component of the dorsal root mediating vasodilation and the Sherrington contracture. *Am. J. Physiol.* **99**, 679–689.

Höyges A. (1878) Beitrage zur physiologischen Wirkung der Bestandteile des Capsicum Annuum. *Arch. Exper. Pathol. Pharmakol.* **9**, 117–130.

Iggo A. (1974) Cutaneous receptors. In: Hubbard J. I. (ed.) *The Peripheral Nervous Systems*, Ch. 12, 347–404. New York: Plenum Press.

Janscó G., Király E. and Janscó-Gábor A. (1977) Pharmacologically induced selective degeneration of chemosensitive primary sensory neurones. *Nature* **270**, 741–743.

Janscó G., Király E. and Janscó-Gábor A. (1980) Chemosensitive pain fibres and inflammation. *Int. J. Tiss. Res.* **2**, 57–66.

Janscó G., Hökfelt T., Lundberg J. M. et al. (1981) Immunohistochemical studies on the effect of capsaicin on spinal and medullary peptide and monoamine neurones using antisera to substance P, gastrin/CCK, somatostatin, VIP, enkephalin, neurotensin and 5-hydroxytryptamine. *J. Neurocytol.* **10**, 963–980.

Janscó N. (1960) Role of the nerve terminals in the mechanism of inflammatory reactions. *Bull. Millard Fillmore Hosp., Buffalo, New York* **7**, 53–77.

Janscó N., Janscó-Gábor A. and Szolcsányi J. (1967) Direct evidence for neurogenic inflammation and its prevention by denervation and by pretreatment with capsaicin. *Br. J. Pharmacol.* **31**, 138–151.

Janscó N., Janscó-Gábor A. and Szolcsányi J. (1968) The role of sensory nerve endings in neurogenic inflammation induced in human skin and in the eye and paw of the rat. *Br. J. Pharmacol.* **33**, 32–41.

Jessel T. M., Iversen L. L. and Cuello A. C. (1978) Capsaicin induced depletion of substance P from primary sensory neurones. *Brain Res.* **152**, 183–188.

Kenins P. (1982) Responses of single nerve fibres to capsaicin applied to the skin. *Neurosci. Lett.* **29**, 83–88.

Lembeck F. (1983) Mediators of vasodilation in the skin. *Br. J. Dermatol.* **119**, Supp. 25, 1–9.
Lewis T. and Grant R. T. (1924) Vascular reactions of the skin to injury. *Heart* **11**, 209–265.
Lewis T. and Pochin E. E. (1937) The double pain response of the human skin to a single stimulus. *Clin Sci.* **3**, 67–76.
Otten U., Lorez H. P. and Businger F. (1983) Nerve growth factor antagonizes the neurotoxic action of capsaicin on primary sensory neurones. *Nature* **301**, 515–517.
Petsche U., Fleischer E., Lembeck F. et al. (1983) The effect of capsaicin application to a peripheral nerve on impulse conduction in functionally identified afferent-nerve fibres. *Brain Res.* **265**, 233–240.
Porszasz J. and Jansco N. (1959) Studies on the action potentials of sensory nerves in animals desensitized with capsaicin. *Acta Physiol. Acad. Sci. Hung.* **15**, 231–235.
Price D. D. and Dubner R. (1977) Neurones that subserve the sensory-discriminative aspects of pain. *Pain* **3**, 307–338.
Ramage A. G. (1977) *An investigation of the effects of chemical irritants on sensory nerves of the cat skin.* PhD thesis, University of Manchester.
Szolcsanyi, J. (1977). A pharmacological approach to elucidation of the role of different nerve fibres and receptor endings in mediation of pain. *J. Physiol.* (Paris) **73**, 251–259.
Szolcsanyi J. and Jansco-Gabor A. (1975) Sensory effects of capsaicin congeners. I. Relationship between chemical structure and pain producing potency of pungent agents. *Arzneim-Forsch.* (*Drug Res.*) **25**, 1877–1881.
Szolcsanyi J., Jansco-Gabor A. and Joo F. (1975) Functional and fine structural characteristics of the sensory neuron blocking effect of capsaicin. *Naunyn-Schmiedeberg's Arch. Pharmac.* **287**, 157–169.
Torebjork H. E. (1974) Afferent C units responding to mechanical, thermal and chemical stimuli in human non-glabrous skin. *Acta Physiol. Scand.* **92**, 374–390.
Torebjork H. E. and Hallin R. G. (1974) Identification of afferent C units in intact human skin nerves. *Brain Res.* **67**, 387–403.
Weston K. M. (1982) *Chemical irritation, accessed using some exteroceptors of the leech, guinea-pig and man.* PhD thesis, University of Manchester.

Chapter 3

Ototoxicity: Morphological and Functional Correlations between Experimental and Clinical Studies

E. S. Harpur

Although we still know little about the mechanisms by which drugs and other chemicals damage the ear, i.e. are ototoxic, a considerable fund of knowledge has accumulated, particularly during the past decade, about the sites and nature of the lesions caused by ototoxic substances. Since the vast majority of studies have been directed toward an understanding of the ototoxic effects of drugs, no consideration is given in this chapter to the ototoxicity of industrial or environmental chemicals. Refinements in histopathological, electrophysiological and behavioural methodologies have facilitated the detailed examination of both the morphological and functional changes resulting from ototoxic drug administration. There are now sufficient data regarding the effects of ototoxic drugs in animals and man to permit comparisons to be made. It is therefore possible to attempt an assessment of the validity of animal models for the prediction of effects in man.

THE DRUGS INVOLVED

A large number of drugs are now known to exert some harmful action on the inner ear (see Harpur (1983) for full list). Some of these ototoxic drugs produce effects which are reversible. For example, intravenous administration of large doses of loop diuretics, such as frusemide, can cause loss of hearing which is rapid in onset and of short duration. Although permanent hearing loss can occur (Gallagher and Jones, 1979), this would seem to be an infrequent event. A permanent cochlear lesion has been shown to result from administration of a single dose of loop diuretic with a single dose of an aminoglycoside antibiotic in animal studies (Brummett et al., 1975), but this interaction may have little relevance to the normal clinical use of the two groups of drugs in combination (Smith and Lietman, 1983). Non-steroidal anti-inflammatory drugs, particularly salicylates, also cause hearing impairment, with associated tinnitus, but in almost all patients these effects are reversible when the therapy is stopped.

Permanent loss of hearing or vestibular function is quite frequently encountered with aminoglycoside antibiotic therapy. This group of drugs includes streptomycin, neomycin, kanamycin, gentamicin, tobramycin, sisomicin, netilmicin and dibekacin. The anti-tumour agent *cis*-platinum is also prone to cause permanent damage to the inner ear, usually manifest as hearing loss. Together, these drugs account for the great majority of permanent ototoxic lesions observed in patients. They are also the only drugs to have been extensively studied in patients. As a result, it is only with these drugs that it is feasible to compare the results of experimental studies in animals with clinical findings in patients.

MICROANATOMY OF THE INNER EAR

Since much of what follows is a comparison of the morphological changes induced by ototoxic drugs in animals and man, the inclusion of a brief description of the microanatomy of the inner ear is likely to benefit the reader with little specialized knowledge of this organ.

The inner ear, surrounded by the temporal bone, comprises the cochlea, or organ of hearing, and the vestibular structures, the organs of balance (*Fig.* 3.1).

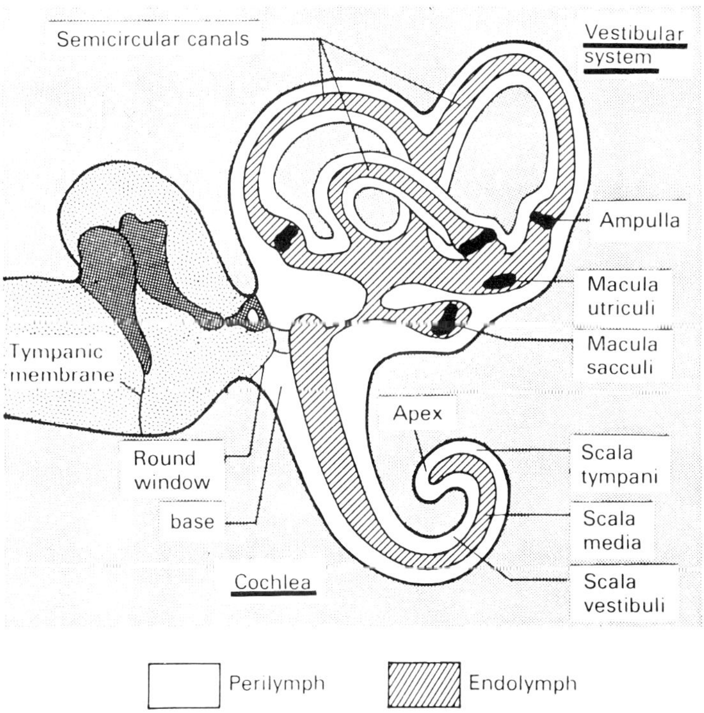

Fig. 3.1. Schematic representation of the middle and inner ear. There are five sensory structures in the vestibular system: the three cristae ampullaris and the two maculae of the utricle and saccule. In the cochlea, the organ of hearing, or organ of Corti, rests on the basilar membrane and divides the scala tympani from the scala media.

It is appropriately named the labyrinth, since it consists of a series of fluid-filled canals which are subdivided into several compartments by membranous partitions. The elements of the vestibular system are the three cristae ampullaris within the semicircular canals, and the two maculae of the utricle and the saccule. In each of these five structures are located the sensory cells, the vestibular hair cells (HCs), so called because a tuft of stereocilia or hairs projects from the surface of each cell. These cells are responsive to movements of the head, and send information to the vestibular nuclei in the brainstem via the primary afferent neurones with which they synapse.

The cochlea is a helical structure, making several turns from base to apex (the actual number of turns varies between species) around a central bony spindle which contains the nerve supply to the sensory structures. The subdivision of the bony cochlear canal into three fluid-filled compartments by the basilar membrane, and by Reissner's membrane, is readily seen in a transverse section (*Fig.* 3.2). The transduction of sound takes place in the organ of Corti, which is located on the basilar membrane and contains the sensory cells, or hair cells (HCs), and various supporting cells (*Fig.* 3.3). The cochlear HCs are arranged in orderly rows, a single row of inner hair cells (IHCs), and three to five rows of outer hair cells (OHCs), depending on the species. The HCs are activated by the displacement of the hairs which project from their surfaces toward the tectorial membrane. The organ of Corti is innervated by both afferent and efferent neurones, the cell bodies of the former being in the spiral ganglion (*Fig.* 3.2).

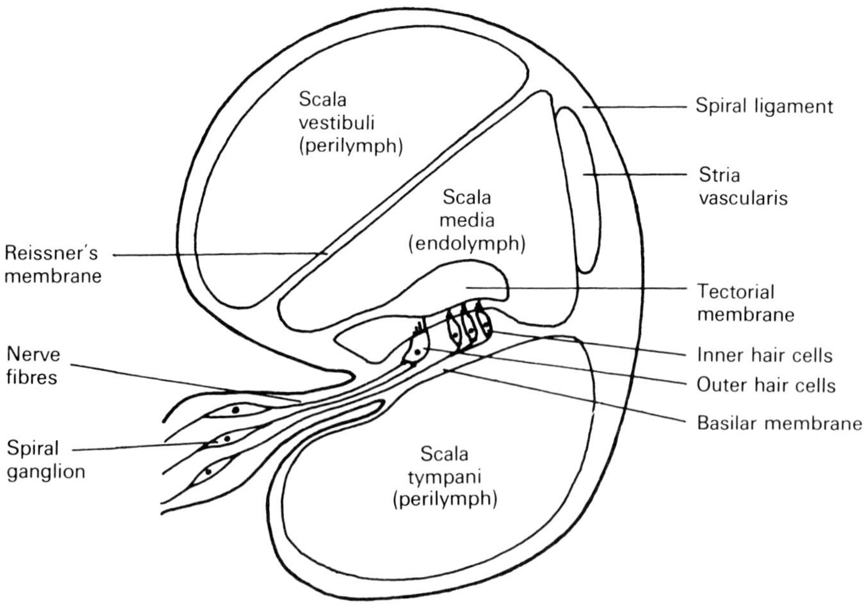

Fig. 3.2. Simplified drawing of a transverse section through one turn of the cochlea, showing the division by membranous partitions into three compartments filled either with perilymph or potassium-rich endolymph.

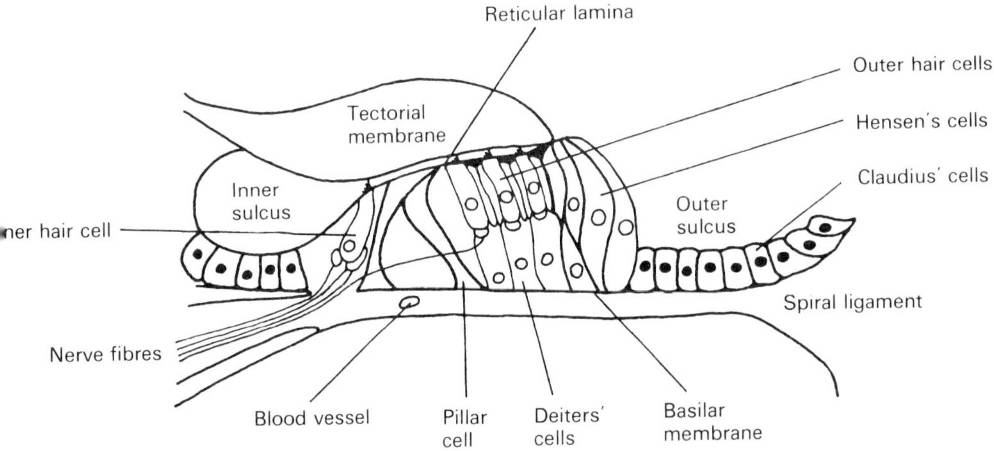

Fig. 3.3. Relationship of the various cell populations within the organ of Corti.

METHODS OF STUDY

A comprehensive array of histopathological methods for the study of cochlear and vestibular tissues has been developed and refined over the past two decades. These techniques may be applied with suitable modification to the study of inner ear tissue in a variety of species, including the human. Good use has been made of technical innovations, such as interference contrast microscopy and scanning electron microscopy. The labyrinth may be fixed by perfusion, followed by conventional processing, including decalcification and embedding. This is a slow process, and subsequent hitopathological assessment by serial sectioning is tedious, although it offers the advantage of simultaneous examination of the different tissues in their normal juxtaposition. In the case of the cochlea, one alternative to reconstruction from serial sections is to estimate the overall HC damage by examining a single mid-modiolar section, and integrating the score allotted to each individual cell according to its degree of integrity (Gregory, 1986). This technique has not gained wide acceptance, and most workers have used some variation of the 'surface preparation' (Engstrom et al., 1966; Hawkins and Johnsson, 1975). In this method, the cochlear bone is broken away, after thinning if necessary, and the underlying tissues are carefully removed by microdissection. The tissue fragments, free of bone, may be embedded, and thick sections cut for light microscopy, or thin sections cut for electron microscopy. The fragments of the organ of Corti, each approximately half a turn in length, may be mounted as a surface preparation and viewed using either phase contrast or interference contrast microscopy. Alternatively, after removal of the tectorial membrane and further preparation, the specimens can be examined using scanning electron microscopy. The examination of the dissected organ of Corti as a surface preparation is an appropriate and rapid technique for quantifying HC damage. Missing cells can be counted easily because of the highly organized arrangement of the HCs (*Fig*. 3.4). Some workers, e.g. Ylikoski (1974), have used a technique which facilitates the study of the organ of Corti as a surface preparation, and yet preserves the relationship of the various cochlear tissues for subsequent study in transverse section. In this 'block-surface' technique (Spoendlin and Brun, 1974), the embedded cochlea is cut into two halves along a mid-modiolar plane, and each cochlear half turn is sawn off in the form of a small disc.

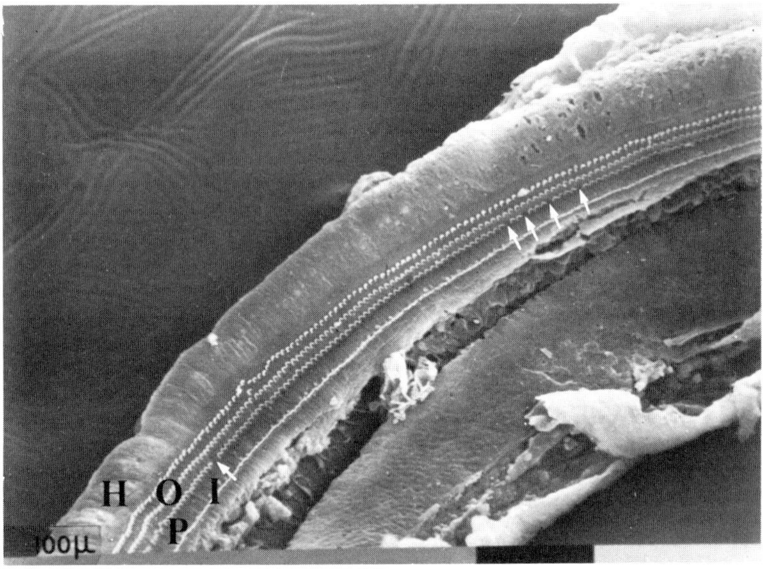

Fig. 3.4. Scanning electron micrograph of the surface of the organ of Corti of a guinea-pig, showing the regular arrangement of the inner (I) and outer (O) HCs, the inner pillar cells (P) and Hensen's cells (H). Occasional missing first row OHCs are arrowed. Middle turn; gentamicin, 140 mg kg^{-1} day^{-1} for 14 days; survival time, 7 days. (Reproduced with permission from Harpur and Bridges, 1979.)

Although the vestibular sensory structures can be dissected out and mounted as surface preparations (Hawkins and Johnsson, 1975), they are not well suited to this method of study because of their thickness, and the dark background caused by the heavy straining of the underlying myelinated nerve fibres (Hawkins and Johnsson, 1981; Aran et al., 1982). A further problem is created by the lack of a regular arrangement of the HCs such as is found in the cochlea (Aran et al., 1982); thus, only remaining HCs can be counted. Consequently, the vestibular tissues are best embedded and cut in thick sections for examination in the light microscope.

Methods available for the assessment of cochlear and vestibular function in animals and man are so numerous and diverse that it would be quite unrealistic to attempt to summarize them here. A general review of methods which have applications in ototoxicological studies in animals is available (Harpur, 1981). More specific reviews of behavioural and electrophysiological assessment of cochlear and vestibular toxicity in animals, as well as descriptions of appropriate methodology for ototoxicological assessment in man, may be found in Lerner et al. (1981).

EXPERIMENTAL STUDIES

Histopathological Changes

Cochlea

The pattern of HC degeneration in the guinea-pig cochlea is similar with the various aminoglycoside antibiotics. Furthermore, although the ototoxicity of *cis*-platinum in the guinea-pig has not been systematically studied, there is evidence to show that *cis*-platinum-induced cochlear damage is essentially the same as that caused by aminoglycosides. Consequently, it is possible to state certain generalia. The OHCs are usually more sensitive than the IHCs, and the first row of OHCs appears to be the most vulnerable of all. HC damage is usually first seen in the basal coil, and then progresses in an apical direction, depending on the dosage of the drug and the duration of the treatment. Long-term administration of low doses of aminoglycosides is reported to lead to scattered degeneration over large areas of the cochlea, whereas short-term administration of high doses tends to cause damage which is localized in the basal part of the cochlea (Wersall, 1981).

The fine detail of cochlear HC degeneration has been described by a number of authors and summarized by Wersall (1981). The sequence of intracellular changes is similar in both OHCs and IHCs, although degeneration of the IHCs is usually much delayed relative to the OHCs. One of the earliest signs of HC damage is the appearance of membrane-bound dense lamellar structures in the subcuticular region of the cells. At least some of these structures are identified as phagolysosomes, indicating the capacity of the HCs to digest degenerating cell structures during the early phase of ototoxic damage. Coincident with the appearance of phagolysosomes, is the occurrence of disruption of the lateral membranes of the HCs. There follows mitochondrial damage, a decrease in ribosomal content, nuclear swelling, vacuolation of the cytoplasm, and finally rupture of the plasma membrane. Surface changes such as fusion of stereocilia, or decrease in their number, or protrusion of the cuticular plate also occur. However, these changes are seen during the late stages of degeneration (*Fig* 3.5), and the cuticular plate and stereocilia may appear normal in cells which are otherwise in an advanced state of degeneration (Harpur and Bridges, 1979). As the cuticular plate and stereocilia disintegrate, cell debris can be observed in the endolymphatic space. A role for the cells of the outer sulcus, and of Reissner's membrane, in engulfment and digestion of the remnants of HCs has been proposed by Duvall and Quick (1969).

The observation that HCs at an advanced state of degeneration may have normal stereocilia and cuticular plates has significant implications. Such cells would appear normal in surface view. This must be borne in mind when using light microscopy or scanning electron microscopy to evaluate HC loss in a surface preparation. It is essential to allow sufficient time between the end of ototoxic drug administration and death, in order that all irreversibly damaged cells will have fully disintegrated. This is particularly important when scanning electron microscopy is used (Hunter-Duvar, 1978; Astbury and Read, 1982). If light microscopy is used, then phase contrast or, ideally, interference contrast methodology, will allow the observer to focus at different levels within the cell. Thus, it should be possible at least to identify damaged cells with swollen nuclei.

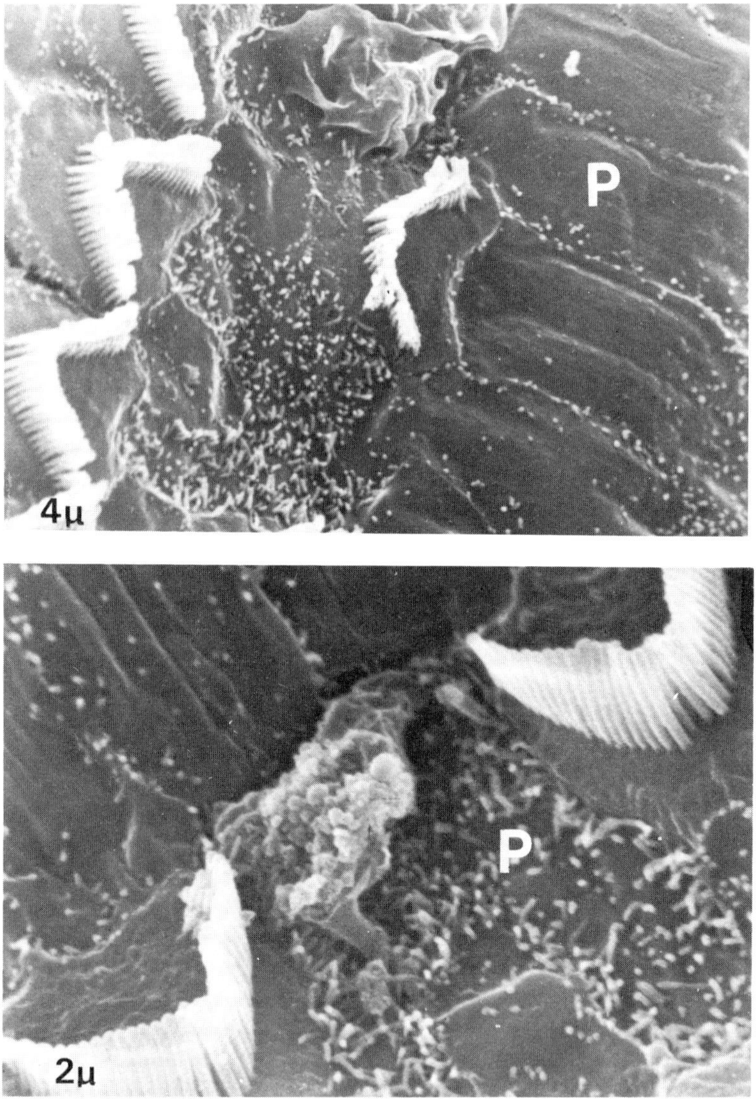

Fig. 3.5. *a*. Various stages in the surface degeneration of first row OHCs seen to the left of the pillar cells (P). A degenerated HC, at the bottom, has been replaced by expansion of the heads of adjacent supporting cells. Recent evidence suggests that both the outer pillar cells and Deiter's cells are involved in the replacement of the first row of OHCs. The hairs and cuticular plates of the two HCs at the top are formed into a fused mass; the cell between shows some disorganisation of the hair pattern. The second row of OHCs look normal. Guinea-pig cochlea; upper basal, turn; scanning electron micrograph (Drug administration and source as for *Fig*. 3.4.) *b*. First row OHC in final stage of degeneration. The hairs have fused and disintegrated into a clump and, together with the cuticular plate, are about to be shed into the endolymph. Already the head of the outer pillar cell and the phalangeal plate of the neighbouring Deiter cell (P) have expanded to fill the space left by the degenerating HC, thus preserving the integrity of the reticular lamina. Guinea-pig cochlea; middle turn; scanning electron micrograph. (Drug administration and source as for *Fig*. 3.4.)

The space left by the disintegrating HC is filled by an expansion of the head plate of an adjacent supporting cell (*Fig.* 3.5). As a consequence, Wersall (1981) commented that it is unlikely that any defect would appear in the reticular lamina during the process of HC degeneration. This is an important observation, since the reticular lamina or surface of the organ of Corti (*Fig.* 3.3) comprises the heads of the HCs and supporting cells which are separated by tight junctions. This appears to form a permeability barrier between the endolymph of the scala media and the perilymph present in the scala tympani and the fluid spaces between the cells of the organ of Corti (*Fig.* 3.6). Ototoxic drugs can, at certain dosages, result in a small restricted area of HC damage. It is unlikely that this damage could be confined to a small area if the integrity of the reticular lamina were not maintained. For example, the progressive loss of supporting cells and nerve fibres which follows acoustic trauma might be a consequence of the occurrence of perforations in the reticular lamina (Bohne and Rabbitt, 1983). In such circumstances, the exposure of the lateral membranes of the HCs to the potassium-rich endolymph may contribute to the spread of HC damage.

Considerable structural reorganization is required to take place within the organ of Corti for the supporting cells to replace the missing HCs. With further progression of the damage, the supporting cells also start to degenerate with concomitant contraction of the organ of Corti. Eventually, the entire organ of

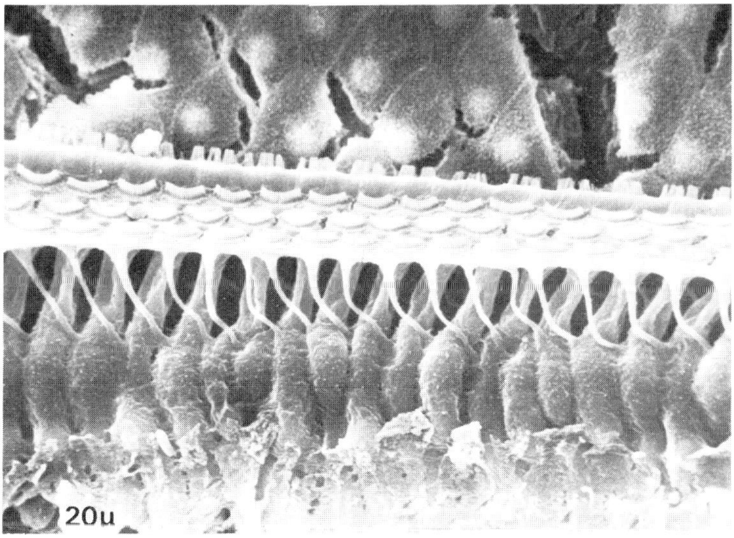

Fig. 3.6. Axial view of a basal turn of guinea-pig organ of Corti. Hensen's cells have been removed to reveal the internal arrangement of the sensory and supporting cells. In the foreground, the outermost Deiter's cell bodies can be seen to give rise to angled processes which expand to form head plates on the surface of the organ of Corti. Behind these Deiter's cells are seen the tall cylindrical bodies of the third row of OHCs. The extensive fluid spaces between the cells is readily apparent, although these are accentuated by some shrinkage of the HCs which has occurred during the drying process. The head plates of the Deiter's cells and the cuticular plates of the HCs interlock to form an impermeable barrier between the endolymph of the scala media and the perilymph of the fluid spaces within the organ of Corti. Scanning electron micrograph.

Corti, both sensory and supporting cells, may be totally destroyed and replaced by a layer of flat, relatively undifferentiated cells, resembling the cells of the inner and outer sulcus (*Fig.* 3.7) This total replacement of the organ of Corti may initially be patchy, but ultimately in extreme cases may extend to long portions of the basilar membrane. Degeneration of the afferent nerve endings occurs soon after the degeneration of the HCs (Wersall, 1981). That the degeneration of the nerve fibres and the ganglion cells begins at the nerve endings, and progresses retrogradely toward the ganglion cells, has been demonstrated very clearly by Ylikoski (1974).

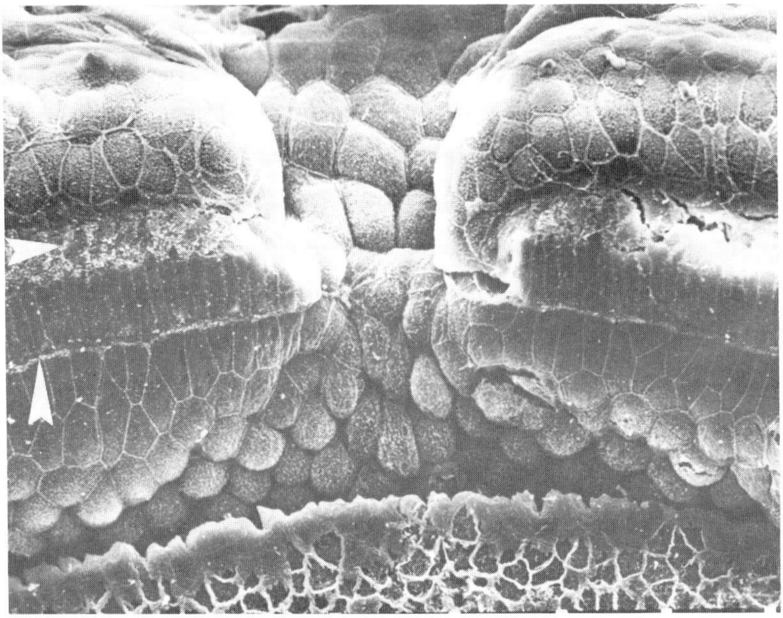

Fig. 3.7. Guinea-pig organ of Corti severely damaged by administration of kanamycin, 500 mg kg^{-1} day^{-1} for 10 days; survival time, 30 days. All the IHCs and OHCs have degenerated (vertical and horizontal arrows respectively). The heads of some of the inner pillar cells may still be seen between the remnants of the IHCs and OHCs. In the centre, a short portion of the organ of Corti has totally degenerated, including the supporting cells, and has been replaced by flat cells resembling those of the inner or outer sulcus. Upper basal turn; scanning electron micrograph.

Observations of damage caused by aminoglycoside antibiotics to cochlear tissues other than those in the organ of Corti, such as Reissner's membrane, the cells of the outer sulcus, the spiral ligament, or the stria vascularis (Hawkins et al., 1972; Johnsson and Hawkins, 1972), have prompted the suggestion that degeneration of the HCs in the organ of Corti might occur secondary to drug effects at these other sites (Hawkins, 1973a,b). However, the exact time sequences of the damage to these tissues and HC degeneration is unknown (Hawkins, 1973a), so that a cause and effect relationship is speculative.

Vestibular System

As in the cochlea, the sensory cells in the vestibular system are much more sensitive to damage caused by ototoxic substances than are the supporting cells. Degeneration of HCs in the cristae ampullaris precedes that in the maculae of the utricle and saccule. Of the two types of HC, the type I cells are more vulnerable than type II. Thus, the degeneration begins at the tip of the cristae, where the type I cells are predominant, and then spreads toward the sides of the cristae as the type II cells are affected. The initial selectivity for the type I cells is also seen in the utricle and saccule.

The pattern of degeneration of individual cells in the vestibular system is reportedly very variable depending upon the drug, the dose schedule, the total dose, or even the route of administration (Wersall, 1981). However, although intracellular changes occur resembling those seen in cochlear HCs, surface changes such as fusion of the stereocilia and ballooning of the plasma membrane are frequently seen during the early stages of degeneration. Ultimately, the debris which results from disintegration of the cell is either taken up by the phagocytic activity of the neighbouring cells in the sensory epithelium, or it is ejected into the endolymph. When the HCs degenerate completely, the supporting cells take their place and seem to remain intact, even in severely damaged vestibular structures. The nerve fibres remain in the vestibular epithelia for several weeks following HC degeneration, but then degenerate in a retrograde manner.

Functional Changes

Cochlea

There is abundant evidence to show that the pattern of cochlear HC loss caused by ototoxic drugs is paralleled by a hearing loss which initially affects only high frequencies, but eventually progresses to affect low frequencies. The function of the cochlea can be assessed in a variety of ways, and ultimately, the only true measure of auditory acuity is the behaviourally determined auditory threshold. However, valuable information can also be obtained by using electrodes placed on or inside the cochlea to record the electrical response of the HCs or the cochlear nerve fibres to sound stimuli; these responses are known as the a.c. cochlear potential or cochlear microphonic (CM) and the compound action potential (CAP).

The CM correlates very closely with the presence of OHCs (Dallos and Wang, 1974; Dallos and Cheatham, 1976), and amplitude of the CM response as a function of the frequency of the stimulating tone has been used to monitor the ototoxic effect of aminoglycosides (Brummett and Fox, 1982). However, Aran (1981) has pointed out that the CM response provides little information about the IHCs, and he advocates the use of CAP threshold determinations to assess ototoxicity. A frequency threshold curve for CAP can be measured using filtered clicks or tone pips. Aran (1981) has also indicated that the CAP response latency provides information about its point of origin on the basilar membrane. Threshold elevations of CAP at high frequencies correspond to a lesion in the basal turn of the cochlea. As the HC loss spreads along the cochlea, so CAP threshold becomes elevated at lower frequencies. Most electrophysiological recordings from drug damaged cochleas are done as terminal procedures in anaesthetized animals following a period of drug administration. Although it is technically difficult, it is possible to implant electrodes and make serial recordings from individual animals at appropriate intervals during and following drug administration. Such studies as have been done demonstrate very clearly the evolution of threshold changes in CAP, beginning at high frequencies and gradually spreading to involve low frequencies (Aran, 1981).

Behavioural methods for assessing hearing in animals also offer the advantage that they can be used serially in conscious animals. Once again, there is very clear evidence that chronic administration of cochleotoxic aminoglycosides causes the gradual development of a hearing impairment, affecting high frequencies first, and subsequently spreading to affect lower frequencies (Stebbins et al., 1981). The correspondence between a hearing loss affecting high frequencies and a lesion in the organ of Corti confined to the basal turns is striking (Stebbins and Coombs, 1976).

Vestibular System

Although the gradual development of a vestibular lesion caused by aminoglycosides is associated with a characteristic loss of HCs in the vestibular end-organs, it is not possible to correlate the functional and morphological changes with any degree of precision. Objective testing of vestibular function is difficult to do in animals, and has been attempted infrequently in ototoxic studies (e.g. Aran et al., 1982). Some of the most sensitive methods for assessing vestibular function involve testing an animal's righting reflex (Igarashi and Jensen, 1981), or its ability to perform a complex motor task which depends on the integration of sensory information from the vestibular end-organs with other sensory inputs (Igarashi et al., 1971). One cannot readily attribute a deficit in complex behavioural responses to a lesion at a particular site in the vestibular system. Even the nystagmic eye movements, which may be objectively recorded following rotational stimulation of the vestibular end-organs, are the product of both peripheral and central mechanisms. Furthermore, the difficulties in quantifying HC loss in the vestibular end-organs have been emphasized (see p. 46). Thus, any precise correlation of vestibular dysfunction with vestibular HC damage must await the development of better methods for assessing the function of the different portions of the vestibular neuroepithelia.

Differences Between Drugs

Differences in Effect on the Cochlea and the Vestibular System

Aminoglycoside antibiotics have the potential to damage both the cochlea and the vestibular system, but some show a marked predilection for one or other sensory system. Thus, it has been a consistent finding in animal studies that the ototoxic action of streptomycin is directed almost exclusively against the vestibular end-organs. In contrast, neomycin and kanamycin are usually found to be primarily cochleotoxic. Drugs such as gentamicin and tobramycin damage both the cochlea and the vestibular epithelia although to different degrees. The propensity of amikacin to affect the cochlea rather than the vestibular system has been noted in several studies using animals. This was demonstrated very strikingly by the work of Cazals et al. (1983) who showed that administration of large doses of amikacin could result in total destruction of the cochlea with preservation of the vestibular HCs. One of the newer aminoglycosides, dibekacin, has been shown to have quite a low ototoxic potential. Nevertheless, it shows a predilection for the vestibular system. In one study, it had a negligible effect on the cochlea, but a definite toxicity on the vestibular system (Aran et al., 1982).

Quantitative Differences

Since problems of bacterial resistance to the effect of streptomycin first emerged and gave impetus to the search for alternative antibiotics, a great many new aminoglycosides have been isolated or synthesized, particularly in the last two decades. In the early development of aminoglycosides, the main objectives in introducing new drugs were to improve the antibacterial spectrum, and to overcome the problems of bacterial resistance. In recent years, as the number of highly effective aminoglycoside antibiotics grew, attention was increasingly focussed on the comparative toxicity of the compounds, nephrotoxicity as well as ototoxicity. Thus, the recent literature contains a considerable number of reports of controlled studies in animal models to evaluate the comparative ototoxicity of aminoglycosides. It would be too much to expect universal agreement, but there is at least a consensus emerging about the relative ototoxicity of the various compounds.

Neomycin is almost certainly the most ototoxic aminoglycoside in current clinical use. Indeed it has long been considered too ototoxic for anything other than oral or topical use. Time, the changing character of patients and procedures, and bacterial evolution with the selection of resistant strains has led to the virtual eclipse of streptomycin and kanamycin (Jackson, 1984), although streptomycin is still used in the treatment of tuberculosis. Following the introduction of gentamicin in 1962, it rapidly became established as the drug of first choice in the treatment of life-threatening sepsis (Noone, 1982). Consequently, most studies of the relative toxicities of aminoglycosides have been conducted recently using gentamicin as the standard for comparison. Gentamicin is itself a mixture of three components, gentamicin C_1, gentamicin C_{1a} and gentamicin C_2, which differ in their ototoxic potential in guinea-pigs. However, although gentamicin C_1 was less cochleotoxic than gentamicin (Fox et al., 1980), any therapeutic advantage was likely to be negligible because of its lesser antibacterial potency (Brummett and Fox, 1982).

Brummett et al. (1972, 1978a) have consistently found tobramycin to be less cochleotoxic than gentamicin in guinea-pigs, although any advantage of tobramycin compared with gentamicin was seen to be very slight in two other studies (Aran et al., 1982; Parravicini et al., 1982). However, tobramycin was significantly less vestibulotoxic than gentamicin in one of these latter studies (Aran et al., 1982). When compared at equitherapeutic doses, amikacin appears to have similar cochleotoxic potential to gentamicin (Brummett and Fox, 1982; Parravicini et al., 1982). Reference has already been made to the selectivity of amikacin for the cochlea. Thus, amikacin seems to be very much less toxic to the vestibular system than gentamicin, both in the cat (Christensen et al., 1977), and the guinea-pig (Cazals et al., 1983). Aran et al. (1982) found that the cochlear toxicity of dibekacin was minimal, much less than that of tobramycin or gentamicin, and its vestibular toxicity was much less than that of gentamicin, but comparable to tobramycin. One of the most universally consistent findings of animal studies is that netilmicin is less toxic for both the cochlea and the vestibular system than all the other aminoglycosides it has been compared with (Miller et al., 1976; Brummett et al., 1978b; Igarashi et al., 1978; Wersall, 1980; Parravicini et al., 1982, 1983).

Thus, summarizing the animal data, one might predict very little difference between the cochlear toxicities of gentamicin and tobramycin or amikacin. Dibekacin and, particularly, netilmicin should be significantly less cochleotoxic than any of the three preceding drugs. Tobramycin and dibekacin should offer advantages of reduced toxicity against the vestibular system compared with gentamicin; amikacin and netilmicin should have very low vestibular toxicities.

Qualitative Differences in Cochlear Toxicity

As stated earlier, OHC damage generally begins in the basal turns of the cochlea and precedes IHC damage. However, if large numbers of animals are used and the entire organ of Corti is examined in detail, then differences emerge in the pattern of HC degeneration caused by different aminoglycosides. Such a study was conducted by Ylikoski (1974) using guinea-pigs which were administered gentamicin, kanamycin or neomycin in various dosage regimens. At an early stage, neomycin destroyed only the OHCs at the extreme basal end and those in the upper coil, the area between showing little damage. Eventually, with each of these drugs, all the OHCs in the basal coil were destroyed, and with gentamicin and kanamycin this was followed by loss of IHCs at the base of the cochlea. With neomycin, IHC damage was more prominent at the apex, even when many of the apical OHCs were present. Ylikoski never saw more extensive IHC damage at the apex of the cochlea compared with the base in animals administered gentamicin, and only in one case following kanamycin administration. This contrasts with the work of Kohonen (1965), who had reported that IHC loss in the guinea pig caused by both neomycin and kanamycin started at the apex of the cochlea and progressed towards the base.

Similarities and Differences Between Species

Hawkins and Johnsson (1981) have described some subtle differences in the pattern of cochlear HC degeneration caused by aminoglycosides in different laboratory animals. For example, lesions involving both IHCs and OHCs, but confined to the basal end of the cochlea, were observed in the macaque monkey, whereas selective loss of HCs, particularly OHCs, in the upper basal and lower middle turns was sometimes found in guinea-pigs. Hawkins and Johnsson drew two conclusions. First, although in the guinea-pig aminoglycosides (notably kanamycin) could differentiate between IHCs and OHCs, discreetly damaging the OHCs, in macaque monkeys, both types of HC were almost equally vulnerable. Secondly, although HCs at the extreme basal end of the cochlea are usually the first to be affected by aminoglycosides, followed by an orderly progression of the damage from base to apex, this pattern of damage is not invariable among species.

However, it should be appreciated that conclusions about species differences based on observations made in small numbers of animals might be misleading since individual animals may also vary greatly in their response to an ototoxic drug (Ylikoski, 1974), particularly if more than one dosage regimen is used. The pattern and extent of damage may also be related to the length of time which elapses between the end of the drug administration and the death of the animal. Toyoda et al. (1977) administered 400 mg/kg kanamycin to guinea-pigs by daily injection for 7, 10 or 14 days, and killed the animals after five different time intervals, ranging from 1 day to 6 months. They identified seven different patterns of cochlea HC damage, including the two extremes where all or none of the HCs were damaged. Three of the intermediate patterns were represented by OHC loss in the basal turns, accompanied by normal IHCs or IHC loss, either predominantly in the basal turns or the apical turns. The two other patterns were described as HC loss scattered throughout the cochlea and OHC loss, with or without IHC loss, which was confined to the apical turns. This last pattern of HC loss was the most common in animals given the drug for just 7 days, which led Toyoda et al., to conclude, contrary to the findings of the great majority of other workers, that HC degeneration began in the upper turns, even if eventually the HCs in the lower turns were more severely affected. Although the interval between the last injection and death of these animals varied from 1 day to 6 months, it would appear that this did not greatly influence the extent of HC damage, since Toyoda et al. concluded that there was no progression of the damage beyond 1 week. Therefore, it would seem that the differences between the animals in the sites of maximal HC degeneration were attributable mainly to the different periods for which the drug was given. Since the pattern of HC damage in animals of the same species can show great variability according both to the drug given and the dose, it is evident that caution must be exerted when attempting to interpret the results of studies in different species.

Kanamycin is often used to produce ototoxic lesions in electrophysiological studies of cochlear function, and therefore is probably the aminoglycoside which has been given to the largest number of different species. There is a considerable degree of consistency in the descriptions of the effects of kanamycin on the cochlea of different animal species. Behavioural techniques for assessment of auditory thresholds in animals have shown close similarities in the response of different species to kanamycin. Thus, the progress of hearing loss after chronic administration of kanamycin was similar in the cat, the guinea-pig and the macaque monkey, even though the dosage schedules differed (Stebbins et al., 1981). In all cases, high frequencies were first affected and, following the onset of a threshold shift at any frequency, the decline in hearing was very rapid. However, there were also some differences. There was some residual hearing at high frequencies in the guinea-pig, but not in the monkey. In the monkey, the total loss of hearing at high frequencies was correlated with a total absence of both OHCs and IHCs in the basal turn of the cochlea. In the guinea-pig, missing OHCs with intact normal-appearing IHCs in the basal part of the cochlea correlated with a partial hearing loss (50–60 dB) at higher frequencies.

The rabbit and the chinchilla have seldom been used in ototoxicological investigations, but two studies have demonstrated that the cochlear damage caused by kanamycin in these animals primarily involves OHCs at the base of the cochlea (Ryan et al., 1980; Ohtani et al., 1982). In the chinchilla, as Stebbins et al. (1981) observed in the guinea-pig, threshold shifts of 40–60 dB at high frequencies were correlated with complete loss of OHCs and a slight loss of IHCs in the basal-most portion of the organ of Corti (Ryan et al., 1980).

Most of the preceding discussion relates to comparisons made between species in an attempt to identify what might be described as qualitative differences in the effects of ototoxic drugs, e.g. comparisons of the primary site of the lesion. If quantitative comparisons are to be made, then it is imperative that like is compared with like, i.e. that the drug is administered in the same way and at the same dose in the two species. Two studies of kanamycin ototoxicity, that of Bamonte et al. (1980) using albino guinea-pigs, and that of Astbury and Read (1982) using the Wistar albino rat, appear to be directly comparable. In both studies, the drug was given daily by a single s.c. injection. Bamonte et al. administered the drug for 21 days and allowed the animals to survive for between 7 and 14 days. Astbury and Read killed some of their animals 20 days following the last of 20 injections. The dose response curve for kanamycin ototoxicity in the guinea-pig was very steep. The small degree of HC loss caused by a dose of 178 mg/kg was not significantly greater than that seen in control animals, whereas a dose of 267 mg/kg destroyed all the IHCs and OHCs along the entire cochlea (Bamonte et al., 1980). In contrast, a dose of 400 mg/kg in the rat damaged 70–80% of OHCs, but all IHCs were present except in a small portion of the upper basal turn (Astbury and Read, 1982). All the OHCs were destroyed at a dose of 600 mg/kg, but many IHCs were still present in the apical turns. Only at doses of 800 mg/kg and above were all the cochlear HCs destroyed in the rat.

The foregoing results suggest that the guinea-pig is more sensitive to ototoxic drug effects than the rat, at least in the case of kanamycin. Although the ototoxic damage caused by kanamycin can progress long after the drug administration has been stopped (Gonzalez et al., 1972), the difference in ototoxic susceptibility between the rat and the guinea-pig as described above cannot be attributed to the differences between the studies in survival time, since the rats were permitted the longer survival time, but displayed the lesser toxicity.

The lack of sensitivity of the rat to aminoglycoside-induced ototoxicity has been noted by other workers. Hawkins (1959) presented data to show that the rat was less susceptible to kanamycin than either the cat or the guinea-pig. Vernier and Alleva (1968) reported that the ototoxic potency of kanamycin in the cat and the guinea-pig was about 3 to 4 times greater than in the rat. Neomycin was about 1·5 to 3 times more potent in the cat and the guinea-pig than in the rat.

Two aminoglycosides with closely similar structures, streptomycin and dihydrostreptomycin, provide some of the most notable illustrations of species differences in susceptibility to ototoxic drugs. The early success with streptomycin in the treatment of tuberculosis was clouded by recognition of the vestibulotoxicity of this drug in man. The first studies of dihydrostreptomycin in animals suggested that it was less vestibulotoxic than streptomycin, and this was borne out in clinical use (Hinshaw et al., 1948). However, it soon became apparent that dihydrostreptomycin was significantly cochleotoxic in man (Glorig, 1951; Cohen et al., 1953; Liden, 1953; Mahady et al., 1953) to the extent that it was considered unsuitable for clinical use. Subsequent experimental studies have shown that the cochlear damage caused by dihydrostreptomycin in man cannot be easily reproduced in animals. The cochlear toxicity of dihydrostreptomycin was said to be minimal in the rat and the guinea pig (Vernier and Alleva, 1968). Cats did show some cochlear damage with dihydrostreptomycin, but only after prolonged administration (Hawkins and Lurie, 1953; McGee and Olszewski, 1962). The damage was much less than that caused by smaller doses of neomycin and, surprisingly, less than that caused by streptomycin (Hawkins and Lurie, 1953), whereas the reverse was true in man. The cat, which is susceptible to the vestibulotoxicity of streptomycin, is one of the few species to display any cochlear sensitivity to streptomycin. Rodent species, such as the rat and the guinea-pig, appear to parallel man in being sensitive to the vestibulotoxic effects of streptomycin, but resistant to its cochleotoxic action.

One of the most striking differences between species is illustrated by the responses of the patas and macaque monkeys to aminoglycosides (Hawkins et al., 1977; Hawkins and Johnsson, 1981; Stebbins et al., 1981). To date, the patas monkey seems to be the only laboratory animal with a cochlea which is sensitive to the toxic action of dihydrostreptomycin—in a manner similar to the response of the guinea-pig to kanamycin. Missing OHCs and normal IHCs in the basal portions of the cochlea correlate with a 60–70 dB hearing loss at high frequencies. A significant feature of the response of the patas monkey to dihydrostreptomycin (Hawkins et al., 1977) is the fact that the hearing loss progresses long after the cessation of drug administration, resembling the situation in man. Indeed, the sensitivity of the patas monkey to doses as low as 20 mg/kg is greater than that which was seen when dihydrostreptomycin was used in man. Streptomycin also produces hearing loss in patas monkeys when given at a daily dose of 20 mg/kg, a dose which has been shown not to be toxic in man when administered for prolonged periods (Hawkins and Johnsson, 1981). However, in the macaque monkey treated with daily doses of 100 mg/kg of dihydrostreptomycin for as long as eight months, there was only a very modest shift in threshold at the highest frequency tested (40 kHz), and less than 10% of the HCs were absent at the basal end of the cochlea (Hawkins et al., 1977). The macaque had earlier been shown to be sensitive to the ototoxic effects of kanamycin and neomycin (Stebbins et al., 1969).

CLINICAL STUDIES

Histopathological Changes

From the preceding sections, it is evident that studies in animals have provided general information on the pattern of sensory cell degeneration in response to ototoxic drug administration. There are notable similarities between the effects of different drugs and, indeed, between the effects of drugs and of other ototoxic trauma, such as noise (Hawkins, 1973b). However, there are also qualitative and quantitative differences in effect both between various ototoxic drugs, even those which are chemically similar, and also between species in their response to the same ototoxic agent. Individual variability among animals of the same species and strain in response to an ototoxic agent has also been recorded. Much of this latter variability seems to be attributable to differences in dosage regimens, and in the time which elapses between the end of drug administration and the examination of inner ear structures. In human studies, these factors must inevitably be important sources of variability. A further complication in the interpretation of the findings of inner ear histopathology in the human arises if the subject has a history of prior or concurrent exposure to ototoxic trauma other than the drug.

Given these problems, and the fact that opportunities for histopathological examination of the drug-damaged human cochlea are limited, it is remarkable that so many similarities have been observed between the patterns of damage in man (outlined below) and those seen in animals.

Streptomycin

In two patients who had both experienced symptomatic vestibular dysfunction after treatment with streptomycin (Nadol, 1981), there was extensive HC loss in vestibular structures, particularly at the tips of the cristae ampullaris, i.e. type I cells. There was little or no HC loss in the maculae utriculi and sacculi, and no HC loss in the cochlea.

Neomycin

Although neomycin is considered to be too toxic for systemic use, there are a number of reports in the literature of deafness resulting from its oral or topical use (see Harpur, 1977, for summary). Nadol (1981) and Johnsson et al. (1981) studied the damage to inner ear tissues caused by neomycin administered either orally or by irrigation of body cavities. In four of the five cases reported, both ears were examined and the histopathological changes were either identical or very similar in each ear. Profound hearing loss was generally associated with extensive cochlear HC loss, most marked in the basal turns. In regions where HC loss was total, there was also degeneration of supporting cells and nerve cells.

Johnsson et al. (1981) reported a good correlation between the presence of supporting cells and the presence of nerve fibres. Atrophy of the stria vascularis, and even Reissner's membrane, accompanied degeneration of the organ of Corti in some ears (Nadol, 1981), although in two specimens where all HCs had degenerated, the slight degree of strial atrophy present was consistent with age-related changes. In some cases, the entire cochlear HC population had degenerated, or only a few HCs remained at the apex.

In one case, Johnsson et al. (1981) also examined the vestibular neurosensory epithelia and found bilateral extensive HC loss, notable among the type I cells on the maculae of the utricle and saccule (the patient had not shown any vestibular symptoms). However, in all of the three cases described by Nadol (1981), the vestibular HC and neuronal populations appeared normal.

Kanamycin

The pattern of inner ear damage after parenteral kanamycin therapy has been described by Nadol (1981). Where cochlear HC loss was incomplete, it was seen to be most advanced in the basal turns. Damage within a cochlea ranged from total loss of IHCs and OHCs at the very base of the cochlea, through about 50% loss, mainly of OHCs, in the middle turns, to complete preservation of HCs at the apex. HC loss was occasionally accompanied by limited loss of supporting structures, but generally, even when HC loss was total throughout the entire cochlea, both supporting structures and cochlear neuronal populations were normal. This is a significant observation, although it cannot be discounted that the time interval between the kanamycin therapy and death of the patients studied by Nadol (1982) was not sufficiently long (maximum three months) to allow progression of secondary neuronal degeneration. In two cases studied by Nadol (1981), vestibular sensory and neuronal structures were normal.

Amikacin, Tobramycin and Gentamicin

Johnsson et al. (1981) described one case of amikacin-related ototoxicity, although this patient had also received a course of gentamicin therapy about one month prior to death. Pretreatment audiograms were normal, and a mild hearing loss which developed during the aminoglycoside therapy, particularly at high frequencies, was attributed to ototoxicity. Only the left temporal bone was examined and shown to have scattered HC loss throughout the cochlea, most severe in the second and third rows of OHCs at the basal end. In this region there was also a slight nerve degeneration. The stria vascularis displayed an unusual form of pathology—numerous small areas of relatively diffuse atrophy scattered along its entire length. Although no audiograms were recorded, a second patient almost certainly had ototoxic hearing loss attributable to therapy with tobramycin and gentamicin. An eleven week course of tobramycin therapy immediately prior to death had been preceded by a five week course of gentamicin, and even a few doses of streptomycin and kanamycin. It is likely that the gentamicin, but not the streptomycin or kanamycin, contributed to ototoxic damage. There was HC loss in both ears, but the degree of loss was markedly asymmetrical. In the left ear, there was almost total loss of OHCs and extensive loss of IHCs in the lower third of the cochlea, but preservation of most of the sensory cells above this region. In the right ear, there was severe to complete loss of OHCs throughout the cochlea with 10–30% remaining only in the middle turns. A varying degree of inner hair cell loss was observed throughout the cochlea, most severe at the basal end. Supporting cells were absent in regions of complete loss of sensory cells, but there was only minimal evidence for nerve degeneration, and only mild changes in the stria vascularis.

Gentamicin was the only aminoglycoside antibiotic known to have been given to a third patient who developed a mild hearing loss as a consequence. In the right temporal bone, the only side examined, there was light scattered HC loss throughout the cochlea. The greatest loss was in the third row of OHCs at the base and the apex of the cochlea. The pattern of HC loss and the slight degree of nerve degeneration at the very base were similar to the changes found in the patient who had been treated with both amikacin and gentamicin, and could have been 'normal' age-related changes.

Tange and Huizing (1980) have described what unequivocally appeared to be gentamicin-induced ototoxicity in a young woman (aged 24). The subject had normal hearing prior to an approximately 12 week course of gentamicin. Severe hearing loss developed during the gentamicin therapy, and progressed following the end of treatment until it stabilized after about eight months. Caloric testing revealed bilateral absence of vestibular function. Eight years later the subject died of an infection for which she had been given tobramycin over a five day period. The right cochlea was examined histopathologically and found to have no HCs or supporting cells except in the first three millimetres at the apex, where there was about 60% of the IHCs and a very small percentage of the OHCs. In the lower half of the cochlea, the organ of Corti was replaced by a layer of flat, polygonal cells resting on the basilar membrane. A normal number of nerve fibres and ganglion cells were present only at the very apex, and their population diminished rapidly so that there were none present in the lower half of the cochlea. The stria vascularis was normal only at the apex; elsewhere it was cystic, and in the basal coil it was markedly atrophied.

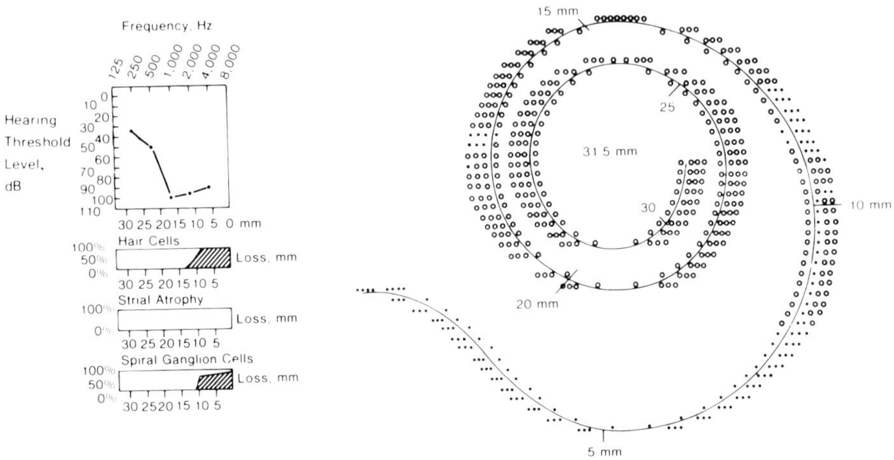

Fig. 3.8. Graphic reconstruction of cochlear neuroepithelium from a patient who experienced hearing loss associated with gentamicin therapy. HC and spiral ganglion cell loss was found mainly in the basal turn with additional loss of the first row of OHCs in the zone between 8 and 10 mm. Open circles indicate HCs present; filled circles, HCs missing. The damage to the basal turn of the cochlea was accompanied by a hearing loss which was most severe at high frequencies. (Reproduced with permission from Keene et al., 1982.)

A further case of gentamicin-related ototoxicity has been described by Keene et al. (1982). The patient, who was anephric and was undergoing haemodialysis, had a history of slowly progressive hearing loss, but without symptoms of vestibular dysfunction. Following therapy with gentamicin, there was a rapid deterioration in hearing function, particularly at high frequencies, with the simultaneous onset of vertigo. When the patient died one month later, the left temporal bone was removed for histopathological examination. In all sections of the vestibular neurosensory epithelia there was damage to the HCs, principally vacuolization, and clubbing of the stereocilia. In the ampullae, the damage was most severe at the base of the cristae. In the cochlea there was total loss of HCs and some loss of neural cells in the spiral ganglion in the lower basal turn (*Fig.* 3.8). In the upper basal turn there was a small region of total loss of OHCs, otherwise the loss was confined to the first row of OHCs.

Cis-platinum

It is not surprising, in view of the drug's relatively short history, that few reports of histopathological examination of *cis*-platinum ototoxic damage have appeared in the literature. However, Wright and Schaefer (1982) examined the temporal bones of five patients who had received therapy with *cis*-platinum. The problems of interpretation of the observed damage are well illustrated by these cases. In two subjects, histological evaluation proved difficult because of the presence of postmortem artefact. Pretreatment audiograms showed that all five individuals had some degree of bilateral sensorineural hearing loss prior to chemotherapy. Cochlear hair cell losses were therefore expected in association with ageing—the average age of the subjects was 59 years—and other influences unrelated to the therapy with *cis*-platinum. In view of this, scanning electron microscopy—which permits assessment of subtle morphological changes not easily recognized by light microscopy—was used to identify signs of fresh sensory cell injury that would correlate with the relatively recent drug treatment.

The most pronounced damage was seen in the OHCs, although some IHC degeneration was also seen, particularly in one individual with a severe hearing impairment which was worst at high frequencies, but also marked at low frequencies. Degenerating IHCs were prominent in the basal and apical regions —where OHC loss was greatest. In several cases, there was very extensive or total loss of all sensory cells at the lower end of the basal turn, and associated loss of nerve fibres. In areas where there was less OHC loss, the IHCs appeared essentially normal. Evidence of fresh degeneration in the apical turns, e.g. fusion of stereocilia, disruption of the cuticular plates and extrusion of apical cytoplasm, appeared to correlate with a dramatic decline in low frequency hearing during the course of chemotherapy.

One of the five patients developed symptoms of vestibular toxicity during *cis*-platinum therapy. Although vestibular hypofunction had been evident before treatment, there was no response to caloric stimulation (see next section) in either ear following treatment. Histological examination showed almost total HC loss in the cristae ampullaris and extensive HC loss in the maculae.

Wright and Schaefer (1982) commented that the HC loss they observed in their subjects must represent a combination of pre-existing loss and ototoxic damage. Since lesions involving the loss of both HCs and nerve fibres in the extreme basal turn are frequently seen in the cochleae of older persons who have not been exposed to ototoxic drugs, these changes were probably also age-related in the subjects treated with *cis*-platinum. However, the presence in other parts of the cochlea of large numbers of HCs which were in the process of degeneration was indicative of drug-related damage. The observation, in one case, of acute degenerative changes in HCs several months after the last course of *cis*-platinum suggested that the ototoxic damage might progress long after the drug administration was terminated.

The problems exemplified by the material studied by Wright and Schaefer illustrate the value of obtaining postmortem material from young subjects. Strauss et al. (1983) have described the temporal bone histopathology in a 9-year-old boy who died four weeks after receiving a short course of *cis*-platinum therapy. The child had developed a moderately severe bilateral hearing loss, most marked at high frequencies. The vestibular neurosensory epithelia were well preserved. In the left cochlea, there was extensive loss of OHCs, particularly in the basal coil where all three rows were absent. Least damage was present in the apical coil where only the first row of OHCs was absent. Some IHC damage was present, mainly in the basal and middle turns. The supporting cells appeared well preserved throughout the organ of Corti, but there was degeneration of the nerve cells in the spiral ganglion. Loss of HCs was more extensive in the right cochlea, and the myelinated nerve fibres and spiral ganglion cells were severely degenerated in the basal and middle turns. There was also axonal degeneration in the cochlear nerve, but not in other cranial nerves, in the spinal roots, or the peripheral nerves. Strauss et al. commented that it was unusual to see degenerative changes in the spiral ganglion and cochlear nerve when the supporting cells in the organ of Corti were well preserved. Experience of mechanical injury or aminoglycoside toxicity has shown that cochlear nerve changes occur only when damage within the organ of Corti extends to the supporting cells. Strauss et al. were uncertain, therefore, whether their findings indicated a dual mode of *cis*-platinum ototoxicity with simultaneous involvement of the cochlea and its nerve, or whether the neural changes were secondary to HC damage.

Functional Changes

Reference was made earlier to the problems associated with assessment of vestibular function in animals, in particular the problem of trying to correlate some measure of dysfunction with a lesion at a particular site in the vestibular end-organs. It is also extremely difficult to obtain reliable quantitative information about the extent of any vestibular dysfunction in a patient treated with an ototoxic drug. Frequently, a diagnosis is based on the patient's account of symptoms, such as nausea and vertigo, or the results of simple clinical tests of posture and gait. Objective tests of vestibular function, such as the recording of eye movements (nystagmus) in response to caloric (thermal) or rotational stimulation of the labyrinth, rarely serve any purpose other than to diagnose or confirm the presence of a lesion in the peripheral vestibular structures. In theory, it is possible to perform the caloric test of vestibular function on a sick patient in a hospital ward using portable equipment. In practice, this is extremely difficult for a variety of reasons, not least because the test requires an alert subject who is both willing to cooperate and to endure some discomfort. Furthermore, the test is insensitive and shows such large inter-test variability within subjects that it is not suited to serial monitoring of vestibular function (Davey et al., 1982a; Brask et al., 1984). As a result of these difficulties of assessing vestibular function in animals and in man, it is unrealistic to do more than compare, between animals and man, the general tendency of a drug to cause vestibular impairment (see next section).

In contrast to the problems associated with tests of vestibular function, pure-tone audiometry is an accurate and reliable technique for assessing auditory function and, if reasonable precautions are taken, can even be used to test patients in a hospital ward where background noise levels can be quite high (Davey et al., 1982b, 1983).

When cochlear function has been prospectively assessed using audiometric methods, the hearing loss in patients caused by aminoglycoside therapy has almost invariably been reported to occur first at high frequencies (8 kHz is usually the highest frequency tested), with a gradual involvement of lower frequencies. However, the possibility of selective involvement of lower frequencies cannot be totally discounted since Fee (1980) observed that 6 of 22 patients who developed cochlear toxicity associated with gentamicin or tobramycin therapy had a hearing loss involving frequencies in the 1–4 kHz range, with unchanged responses at 6 and 8 kHz. If hearing function is not objectively assessed using audiometry, there is a risk that a hearing loss may not be detected before the speech frequencies are involved and the patient complains of deafness. Consonant with the results of studies in animals, a progression of the degree of hearing loss at high frequencies and the involvement of lower frequencies is sometimes seen, even after the therapy has been stopped. This was a particular characteristic of some of the earlier aminoglycosides, such as neomycin and dihydrostreptomycin, which, in man at least, had a marked predilection for the cochlea. With the newer aminoglycosides, such as gentamicin, amikacin and netilmicin, the hearing loss may not extend beyond a high frequency deficit, and has even been reported to reverse after stopping the drug therapy (Black et al., 1976; Bock et al., 1980; Fee, 1980). As is the case in animals, the high frequency hearing loss in man seems to be correlated with a loss of HCs predominantly at the basal end of the cochlea (*Fig*. 3.8).

With *cis*-platinum, the hearing loss also seems first to occur and to be most severe at high frequencies. For example, of 17 patients who developed a hearing impairment associated with *cis*-platinum, 12 had a loss confined to frequencies in the range 4–8 kHz, and in 5 patients the loss extended to frequencies below 2 kHz. In no case was an isolated low frequency loss present.

Although human subjects can hear frequencies as high as 20 kHz, these high frequencies have little relevance for the ability of the person to communicate normally, and rarely are high frequency thresholds measured audiometrically. However, if the pattern of ototoxic lesions in animals are closely paralleled in humans, then one would predict that the first threshold elevations would be seen at the highest frequencies. Interest in performing high-frequency audiometry has been aroused recently in several centres with a view to its application in detecting drug-induced ototoxicity (Fausti et al., 1979). There are numerous problems to be overcome, both technical and also associated with the difficulty of performing the test on patients under less than ideal conditions in a noisy hospital ward. Patients receiving *cis*-platinum are often well enough to go to a specialized sound-proofed laboratory to be tested, and Fausti et al. (1984) have studied ototoxicity caused by *cis*-platinum using audiometric testing up to 20 kHz. Fausti et al. found that significant increases in threshold often occurred first at frequencies above the conventional test range. When threshold elevations were also present in the conventional range, the magnitude of the change was characteristically greater in the high frequency range (8–20 kHz).

These data appear to provide confirmation that, in human subjects, ototoxic drugs characteristically cause hearing impairment with a selectivity for high frequencies which closely resembles that seen in animals. The limited amount of histopathological data on humans also appears to confirm that this predominantly high frequency hearing loss is correlated with HC loss at the base of the cochlea.

Comparative Assessment of Aminoglycoside Ototoxicity in Man—Correspondence with Animals Studies

Consideration of the results of ototoxicological testing of aminoglycoside in animals and man leads to the conclusion that the only conspicuous anomaly has been the failure of most animal models to reproduce the cochlear toxicity of dihydrostreptomycin, which was very evident in patients. Generally, the results of studies in animals and man are in agreement. Thus, streptomycin shows a marked predilection for the vestibular system both in animals and in man. Neomycin, which in early clinical studies was found to cause rapid and profound loss of hearing, has been shown to be one of the aminoglycosides most toxic to the cochlea in animals.

Most of the newer aminoglycosides are less ototoxic, and also show a less distinct selectivity for one or other part of the inner ear. With these drugs, the parallels between animal and clinical studies, although still apparent, are less clear cut. The initial clinical use of gentamicin revealed that it was toxic to both the cochlea and the vestibular system, although there is a higher incidence of effects on vestibular function (Jackson and Arcieri, 1971). The dual toxicity of gentamicin has been confirmed in numerous clinical studies, and it is quite evident from animal studies that gentamicin is toxic to both divisions of the inner ear (e.g. Aran et al., 1982).

The data from animal studies, although not entirely uniform, would seem to predict very little difference between the cochlear toxicities of gentamicin and tobramycin (Aran et al., 1982; Parravicini et al., 1982), and the results of clinical studies confirm this (Fee, 1980; Smith et al., 1980). Any advantage of tobramycin over gentamicin in animal studies was probably confined to the vestibular system (Aran et al., 1982), and given the problems of assessing vestibular function in patients, it is not difficult to see why a subtle difference between the vestibular toxicity of gentamicin and tobramycin would be difficult to detect. Nevertheless, Fee (1980) did conclude that the incidence of vestibular toxicity was lower with tobramycin than gentamicin.

At high doses in animals, amikacin shows a marked selectivity for the cochlea (Cazals et al., 1983). However, it is no more cochleotoxic than gentamicin or tobramycin when compared to these drugs at doses proportional to their therapeutic doses (Brummett and Fox, 1982; Parravicini et al., 1982). Thus, the selectivity of amikacin for the cochlea in animals probably reflects a very low vestibulotoxic potential rather than a marked cochleotoxic potential. These distinctions have not been readily apparent in man, probably because the incidence of ototoxicity at clinical doses is low. However, a review of clinical studies of ototoxicity does at least suggest that amikacin has a predilection for the cochlea in man (Kahlmeter and Dahlager, 1984). Amikacin was associated with a higher average incidence of cochlear toxicity than gentamicin, tobramycin or netilmicin, while the incidence of vestibular toxicity was very low with all four drugs.

Netilmicin has consistently been found to have a very low toxicity for the cochlea and the vestibular system in animal studies, and compared favourably with all the other aminoglycosides against which it was tested. The low ototoxic potential of netilmicin seemed to be confirmed in the first clinical studies (Nordstrom et al., 1979; Tjernstrom, 1980; Vesterhauge et al. 1980). However, the clear advantage displayed by netilmicin compared with other aminoglycosides in ototoxicological studies in animals has been difficult to confirm in clinical use of the drug. There are undoubtedly many reasons why it is very difficult to establish unequivocally whether one aminoglycoside is more or less ototoxic in man than another—these reasons have been discussed elsewhere (Harpur, 1985). One overriding reason is that the incidence of ototoxicity with all these drugs is quite low, so that large populations would be required to detect any differences. Smith and Lietman (1982) reviewed the English language literature on comparative clinical trials of aminoglycosides until the end of 1979. They calculated that the mean frequency of ototoxicity with gentamicin was 8%. Given that the average number of patients in a group was 35, they concluded that it would be impossible to show a statistically significant advantage of another aminoglycoside compared with gentamicin, even if the incidence of ototoxicity with the second drug was zero. Despite these reservations, it should be stated that the clinical ototoxicity of netilmicin, both for the auditory and vestibular systems, seems invariably to be lower than that of any other aminoglycoside with which it has been compared, even if the differences are rarely statistically significant (Barza et al., 1980; Bock et al., 1980; Lerner et al., 1983).

CONCLUSION

There is a remarkable degree of accord between the qualitative effects of ototoxic drugs in animals and in the human. With few exceptions, e.g. dihydrostreptomycin, the effects of ototoxic drugs in the human can be modelled by experimental studies in guinea-pigs. In the case of dihydrostreptomycin, its cochlear toxicity appears to be evident to any significant extent only in the human and the patas monkey. Problems in correlating the vestibular effects of ototoxic drugs between species arise because of the lack of sensitive objective methods of study of the function of each of the vestibular sensory organs, and of an entirely satisfactory method for quantifying vestibular HC loss. When drugs are compared on a quantitative basis, the relative magnitudes of their effects in animals and man also show reasonable agreement. It is probably the infrequency of ototoxicity at low doses of the drugs which frustrates the demonstration of a better correspondence between experimental and clinical studies. Thus, it is necessary to extrapolate from high dose use in animals to low dose in humans. Although ototoxic effects seem invariably to be dose related, there is insufficient information about the slopes of the dose-response curves of different drugs to be certain that predictions of the comparative ototoxicity of drugs will be entirely valid. Further problems are created by the considerable difficulties of quantitatively assessing ototoxicity in patients.

The development and application of improved methods of studying the effects of ototoxic drugs, particularly their effects on vestibular function, is likely to provide confirmation of the general agreement between the effects in animals and in man. However, it may also be predicted that better methods of testing will reveal more of the subtle differences in effect which have already been observed both between species and between individuals.

ACKNOWLEDGEMENTS

The author thanks Beci Holt for preparing the figures, and Janet Bramble for typing the manuscript.

REFERENCES

Aran J-M. (1981) Electrophysiology of cochlear toxicity. In: Lerner S. A., Matz G. J. and Hawkins J. E. Jr (ed.) *Aminoglycoside Ototoxicity*, 31–47 Boston: Little, Brown.

Aran J-M., Erre J-P., Guilhaume A. et al. (1982). The comparative ototoxicities of gentamicin, tobramycin and dibekacin in the guinea-pig. A functional and morphological cochlear and vestibular study. *Acta Otolaryngol. Suppl.* **390**, 1–30.

Astbury P. J. and Read N. G. (1982) Kanamycin induced ototoxicity in the laboratory rat. A comparative morphological and audiometric study. *Arch. Toxicol.* **50**, 267–278.

Bamonte F., Parravicini L. and Arpini A. (1980) Histological evaluation of ototoxic reaction due to some aminoglycoside antibiotics. *Arch. Otorhinolaryngol.* **228**, 163–170.

Barza M., Lauermann M. W., Taly F. P. et al. (1980) Prospective, randomized trial of netilmicin and amikacin with emphasis on eight-nerve toxicity. *Antimicrob. Agents Chemother.* **17**, 707–714.

Black R. E., Lau W. K., Weinstein R. J. et al. (1976) Ototoxicity of amikacin. *Antimicrob. Agents Chemother.* **9**, 956–961.

Bock B. V., Edelstein P. H. and Meyer R. D. (1980) Prospective comparative study of efficacy and toxicity of netilmicin and amikacin. *Antimicrob. Agents Chemother.* **17**, 217–225.

Bohne B. A. and Rabbitt K. D. (1983) Holes in the reticular lamina after noise exposure: implication for continuing damage in the organ of Corti. *Hearing Res.* **11**, 41–53.

Brask T., Møller K., Leth S. et al. (1984) The reproducibility of caloric-induced nystagmus in normal persons. *Act Otolaryngol. Suppl.* **412**, 61–63.

Brummett R. E. and Fox K. E. (1982) Studies of aminoglycoside ototoxicity in animals models. In: Whelton A. and Neu H. C. (eds.) *The Aminoglycosides. Microbiology, Clinical Use and Toxicology*, 419–451. New York: Dekker.

Brummett R. E., Fox K. E., Bendrick T. W. et al. (1978a) Ototoxicity of tobramycin, gentamicin, amikacin and sisomicin in the guinea-pig. *J. Antimicrob. Chemother. Suppl. A* **4**, 73–83.

Brummett R. E., Fox K. E., Brown R. T. et al. (1978b) Comparative ototoxic liability of netilmicin and gentamicin. *Arch. Otolaryngol* **104**, 579–584.

Brummett R. E., Himes D., Saine B. et al. (1972) A comparative study of the ototoxicity of tobramycin and gentamicin. *Arch. Otolaryngol.* **96**, 505–512.

Brummett R. E., Traynor J., Brown R. et al. (1975) Cochlear damage resulting from kanamycin and furosemide. *Acta Otolaryngol.* **80**, 86–92.

Cazals Y., Aran J-M., Erre J-P. et al (1983) Vestibular acoustic reception in the guinea pig: a saccular function? *Acta Otolaryngol.* **95**, 211–217.

Christensen E. F., Reiffenstein J. C. and Madissoo H. (1977). Comparative ototoxicity of amikacin and gentamicin in cats. *Antimicrob. Agents Chemother.* **12**, 178–184.

Cohen S. S., Johnsen L., Lichtenstein M. R. et al (1953) A comparative study of streptomycin and dihydrostreptomycin in pulmonary tuberculosis. *Am. Rev. Tuberc.* **68**, 229–237.

Dallos P. and Cheatham M. A. (1976) Production of cochlear potentials by inner and outer hair cells. *J. Acoust. Soc. Am.* **60**, 510–512.

Dallos P. and Wang C. Y. (1974) Bioelectric correlates of kanamycin intoxication. *Audiology* **13**, 277–289.

Davey P. G., Harpur E. S., Jabeen F. et al (1982a) Variability and habituation of nystagmic responses to hot caloric stimulation of normal subjects. Evidence that this test may be inapplicable to monitoring drug-induced vestibular toxicity. *J. Laryngol.* **96**, 599–612.

Davey P. G., Jabeen F., Harpur E. S. et al. (1982b) The use of pure-tone audiometry in the assessment of gentamicin auditory toxicity. *Br. J. Audiol.* **16**, 151–154.

Davey P. G., Jabeen F., Harpur E. S. et al. (1983) A controlled study of the reliability of pure-tone audiometry for the detection of gentamicin auditory toxicity. *J. Laryngol.* **97**, 27–36.

Duvall A. J. and Quick C. A. (1969) Tracers and endogenous debris in delineating cochlear barriers and pathways. An experimental study. *Ann. Otol.* **78**, 1041–1057.

Engstrom H., Ades H. W. and Anderson A. (1966) *Structural Pattern of the Organ of Corti.* Stockholm: Almqvist and Wiksell.
Fausti S. A., Frey R. H., Erickson D. A. et al. (1979) A system for evaluating auditory function from 8000–20 000 Hz. *J. Acoust. Soc. Am.* **66**, 1713–1718.
Fausti S. A., Schechter M. A., Rappaport B. A. et al. (1984) Early detection of *cis*-platin ototoxicity. *Cancer* **53**, 224–231.
Fee W. E. (1980) Aminoglycoside ototoxicity in the human. *Laryngoscope Suppl. 24* **90**, 1–19.
Fox K. E., Brummett R. E., Brown R. et al. (1980) A comparative study of the ototoxicity of gentamicin and gentamicin C_1. *Arch. Otolaryngol.* **106**, 44–49.
Gallagher K. L. and Jones J. K. (1979) Furosemide-induced ototoxicity. *Ann. Intern. Med.* **91**, 744–745.
Glorig A. (1951) The effect of dihydrostreptomycin hydrochloride and sulphate on auditory mechanism. *Ann. Otol.* **60**, 327–335.
Gonzalez G., Miller N. and Wasilewski V. (1972) Progressive neuroototoxicity of kanamycin. *Ann. Otol.* **81**, 127–131.
Gregory M. H. (1986) *Personal Communication.*
Harpur E. S. (1977) Neomycin and deafness. *Pharm. J.* **218**, 494–495.
Harpur E. S. (1981) Ototoxicological testing. In: Gorrod J. W. (ed.) *Testing for Toxicity*, 219–240. London: Taylor and Francis.
Harpur E. S. (1983) Disorders of the ear. In: D'Arcy P. F. and Griffin J. P. (eds) *Iatrogenic Diseases*, 2nd. ed. update, 169–180. Oxford: Oxford University Press.
Harpur E. S. (1985) Disorders of the ear. In: D'Arcy P. F. and Griffin J. P. (ed.) *Introgenic Diseases*, 3rd ed. in press. Oxford: Oxford University Press.
Harpur E. S. and Bridges J. B. (1979) An evaluation of the use of scanning and transmission electron microscopy of the gentamicin-damaged guinea-pig organ of Corti. *J. Laryngol.* **93**, 7–23.
Hawkins J. E. Jr (1959) The ototoxicity of kanamycin. *Ann. Otol.* **68**, 698–715.
Hawkins J. E. Jr (1973a) Ototoxic mechanisms. *Audiology* **12**, 383–393.
Hawkins J. E. Jr (1973b) Comparative otopathology: ageing, noise and ototoxic drugs. *Adv. Otorhinolaryngol.* **20**, 125–141.
Hawkins, J. E. Jr and Johnsson L-G (1975) Microdissection and surface preparations of the inner ear. In: Smith C. A. and Vernon J. A. (eds) *Handbook of Auditory and Vestibular Research Methods*, 5–52. Springfield, Illinois: Thomas.
Hawkins J. E. Jr and Johnsson L-G. (1981) Histopathology of cochlear and vestibular ototoxicity in laboratory animals. In: Lerner S. A., Matz G. J. and Hawkins J. E. Jr. (ed.) *Aminoglycoside Ototoxicity*, 175–195. Boston: Little, Brown.
Hawkins J. E. Jr, Johnsson L-G and Preston R. E. (1972) Cochlear microvasculature in normal and damaged ears. *Laryngoscope* **82**, 1091–1104.
Hawkins J. E. Jr and Lurie M. H. (1953) The ototoxicity of dihydrostreptomycin and neomycin in the cat. *Ann. Otol.* **62**, 1128–1148.
Hawkins J. E. Jr, Stebbins W. C., Johnsson L-G. et al. (1977) The patas monkey as a model for dihydrostreptomycin ototoxicity. *Acta Otolaryngol.* **83**, 123–129.
Hinshaw H. C., Feldman W. H., Carr D. T. et al. (1948) The clinical administration of dihydrostreptomycin in tuberculosis: a preliminary report. *Am. Rev. Tuberc.* **58**, 525–530.
Hunger-Duvar I. M. (1978) Reissner's membrane and endocytosis of cell debris. *Acta Otolaryngol. Suppl.* **351**, 24–32.
Igarashi M. and Jensen D. W. (1981) Vestibulotoxicity experiments in animals. In: Lerner S. A., Matz G. J. and Hawkins J. E. Jr (eds) *Aminoglycoside Ototoxicity* 127–134. Boston: Little, Brown et al.
Igarashi M., Levy J. K. and Jerger J. (1978) Comparative toxicity of netilmicin and gentamicin in squirrel monkeys. *J. Infect. Dis.* **137**, 476–480.
Igarashi M., Lundquist P-G., Alford B. R. et al. (1971) Experimental ototoxicity of gentamicin in squirrel monkeys. *J. Infect. Dis. Suppl.* **124**, S114–S129.
Jackson G. G. and Arceieri G. (1971) Ototoxicity of gentamicin in man: a survey and controlled analysis of clinical experience in the United States. *J. Infect. Dis. Suppl.* **124**, 130–137.
Johnsson L-G. and Hawkins J. E. Jr (1972) Strial atrophy in clinical and experimental deafness. *Laryngoscope* **82**, 1105–1125.
Johnsson L-G., Hawkins J. E. Jr, Kingsley T. C. et al (1981) Aminoglycoside-induced cochlear pathology in man. *Acta Otolaryngol. Suppl.* **383**, 1–19.
Kahlmeter G. and Dahlager J. I. (1984) Aminoglycoside toxicity—a review of clinical studies published between 1975 and 1982. *J. Antimicrob. Chemother. Suppl. A* **13**, 9–22.

Keene M., Hawke M., Barber H. O. et al. (1982) Histopathological findings in clinical gentamicin ototoxicity. *Arch. Otolaryngol.* **108**, 65–70.
Kohonen A. (1965). Effect of some ototoxic drugs upon the pattern and innovation of cochlea sensory cells in the guinea pig. *Acta Otolaryngol. Suppl.* **208**, 9–70.
Lerner S. A., Matz G. J. and Hawkins J. E. Jr (eds) (1981) *Aminoglycoside Ototoxicity*. Boston: Little, Brown
Lerner A. M., Reyes M. P., Cone L. A. et al. Randomized controlled trial of the comparative efficacy, auditory toxicity, and nephrotoxicity of tobramycin and netilmicin. *Lancet* **i**, 1123–1126.
Liden G. (1953) Loss of hearing following treatment with dihydrostreptomycin or streptomycin. *Acta Otolaryngol.* **43**, 551–572.
McGee T. M. and Olszewski J. (1962) Streptomycin sulfate and dihydrostreptomycin toxicity. Behavioural and histopathological studies. *Arch. Otolaryngol.* **75**, 295–311.
Mahady S. C. F., Armstrong F. L., Beck F. et al. (1953) A comparative study of streptomycin and dihydrostreptomycin in pulmonary tuberculosis. *Am. Rev. Tuberc.* **68**, 238–248.
Miller G. H., Arcieri G., Weinstein M. J. et al. (1976) Biological activity of netilmicin, a broad-spectrum semisynthetic aminoglycoside antibiotic. *Antimicrob. Agents Chemother.* **10**, 827–836.
Nadol J. B. Jr (1981) Histopathology of human aminoglycoside ototoxicity. In: Lerner S. A., Matz G. J. and Hawkins J. E. Jr. (ed.) *Aminoglycoside Ototoxicity*, 409–434. Boston: Little, Brown.
Nordstrom L., Cristensson P., Haeger K. et al. (1979) Netilmicin: clinical evaluation of efficacy and toxicity of a new aminoglycoside. *J. Int. Med. Res.* **7**, 117–125.
Ohtani I., Ohtsuki K., Aikawa T. et al. (1982) Individual variation and mechanisms of kanamycin ototoxicity in rabbits. *Acta Otolaryngol.* **94**, 413–419.
Parravicini L., Arpini A., Bamonte F., et al. (1982) Comparative ototoxicity of amikacin, gentamicin, netilmicin and tobramycin in guinea-pigs. *Toxicol. Appl. Pharmacol.* **65**, 222–230.
Parravicini L., Forlani A., Marzanatti M. et al. (1983) Comparative ototoxicity of dibekacin and netilmiccin in guinea-pigs. *Acta Pharmacol. Toxicol.* **53**, 230–235.
Ryan A. F., Woolf N. K. and Bone R. C. (1980) Ultrastructural correlates of selective outer hair cell destruction following kanamycin intoxication in the chinchilla. *Hearing Res.* **3**, 335–351.
Smith C. R. and Lietman P. S. (1982) Comparative clinical trials of aminoglycosides. In: Whelton A. and Neu H. C. (ed.) *Thge Aminoglycosides. Microbiology, Clinical Use and Toxicology*, 497–509. New York: Dekker.
Smith C. R. and Lietman P. S. (1983) Effect of furosemide on aminoglycoside-induced nephrotoxicity and auditory toxicity in humans. *Anbtimicrob. Agents Chemother.* **23**, 133–137.
Smith C. R., Lipsky J. J., Laskin O. L. et al. (1980) Double-blind comparison of the nephrotoxicity and auditory toxicity of gentamicin and tobramycin. *N. Engl. J. Med.* **302**, 1106–1109.
Spoendlin H. and Brun J-P. (1974) The block-surface technique for evaluation of cochlear pathology. *Arch. Otorhinolaryngol* **208**, 137–145.
Stebbins W. C. and Coombs S. (1976). Behavioral assessment of ototoxicity in nonhuman primates. In: Weiss B. and Laties V. F. (ed.) *Behavioral Toxicology*, 401–427. New York: Plenum.
Stebbins W. C., McGinn C. S., Feitosa M. A. G. et al. Animal models in the study of ototoxic hearing loss. In: Lerner S. A., Matz G. J. and Hawkins J. E. Jr (ed.) *Aminoglycoside Ototoxicity*, 5–25. Boston: Little, Brown.
Stebbins W. C., Miller J. M., Johnsson L-G. et al. (1969) Ototoxic hearing loss and cochlear pathology in the monkey. *Ann. Otol.* **78**, 1007–1025.
Strauss M., Towfighi J., Lord S. et al. (1983) *Cis*-platinum ototoxicity: clinical experience and temporal bone histopathology. *Laryngoscope* **93**, 1554–1559.
Tange R. A. and Huizing E. H. (1980) Hearing loss and inner ear changes in a patient suffering from severe gentamicin ototoxicity. *Arch. Otorhinolaryngol.* **228**, 113–121.
Tjernstrom O. (1980) Prospective evaluation of vestibular and auditory function in 76 patients treated with netilmicin. *Scand. J. Infect. Dis. Suppl.* **23**, 122–125.
Toyoda Y., Saito H., Matsuoka H. et al. (1977) *Acta Otolaryngol.* **84**, 202–212.
Vernier V. F. and Alleva F. R. (1968) The bioassay of kanamycin auditory toxicity. *Arch. Int. Pharmacodyn.* **176**, 59–73.
Vesterhauge S., Johnsen N. J., Thomsen J. et al (1980) Netilmicin treatment followed by monitoring of vestibular and auditory function using highly sensitive methods. *Scand. J. Infect. Dis. Suppl.* **23**, 117–121.
Wersall J. (1980) The ototoxic potential of netilmicin compared with amikacin. An animal study in guinea pigs. *Scand. J. Infect. Dis. Suppl.* **23**, 104–113.

Wersall J. (1981) Structural damage to the organ of Corti and the vestibular epithelia caused by aminoglycoside antibiotics in the guinea-pig. In: Lerner S. A., Matz G. J. and Hawkins J. E. Jr. (ed.) *Aminoglycoside Ototoxicity*, 197–214. Boston: Little, Brown.

Wright C. G. and Schaefer S. D. (1982) Inner ear histopathology in patients treated with *cis*-platinum. *Laryngoscope* **92**, 1408–1413.

Ylikoski J. (1974) Correlate studies on the cochlear pathology and hearing loss in guinea pigs after intoxication with ototoxic antibiotics. *Acta Otolaryngol. Suppl.* **326**, 5–62.

Chapter 4

Xenobiotic-Induced Rhabdomyolysis

Bryan Ballantyne

INTRODUCTION

Rhabdomyolysis is a word applied to a variety of aetiologic conditions which result in skeletal muscle injury and necrosis, with myofibril disruption and the release of muscle fibre contents into the circulation. The nature and absolute amount of substances released depends on the degree and extent of skeletal muscle tissue injured. Whilst their quantitative detection in blood or urine may be of value in confirming a clinical diagnosis and assist in defining prognosis, they may cause or contribute to secondary pathophysiological effects and complications. Particularly important in these respects are the respiratory pigment myoglobin, muscle enzymes (notably creatinine phosphokinase, transaminases, lactate dehydrogenase and aldolase), electrolytes (K^+ and phosphate), creatinine and purines. In contrast with haemoglobin, myoglobin does not bind to haptoglobulin, and because of this and its lower molecular weight (17 000 daltons), at a low plasma threshold myoglobin appears in the urine to which it imparts a red or brown discoloration when the concentration is sufficiently high. Although the clinical syndrome of muscle weakness, myalgia, and brown urine has been referred to as Meyer-Betz disease (Meyer-Betz, 1911), it has been stressed by Knochel (1982) that the descriptive terms rhabdomyolysis and myoglobinuria are more appropriate.

Depending on the degree of muscle injury, the clinical and laboratory features of rhabdomyolysis cover a spectrum ranging from a subject having mild muscle ache and the presence of low concentrations of myoglobin in their urine, to a severely ill patient with marked metabolic disturbances and life-threatening complications. The most significant biochemical and functional abnormalities include hyperkalaemia, hypo- or hypercalcaemia, acute renal failure (anuric, oliguric, and non-oliguric), disseminated intravascular coagulation syndrome, and cardiac arrhythmias and conduction defects. Local complications of rhabdomyolysis include mineralization of the injured muscle and, as a result of increased osteofascial compartment pressure, peripheral neuropathies and vascular compression leading to gangrene may occur. Although rhabdomyolysis has been defined in terms of skeletal striated muscle injury, in some instances there may also be direct involvement of the myocardium.

This essay will review some major and general features of rhabdomyolysis before discussing skeletal muscle injury induced by xenobiotics.

GENERAL FEATURES OF RHABDOMYOLYSIS

The following section will review the essential biochemistry of myoglobin, the causes of rhabdomyolysis, clinical features, the pathophysiology and pathogenesis of local and systemic complications, laboratory findings, diagnostic aids and management.

Myoglobin

Myoglobin is a haem-containing protein found in skeletal and cardiac myocytes, and normally constitutes 1–2% the wet weight of skeletal muscle. However, the myoglobin content may depend on the degree of physiological conditioning; for example, highly trained subjects may have muscle myoglobin approaching 3–5% wet weight (Perkoff and Tyler, 1958). Myoglobin consists of a single polypeptide chain of 153 residues, has a compact structure with about 75% of the main chain in a α-helical configuration, with the Fe atom of haem being bonded to residue F8. The molecular and biochemical features of myoglobin have been concisely reviewed by Stryer (1981).

The function of myoglobin is to bind oxygen and facilitate its transport to sites of muscle oxidative metabolism. Myoglobin has a much greater binding affinity for oxygen than has haemoglobin. For example, the ambient plasma pO_2 for a haemoglobin P_{50} at pH 7·4 and 37 °C is 26 mm Hg compared with a myoglobin P_{50} of 3 mm Hg. This permits myoglobin to function as an O_2 shuttle under the low pO_2 conditions which operate with working skeletal muscle (Knochel, 1982).

In contrast with haemoglobin, myoglobin is not bound to haptoglobin and hence is found in urine at relatively low plasma concentrations. Thus, with haemoglobin there is a haptoglobin binding capacity up to 100 mg dl^{-1} of plasma, but with myoglobin only up to 1·5 mg dl^{-1} may become bound to a molecular fraction between 50 000 and 300 000 daltons and above which it is excreted in urine (Knochel, 1982). According to Rowland and Penn (1972) injury to about 200 g of skeletal muscle is required to reach this plasma threshold for renal excretion. Also, because of its comparatively low MW of 17 000 daltons, the renal clearance of myoglobin is approximately 75% that of creatinine. The absence of significant quantitative plasma binding of myoglobin and its high renal excretion ratio results in its rapid appearance and excretion in the urine.

Causes and Classification of Rhabdomyolysis

As a consequence of the numerous mechanisms by which rhabdomyolysis may be produced, and contrary to some viewpoints, it is a relatively common condition. The causes of rhabdomyolysis may be generally grouped as follows: direct physical injury to muscle, ischaemia, excessive muscle activity, metabolic disorders (both pathophysiological and genetic variants), certain myoimmunological diseases, infections, certain animal toxins and xenobiotics. This generalized aetiological classification for rhabdomyolysis is shown in *Table* 4.1. It will be appreciated, however, that there is considerable functional overlap between the groups. For example, with some xenobiotics the rhabdomyolysis is secondary to a compression effect due to xenobiotic-induced coma, or the rhabdomyolysis seen in certain infections may be mainly a consequence of pyrexia and convulsions. Thus, several subcategories could appear in the different major aetiological classes, and the classification shown in *Table* 4.1 is merely one of descriptive convenience that encompasses many undeclared functional interrelationships. Although it has been general practice in several texts to refer to rhabdomyolysis as being traumatic or non-traumatic in type, there may be a significant contribution from locally induced muscle injury to some cases described as 'non-traumatic' rhabdomyolysis. For example, when coma is induced by certain xenobiotics the resultant muscle injury may be caused mainly be compression which produces ischaemic myonecrosis, and any direct myotoxicity may be minimal. Thus, whilst the term traumatic rhabdomyolysis can be clearly used for some cases of rhabdomyolysis, the use of the word non-traumatic may be misleading from a functional point of view. Aspects of the various general causes of rhabdomyolysis listed in *Table* 4.1 are discussed below.

Table 4.1. An aetiologic classification of rhabdomyolysis.

Major cause	*Examples*
Acute direct physical injury	Trauma (crush injury) Burns (thermal and electrical)
Ischaemia	Muscle compression Arterial occlusion Sickle-cell disease
Excessive muscle activity	Sports (contact and non-contact) Severe exercise Convulsions Status asthmaticus
Metabolic disorders	Hypokalaemia Hypophosphataemia Hyponatraemia Diabetic ketoacidosis
Immunological diseases	Dermatomyositis Polymyositis
Genetic enzyme deficiencies	McCardle's syndrome Tauri's syndrome Carnitine deficiency Carnitine-palmityl-transferase deficiency
Infections	Viral Bacterial Parasitic
Animal toxins	Snake bites Insect bites
Xenobiotics	See *Tables* 4.2 and 4.3

Acute Direct Physical Trauma

The most obvious example of traumatic rhabdomyolysis is that involving direct physical injury to skeletal muscle, particularly crush injuries involving the limbs. Particular attention was drawn to crush injuries, and the recognition of an association between them and the subsequent development of acute renal failure, as a result of the barbaric bombing of civilian populations during the World War II (Bywaters and Beall, 1941; Bywaters et al., 1941; Bywaters, 1944). Thermal injury to muscle will also cause clinical and biochemical features of rhabdomyolysis. One special example of this is myocardial and skeletal muscle injury resulting from lightning strikes on the body. As the electrical current flows through the tissues the energy is converted to heat that may injure muscle, producing increased muscle-specific enzyme activity in serum and myoglobinuria (Yost and Holmes, 1974; Tribble et al., 1985). In addition to muscle-specific creatinine phosphokinase (CPK-MB) increases, the serum (*s*) activity of brain-characteristic CPK (*s*CPK-BB) activity may be increased as a result of cerebral anoxia (Harwood et al., 1978; Scheulen and Munster, 1983).

A particular cause of traumatic rhabdomyolysis which may require to be differentiated from myotoxic rhabdomyolysis is that following the intramuscular (im) injection of therapeutic substances. For example, Meltzer et al. (1970) found that *s*CPK activity increase was measured in 6 of 14 patients receiving a single im injection of chlorpromazine, but not when given perorally. Experimentally it was also found that chlorpromazine measured *s*CPK activity given im but not by intraperitoneal injection. Also, no effect was seen *in vivo* or *in vitro* on CPK activity of human or rat muscle, or purified rabbit CPK. Hence, it is reasonable to conclude that the effect of im chlorpromazine is due to local muscle trauma. Thus, during investigational procedures, local trauma from im injections needs to be excluded as a source of modest increases in *s*CPK activity.

Muscle damage, producing typical clinical and biochemical findings for rhabdomyolysis, has been described as a complication of exposure of the limbs to cold (Raifman et al., 1978).

Ischaemia

Regional rhabdomyolysis may be produced by proximal arterial compression, or by arterial embolus or thrombosis, resulting in hypoxic muscle injury. Rhabdomyolysis may be a feature of the sickle-cell crisis due to microvascular occlusion of muscle capillaries by sickled cells with resultant ischaemia. Devereux and Knowles (1985), for example, described the case of a black 25 year-old male with homozygous sickle-cell disease and acute renal failure (ARF) associated with a severe sickling episode, probably precipitated by infection and dehydration. The *s*CPK was >5 000 000 U l^{-1}, and they believe that the pathogenic mechanism was probably massive muscle ischaemia secondary to intramuscular sickling. The cause of ARF associated with sickle cell disease may be difficult to determine if microvascular occlusion due to sickling occurs both in the kidney and skeletal muscle, and clearly the demonstration of myoglobinuria may aid in defining if a contribution from rhabdomyolysis is a possibility (Lewin, 1985). The occurrence of rhabdomyolysis in sickle-cell trait appears more variable. Thus, George et al. (1979) reported three cases of anuric rhabdomyolysis in patients with sickle-cell trait, with a history in each case of abnormal muscle exercise. However, in a study of the biochemical determinants of rhabdomyolysis in marine recruits, Olerud et al. (1976) did not find that individuals with a sickle-cell trait had a greater incidence of rhabdomyolysis due to exercise than other black members of the population studied.

Excessive Muscle Activity

Rhabdomyolysis has been described in a large variety of contact and non-contact sporting activities including, for example, marathon running, karate, American football, calisthenics and ice skating (Morton and Waldek, 1985; Ono, 1953; Schiff et al., 1978). Rhabdomyolysis resulting from exertion is well documented, and known to cause myoglobinaemia, myoglobinuria and, occasionally, ARF. It is frequently diagnosed in untrained military recruits (Greenberg and Arneson, 1967). Olerud et al. (1976) investigated the incidence of acute exertional rhabdomyolysis amongst marine recruits during the first six days of regularly scheduled training. Substantial increases in *s*CPK, lactate dehydrogenase (LDH) and aspartate aminotransferase (AST) were measured throughout the period studied; 39·2% had serum myoglobin ranging 0·37 to 21·9 μm ml^{-1} and 6 had levels consistent with clinical cases of acute exertional rhabdomyolysis (>4·5 μg ml^{-1}). It is of interest to note that, in the black recruits, neither the presence of sickle-cell trait nor glucose-6-phosphate dehydrogenase deficiency resulted in a greater degree of biochemical evidence of rhabdomyolysis than other blacks. Demos et al. (1974) prospectively studied 21 marine corps recruits for one week for the presence of myoglobinaemia and the development of clinical rhabdomyolysis during exercises. Myoglobin was found in the serum of two-thirds of the recruits at least once during the study period despite the absence of clinical rhabdomyolysis; values ranged 0·3 to 3·6 μg μl^{-1}. Mean serum enzyme activities were: *s*CPK 1413 mU ml^{-1} (normal 0–230), *s*AST 69 Karmen units (normal 0–59), and *s*LDH 246 mU ml^{-1} (normal 133–288).

Schiff et al. (1978) described myoglobinaemia in 25 of 29 runners completing a 99 km marathon, together with marked increases in lactate and *s*CPK, *s*AST and *s*ALT. There was a linear correlation between serum myoglobin and enzyme activities. Very high serum myoglobin concentrations and CPK activities may occur as a result of severe exercise. For example, in a study by Ross et al. (1986) involving observation of healthy males on a three-day schedule of severe exercise, the serum myoglobin increased from 17·9 ± 5.7 SD μg l^{-1} to 1108 ± 829 μg l^{-1}, and *s*CPK from 199 ± 130 iu l^{-1} to 6929 ± 8119 iu l^{-1}. In athletes having myoglobinaemia, myoglobinuria and dehydration, ARF can be aborted by prompt diuresis (Schiff et al., 1978). A fatality in a marathon runner has been ascribed to rhabdomyolysis (Lonka and Pederson, 1987). The subject, a 27-year-old male, was hospitalized within 30 minutes of collapsing after an 8 km run. Some 45 hours later he was transferred to a renal unit because of the development of acute oliguric renal failure. At this time he had diffuse myalgia with *s*CPK 3500 U l^{-1} and *s*[myoglobin] of 3000 nmol l^{-1}; he also had severe DIC. Haemodialysis only partially corrected the metabolic acidosis, and consciousness and pulmonary function deteriorated and *Staphylococcus aureus* septicaemia developed. He died 6 days after collapsing. Commenting on this case, Boyd (1987) questions whether the runner could have been incubating a viral infection, which could have been aggravated by the marathon run. He suggests that subclinical infection may predispose to the development of strenuous exercise-induced rhabdomyolysis.

Slight to moderate increases of *s*CPK activity occur in classical heatstroke, but in the absence of exertion this is not usually associated with ARF or hyperkalaemia (Hart et al., 1982). However severe rhabdomyolysis may be a major complication of exertional heatstroke (Anderson et al., 1980, 1983), and the agitated hyperthermic state associated with delirium tremens. ARF may occur in up to 30% of victims of exertional heatstroke, often being referred to as 'heat stress nephropathy' (Schrier et al., 1967; Knochel et al., 1974; Hart et al., 1982). Demos et al. (1974) subdivided acute exertional rhabdomyolysis into the following three categories.

1. Asymptomatic acute exertional rhabdomyolysis (exercise myoglobinaemia) with small increases in serum myoglobin and a normal physiological response to exercise.
2. Subclinical exertional rhabdomyolysis, with increases in serum myoglobin concentrations significantly above those associated with exercise myoglobinuria but without clinical signs or symptoms.
3. Clinical exertional rhabdomyolysis, where there is myalgia, induration, swelling and weakness of affected muscle groups, with significant increases in serum myoglobin and muscle-specific enzymes, and ARF may be a complication.

Demos et al. (1974) compared asymptomatic recruits with exercise myoglobinaemia with others hospitalized for clinical exertional rhabdomyolysis, and found the latter group had significantly higher serum myoglobin concentrations and enzyme activities respectively as follows (for average values): myoglobin 0·4 *v.* 20·8 $\mu g\ ml^{-1}$, CPK 1413 *v.* 76 803 $mU\ ml^{-1}$, AST 69 *v.* 1092 Karmen units, and LDH 246 *v.* 1648 $mU\ ml^{-1}$.

The influence of environmental temperature on the severity of rhabdomyolysis and the potential for complications is also reflected in K^+ balance. Thus, severe exercise in a hot environment may be associated with a K^+ deficiency due to its loss in sweat and urine. The kaluresis may be in part due to an associated hyperaldosteronism resulting from renin release associated with shifts of fluid volume. In a cooler environment there may be a more typical increase in serum K^+ due to the rhabdomyolytic process (Knochel and Carter, 1976).

Grand mal convulsions lead to an increase in *s*CPK (Gloetzner et al., 1979), and any cause of severe and prolonged convulsions may result in the clinical and biochemical syndrome typical of rhabdomyolysis, with the possibility for the development of ARF. Also, status asthmaticus has been recorded as a cause of rhabdomyolysis (Chugh et al., 1978).

Metabolic Disorders (*Pathophysiological*)

Disturbances of K^+, Na^+ and phosphate balance may be directly or indirectly causative in some cases of rhabdomyolysis, as may certain metabolic complications of diabetes melliltus. Some major aspects of these factors are summarized below.

HYPOKALAEMIA

There appears to be a relative rarity of rhabdomyolysis in K^+-deficiency studies, which has been postulated by Campion et al. (1972) to be reflection of the generalized weakness or paralysis being sufficient to prevent breakdown of muscle cell integrity. However, rhabdomyolysis has been described in association with the following hypokalaemic conditions:

1. Hyperchloraemic renal tubular acidosis (Campion et al., 1972).
2. Some patients with exertional-heatstroke-induced kaluretic diuresis (Chugh et al., 1979).
3. Xenobiotic-induced hypokalaemia, including liquorice, carbenoxalone sodium and amphotericin.

K^+-loosing states with complications may sometimes result from multiple therapy. For example, Van Horn et al. (1970) described three patients with gastrointestinal and urinary K^+ loss possibly due to therapy with variable collections of laxatives and diuretics. There was hypokalaemia, severe muscle weakness, and marked increases in *s*CPK, adolase and AST. Respective initial K^+ values were *s*CPK 41–1900 U, *s* aldolase 50–78 U, and *s*AST 280–425 U. Skeletal muscle biopsy in two patients showed patchy coagulation necrosis and fragmentation of myofibrils, sarcolemmal cell proliferation, and a phagocytic response. Correction of hypokalaemia resulted in return of muscle strength paralleled by a decrease in serum muscle enzyme activities, suggesting K^+ deficiency as a causative factor in this reversible myopathy. Van Horn et al. (1970) stress that hypokalaemic myopathy should not be confused with hypokalaemic periodic paralysis (Pearson and Kalyanaraman 1983). There may be clear clinical findings to allow a differential diagnosis. Thus periodic paralysis is abrupt in onset, periodic, and persistent, whereas hypokalaemic myopathy may not be abrupt in onset, is not periodic, and not persistent.

Investigations into the influence of K^+ deficiency on muscle function and pathology require the choice of an appropriate animal model. With the rat, dietary deficiency of K^+ leads to reversible renal tubular and myocardial lesions, and generally at low K^+ concentration muscle paralysis or histological changes in skeletal muscle do not occur (Welt et al., 1960). With dogs, the development of a K^+ deficiency state leads to generalized weakness and, at K^+ concentrations less than 1·5 mmol l^{-1}, a syndrome similar to periodic paralysis. Also, in paralyzed dogs there may be focal skeletal muscle degeneration (Smith et al., 1950). Studies on K^+ depleted dogs (Knochel and Carter, 1976), by feeding K^+-deficient diets, showed evidence of weakness when there was a loss of 20% of estimated total body K^+. This was followed by increasing weakness, polydipsia, polyuria, and finally paralysis with death at 25–30% K^+ depletion; a period of 40 days was usually required to produce these effects. Serial measurements of *s*CPK and recording skeletal muscle transmembrane potential difference (E_m) showed an initial (at about 20 to 30 days) increase in E_m from an average of −85·4 mV to −94·6 mV with 10–20% K^+ deficiency. However, as K^+ loss increased to 30% the E_m decreased sharply to abnormally low values and there was a simultaneous increase in *s*CPK activity, indicating loss of skeletal muscle integrity with associated decrease in intracellular K^+ concentration, $[K^+]_i$, and increase in $[Na^+]_i$ and $[Cl^-]_i$. It was postulated that because of the deficiency in K^+ supply, part of the $[K^+]_i$ deficit is replaced by Na^+ and H^+, which could result in the following abnormalities:

1. Impairment of the Na^+-pump, possibly due to intracellular acidosis (Relman, 1972) or decreased availability of Na^+-K^+-ATPase (Leaf, 1970). This would result in a net increase in $[Na^+]_i$ and decrease in E_m.

2. Increased cell permeability to Na^+, leading to increased intracellular osmotic activity, and hence an increase in cellular water and increased total volume.
3. Abnormal synthesis and storage of glycogen could occur, since moderate K^+ deficiency impairs storage of muscle glycogen.

To examine the vulnerability of K^+ deficient muscle to exercise-induced injury, the effect of electrically stimulated contraction of the isolated gracilis muscle was examined in K^+ depleted dogs (Knochel and Schlein, 1972). In normal animals, stimulation of the gracilis nerve was associated with K^+ release and a sharp rise in muscle blood flow. With K^+ deficient animals, although the gracilis responded briskly to electrical stimulation of the motor nerve supply, both K^+ release and blood flow were markedly impaired. Histological examination of muscle from K^+ depleted and stimulated muscle showed extensive necrosis, but normal dogs subjected to the same degree of stimulation showed no evidence of muscle necrosis. Clearly K^+ depletion may predispose muscle to exercise-induced rhabdomyolysis.

DISTURBANCES OF Na^+ BALANCE

Hyponatraemia may occur in a variety of circumstances, including diuretic therapy, use of drugs with antidiuretic properties, adrenal insufficiency, salt-loosing nephritis, osmotic diuresis and water intoxication. However, as judged by the absence of documentation, it would appear that rhabdomyolysis due to hyponatraemia is rare, although it has been reported as a complication of water intoxication (Browne, 1979). Likewise with hypernatraemia, although there are a variety of differing aetiologies for this condition (Bichet et al., 1985), it is only rarely reported as a cause of rhabdomyolysis (Uvila and Nessan, 1973). However, the spasticity and convulsions that may occur as a consequence of the hypernatraemic cerebral dehydration could result in a secondary rhabdomyolytic process.

PHOSPHATE DEPLETION

Several clinical and experimental studies have suggested a relationship between phosphorus depletion and the rapid onset of acute hypophosphataemia and the development of rhabdomyolysis (Knochel, 1985). A considerable amount of the evidence has come from studies directed towards defining the role of hypophosphataemia in alcoholism, in which phosphorus depletion is common. In humans, hypophosphataemia and rhabdomyolysis may occur within a few days of abstinence from alcohol. The rhabdomyolysis associated with ethanol is discussed in detail in the section on xenobiotics.

Fuller et al. (1976) found that phosphate deficiency reduced the E_m, and was associated with increased tissue Na^+, Cl^- and water content, with decreased K^+ content; these effects were reversed on replenishment of phosphate. Also, administration of excess calories to partially starved dogs resulted in a profound hypophosphataemia with sharp increase in *s*CPK and the development of rhabdomyolysis (Knochel et al., 1978). Several studies have suggested that rhabdomyolysis does not occur with acute hypophosphataemia in the absence of pre-existing muscle injury (Knochel, 1985). Skeletal muscle, as well as bone, may act as an endogenous reservoir for phosphorus. Thus when acute hypophosphataemia occurs the muscle phosphorus is rapidly mobilized in order to provide vital supplies. If this occurs in situations where low skeletal muscle ATP exist, as for example in chronic phosphorus depletion, then ATP levels may fall further and cell death occurs (Emmett et al., 1977). The relationship between hypophosphataemia and skeletal muscle injury has been reviewed by Knochel (1985).

DIABETES MELLITUS

The metabolic and osmotic disturbances associated with hyperosmolar non-ketotic coma and ketoacidosis have resulted in the development of rhabdomyolysis (Grossman et al., 1974; Rainey et al., 1963).

Genetically Determined Enzyme Defects of Metabolism

Genetically determined enzyme defects that impair energy utilization, and in particular those with defective carbohydrate and lipid metabolism in skeletal muscle, have been implicated as causing rhabdomyolysis as one of their clinical features. Examples are as follows.

McARDLE'S DISEASE

There is muscle phosphorylase deficiency, as a consequence of which muscle glycogen cannot be utilized during anaerobic exercise. Attempts at strenuous muscle exercise produce painful muscle cramps, but clinically these patients are normal at rest. Myoglobinuria occurs in about half the patients on exercise, and ARF can occur (McArdle, 1951; Howell and Williams, 1983).

TARUI'S SYNDROME

Muscle phosphofructokinase is markedly reduced in this disease, which is possibly inherited as an autosomal recessive. Rhabdomyolysis has been described in a few cases (Tarui et al., 1965; Layzer et al., 1967; Howell and Williams, 1983).

CARNITINE-PARMITYL-TRANSFERASE (CPT) DEFICIENCY

The features of this syndrome are rhabdomyolysis and myoglobinuria, often preceded by exercise, with associated muscle cramps, myalgia and weakness, particularly after fasting. The urine is positive for myoglobin and *s*CPK is high (DiMauro and Melis-DiMauro, 1973; Bank et al., 1975; Cummings et al., 1976). Patten et al. (1979), for example, described a syndrome of recurrent rhabdomyolysis and myoglobinuria in two brothers found to have low (0–14%) muscle CPT activity. Measurements on isolated muscle mitochondria showed 88% of the total measurable CPT activity in this deficiency state was associated with the external membrane. In contrast, normal mitochondria showed a 1 : 1 distribution of CPT activity between the external and internal mitochondrial membranes. Muscle activity was normal for phosphofructokinase, phosphoglucomutase and phosphohexoisomerase.

Infections

Rhabdomyolysis with or without ARF, has been described in a large variety of infective conditions. Bacterial causes have included *Francisella tularensis* (Kaiser et al., 1985), *Clostridia* (Jendrzejewski et al., 1978), *Shigella* bacteraemia (Bowden et al., 1956) *Salmonella typhosa* bacteraemia (Rheingold et al., 1977), *Escherichia coli* septicaemia (Henrich et al., 1980), *Herbicola lathyri* contaminated intravenous fluids (Soule and Cunningham, 1973), *Legionella pneumophila* (Posner et al., 1980; Rodriguez et al., 1983), bronchoalveolar *aspergillosis* (El Nahas et al., 1983), and polymicrobial septicaemia (Kalish et al., 1982). Viral infections in which rhabdomyolysis has been described as a complication include Coxsackie virus (Tang et al., 1974), adenovirus (Wright et al., 1979), echovirus (Jehn and Fink, 1980), Herpes group (Schelesinger et al., 1978), the Epstein-Barr virus of infectious mononucleosis (Kantor et al., 1978), and influenza (Cunningham et al., 1979; Minow et al., 1974).

The pathogenesis of rhabdomyolysis in bacterial and viral infections may be complex and differ according to a given situation. There may be direct myotoxicity, skeletal muscle degeneration due to an invasion of muscle, rigors and pyrexia, and the effects of endotoxin on the cardiovascular system which may result in peripheral vasoconstriction, hypotension and decreased cardiac output.

Animal Toxins

Rhabdomyolysis may be a complication following bites and stings from a variety of reptiles, anthropods, lepidoptera and hymenoptera (Podgorny, 1983). The following two examples highlight the possible severity of the illness which may result from such evenomations.

Logan and Ogden (1985) reported the case of a 40-year-old female who developed rhabdomyolysis and ARF following a bite from the giant desert centipede (Scolopendra heros). Following the bite there developed pyrexia, nausea, breathlessness, blurred vision, and pain and swelling of the leg. When examined 5 days after the bite there was massive swelling of the right leg with decreased sensation, and absence of movement of the toes and ankle. Pertinent laboratory data on admission at this time were: $s[Cl^-]$ 87 mmol l^{-1}, $s[HCO_3^-]$ 15 mmol l^{-1}, blood urea nitrogen 160 mg l^{-1}, serum creatinine 11·4 mg dl^{-1}, uric acid 15·8 mg dl^{-1}, $s[Ca^{++}]$ 7·4 mg dl^{-1}, s[phosphate] 11·2 mg dl^{-1}, sCPK 18 860 iu l^{-1}, pH_a 7·36. A clinical chemistry diagnosis was therefore made of azotaemia with metabolic acidosis, hyperuricaemia, hyperphosphataemia and hypocalcaemia; the patient was haemodialyzed. An anterior compartment tissue pressure of 45 mm Hg was measured on the right and 25 mm Hg on the left, fasciotomy and debridgement were carried out.

Patten et al., (1985) described the case of a 9-year-old boy who was bitten probably by the rough tailed snake, *Tropidechis carinatus*. During the subsequent 24 hours he became progressively weaker and developed limb pains and dark red urine. The clinical picture was of total body paralysis, rhabdomyolysis and ARF. He required artificial ventilation for 10 weeks, and muscle paralysis and paresis persisted for 18 weeks. ARF was present for 18 days and treated with peritoneal dialysis. Initial laboratory findings included sCPK 380 000 iu l^{-1} (normal 1·25–3·25).

An example of basic investigations into the myotoxic potential of snake venoms is provided by crototoxin, a presynaptically active phospholipid isolated from the venom of the South American rattlesnake Crotalus durissus terrificus. It consists of a reversible complex of two sub-units, an acidic peptide (crotopotin, CA) and a basic phospholipase A_2 enzyme (phospholipase A or CB). Although mainly an inhibitor of transmitter release from the skeletal neuromuscular junction (Chang and Lee, 1977), some postsynaptic neuromuscular blockade may occur (Bon and Jeng, 1979). However, crotoxin has also been shown to be myotoxic (Gopalakrishakone et al., 1984). Kouyoumdjian et al. (1986) found that CB caused muscle necrosis in the rat with minor inflammatory response. Although CA was per se inactive, it did potentiate the affect of CB if given in combination; the myotoxic response was both more severe and more widespread.

Clinical Features

With the exception of direct acute physical injury the initial signs and symptoms will usually reflect the primary causative disease process, with subsequent development of signs and symptoms referable to affected skeletal muscle and the complications of rhabdomyolysis.

Muscle involvement may vary from subclinical to severe and producing incapacitation. With clinical indications of rhabdomyolysis there will be weakness, which may cover a spectrum of effects from simple difficulty with writing, through difficulty with walking, to complete paralysis. Muscle pain may be mild to severe and incapacitating, and in general is related to the degree of muscle weakness. Pain may occur in response to attempted minor movements. Muscle tenderness is a characteristic feature and often parallels the degree of muscle pain. Muscle swelling, secondary to intracellular oedema, and local hyperthermia may be present. The pain , myalgia, weakness and swelling decrease as the muscle injury resolves. In a few cases, muscle swelling may not occur until after the administration of intravenous fluids (Gabow et al., 1982). With non-traumatic causes of rhabdomyolysis, the distribution of affected muscles may vary from segments of a limb to involvement of most of the skeletal musculature of the body. In the presence of respiratory muscle involvement, subjects may experience anything from dyspnoea to complete failure of breathing which requires ventilatory support. Second wave phenomena may occur, i.e. resolution of initial signs and symptoms referable to muscle involvement, followed by a recurrence of swelling and tenderness. This may be due to the late fragmentation of intracellular components leading to increased intracellular osmolality and water movement; for example, an increase of only 10 mOs kg^{-1} increases osmotic pressure by about 1·7 mm Hg which is sufficient to produce significant swelling (Quintanilla, 1982). This may lead to a secondary ischaemic necrosis with nerve and vessel compression, and hence possible peripheral neurological complications and gangrene (Knochel, 1976). The second wave phenomena may, in some patients, be initially misdiagnosed as thrombophlebitis, e.g. Homans' sign will be positive.

A variety of complications of rhabdomyolysis may develop to variable degrees of severity and coexistence. The major complications which require management are vascular and peripheral neurological effects due to osteomuscular compartment swelling, mineralization of muscle, disseminated intravascular coagulation, cardiovascular abnormalities and ARF. Electrolyte disturbances are discussed under chemical pathology diagnosis.

Local Compression

Nerve and blood vessel compression may result from increased pressure in osteomuscular compartments as a result of oedema due to muscle fragmentation and an increase in the number of osmotically active particles. As noted above, an increase of 10 mOs kg^{-1} can result in an increase in osmotic pressure by almost 1·7 mm Hg. Such increases are due to direct physical trauma and subsequent degenerative and necrotic effects resulting in acute direct traumatic rhabdomyolysis. In conditions where there is no direct traumatic element, the mechanism of production of rhabdomyolysis may be complex. However, a tentative hypothesis has been constructed to explain the rhabdomyotic process. If the aetiological factor causes an alteration in myocyte membrane integrity, there will be an impairment of the Na^+ pump mechanism and $[Na^+]_i$ increase which results in a disturbance of the Na^+/Ca^{++} exchange mechanism, and $[Ca^{++}]_i$ increases. This, in turn, will activate myofibrillar neural protease and degenerative processes begin to occur intracellularly, leading to fragmentation and necrosis. Experimental support for this proposal is to be found in the fact that calcium ionophores induce muscle damage, and simultaneous administration of drugs to prevent Ca^{++} accumulation (e.g. verapamil) prevent protease activation and rhabdomyolysis (Statham et al., 1976; Publicover et al., 1978; Knochel, 1982).

In a literature review Cadnapaphornchai et al., (1980) found peripheral nerve injury in 16 of 51 (31%) patients with rhabdomyolysis. Akmal and Massry (1983) described 4 out of 40 patients with drug intoxication in whom peripheral nerve damage was present. Evidence of rhabdomyolysis was present in the form of significantly increased *s*CPK activity (> 24 000 iu) and a strong positive ortho-toluidine urine test in the absence of erythrocytes. ARF developed in three, and slight renal insufficiency in the fourth; all recovered. In addition to the influence of increased fascial compartment pressure secondary to muscle damage and swelling, when peripheral neuropathy is present in patients who were comatose, other contributory factors may include direct physical pressure and traction during coma, and a compromised circulation secondary to pressure from immobilization.

Fasciotomy may be essential to prevent permanent neurological sequelae.

Mineralization of Muscle

In experimental animals, calcium is deposited in damaged muscle and the amount increases with the degree of uraemia (Meroney et al, 1957). Radiological evidence of calcium deposition has been obtained in the muscles of patients with non-traumatic rhabdomyolysis and associated ARF, and apparent disappearance of the calcification within one to three months (Clark and Summerling, 1966; Butifkofer and Molleyres, 1968; Grossman and Large, 1968). Patients with drug-induced rhabdomyolysis were studied by Akmal et al (1978) with particular reference to calcium deposition in muscle during the various phases of renal injury. Their patients had muscle swelling and tenderness, with initial hypocalcaemia and hyperphosphataemia and subsequent hypercalcaemia, and muscle calcification appeared to be transient. They detected the presence and progression of calcium deposits by conventional and electron radiography with technetium-99 m scan; the latter was found to be the most sensitive method. All patients were found to have calcium deposits during the oliguric phase, which disappeared on recovery of normal renal function and muscle healing. Possible mechanisms related to the precipitation and resolution of calcium deposits are discussed later together with chemical pathology features.

Disseminated Intravascular Coagulation (DIC)

DIC may occur with major rhabdomyolysis, as evidenced by leucocytosis, the presence of fibrin-split products in serum and urine, thrombocytopenia, hypofibrinogenaemia and increased prothrombin time. DIC may be associated with haemorrhage and marked fluid loss, and endotoxaemia may be contributory or causative in some instances. DIC usually resolves spontaneously within a few hours or days. Possible factors in the production of this coagulopathy include the following:

1. Endotoxaemia when infection is present (Kendrick et al., 1977).
2. Damage to the muscle may release the following active factors:
   a. tissue thromboplastin which activates platelet aggregation and hence fibrin deposition,
   b. CPK, creatine or ADP which may promote platelet aggregation (Meltzer, 1971), and
   c. plasminogen activator from muscle may cause excess fibrinolysis (Berman et al., 1973).

Renal Injury

Rhabdomyolysis may be complicated by the onset of an acute reduction in renal function not attributable to haemorrhage, shock or urine flow obstruction. The probability of developing ARF, and its severity, often reflects the degree of rhabdomyolysis. Gabow et al. (1982) reviewing a series of 77 patients with rhabdomyolysis of differing aetiology found an incidence of ARF amounting to 33%; 6 of their patients died. Koffler et al (1976) reported 24 patients who developed ARF in association with rhabdomyolysis caused in the majority of cases by various overdoses. They found that, although the initial biochemistry was similar to that occurring in other causes of ARF, there was a significant increase in serum creatinine relative to serum urea nitrogen and marked hyperuricaemia. There was an initial hypocalcaemia and hyperphosphataemia, and a subsequent transient hypercalcaemia during the diuretic phase. ARF due to rhabdomyolysis with associated myoglobinuria appears to be much more likely to occur in individuals with large muscle masses (Knochel, 1982).

Determinants for the development of ARF are not totally clear. According to some observers, most patients with myoglobinuria who develop ARF are also compromised in other ways that may influence renal function; these include volume depletion, or loss of plasma volume into damaged tissues with consequent decrease in renal perfusion (Medical Staff Conference, 1976). Knochel (1976) noted that in several patients with 'flu-like' illness and having features of rhabdomyolysis, those patients with volume depletion, secondary to vomiting and diarrhoea, developed ARF. Support for a contribution to ARF from volume depletion comes from an experimental demonstration that volume expansion (e.g. with mannitol) appears to minimize or prevent ARF following myoglobin release (Wilson et al., 1967) and, *in vitro*, hypoxia potentiates the effects of haem pigments on renal cortical slices (Braun, 1970). The influence of volume depletion on the pathogenesis of ARF is particularly marked in exertional heatstroke, when up to 30% of victims may develop ARF. In this situation there is dehydration, fluid sequestration into injured muscle, myoglobinuria, hyperuricaemia and the excretion of large quantities of uric acid into a concentrated urine (Anderson et al., 1983). In many reports the situation is complex and several contributing factors may be present. For example, in the series by Chugh et al., (1979) many of the 17 patients with ARF had fluid and electrolyte loss, vomiting and hypotension.

A variety of mechanisms have been proposed to explain the ARF of rhabdomyolysis; these include tubular obstruction, direct toxicity to the renal tubular epithelium by released muscle substances, renal ischaemia, and decreased glomerular permeability. Some of these factors are discussed below.

HYPERURICAEMIA

The plasma uric acid concentration in rhabdomyolysis appears to be proportional to the degree of myoglobin release (Schiff et al., 1978). Injured muscle releases purine precursors into the circulation which are converted to uric acid in the liver, which is then excreted in the urine. If urine pH is less than 5.0, and particularly if uric acid is highly concentrated and lactate raised, urate may precipitate in the distal tubule. Both urate and lactate are actively excreted by the same transport mechanism across the distal tubular epithelium (Steel and Rieselbach, 1975), and increasing the lactate concentration would inhibit the secretion of urate (Warren et al., 1975). In this manner, hyperuricaemia may be a factor in the pathogenesis of rhabdomyolysis-induced acute renal failure (Klinenberg et al., 1975). Uric acid nephropathy may be particularly significant in some forms of ARF secondary to rhabdomyolysis, and that associated with exertional heatstroke is a particular example (Schrier, 1967; Knochel et al., 1974). These volume depleted patients, in addition to having myoglobinuria, are hyperuricaemic and excrete large quantities of uric acid into concentrated urine (Anderson et al., 1983). As noted above, low pH concentrated urine favours precipitation of uric acid (Knochel, 1976).

Warren et al. (1975) described 7 patients having status epilepticus or recurrent episodes of grand mal seizures, all of whom developed hyperuricaemia (serum uric acid 13 ± 5 SE mg dl^{-1}) with lactate acidosis (serum lactate $7{\cdot}6 \pm 3{\cdot}7$ mmol l^{-1}) and a reversible ARF which required haemodialysis in two patients. Initially, with the exception of two cases, there was normal blood urea, and therefore the hyperuricaemia was not secondary to uraemia. It was considered that the major source of uric acid was from the degradation of released endogenous muscle proteins, and that this may have been potentiated by the severe hypoxia during the seizure period.

In blood and interstitial fluids, at pH 7·4, 95% of uric acid is in the form of monosodium urate monohydrate. At the lower pH of renal tubular fluid and urine there is a marked shift in the (uric acid) : (urate) ratio. At pH 6·0, about 20% uric acid is present, and the proportion rises sharply as the pH decreases. Solubility also decreases with decreasing pH, and an acute hyperuricaemic nephropathy (acute tubular obstruction) may occur (Klinenberg et al., 1975).

MYOGLOBIN

There have been suggestions that myoglobin may be a tubular nephrotoxin responsible, to a variable extent, for the ARF associated with rhabdomyolysis. However, the evidence is not convincing, and in some cases does not support a myoglobin pathogenesis (Fraser et al., 1986). An alternative suggestion is that myoglobin may become crystallized within the renal tubular lumen and produce tubular obstruction. It is known that serum, and therefore tubular fluid, myoglobin concentrations may be very high. For example, Ross et al., (1983) found that in healthy young men taking severe exercise, the serum myoglobin concentrations increased from $17\cdot9 \pm 5\cdot7$ SD $\mu g\,l^{-1}$ to $1108 \pm 929\ \mu g\,l^{-1}$ and *s*CPK increased from 199 ± 130 iu l^{-1} to 6929 ± 8119 iu l^{-1} after 3 days of exercise. Creatinine increased only from $85 \pm 10\ \mu mol\,l^{-1}$ to $104 \pm 12\ \mu mol\,l^{-1}$. The highest concentration of myoglobin was 2400 $\mu g\,l^{-1}$, creatine 132 $\mu mol\,l^{-1}$, and CPK 8840 iu l^{-1}. Changes in myoglobin concentration correlated closely with *s*CPK activity, but not with creatinine.

Experimentally it has been shown that muscle injury in rats resulting from local im glycerol injections leads to acute renal failure characterized by impairment of organic acid (*p*-aminohippurate) and organic base (tetraethylammonium) transport. These findings accord with the results from an *in vitro* renal cortical slice technique in which the uptake of *p*-aminohippurate and tetraethylammonium was significantly decreased by the presence of free haem but not myoglobin in the incubating medium (Braun et al., 1970). Therefore, if myoglobin has a nephrotoxic role in the pathogenesis of ARF in rhabdomyolysis it is likely to be based on degradation of myoglobin to ferrihaemate in the acidic tubular fluid. There may be evidence that with very high myoglobin concentrations, it may play a role in the production of ARF. For example, Ross et al., (1986) described the case of a girl with severe convulsions who died of ARF; serum myoglobin concentrations increased from 157 to 490 000 $\mu g\ l^{-1}$, with *s*CPK activity increasing from 236 to 900 000 iu l^{-1}. Renal histopathology showed tubular necrosis with casts and some glomerular ischaemia. However, as noted by Morris (1981), since many cases of myoglobinaemia and myoglobinuria are not accompanied by ARF, it is likely that other major factors must operate in 'myoglobinuria-associated ARF'. The role of myoglobin, if any, is still unclear.

RENAL ISCHAEMIA

There is experimental evidence, and clinical impression, that renal ischaemia may be a major factor in some cases of rhabdomyolysis-associated renal failure. Ayer et al. (1971) used a ^{133}Xe washout technique to study changes in intrarenal haemodynamics following im glycerol-induced experimental renal tubular failure in the rat. They found a severe progressive and preferential cortical hypoperfusion during the oliguric phase and a normalization of the intrarenal haemodynamics during the recovery phase. They regarded their observations as being in agreement with micropuncture studies showing that the oliguria and renal insufficiency of myohaemoglobinuric-associated renal failure are due to a primary decrease in glomerular filtration rate (GFR), and that this is itself due to an increase in afferent glomerular arteriolar tone. Wilson et al. (1976) investigated the effectiveness of plasma infusion, saline injection, mannitol infusion, and combined treatments with mannitol and saline on the development of intramuscular glycerol-induced ARF in the rat. All methods of treatment decreased azotaemia, and combined treatment with mannitol and saline almost completely prevented the development of azotaemia. The effectiveness of each treatment correlated with the prevention of severe renal ischaemia shortly after im injection of glycerol.

CHANGES IN GLOMERULAR PERMEABILITY

Clarkson et al. (1970) demonstrated fibrin strands ultrastructurally in renal biopsy specimens from myoglobinuric patients with ARF. They suggested that the fibrin deposition decreased GFR and led to acute renal failure. Wardle and Wright (1973) produced ARF in the rabbit by im injections of glycerol, and found evidence for enhanced coagulation activity as deposition of fibrin in the glomerular arterioles, vasa recta, and peritubular vessels; this was enhanced by treatment with E-aminocaproic acid. It is thus possible that intraglomerular fibrin deposits could contribute to ischaemia and impair glomerular permeability, and hence contribute to the pathogenesis of ARF in rhabdomyolysis.

It is likely that no one factor operates solely in the pathogenesis of ARF in rhabdomyolysis, but that there may be variable contributions from hyperuricaemia, myoglobinuria, hypotension, renal ischaemia, dehydration, and other as yet unknown factors.

Cardiovascular Effects

A variety of cardiac irregularities and ECG changes have been described in cases of rhabdomyolysis. These have included ventricular arrhythmias, intraventricular conduction delays, abnormal axis deviation, sinus bradycardia, sinus tachycardia, ischaemic changes, non-specific S-T segment and T-wave changes, and T-wave changes characteristic of hyperkalaemia (Robotham and Haddow, 1976). Primary myocardial damage may occur along with skeletal muscle injury in some cases of rhabdomyolysis, particularly xenobiotic-induced, but in most cases the cardiac abnormalities are explicable on the basis of plasma electrolyte changes.

Investigational Findings and Diagnosis

Myoglobin Determinations

The major biochemical diagnostic feature of rhabdomyolysis is the detection of myoglobin in plasma and urine. Unlike haemoglobin, which has a plasma haptoglobin binding affinity up to 100 mg dl^{-1}, myoglobin has a limited plasma binding of 1·5 mg dl^{-1} to a molecular fraction of 50 000–300 000 daltons. Because of this, and its comparatively low MW, myoglobin appears in the urine at low plasma concentrations (Knochel, 1982). Because of this difference in plasma binding, and the threshold for renal excretion, the colour of plasma is different for conditions producing haemoglobinuria and myoglobinuria. In the case of haemoglobin the serum is coloured pink and the haptoglobulin is low, whereas with myoglobin the serum is clear and the haptoglobulin concentration normal. Urine colouration with myoglobinuria depends on pH; when urine is neutral or alkaline myoglobin confers a pink colour, and when acid the urine has a brown discolouration. A further simple means of indicating the possible presence of myoglobin is the demonstration of a positive *o*-toluidine test with urine in the absence of erythrocytes. However, standard dipstick methods detect the haem radical by the *o*-toluidine reaction, with a sensitivity in the range 1–10 $\mu g\ ml^{-1}$, and thus cannot differentiate myoglobinuria and haemoglobinura. In the absence of sufficient clinical information it may be necessary to confirm specifically the presence of myoglobin. This can be undertaken by absorption spectrophotometry, although the bands are close; more specific methods are by electrophoresis and immunodiffusion. For quantitative measurement of myoglobin in body fluids the sensitivity of the various techniques is as follows (Knochel, 1982): radioimmunoassay $5–10 \times 10^{-3}\ \mu g\ ml^{-1}$; haemagglutination $0{\cdot}3–1{\cdot}0\ \mu g\ ml^{-1}$ immunodiffusion $5–10\ \mu g\ ml^{-1}$; immunoelectrophoresis $5–20\ \mu g\ ml^{-1}$.

The differential diagnosis of pigmenturia involves porphyria, haemoglobinuria, and myoglobinuria. Major factors in differentiating these various causes of pigmenturia, aside from clinical indications, are as follows for uncomplicated cases:

a. *Porphyria*: there is no reaction with haem-detecting agents, and the Watson–Schwartz reaction for porphobilinogen is positive.
b. *Haemoglobinuria*: serum is pink, serum (muscle) enzymes are normal, and serum haptoglobulin is low.
c. *Myoglobinuria*: serum is clear, haptoglobin concentration is normal, and serum (muscle) enzymes are increased.

In march haemoglobinuria there is a susceptibility to traumatic haemolysis because of erythrocyte abnormality or genetically defective haptoglobulin. Thus during physical trauma to the extremities there is haemolysis, and saturation of haptoglobulin occurs with consequent haemoglobinuria (Buckle, 1965; Streeton, 1967). The circumstances may require an initial differentiation of pigmenturia between march haemoglobinuria and the myoglobinuria of exercise-induced rhabdomyolysis.

Serum Enzymes

The most appropriate enzymes for the biochemical diagnosis of rhabdomyolysis are as listed below.

CREATINE PHOSPHOKINASE

(CPK; EC 2.7.3.2; ATP; creatine-N-phosphotransferase). CPK catalyzes the transfer of a phosphate group from ATP to creatine, forming creatine phosphate, the latter serving as a muscle energy store for transfer of phosphate to ADP to yield ATP. CPK is a dimer, with subunits designated M (muscle) and B (brain) which combine to form the following three isozymes:

BB — brain (CPK-1)
MB — myocardium and skeletal muscle (CPK-2)
MM — myocardium and skeletal muscle (CPK-3)

Tsung and Tsung (1986) analyzed CPK activity in a variety of human skeletal muscles and found that substantial activities attributable to CPK-MM were present in all specimens, and CPK-MB in about 44% of them (at approximately 1–6% of total activity). Thus, in skeletal muscle degenerative processes, CPK-MB and CPK-MM may both be increased. Also described are two other CPK isozymes: CPK-MIT, a mitochondrial enzyme which may appear when there is extensive muscle damage, and macro-CT, which appears as a band in the electrophoretogram between CPK-2 and CPK-3 and is bound to IgG. Assay procedures and isozyme fractionation are reviewed by Blick and Liles (1985).

ASPARTATE AMINOTRANSFERASE

(EC 2.6.1.1; AST; originally known as glutamate:oxaloacetate transaminase, GOT). AST is an L-aspartate: 2-oxyglutarate aminotransferase found in cytosol and mitochondria, having highest activities in heart, liver, skeletal muscle and kidney.

ALANINE AMINOTRANSFERASE

(EC 2.6.1.2; ALT; originally known as glutamate:pyruvate transamine, GPT). ALT is an L-alanine:2-oxyglutarate aminotransferase found in high activity in liver, followed by heart, skeletal muscle and pancreas. AST gives a better index of skeletal muscle injury than ALT. Assay procedures for transaminases have been reviewed by Blick and Liles (1985).

LACTATE DEHYDROGENASE

(EC 1.1.1.27; LDH; L-lactate:NAD^+-oxidoreductase). LDH is a cytosolic enzyme which catalyzes the conversion of pyruvate to lactate, with the oxidation of NADH to NAD^+. Found in virtually all tissues, with the highest activity being in skeletal muscle and liver, followed by myocardium. The enzyme is a tetramer, with each tetramer being composed of a combination of two different polypeptide chain subunits, the H (heart) variety and the M (muscle) variety. Five isozymes that have been described are LD-1(H_4), LD-2(H_3M), LD-3(H_2M_2), LD-4(H_1M_3) and LD-5(H_4). Distribution of major activities is as follows: LD-1 and LD-2 in myocardium, erythrocyte and kidney; LD-3 is in many tissues and non-specific; LD-4 and LD-5 in liver and skeletal muscle. Assay procedures for LDH isozymes have been reviewed by Blick and Liles (1985).

Increases in serum activities of all the above enzymes have been described in a large number of reported cases of rhabdomyolysis. The magnitude of the rise in serum enzyme activity depends on the muscle mass of the patient, the physical condition of the patient, the extent of muscle injury, and the time of sampling in relationship to the onset of signs and symptoms. Along with measurements of plasma and urine myoglobin, sequential determination of enzyme activities may be used as an index of the progression and regression of muscle injury. Often in the acute phase, there may be a direct relationship between serum myoglobin concentration and sCPK, *s*LDH and *s*AST activities (Schiff et al., 1978). Also, measurement of *s*CPK may help in differentiating ARF due to rhabdomyolysis from that due to other causes (Chugh et al., 1979). Where it is possible that the myopathic process affects cardiac as well as skeletal muscle, or in circumstances where other cardiac pathology is present, the use of isozyme determinations is particularly useful. Also, and particularly with lesser degrees of rhabdomyolysis, measurement of muscle-specific serum enzyme activities may be a more sensitive index of the presence of injury. For example, in the series by Gabow et al. (1982), 26% of their patients with rhabdomyolysis, as documented by increased *s*CPK activity, had a negative o-toluidine dipstick test for myoglobinuria within 24–48 hours of admission. Thus the relatively slower clearance of *s*CPK may be a more reliable monitor of the rhabdomyolytic process, particularly after a few days.

Serum K^+

Serum K^+ is usually increased in cases of rhabdomyolysis. Two exceptions are, (*a*) when there is exertional heat stroke and significant K^+ losses occur in sweat and urine, and (*b*) when the aetiological cause of rhabdomyolysis is hypokalaemic kaluresis. In other cases the initial hyperkalaemia, due to K^+ release from injured myocytes, may be cardiotoxic.

Muscle fibre $[K^+]$ is around 100 mmol kg^{-1}, and hence an abrupt necrosis of about 150 g skeletal muscle would release about 15 mmol K^+ and increase $s[K^+]$ by about $1{\cdot}0$ mmol l^{-1}. Reported cases show the variability in $s[K^+]$ that may be present in rhabdomyolysis, and that renal function is also an important determinant. For example, in the series by Gabow et al (1982) only 7 of 77 patients (and 87 episodes of rhabdomyolysis) had $s[K^+] > 5.5$ mmol l^{-1} on admission; 6 of these had, or developed, ARF. Reviewing 71 cases from the literature they noted that 43% (47/71) cases on admission had hyperkalaemia ($s[K^+] \geqslant 5{\cdot}5$ mmol ml^{-1}), and of these 47, 13 had admission serum creatinine $< 3{\cdot}0$ mg dl^{-1} or blood urea nitrogen < 50 mg dl^{-1}. However, all but two developed ARF. That renal function is a major determinant of $s[K^+]$ in rhabdomyolysis is supported by the observation of the following $s[K^+]$ values in patients with rhabdomyolysis in the series reported by Cadnapaphornchai et al. (1980): without ARF $4{\cdot}4$ mmol l^{-1}; with non-oliguric ARF $4{\cdot}5$ mmol l^{-1}; and with oliguric ARF $6{\cdot}3$ mmol l^{-1}. Thus Gabor et al. (1982) note that the absence of hyperkalaemia should not deter consideration of a diagnosis of rhabdomyolysis, especially in patients with normal renal function. However, when ARF is present the degree of hyperkalaemia may be life threatening. For example, Koffler et al. (1976) found in 11 of 21 patients with ARF the $s[K^+]$ was in the range 6.0–$8{\cdot}5$ mmol l^{-1}.

Plasma Phosphate

Hyperphosphataemia usually occurs in rhabdomyolysis as a result of its release from injured muscle and because of changes in $s[Ca^{++}]$. It is also found when ARF is present; for example, Koffler et al. (1976) found in 11 patients with ARF the average serum phosphorus concentration was $9{\cdot}3$ mg dl^{-1} (range $8{\cdot}5$–$19{\cdot}0$ mg dl^{-1}).

Uric Acid

Significant increases in uric acid may occur in plasma and be excreted in urine before any oliguria appears. This is due to the release of purine precursors (inosine, xanthine, hypoxathine) from injured muscle, which are then converted in the liver to uric acid. During severe exercise in a hot environment there may be significant increases in the production of uric acid (Knochel et al., 1974). In these studies some had serum uric acid concentrations exceeded 12 mg dl^{-1}. Average uric acid excretion before physical activity was 640 mg per day; by the eleventh day of physical exercise, when indices of muscle injury were highest and $s[K^+]$ at its lowest, the average uric acid excretion had risen to 1031 mg per day. Schiff et al. (1978) found that, with marathon runners, increase in urate was proportionate to that of myoglobin. With exertional rhabdomyolysis in muscular subjects, the serum uric acid concentration may increase as high as 50 mg dl^{-1} (Knochel, 1982). When ARF is present, severe hyperuricaemia may develop. For example, in a series by Koffler et al. (1976) the average serum uric acid was 17.9 mg dl^{-1} (range 16.0–34.5 mg dl^{-1}) at a time when serum creatinine concentration was only slightly increased. Chugh et al. (1979) compared features of ARF in myoglobinuric and non-myoglobinuric patients, and found uric acid concentrations to be significantly higher in those with rhabdomyolysis in comparison with those not exhibiting rhabdomyolysis ($0{\cdot}73 \pm 0{\cdot}20$ mmol l^{-1} versus 0.58 ± 0.09 mmol l^{-1}).

Creatinine

Creatinine excretion may rise considerably in rhabdomyolysis due to its release from injured muscle (Quintanilla, 1982). As a consequence of the increased plasma creatinine, the [blood urea nitrogen/creatinine] ratio (normal 10 : 1–20 : 1) may be less than 10. For example, in the series reported by Patel and Conner (1985) of phenycyclidine-associated rhabdomyolysis, in 29 patients the [urea nitrogen/creatine] ratio averaged 9·3 (range 6–13).

Calcium

Abnormal plasma $[Ca^{++}]$ is frequently recorded in rhabdomyolysis. Hypocalacaemia often occurs in the initial stages of rhabdomyolysis. For example, in the series of 77 patients reported by Gabow et al. (1982) 55 had hypocalcaemia in the early stages. Values as low as 3·5 mg dl^{-1} may occur within 2 to 4 days of the onset of rhabdomyolysis, mainly due to calcium deposition in the injured skeletal muscle. When ARF occurs in association with rhabdomyolysis, hypocalcaemia frequently occurs in the oliguric phase followed by acute hypercalcaemia in the early polyuric phase (Tavill et al., 1964, Segal et al., 1968; Leonard and Eichner, 1972; Grossman et al., 1974; Koffler et al., 1976; Chugh et al., 1979).

It has been considered that hyperphosphataemia and skeletal resistance to the calcaemic action of parathyroid hormone (PTH) are important factors in the pathogenesis of the oliguric phase hypocalcaemia (Somerville and Kaye, 1978, 1979). The pathophysiology of the polyuric phase hypercalcaemia has been the subject of considerable discussion, and principal factors that have been implicated are resolution of soft tissue calcification and increased bone resportion (Tavill et al., 1964; de Torrente et al., 1976; Akmal et al., 1978). For example, Akmal et al. (1978) studied 4 patients with non-traumatic rhabdomyolysis associated ARF by following the progression of calcium deposition in injured skeletal muscle with conventional and electron radiography, and technetium-99m diphosphonate scans. Calcium deposits were demonstrated during the oliguric period, which disappeared on recovery of renal function.

Studies with experimental animals have shown that skeletal resistance to the calcaemic action of PTH may be lessened or overcome by the administration of 1,25-dihydroxycholecalciferol [$1,25(OH)_2D$] (Massry et al., 1978). Llach et al. (1981) studied 6 oliguric patients with rhabdomyolysis-associated ARF who also had marked hyperphosphataemia and hypocalcaemia with low levels of $1,25(OH)_2D$ on admission. During the early polyuric phase, moderate hypercalcaemia was associated with marked increase in plasma $1,25(OH)_2D$ and increase in PTH. During the late polyuric phase the concentrations of serum Ca^{++} and $1,25(OH)_2D$ reverted to normal. The authors concluded that in rhabdomyolysis-associated ARF, the hypocalcaemia of the oliguric phase may be secondary to decreased synthesis of $1,25(OH)_2D$ and skeletal resistance to PTH, and that both may be in part secondary to hyperphosphataemia. The hypercalcaemia in the recovery phase may be related to an increased synthesis of $1,25(OH)_2D$ and increased mobilization of calcium from bone to soft tissue; both may result from secondary hyperparathyrodism and recovery of renal function. Increased serum PTH has been found in the hypercalcaemic diuretic phase by Leonard and Eichner (1970).

Albumin

In severe rhabdomyolysis, the associated capillary injury may lead to loss of circulating albumin and the development of a marked hypoalbuminaemia within a few hours of injury to skeletal muscle. Thus, administration of albumin may aggravate any associated interstitial oedema (Knochel, 1982).

Haematology

Leucocytosis is a frequent finding in cases of rhabdomyolysis. For example, Akmal et al. (1981) described leucocytosis in 25 patients intoxicated with phencyclidine, of whom 10 had ARF and 7 had mild impairment of renal function; the average leucocyte count was 17 345 mm^{-3} (range 10 700–24 900 mm^{-3}). Leucocytosis usually spontaneously resolves within 2 to 8 days. As discussed earlier, transient disseminated intravascular coagulation may develop.

Muscle Biopsy

The histopathological features vary with the site and time of sampling, the cause of the rhabdomyolytic process, and degree of clinically assessed injury. Where microscopic pathology is present this normally takes the form of necrosis, fragmentation and vacuolization of fibres, proliferation of sarcolemmal cells, and the presence of phagocytes. Blood vessels are usually patent and normal. Except with cases of primary metabolic myopathies, histochemistry is usually normal, e.g. phosphorylase, hexokinase, phosphofructokinase, pyruvate kinase and LDH (George et al., 1979).

Treatment

In addition to the management of the patient with respect to the primary aetiologic factor(s), the following may need to be undertaken with specific reference to the rhabdomyolytic process and incipient or established ARF.

1. MAINTENANCE OF FLUID, ELECTROLYTE, AND ACID–BASE BALANCE

In the early stages of rhabdomyolysis, large quantities of fluid may be lost into the injured muscle and replacement is required to maintain and stabilize blood pressure, and minimize the potential for renal hypoperfusion. Treatment may be required for hyperkalaemia, including iv calcium gluconate, insulin and glucose (Greenwood, 1974), and hyperphosphataemia may require correction using phosphate binding antacids perorally. Although hypocalcaemia per se seldom causes effects, it may potentiate the cardiotoxicity of hyperkalaemia. However, since administration of calcium salts may potentiate cellular damage and aggravate rhabdomyolysis, the treatment of hypocalcaemia should be undertaken cautiously (Knochel, 1982). Where hyperuricaemia exists, it has been recommended that alkalinization of the urine be undertaken, together with fluids, in order to prevent tubular crystalluria. If pulmonary oedema is present, or urine alkalinization not possible, haemodialysis is effective (Warren et al., 1975).

2. FASCIOTOMY

Peripheral neurological and vascular complications may occur as a consequence of the osteomuscular compartment increased pressure. This is particularly notable during second wave swelling affecting limb muscles. If undertaken promptly, fasciotomy can relieve the excess pressure and prevent the loss of muscle power and sensation, or the development of distal gangrene (Akmal and Massry, 1983; Finley et al., 1977). Pressure transducer measurements are useful, and it has been proposed that fasciotomy may be necessary if the compartmental pressure exceeds 35 mm Hg (Knochelk, 1982). The value of fasciotomy is emphasized, as an example, by the report of Koffler et al., (1976). In a description of a series of cases of ARF secondary to rhabdomyolysis, there were 3 cases of excessive muscle swelling leading to signs of nerve and blood vessel compression. In 2 patients fasciotomy was undertaken; in the patient not having this procedure, motor and sensory deficit in the affected limb was permanent.

3. PREVENTION OR MANAGEMENT OF ACUTE RENAL FAILURE

Clearly the use of any drugs with known nephrotoxic potential should be avoided in cases of rhabdomyolysis. Fluid volume replacement, and maintenance, is one of the most critical factors in avoiding the development of ARF in rhabdomyolysis (Medical Staff Conference, 1976). If there is a presumptive clinical diagnosis of rhabdomyolysis-induced ARF, it is generally recommended that an iv infusion of mannitol and sodium bicarbonate be given (25 g mannitol and 100 mEq $NaHCO_3$ in 800 ml 5% aqueous dextrose, reconstituted to 1 litre). Alkalinization of the urine is recommended to correct any acidosis and solublize any renal tubular myoglobin. However, Knochel (1982) notes that alkalinization of urine in patients with major rhabdomyolysis is difficult to achieve except if very large quantities of bicarbonate are given, and this may aggravate hypocalcaemia. Mannitol, a volume expander, will improve renal haemodynamics. Infusion rate should be determined by clinical biochemical findings and the rate of urine flow. It should be noted in assessing the degree of intravascular fluid loss that in many cases of rhabdomyolysis there is a sequestration of fluid into damaged tissue, and hypovolaemia may develop with very little weight change, and in such circumstances body weight measurements may give misleading information about fluid balance (Quintanilla, 1982).

There have been some differences of opinion on the use of diuretics in the management of rhabdomyolysis (Medical Staff Conference, 1976). However, many authorities do recommend the use of diuretics in preventing or ameliorating ARF in patients with myoglobinuria. Thus Knochel (1976) notes that by interfering with Na^+ reabsorption, furosemide impairs the concentrating mechanism and may increase renal parenchymal oxygen tension. The osmotic diuretic effect of concomitantly administered mannitol will produce an increase in renal intratubular pressure and a washout effect. With a hypercatabolic ARF both peritoneal dialysis and haemodialysis have been employed, although when there is a rapid rate of catabolism peritoneal dialysis as an alternative may not be appropriate (Knolph, 1969).

RHABDOMYOLYSIS ASSOCIATED WITH XENOBIOTICS

Substances causing rhabdomyolysis cover a wide spectrum of materials used for differing industrial, domestic, medicinal and self-abuse purposes. Thus, rhabdomyolytic substances may be found amongst therapeutic products, domestic and industrial chemicals, and drugs of addiction. Due to the greater ease of documenting, recording and reporting, together with the circumstances of occurrence, information is more readily available on the incidence, clinical features, diagnosis, complications and mechanism of production of rhabdomyolysis for therapeutic products and substances used for self-abuse. A list of substances known or strongly suspected of producing rhabdomyolysis is presented in *Table* 4.2 arranged by the chemical and pharmacological nature of the materials, and in *Table* 4.3 organized by possible major cause(s) of the rhabdomyolytic process.

Xenobiotics that produce rhabdomyolysis may do so by a variety of processes, which include the following:

1. A direct myotoxic action (primary xenobiotic rhabdomyolysis).
2. By producing a disturbance of metabolism and ionic balance which induces a rhabdomyolysis process (secondary metabolic rhabdomyolysis).
3. By inducing coma or otherwise disturbing mobility and allowing compression of skeletal muscle to occur (secondary traumatic rhabdomyolysis).
4. By a combination of causes 1–3 above (multiple aetiology rhabdomyolysis).

Clearly the factors governing the development and severity of the rhabdomyolytic process, the clinical features, diagnosis and management will vary according to the aetiology.

As with other causes of rhabdomyolysis, ARF may be a complication. Indeed,

Table 4.2 Xenobiotic-induced rhabdomyolysis as classified by causative substances.

Category	Class (and examples)
Therapeutic agents	Antifibrinolytics (epsilon-aminocarproic acid)
	Emetics (emetine-containing)
	Antiemetics (metoclopramide)
	Hypolipidaemic agents (clofibrate)
	Antipeptic ulcer agents (carbenoxolone)
	Andrenoceptor antagonists (labetol, propanol oxprenolol)
	Diuretics (benzothiadiazides)
	Cancer chemotherapeutic agents (5-azocytidine, 6-mercaptopurine, adriamycin)
	CNS stimulants (strychnine, xanthines, sympathomimetics)
	Neuroleptics (dibenzoxazepines, phenothiazines, butyrophenones, thioxanthenes)
	Muscle relaxants (suxamethonium)
	Miscellaneous (isotretinoin, diphenhydramine)
Drugs of dependence	Sympathomimetics (amphetamine pheylpropanolamine)
	Opiods (heroin, methadone)
	Psychodelics (phencyclidine, lysergic acid diethylamide)
Commercial products	Liquorice
	Ethanol
Industrial chemicals	Carbon monoxide
	Methanol
	Toluene
	Methylene chloride
	p-phenylenediamine
	Organophosphrous anticholinesterases
	Hexachlorocyclohexane
	Triethylene tetramine
	Mercuric chloride
	Potassium cyanide

drug-induced renal toxicity in general is becoming one of the most common causes of ARF (Robinson, 1984; Gutman 1986). For example, it has been estimated that 24% of ARF patients and 10% of all renal consultations are associated with nephrotoxicity (Porter and Benett, 1981). In the context of rhabdomyolysis-associated ARF, renal injury may be seen with materials falling into the following categories:

1. Myotoxic, non-nephrotoxic materials where ARF is due to the rhabdomyolysis process.
2. Non-myotoxic, non-nephrotoxic materials where ARF is due to rhabdomyolysis secondary to muscle compression.
3. Non-myotoxic materials where ARF is associated with secondary (compressive) rhabdomyolysis and intrinsic nephrotoxicity.
4. Materials having both myotoxic and nephrotoxic potential where ARF is due to a combination of rhabdomyolysis and intrinsic nephrotoxicity.

Specific xenobiotics and classes of materials producing rhabdomyolysis by various means are discussed below, followed by a general discussion on xenobiotic-induced rhabdomyolysis based on the consideration of specific rhabdomyolytic materials.

Table 4.3. Xenobiotic rhabdomyolytics classified according to possible mode of action.

Major class and division	*Examples*
Primary (direct) rhabdomyolytics	Epsilon-aminocaproic acid
	Emetine-containing emetics
	Opioids (heroin and methadone)
	p-phenylenediamine
	Cancer chemotherapeutic agents (adriamycin, 6-mercaptopurine, 5-azocytidine)
	Suxamethonium
	Ethanol
Secondary (indirect) rhabdomyolytics:	
a. Metabolic aberration	Hypokalaemia (liquorice, carbenoxolone, benzothiadiazide diuretics, amphotericin B)
b. Hypoxia (cytotoxic)	Carbon monoxide
c. Coma and compression	Toluene
d. Hyperkinetic movements	Strychnine
	gamma-hexachlorocyclohexane
	Potassium cyanide
	Antiemetics (?)
e. Isometric contractions	Psychomimetics (phencyclidine, LSD)
Combined effects:	
a. Myotoxicity and convulsions	CNS stimulants (xanthines, sympathomimetics)
b. Myotoxicity and coma	Opioids (heroin, methadone)
c. Hypokalaemia and convulsions	Theophylline (+ possible direct myotoxicity)
Unknown	Adrenoceptor antagonists
	Diphenhydramine
	Isotretonoin
	Methanol
	Methylene chloride
	Mercuric chloride
	Neuroleptics
	Triethylene tetramine

THERAPEUTIC SUBSTANCES

Fibrinolysis Inhibitors

Epsilon-aminocaproic acid (EACA), an inhibitor of fibrinolysis, is used to prevent the dissolution of preformed blood clots. It acts by competitive inhibition of the activator enzyme converting inactive plasminogen to active proteolytic plasmin. Around 60–90% of EACA is excreted unmetabolized at approximately 75% of the GFR (Bergin, 1966). Blood levels required to inhibit plasminogen are around 13 mg dl^{-1}, which can usually be achieved if renal function is normal by a dose of 24 g per day after priming at a higher dose of around 36 g per day (Brodkin, 1980; Geronemus et al., 1974). EACA has found particular use in the preoperative management of subarachnoid haemorrhage, by reducing the incidence of recurrent haemorrhage (Nibbelink et al., 1975; Chowdhury et al., 1979). It has also been used in the management of hereditary angioneurotic oedema (Korsan-Bengtsen et al., 1969). Side effects of treatment include nausea, nasal stuffiness, vomiting, allergic reactions, diarrhoea and postural hypotension; these are usually mild and disappear on drug withdrawal (Brown et al., 1983). More serious effects include thromboembolism (Bergin, 1966; Sontag and Stein, 1974) and the rhabdomyolysis discussed below.

Rhabdomyolysis has been well documented as a complication of EACA therapy. Typically there is a delay to onset of signs and symptoms following the start of treatment. For the various cases described the dosage range has covered 10 to 36 g per day, with symptoms starting after 5–35 days of treatment, with the longer periods usually being associated with the lower doses. Signs and symptoms may not spontaneously disappear on discontinuance of therapy, and may increase and take several weeks to resolve. There may be no obvious precipitating factors, although there may be preceding exercise in a few cases. The profiles of the elevated serum (muscle) enzyme activities, notably CPK, AST and LDH, are typical of other causes of rhabdomyolysis. Although muscle injury with EACA is predominantly to skeletal muscle, myocardial injury may occur in a few cases. Some typical case reports are summarized below.

Britt et al., (1980) described a 20-year-old female who had experienced several subarachnoid haemorrhages due to A-V malformation involving the mesencephalon, thalamus and splenium of the corpus callosum. On her most recent admission she was given oral EACA, 2 g 4 hourly, which was continued after her discharge. After 5 weeks of treatment she had started to complain of pain and swelling of the calves, and noted fever and dark urine for one day. On examination she had warm, swollen, tender calf muscles. Results of investigation included: Hb 13·8 g dl^{-1}; WCC 12 700 mm^{-3}; serum creatinine 0·8 mg dl^{-1}; blood urea nitrogen (BUN) 12 mg dl^{-1}; *s*AST 1592 iu l^{-1} (normal < 20); *s*ALT 529 iu l^{-1} (normal < 20); *s*LDH 2443 iu l^{-1} with increase of all fractions but predominantly skeletal muscle isozyme; *s*CPK 25 620 iu l^{-1} (normal < 75) with both skeletal muscle and myocardial fractions present. The ECG showed S-T segment depression and T-wave inversion anteriorly and inferiorly. EACA was discontinued on admission, and by 5 days the following chemical pathology was measured: *s* creatinine 4·1 mg dl^{-1}; BUN 52 mg dl^{-1}; *s*CPK 58 235 iu l^{-1}; and myoglobin was present in the urine. There was a progression of S-T depression and T-wave inversion, but after one month only diffuse T-wave inversion. The ECG changes and serum enzyme profile suggest some cardiotoxic effect may have occurred. Myalgia spread to the proximal lower limbs, shoulders and paraspinous muscles. Because of hyperkalaemia and vomiting, peritoneal dialysis was carried out on the tenth day after admission, but was required a further three times over the ensuing two weeks. On the fourteenth day after admission, a biopsy of the left gastrocnemius muscle showed a large number of randomly degenerating fibres, and some vacuolated necrotic fibres were undergoing myophagocytosis; also there were numerous regenerating myofibres with basiphilic cytoplasm and large vesicular nuclei. There was no abnormal PAS-positive material, and examination for NAD tetrazolium reductase and ATPase suggested that intact fibres were Type II. The endomysial connective tissue was oedematous but had few inflammatory cells; blood vessel walls were intact and lumens patent. At 6 weeks, renal function had returned to normal but weakness was still present in the lower limbs, but some improvement had occurred by 10 weeks.

Morris et al., (1983) reported a 20-year-old female who presented with dyspnoea, weakness, dizziness and chronic pelvic infection, and who was found to be markedly anaemic (Hb 4·5 g dl^{-1}) with an absence of haematopoietic cells on bone marrow examination. She was treated with benzylpenicillin, metronidazole and tobramycin for pelvic sepsis and otitis externa. She developed recurrent epistaxis which was treated with prednisolone, transfusion of washed irradiated erythrocytes, and allogenic platelets. She was started on 3 g EACA, 3 hourly, to control local bleeding. By two weeks all infection had cleared, but the marrow had not regressed. She was thus given a marrow transplant after receiving cyclophosphamide 50 mg kg^{-1} on 4 consecutive days. At 72 hours posttransplant she complained of generalized leg pains, which became more severe and tenderness developed over the next 24 hours, and by 72 hours there was a rapid deterioration in power. Medication was withdrawn (EACA at this stage had been taken for 27 days), and slow recovery occurred but with total muscle power not recovering for about 30 days. A pretreatment increased *s*CPK suggested a subclinical muscle disease (? precipitating factor). At the onset of clinical myopathy the presence of myoglobin was confirmed; there were increases in *s*CPK, LDH, AST and ALT, respectively, to 5115, 745, 250 and 52 iu l^{-1}). The serum enzyme activities gradually decreased and near normal levels occurred within a month. A mild hyperbilirubinaemia was present (maximum 26 μmol l^{-1}). Histology of a rectus femoris biopsy at 27 days after the onset of clinical myopathy showed widespread degenerative and necrotic changes in muscle fibres, some fibres contained macrophages, others were calcified. Also, there was evidence of regressed fibres in the form of nucleolated vesicular nuclei and RNA-rich basiphilic cytoplasm. There were focal accumulations of mononuclear cells, but no evidence of vasculitis and blood vessels were patent.

Brown et al. (1982) presented the case of a 72-year-old female admitted with subarachnoid haemorrhage who was treated with EACA 36 g per day, reduced to 24 g per day perorally. Therapy was stopped because of orthostatic hypotension after about 4 weeks, and several days later she developed shoulder and arm pains, with general weakness, and a reduced output of dark urine. Almost one week later she developed bilateral tenderness of the limb muscles. Investigations at this time showed BUN 59 mg dl^{-1}, creatinine 4·7 mg dl^{-1}, *s*CPK 29 800 iu l^{-1}, *s*LDH 415 iu l^{-1}, *s*AST 1023 iu l^{-1}, *s*ALT 627 iu l^{-1}. The electromyogram (EMG) showed marked irritability and pseudomyotonic discharges. A right gastroenemius muscle biopsy showed necrosis with macrophage-filled fibres. She was treated by fluid restriction and prednisolone. Urine output gradually returned to normal, followed by resolution of clinical symptoms at about 5 weeks after stopping treatment, and normal *s*CPK by 8 weeks.

Korsan-Bengtsen et al. (1969) reported a case of 31-year-old male with hereditary angioneurotic oedema, treated with EACA 30 g daily in two episodes. After 5 and 7 weeks he complained of pain in the thighs and calves together with difficulty in walking, and the passage of dark brown urine. Muscle biopsy revealed hyaline degeneration of fibres with no vascular pathology.

Brodkin (1980) described a 51-year-old female who was diagnosed as having a subarachnoid haemorrhage, but no aneurysm was seen on arteriography. EACA was started in at 38 g per day for 28 days, then 24–36 g per day for 21 days. After 36 days dark urine appeared with the development of muscle weakness and tenderness, EACA was discontinued after 41 days, when a total of 1·43 kg of material had been given. The *s*CPK was 1544 iu (normal 0–70), with no myocardial fraction, and urine myoglubin was confirmed by immunoassay. Muscle biopsy showed atrophy and vacuolization with little inflammation and no evidence of vascular thrombosis. Recovery began in about one week, myoglobin disappeared about two weeks after discontinuing EACA, and *s*CPK activity was normal within two months.

Rizza et al. (1976) reported a 24-year old female who had several courses of EACA therapy for recurrent painful subcutaneous haemorrhage. After the current course of 6 g every 6 hours for 4 weeks, there was an onset of progressive weakness of limb muscles with myalgia and followed, after 2 days, by the appearance of dark urine. On admission the serum creatine was 0·8 mg dl^{-1} and *s*CPK 48 600 iu l^{-1}.

Biswas et al. (1980) presented a case of a 20-year-old female admitted with subarachnoid haemorrhage due to right-sided A-V malformation. She was given EACA at a dose of 30 g per day over a period of 7 weeks. After 6 weeks she developed myalgia, haematuria and proteinuria, which progressed to profound muscle weakness with respiratory impairment, and the development of ARF. Chemical pathology was as follows: serum urate 0·57 mmol l^{-1} (9·6 mg dl^{-1}) [Na^+] 116 mmol l^{-1}, BUN 44 mmol l^{-1} (265 mg dl^{-1}), [K^+] 5·4 mmol l^{-1}, creatinine 610 mmol l^{-1} (6·9 mg dl^{-1}). Muscle biopsy showed acute massive muscle necrosis, with no evidence of polymyositis, polyarteritis, or any occlusive or thrombotic disease. After 4 weeks renal failure recovered, and muscle power was almost normal by 3 months. The presence of proteinuria was taken as evidence of possible direct nephrotoxicity since it disappeared on withdrawal of the drug.

MacKay et al. (1978) reported two cases of rhabdomyolysis in six patients receiving EACA for subarachnoid haemorrhage. The first, a 44-year-old male with subarachnoid haemorrhage received 3 g EACA every 2 hours, initially iv and then orally, and at this time had normal chemical pathology, including enzyme activity. After 2 months he began to complain of progressive myalgia and discoloured urine for several days (for 2 weeks before this admission he had 6 g EACA thrice daily for the first week, and 2 g thrice daily for the second week). The myalgia affected principally the thigh and calf, although the upper limbs were affected to some extent. Abnormal findings were as follows: ESR 48 mm h^{-1}, *s*CPK 5000 iu l^{-1}, *s*AST 1050 iu l^{-1}, *s*LDH 1000 iu l^{-1}, *s* alkaline phosphatase 100 iu l^{-1}. The drug was discontinued and diuresis started. At 10 days the *s*CPK was > 5000 iu l^{-1}, the IVP normal, and gradual recovery occurred. The second case was a 64-year-old female, also diagnosed as subarachnoid haemorrhage, who received EACA 3 g every 2 hours. After about 8 weeks the EACA was decreased and stopped over 3 days. She began complaining of myalgia, and previously normal chemical pathology values became abnormal as follows: *s*ALT 250 mU ml^{-1}, *s*LDH 350 mU ml^{-1}, and alkaline phosphatase 200 mU ml^{-1} with normal bilirubin. Serial serum enzyme analysis showed maximum activities of CPK 7500 iu, AST 1000 mU ml^{-1}, LDH 1250 mU ml^{-1}. Cardiospecific CPK isozyme was not detected, and the ECG was unchanged. Also associated with these enzyme changes were decreased haematocrit (35 to 31%), ESR 48 mm h^{-1}, but screening for disseminated intravascular coagulation syndrome, complement, and glucose-6-phosphate dehydrogenase deficiency were negative. Myalgia improved and enzyme activities returned to normal.

Although it has been suggested that EACA-induced rhabdomyolysis is due to intravascular thrombosis (MacKay et al., 1978), the absence of vascular abnormalities and of multiple organ system disease suggests that intravascular thrombosis is an unlikely cause (e.g. Britt et al., 1980; Brodkin, 1980; Morris et al., 1983). It has been shown that 5, 10 and 15 mM EACA produces a 10, 23 and 58% inhibition, respectively, of myofibrillar proteinase or calcium-activating factor in freshly excised skeletal muscle from rats (Morris et al., 1983). They suggest that a surface protease on muscle membrane may be involved rather than an intracellular enzyme. However, Kennard et al. (1980) did not find the rat a suitable model for EACA-induced myopathy *in vivo*. Also, Iannaccone and Griggs (1981) studied EACA toxicity in guinea-pigs, to whom they gave an average of 1·63 g kg^{-1} day^{-1} in drinking water and then sacrificed at intervals of one to two weeks over a 20 week period. None became weak, there were no effects on *s*CPK activity, and no myoglobin was detected in urine. Muscle histology was generally normal. Thus, the guinea-pig appears not to be a good model for EACA-induced myopathy.

Emetics

Rhabdomyolysis has been described particularly after the use of ipecac, which contains the two alkaloids cephaeline and emetine, and is obtained from the root of *Cephanlis ipecacuanha*. The alkaloid content and the relative amounts of cephaeline and emetine varies with the species. For example, Matto Grosso ipecacuanha contains 2–2·4% alkaloids, of which 60–75% is emetine and about 20% cephaeline (Martindale, 1977). Ipecac is used extensively for the pharmacological induction of vomiting in cases of acute peroral poisoning, and emetine has a prolonged history of use for treating amoebiasis (Woolfe, 1965), and in the latter condition it has been estimated that myopathy may develop in 50–60% of patients given the drug (Fewings et al., 1973). The neuromuscular manifestations of ingestion of emetine are weakness, aching, tenderness and stiffness of skeletal muscles, affecting particularly the neck and proximal extremities (Ratnesar and Pobee, 1962; Manno and Manno, 1977). Most cases of ipecac-induced rhabdomyolysis appear to be associated with the binge-purge eating disorders anorexia nervosa and bulimia nervosa, in which patients consume high calorific foods and then purge themselves with a variety of procedures, including mechanically and pharmacologically induced vomiting. Some illustrative examples are given below.

Mateer et al., (1985) describe a three-year abuse of ipecac syrup by a 27-year-old female, who developed painless proximal limb weakness over a period of 6 to 9 months. On examination there was hyperreflexia, non-fatiguable weakness of the proximal muscles of the upper and lower extremities, and no atrophy or fasiculations. Clinical pathology revealed normal electrolytes, *s*CPK, *s*AST and *s*LDH. An EMG showed scattered fibrillation potentials, brief duration, small amplitude, polyphasic and sharp motor unit potentials. Biceps biopsy revealed Type II-B fibres were generally rounded and more atrophic than other fibres. Type II fibres seemed to be depleted in numbers. Scattered large fibres with vesicular nuclei and prominent nucleoli were present. Following the discontinuation of ipecac, the weakness and EMG abnormalities improved.

Palmer and Guay (1985) described a reversible myopathy associated with the long-term use of ipecac in two patients having a binge-purge behaviour. The first patient, a 21-year-old 46 kg female, had generalized muscle weakness. She admitted ingesting several 30 ml vials of ipecac each day for the past 4 months, but less recently; a 30 ml vial contains about 21 mg emetine. Serum enzyme activities were as follows: AST 102 $iu\,l^{-1}$ (normal 8·3–57), LDH 455 $iu\,l^{-1}$ (normal 125–275), and CPK 512 $iu\,l^{-1}$ (normal 10–100). EMG was normal for motor and sensory conduction velocities, but increased insertional activity, occasional fibrillations, and myopathic unit potentials were observed in the proximal muscles. Muscle biopsy showed the average fibre diameter was slightly decreased, but clearly atrophic fibres were not present. During hospitalization, muscle strength gradually improved and enzyme activities returned to normal. The second case was that of a 24-year-old female of weight 51 kg who presented with diffuse muscle weakness, most pronounced in the proximal muscles, normal chemical pathology, serum enzymes, electrolytes and rheumatoid factor. At the age of 20 she had started taking ipecac at least twice a week. After stopping ipecac, muscle strength was regained.

Other cases of myopathy caused by the long-term abuse of ipecac have been described by Bennett et al., 1972, Brotman et al., 1981, and Friedman, 1984. The total dosage of ipecac consumed before clinical evidence of myopathy varies considerably from as low as two doses a week to several doses a day for months or years. Palmer and Guay (1985) calculated that in the various cases reported up to, and including their own, between 500 and 36 000 mg was ingested over a long period of time before any diagnosis of myopathy was established. In general, the muscle biopsy shows normal blood vessels with little cellular infiltration, a predominance of Type I fibres, a slight decrease in average muscle fibre diameter, and isolated necrotic granular basiphilic fibres. Emetine- and ipecac-induced myopathy is reversible, and strength gradually returns over a period of weeks or months. One factor in the slow recovery of muscle function is the slow rate of emetic excretion, presumably due to binding to muscle. The most notable toxicity of emetine is related to its effects on the cardiovascular system, which include precordial pain, tachycardia, dyspnoea, hypotension, and ECG abnormalities which include T-wave flattening or inversion, QRS alterations, Q-T and P-R interval prolongation, and S-T segment abnormalities. Death may occur from cardiac arrest due to asystole and ventricular fibrillation, usually preceded by atrial fibrillation or premature beats (Manno and Manno, 1977; Yang and Dubick, 1980; Friedman, 1984).

Biochemical abnormalities induced by emetine include inhibition of protein synthesis, depression of glycolysis, inhibition of the Krebs cycle, and depression of the incorporation of leucine into actomysin (Lietman, 1971; Pearce et al., 1971; Entner and Grollamn, 1973; Hwang et al., 1974; Rollo, 1980). Although it has been suggested that emetine may produce a neuromuscular block by a tubocurarine-like action (Salako, 1970), EMG studies on patients with ipecac-induced myopathy do not confirm a neuromuscular block (Mateer et al., 1985., Palmer and Guay, 1985).

Emetine myopathy has been studied experimentally in the rat by Duane and Engel (1970), who gave 1·25 mg/kg daily for up to 15 days. All rats lost weight, and after 10 days showed decreased spontaneous activity and muscle tone, and after 15 days the animals walked slowly and climbed with difficulty. Throughout the study period the soleus was more affected than the gastrocnemius. Loss of cross striations occurred by 5 days in small areas of the soleus. By 15 days, an average of 50% of soleus fibres showed multiple lesions, but less than 10% of gastrocnemius fibres displayed lesions. Enlarged and vesicular nuclei appeared in muscle fibres from day 5, and necrotic fibres, some with phagocytosis, were found at day 15. Decreases in mitochondrial oxidative enzyme activity (succinic dehydrogenase, dihydronicotinamide adenine dinucleotide dehydrogenase, and cytochrome oxidase) occurred in circumscribed areas, and was associated with loss in cross striations. Bradley et al. (1976) studied the effect of (-)-emetine on the histology and physiology of skeletal muscle in the rat, and concluded that the myopathy is due to a direct subcellular effect on muscle fibres, and found no evidence for denervation in the aetiology of emetine myopathy. Thus, at doses in the range of 0·25–1·0 mg/kg ip for up to 220 days, weight gain was reduced and marginal changes in muscle physiology occurred, i.e. a small decrease in resting membrane potential and maximum rate of rise of action potential; there was no atrophy or loss of muscle fibres. There was focal loss of myofibrillar ATPase, NADH-tetrazolium reductase in Type II and III fibres but not Type I. At 2·0 mg/kg, animals had weight loss and were weak and emaciated, muscles were severely atrophied, and total muscle weight was reduced by about 20%. *In vitro* direct stimulation showed decreased strength of contraction, both absolute and tension developed per unit weight. In the extensor digitorum longus and soleus there was necrosis, hyalinization and splitting of fibres, and loss of myofibrillar ATPase and NADH-tetrazolium reductase activity in Type I, II and III fibres, suggesting a localized disruption of myosin filaments and mitochondrial damage. There was a marked fall in resting membrane potential and reduction in maximum rate of rise of action potential. In the more severely affected animals there was an increase in the threshold for action potential generation, by approximately 10 mV, from −50 mV (normal) to −40 mV (at 2.0 mg/kg). Even in the animals receiving the highest dose, neuromuscular function was not impaired as evidenced by the presence of miniature end-plate potentials and normal EMG.

Bindoff and Cullen (1978) studied the ultrastructural changes in rat extensor digitorum longus and soleus in experimental (-)-emetine myopathy using a dose of 2 mg kg^{-1} day^{-1}, for 5 days a week for 1 to 4 weeks. Changes were seen between 1 and 2 weeks, and were progressive. They included Z-line streaming, rod formation, myofilament loss and contraction clumping. There was mitochondrial degeneration, and the most striking feature was extensive membrane proliferation which was probably due to an increase in sarcoplasmic reticulum. The ultrastructure of the motor end-plate appeared normal.

All the above experimental observations are consistent with the primary cause of emetine myopathy as that of direct myotoxicity.

Antiemetics

Abnormal movements have been described as an adverse effect of metoclopramide, which is a benzamide derivative of methyldopa and acts as a dopamine antagonist in the corpus striatum (Ahte and Buncum, 1974). It is widely used as an antiemetic (Schulze-Delrieu, 1981) and particularly for controlling the nausea and vomiting that occurs in uraemia, gastrointestinal malignancies, irradiation sickness, gastritis and peptic ulcer. A variety of induced abnormalities of movement have been described including acute dystonic reactions and a parkinsonian-like state (Robinson, 1973; Indo and Ando, 1982). Bateman and Gokal (1980) demonstrated reduced clearance of metoclopramide in renal failure, and hence such patients may be more susceptible to induced abnormal movements.

Hyser and Drake (1983) described multifocal myoclonic movements as a complication of metoclopramide in a 31-year-old male treated for progressive nausea and vomiting. A dose of 3×10 mg per day produced, after 4 days, coarse resting tremors of the head and upper extremities and difficulties in speaking because of intermittent jerking of respiratory muscles. After cessation of therapy, the involuntary movements subsided. Although rhabdomyolysis, *per se*, has not been described as an adverse effect of metoclopramide, the potential exists for involuntary movements.

Hypolipidaemic Agents

Myopathy and myotomia have been described with several hypolipidaemic agents including diazacholesterol (Somers and Winer, 1976), but the majority of recorded cases have been associated with clofibrinate.

Clofibrate (ethyl-2-α-chlorophenoxyisobutyric acid) decreases plasma triglyceride concentrations, and is indicated for Types III, IV and V primary hyperlipoproteinaemias. It lowers concentrations of very light density lipoproteins (VLDL) within 2 to 5 days of starting treatment. In the majority of patients plasma cholesterol and LDL are lowered in addition to VLDL. However, a very large decrease in VLDL may be accompanied by increased LDL and hence the net effect on plasma cholesterol may be slight. Clofibrate is readily absorbed after oral dosing, with peak concentrations about 4 hours postdosing. Absorption is followed by rapid and complete hydrolysis to chlorophenoxy isobutyrate (CPIB), which has a plasma half-life of about 12 hours, and about 60% is conjugated to produce a glucuronate which is excreted in the urine. Clofibrate is also used in the treatment of diabetes insipidus, the basis being a direct release of residual neurohypophysial vasopressin stores (Bonnici, 1973).

During early clinical trials with clofibrate small numbers of side effects were noted, including nausea, diarrhoea, weight gain, skin rash, drowsiness and weakness (Best and Duncan, 1966; Green and Margetts, 1967; Orgain et al., 1967; Dukes, 1980). Increases in *s*ALT and *s*AST were frequently seen in these early clinical trials (Walton et al., 1967; Green and Margetts, 1967; Orgain et al., 1967). In a detailed study of 60 clofibrate-treated hyperlipoproteinaemic patients, Langer and Levy (1968) found 5 cases of increased *s*ALT, *s*AST and *s*CPK activities, of whom two developed muscle weakness and myalgia. Abourizk et al. (1979) described a detailed investigation of a case of a 34-year-old female on clofibrate, 2–2·5 g a day for diabetes insipidus, who developed myalgia after 8 days of treatment. There was increased *s*CPK which decreased along with disappearance of symptoms on removal from clofibrate. Light microscopy of a muscle biopsy showed an increase in the number of lipocytes, with round cell perivascular infiltration. Degenerative changes shown in the muscle fibres were fragmentation of myofibrils and Z-bands, central nucleation, hyalinization to complete disintegration and appearance of ghost fibres with pyknotic nuclei, and myofibrillar debris. Electron microscopy showed myofibrillar disorganization and loss of Z-lines, dilated sarcoplasmic reticulum, swollen mitochondria with variable degrees of disarrangement of cristae, macrophage invasion of fibres, and discontinuance and irregularities of the sarcolemma. Thus, both the light and ultrastructural pathology was not unique, but characteristic of a degenerative process.

Two typical cases are as follows. Geltner et al. (1975) desribed a 49-year-old male on 1·5 g clofibrate per day who, after several weeks, developed limb weakness and severe muscle pain. Although the *s*CPK and *s*AST were within normal limits, the EMG showed (unspecified) myopathic changes. Following the cessation of clofibrate the symptoms disappeared and the EMG returned to normal within two weeks. Three months later, clofibrate was started for hypertriglyceridaemia and after ten days, although the patient was asymptomatic, EMG changes returned and *s*CPK increased from 38 to 90 iu; both the EMG and CPK returned to normal after cessation of therapy.

Smalls et al. (1978) described a 16-year-old male who was given clofibrate 4×500 daily. Within 4 days he developed severe muscle pains with difficulty in walking and myalgia. Serum chemistry showed AST > 400 iu l^{-1}, ALT > 75 iu l^{-1}, LDH 1650 iu l^{-1}, and CPK 12 000 iu l^{-1}. Myoglobin was present in the urine and serum. The ECG showed precordial S-T segment depression compatible with cardiomyopathy. Following cessation of clofibrate therapy ECG and serum enzyme activities reverted to normal within 4 days and 4 weeks respectively.

Kwiecinski (1978) was able to induce myotonia in rats with clofibrate given as 0·4 g kg^{-1} day^{-1}. Myotonic discharges were recorded by EMG from the extensor digitorum longus, tibialis anterior, and gastrocnemius muscles after 4 days of clofibrate treatment. In the soleus, the first myotonic discharges appeared within 11 days. Myotonic activity was also demonstrated in denervated muscle. The myotonic discharges were seen on insertion or slight displacement of the electrode, or after light tapping of the muscle, but rarely spontaneously. The discharges were usually fusiform in shape; extinction was gradual through reduction of amplitude and frequency of the component potentials. Repetitive stimulation to the muscle nerve or directly to the muscle resulted in a decline in muscle electrical response.

In addition to possible renal consequences of clofibrate-induced rhabdomyolysis, muscle effects may be a special risk in nephrotic patients and those with chronic renal failure, in whom up to 18% of circulating clofibrate may be unbound because of low plasma albumin (Dukes, 1980). For example, in one series, 4 of 6 nephrotic patients developed myalgia within three days of starting clofibrate therapy for hyperlipoproteinaemia (Bridgeman et al., 1972). Also Pierides et al. (1975) described muscle weakness and tenderness with increased sCPK in 5 uraemic patients treated with 1–2 g clofibrate daily; the muscle effects developed within 4 days to 2 weeks. Excessive accumulation of free and total serum CPIB, the active circulating metabolite, was found in 3 patients in whom it was sought. They suggest that chronic renal failure be regarded as a contraindication to clofibrate therapy for coexisting hyperlipidaemia. However, if required the patient should be cautiously started at low dosages and monitored regularly by measurement of *s*CPK activity and total free CPIB.

Peptic Ulcer Therapy

Rhabdomyolysis has been specifically associated with carbenoxolone sodium [biogastrone; disodium 3β-(3-carboxypropionyl)-11-oxo-olean-12-en-oate] which is used in the treatment of chronic duodenal and gastric ulceration. It is synthesized from glycyrrhetinic acid, which is obtained from the liquorice root. A possible mode of anti-ulcer action is by enhancement of mucous secretion which provides a protection to the ulcerated area and prolongs the life span of the gastric mucosal cells. Carbenoxolone also selectively inhibits the synthesis of prostaglandin $F_{2\alpha}$ (Harvey, 1980). It causes salt and water retention in about 25% of patients, and a slight decrease in $s[K^+]$ and hypotension, related to a mineralocorticoid activity. The electrolyte imbalance produced by carbenoxolone is completely blocked by the aldosterone antagonist, spironolactone, but this also inhibits the ulcer-healing activity. Whilst the Na^+-retaining effect is blocked by thiazide diuretics, and the ulcer-healing properties remain, kaluresis and hypokalaemia may still be present (Langman, 1980). The effect of carbenoxolone on electrolyte balance is probably due to direct intracellular binding as agonist with specific mineralocorticoid receptors and displacement of aldosterone from non-specific receptor sites. Carbenoxolone kaluresis may be enhanced by thiazide diuretics.

Absorption of carbenoxolone is mainly from the stomach, and may be delayed if $pH > 2$ (Martindale, 1977). A variety of cases of rhabdomyolysis have been reported as complications of carbenoxolone therapy, typical of which are the following. Mohamed et al. (1966) described a case of hypokalaemia, paresis, and myoglobinuria in a 58-year-old man receiving carbenoxolone over a 38 day period. Descamps et al. (1977) reported the case of a 61-year-old male receiving carbenoxolone sodium, 300 mg per day, for the treatment of gastric ulceration. After 7 weeks he developed progressive muscle weakness and became disoriented. About one week later he developed a rapidly progressive anuria. He was found to have hypokalaemic alkolosis ($s[K^+]$ 1·4 $mmol\,l^{-1}$) with *s*CPK and *s*AST markedly elevated at 4400 $iu\,l^{-1}$ and 550 $iu\,l^{-1}$, respectively. Muscle biopsy showed focal muscle necrosis. Barnes and Leonard (1971) reported the case of a 75-year-old man given carbonoxolone sodium, 50 mg thrice daily, for dyspepsia. After six weeks he began to notice pains in the lower limbs with weakness and tiredness. The muscle effects became severe and urine became darkened. On admission his $s[K^+]$ was 1·9 $mmol\,l^{-1}$, *s*CPK 310 $iu\,ml^{-1}$ (normal 0–12), *s*AST 520 $iu\,ml^{-1}$, *s*ALT 115 $iu\,ml^{-1}$, and aldolase 68 units ml^{-1} (normal 3–12 units ml^{-1}). Urine was positive for myoglobin. Muscle biopsy showed foci of acidophilic muscle fibres and a few regenerating fibres, but blood vessels appeared normal. He was treated by withdrawal of carbenoxolone and given K^+ iv and orally, resulting in rapid improvement.

Autonomic Adrenoceptor Antagonists

A few isolated case reports have been presented on muscle pathology induced by adrenoceptor antagonists. However, this has a very low incidence relative to other known adverse effects. For example, myopathology was not mentioned in an extensive review of adverse reactions to β-adrenoceptor blocking drugs (Lewis and McDevitt, 1986). It is also of interest to note that rhabdomyolysis appears not to have been described as an adverse reaction to β_2-agonists, although skeletal muscle tremor is one of their major adverse reactions (Lulich et al., 1986). Rhabdomyolysis has been described with the following adrenoceptor antagonists.

Labetalol

Labetalol is an α- and β-adrenoceptor antagonist, for which instances of muscle pain have been described during treatment (Andersson et al., 1976; Bolli and Wool-Manning, 1977). Teicher et al. (1981) described the case of a 27-year-old male receiving 600 mg of labetalol daily who complained of muscle pain, particularly in the legs. The *s*CPK (MM) was high at around 240 iu l^{-1}, LDH at 350 iu l^{-1}, and aldolase at 170 iu l^{-1}. Light microscopic examination of a deltoid muscle biopsy showed no abnormal histology or histochemical typing of muscle fibres. Electron micropsy showed variable sized vacuoles in the subsarcolemmal sarcoplasm. On cessation of treatment with labetalol, muscle pain disappeared and enzyme activity returned to normal. When labetalol was restarted, this led to a return of pain and increased enzyme activity.

Although rhabdomyolysis with adrenoceptor blockers is usually not severe enough to produce ARF, renal insufficiency may develop from drug-induced effects on the kidney. Thus, Smit et al. (1986) described a case of oliguric ARF in a 19-year-old female who ingested 16 g of labetalol, and in whom myoglobinuria and interstitial nephritis were excluded. They postulated that a fall in postglomerular resistance induced by labetalol, coupled with a renal vasodilator effect to therapeutically administered dopamine, may have been responsible for the filtration failure.

Propranolol

Propranolol is a non-selective β-adrenoceptor blocking agent. Blessing and Walsh (1977) reported a 39-year-old male who developed myotonia whilst taking propranolol, 80 mg per day, and which disappeared on cessation of therapy. There was elevation of *s*CPK (muscle type) during therapy. He complained of general muscle aching and occasional right calf cramps. EMG demonstrated diffuse myotonia. On cessation of treatment with propranolol there was a decrease in *s*CPK activity and subsidence of muscle aching and clinical myotonia. A muscle biopsy was histopathologically characterized as dystrophia myotonica, and hence suggested a possibility that there was a drug-aggravated pre-existing myotonia. Thus, there is a potential for predisposition of myotonic patients to drug-induced rhabdomyolysis.

Forfar et al. (1979) also described a case of muscle weakness in a 68-year-old female receiving propranolol 40 mg, 8 hourly. Weakness was in the arms and legs, particularly in the proximal muscles. Following cessation of propranolol, the weakness rapidly resolved and *s*CPK decreased. Following restart of propranolol, 80 mg 8 hourly, the weakness returned and *s*CPK increased.

Oxprenolol

Schofield et al. (1985) reported a case of definitive rhabdomyolysis in a 27-year-old female found unconscious on the bedroom floor after an overdose of oxprenolol. She required iv pressor therapy. The serum oxprenolol concentration was found to be $9 \cdot 5$ mg l^{-1}. On transurethral catheterization, chocolate coloured urine was obtained which was positive for myoglobin. The *s*CPK activity was 73 000 iu l^{-1} (normal 24–190), serum urea was 10 mmol l^{-1}, serum creatinine 263 mol l^{-1}, the urea and creatinine rose, respectively, to 58 and 1187, but the patient did not become oliguric. During the course of her recovery, she developed a transient left lateral peroneal palsy due to a compartment pressure syndrome. The authors do not speculate as to the cause of the rhabdomyolysis, i.e. limb compression or direct myotoxicity.

Cancer Chemotherapeutic Agents

Myotoxicity has been associated clinically or experimentally with the following cancer chemotherapeutic agents.

5-azacytidine

Koeffler and Haskell (1978) reported the case of a 26-year-old female with acute myelogenous leukemia who received 5-azacytidine iv 300 mg m^{-2} day^{-1} as 3 divided doses, over 5 days. On the second day of chemotherapy she complained of painful generalized muscle weakness and tenderness. *s*CPK rose from 2 iu l^{-1} on day 2 to > 3000 iu l^{-1} on day 5 (normal < 120 iu l^{-1}); serum creatinine rose from $0 \cdot 6$ to $2 \cdot 0$] mg dl^{-1}; urine myoglobin was detected. By the fifth posttherapy day the muscle tenderness had markedly diminished, the *s*CPK returned to normal, and serum creatinine decreased to $1 \cdot 0$ mg dl^{-1}.

6-mercaptopurine

6-mercaptopurine (6-MP) has been used as a cancer chemotherapeutic agent, particularly as an acute antileukaemic, as an immunosuppressive to prevent rejection of organ transplant, and for the treatment of certain autoimmune diseases resistant to other and conventional therapy. 6-MP, a purine antagonist, requires to be converted to a nucleotide to be active, and interferes with the *de novo* synthesis of nucleic acids at a number of steps, and is incorporated into DNA in the form of deoxythioguanosine. The selectivity of 6-MP with respect to leukaemic cells appears to relate to quantitative differences in enzyme activities in leukaemic compared with normal cells, differences in metabolite pool sizes, and differences in catabolic reactions (Elion, 1986). A considerable amount of experimental evidence indicates that 6-MP causes skeletal muscle toxicity, but currently there is no evidence that 6-MP produces a myopathy in humans (Balazs, 1986).

Alleva et al. (1981) demonstrated that 6-MP administered to neonatal rats produced a delayed hind limb paralysis, due to severe atrophic degeneration. The first signs of muscle atrophy were apparent at 12 months by flattened croup, and 16 months by light microscopy, following 2 mg base/kg subcutaneously from day

2 to day 22 of age. Subsequently, Allera et al. (1986), using the same treatment regime in Sprague–Dawley rats, found that the first signs of muscle atrophy was at 2 months by light microscopy, and by 4 months atrophy could be detected grossly. In other experiments involving treatment of Sprague-Dawley rats with large doses at later stages (22 to 45 days) there was no myopathy. Additionally, when 6-MP was given at days 2 to 22 to Wister rats, mice and hamsters, myopathy occurred in rats but not mice or hamsters. These results suggest that muscle atrophy induced by 6-MP occurs only after treatment in the neonatal period and may be species-specific. In general it appears that major muscle groups of the thigh, gluteal and lumbar regions are mostly affected, and that 6-MP affects both fast and slow twitch proximal muscle fibers, but not distal fast-twitch muscles in the hind limbs (Jaweed et al., 1986a).

Slaughter et al. (1986) have shown that the gross appearances are of markedly atrophic and pale muscles, and histologically there is a degenerative myopathy with replacement of myofibers by adipocytes, without involvement of blood vessels or nerves. The earliest damage was seen ultrastructurally with disorganization at the Z-bands and excess of Z-band-like material and loss of myofibrils. In the most extensive lesions there was vacuolated disorganization of fibres (Abraham et al., 1986). That muscle degeneration is not neurogenic in origin is suggested by the finding of normal sciatic nerve conduction to the soleus of 6-MP myopathic rats (Jaweed et al., 1986b). Also Abraham et al. (1986) found no light or electron microscopic evidence of pathological changes in the sciatic nerve of 6-MP myopathic rats. *In vitro* studies of 6-MP treated differentiating cells showed that 6-MP is cytotoxic to cultures of myotubes, but not myoblasts, producing necrosis, inhibition of myotube formation, and the appearance of intracellular vacuoles (Yander and Kaji, 1984; Yander et al. 1986).

All the above evidence suggests that the experimental myopathy is due to a myotoxic effect of 6-MP.

Adriamycin

Adriamycin (doxorubicin) is an antineoplastic antibiotic, with a broad spectrum of therapeutic activity in the treatment of haematogenous malignancies, and solid tumours of breast, lung, thyroid and ovary (Carter, 1975). A major dose-related cardiomyopathy may limit the use of adriamycin (Lenaz and Page, 1986). The cardiomyopathy is seen in both humans (Ferrans, 1978) and experimental animals (Jaenke, 1974; Doroshaw et al. 1981). The myocardial histopathology takes the form of vacuolar degeneration of sarcoplasmic reticulum, swelling of cardiac mitochondria and disorganization of cristae, interstitial oedema, and focal myocytolysis (Ferran, 1978). Associated functional changes are alterations in the control of myocardial Ca^{++} transport and mitochondrial electron transport (Ferrero et al., 1976; Revis and Marusic, 1979). The cardiotoxicity of adriamycin may require the enzymic activation to a reactive intermediate in mitochondria and sarcoplasmic reticulum (Thayer, 1977; Doroshow, 1983).

Doroshow et al. (1985) found that adriamycin also induces degeneration in skeletal muscle of the rat diaphragm, which is apparent within 4 days of an ip injection of 20 mg kg^{-1}. Changes were similar to those observed in the myocardium, i.e. vacuolation of the sarcoplasmic reticulum, myofibrillar degeneration, interstitial oedema, and degradation of mitochondrial membranes; these effects were seen in all fibre types. A gradation of injury was seen across the diaphragm, with the most severe effects being seen on the abdominal side. Milder effects were seen in the gastrocnemius muscle, taking the form of an increase in the size and number of lipid droplets in red fibres. The differential damage was reflected in the relative tissue adriamycin concentrations, being 7- and 50-fold higher in diaphragm than in myocardium and gastrocnemius respectively.

Balducci et al. (1986) studied skeletal and cardiac myotoxicity of adriamycin in rats given 2 mg kg^{-1} $week^{-1}$. Minor changes were present at 6 weeks and more severe at 10 weeks. Since the skeletal muscle injury paralleled the cardiac muscle injury, they suggested that it may be possible to monitor for patients at risk from adriamycin cardiotoxicity by examination of serial skeletal muscle biopsies.

Diuretics

As discussed earlier (under peptic ulcer therapy) thiazide diuretics may potentiate the myotoxicity of materials producing rhabdomyolysis by hypokalaemic mechanisms. However, a few cases of rhabdomyolysis have been ascribed directly to diuretics. Examples are considered below for three benzothiadiazides: chlorothiazide, chlorotalidone, and clopamide.

Clugh et al. (1979) described a case of rhabdomyolysis with ARF in a patient with malignant hypertension following the inappropriate use of chlorothiazide with K^+-supplementation. The patient developed a severe hypokalaemia (1·5 mmol l^{-1}).

Jensen et al. (1967) described two cases of hypokalaemia due to diuretic therapy for arterial hypertension, in which there were increases in serum enzyme activity characteristic of rhabdomyolysis. One patient received chlortalidone, and the other had clopamide. Both patients were hospitalized because of muscle weakness and tenderness and demonstrated hypokalaemic alkalosis. Relevant chemical pathology showed maximum departures from normal as follows. For the patient receiving chlortalidone: $s[K^+]$ 1·6 mmol l^{-1}, *s*CPK 8000 iu l^{-1}, *s*LDH 16 000 iu l^{-1}, *s*ALT 800 iu l^{-1}, with positive benzidine test in the absence of erythrocyturia. For the patient receiving clopamide $s[K^+]$ 1·2 mmol l^{-1}, *s*CPK *c*. 3000 iu l^{-1}, *s*ALT *c*. 300 iu l^{-1}, *s*LDH *c*. 600 iu l^{-1} (these values were obtained at 3 days after admission, whereas those for the patient receiving chlortalidone were from admission blood samples). After iv KCl and NH_4Cl, serum electrolytes returned to normal; *s*CPK and ALT activities returned to normal by 14 days, at which time *s*LDH was still elevated (*c*. 2000 iu l^{-1}). Muscle biopsies taken during the acute phase showed necrotic foci with vacuolation and phagocytosis.

Central Nervous System Stimulants

Although they have a variety of other target pharmacological effects, it is descriptively convenient to consider xanthines and sympathomimetic drugs under the collective heading of CNS stimulants. Both these groups have been noted to produce rhabdomyolysis as an adverse effect.

Xanthines

The major xanthine reported to cause rhabdomyolysis is theophylline, and many reported cases are due to deliberate overdosing.

Rumpf (1985) described a case of a 22-year-old female who took an overdose of theophylline (38.5 g) together with 1·0 mg clenbuterol (a β_2-agonist). Chemical pathology on admission was $s[K^+]$ 2·3 mmol l^{-1}, *s*CPK 615 iu l^{-1} (normal up to 70), serum theophylline 40·5 mg l^{-1} (therapeutic 20). Immediate management was by gastric lavage, peroral charcoal, and $MgSO_4$. Over the subsequent 8 hours she developed *grand mal* seizures (resistant to diazepam, clonazepam, and phenytoin) and ventricular fibrillation for which defibrillation was undertaken. At this time the *s*CPK was 19 910 iu l^{-1} and theophylline 279 mg l^{-1}. Myoglobin, by radioimmunoassay, for plasma was 58 900 μg l^{-1} (normal 70) and for urine 405 000 μg l^{-1} (normal 50). Haemoperfusion and forced diuresis produced a rapid fall (over 2 to 3 days) of serum theophylline and myoglobin.

Several cases, summarized below, have occurred with slow-release theophylline preparations. Lagger et al. (1984) describe a 20-year-old female who took 100 × 25 mg slow release theophylline capsules. On admission, 12 hours later, she was comatose and having seizures. The serum theophylline concentration was 236 mg l^{-1}, *s*CPK 5·94 iu l^{-1}, $s[K^+]$ 3·4 mmol l^{-1}. Management was by gastrointestinal lavage with iso-osmotic fluid containing activated charcoal, and continuous infusion of thiopentone (200 mg h^{-1}). This was followed by activated charcoal haemoperfusion. After 20 hours she was well and cooperative.

MacDonald et al. (1985) described the case of a 19-year-old female who had taken 50 slow-release 225 mg aminophylline tablets. She presented with headache, nausea, vomiting, followed by restlessness and confusion; she developed pneumomediastinitis and anuria. On admission the serum creatinine was 285 μmol l^{-1}, $s[K^+]$ 1·8 mmol l^{-1}, $s[Ca^{++}]$ 2·3 mmol l^{-1}, and serum theophylline 770 μmol l^{-1}. By 48 hours the serum creatinine increased to 700 μmol l^{-1} and $s[Ca^{++}]$ fell to 1·5 mmol l^{-1} with $s[K^+]$ at 4·7 mmol l^{-1} and inorganic phosphorus 6·0 mmol l^{-1}. Serum theophylline decreased to 110 μmol l^{-1} at 48 hours. The *s*CPK rose from an admission value of 2800 iu l^{-1} to 186 000 iu l^{-1} (at 48 hours) with a serum myoglobin concentration of *c.* 25 000 μg l^{-1} (normal 6–85). She was haemodialyzed for oliguric ARF; renal function gradually returned to normal. During the anuric phase there was a low $s[Ca^{++}]$ with high PTH and low $1,25(OH)_2D$.

Modi et al. (1985) described the case of a 79-year-old man who was admitted after ingesting 4·5 g of slow-release theophylline preparation. He was hyperventilating, drowsy and disoriented. Hypokalaemic acidosis was present ($s[K^+]$ 2·7 mmol l^{-1}, $s[Cl^-]$ 111 mmol l^{-1}, and $s[HCO_3^-]$ 16 mmol l^{-1}, pH 7.24). Seizures developed and the management included prolonged charcoal haemoperfusion. Before haemoperfusion the *s*CPK (MM) was 12 400 iu l^{-1}, suggesting the occurrence of rhabdomyolysis. They make mention of a second patient with theophylline overdose who had a *s*CPK(MM) of 77 000 iu l^{-1} and status epilipticus for 3 hours; this patient developed clinical rhabdomyolysis and ARF.

The development of rhabdomyolysis is probably due in many cases to a combination of hypokalaemia and the development of convulsions. If it were due to hypokalaemia alone, then the incidence of myopathy would be expected to be higher. For example, Olson et al. (1985) found that hypokalaemia is frequent in acute peroral theophylline overdoses; in 27 patients the low $s[K^+]$ ranged $1{\cdot}8$–$4{\cdot}1$ mmol l^{-1}. Also, Wright et al. (1987) described a fatal case of a 16-year-old female who developed rhabdomyolysis and hyperkalaemia following an overdose of aminophylline. The peak $s[K^+]$ was $12{\cdot}0$ mmol l^{-1}, and there was clear biochemical evidence for rhabdomyolysis in the form of markedly increased serum myoglobin and creatinine. Diffuse widespread early muscle necrosis was seen histologically in specimens taken at autopsy. The authors believe that a direct myotoxicity by theophylline may have been a significant factor in the production of rhabdomyolysis in this case. They cite as evidence for this conclusion that the degree of rhabdomyolysis seen histologically and the *s*[myoglobin] were in excess of those usually recorded following *grand mal* convulsions and, more convincingly, that the *s*[myoglobin] was raised before the first convulsions. However, interpretation of the later chemical pathology and the autopsy findings is complicated by occurrence of several *grand mal* seizures, episodes of cardiac arrest, and terminal management by cardiopulmonary bypass, haemodialysis and exchange transfusion.

Sympathomimetics

There are several reports of amphetamine and amphetamine-like substances causing rhabdomyolysis, and with the subsequent development of ARF. However, care may be needed in ascribing ARF to rhabdomyolysis in some cases, since occasional instances are recorded where there are no indications of rhabdomyolysis and a direct nephrotoxic effect may occur. For example, Foley et al. (1984) describe the case of 32-year-old male who was an amphetamine abuser, and who developed acute interstitial nephritis from which recovery occurred. There was no clinical or biochemical evidence for rhabdomyolysis and pyrexia did not develop. The following summaries are of descriptions of rhabdomyolysis attributable to methamphetamine, phenmetrazine, phenylpropanolamine, and D-norpseudoepinephrine.

Black and Murphy (1984) described a case of a 16-year-old male who ingested 18×75 mg tablets of Preludin (phenmetrazine), and 3 days later complained of epigastric pain, weakness, malaise, nausea and vomiting. On the fourth day the blood pressure was 180/110 mm Hg, leucocyte count 20 900 mm^{-3}, and the urine contained occult blood, protein and pigmented granular casts. Other aspects of the chemical pathology were BUN 65 mg dl^{-1}, serum creatinine $15{\cdot}1$ mg dl^{-1}, $s[Ca^{++}]$ $8{\cdot}8$ mg dl^{-1}, serum phosphate $6{\cdot}9$ mg dl^{-1}, serum uric acid $11{\cdot}7$ mg dl^{-1}. On the fifth day he became anaemic and required haemodialysis; renal function and muscle pain improved.

Kendrick et al. (1977) reported 5 patients, with long histories of iv drug abuse, who had iv injections of phenametrazine (4 patients) and methamphetamine (1 patient). This resulted in prostration, disseminated intravascular coagulation syndrome, rhabdomyolysis and azotaemia. There was shaking, sweating, nausea, vomiting, diarrhoea and, within hours, myalgia, paraesthesia and orthostasis. Four subjects had diffuse muscle tenderness and myoedema, and all had hypotension and tachycardia. Oliguria developed and all had leucocytosis (range 25 200–44 680 mm^{-3}) and a positive *o*-toluidine test in the presence of clear serum and normal haptoglobulin. Other chemical pathology was (as range): BUN

44–100 mg dl^{-1}, serum creatinine 2·9–8·7 mg dl^{-1}, *s*CPK 505–5842 iu l^{-1}. The main lines of management were volume replacement to avert ARF, prophylaxis against hyperkalaemia, and frusemide and mannitol for diuresis. Although acidification of urine enhances the rate of renal excretion of amphetamines, they discourage treatment with NH_4Cl as a possible nephrotoxic potentiating procedure in myoglobinuric individuals. They believe that the fasciculations and fever, in the presence of a circulating volume deficit and shock, lead to rhabdomyolysis, and the presence of pyrexia, disseminated intravascular coagulation, and volume depletion predispose to ARF.

Hampel et al. (1983) described a case in which a 40-year-old female self poisoned with D-norpseudoepinephrine (an isomer of phenylpropanolamine), and developed nausea, vomiting, general malaise and convulsions. Because of hypotension (BP 70/40 mm Hg), and over 2 days, she became oliguric with dark urine. There was hypocalcaemia (1·98 mmol l^{-1}), and hypophosphataemia (0·59 mmol l^{-1}), with uric acid (535 μmol l^{-1}), urea (53 μmol l^{-1}), creatinine (838 μmol l^{-1}), *s*ALT (37 iu l^{-1}), *s*AST (518 iu l^{-1}) and *s*CPK (50 100 iu l^{-1}); all values returned to normal over 3 weeks. On day 3, the serum myoglobin was 18 000 ng ml^{-1} and urine myoglobin 85 470 ng ml^{-1}. Haemofiltration was required and recovery occurred.

Rumpf et al. (1983) reported the case of a 46-year-old male who overdosed on cathine HC1 (D-norpseudoepinephrine) and who developed drowsiness, vomiting and oligoanuria. Admission chemical pathology was as follows: *s*CPK 50 100 iu 1^{-1}, and serum uric acid 535 μmol 1^{-1}, which rose to a maximum of 838 μmol 1^{-1} over the next 4 weeks following haemofiltration. Initial radioimmunoassay of myoglobin was 18 600 μg 1^{-1} (normal < 70) and urine 85 470 μg 1^{-1} (normal < 70); normal values were attained within 3 weeks.

Swensen et al. (1982) reported two cases of rhabdomyolysis following the ingestion of phenylpropanolamine (PPA) in diet pills (*Lancet*, 1982). Both patients had muscle weakness, myalgia, and increased serum enzyme activities. Case 1 followed a three-week period of ingestion of PPA, and in Case 2 there was ingestion of 9 quarts of (unspecified) malted beverages and 30 to 50 appetite suppressant pills (each contained 50 mg PPA and 200 mg caffeine). Chemical pathology in Case 2 was *s*CPK 9000 iu l^{-1}, *s*ALT 177 iu l^{-1}, serum myoglobin 790 ng ml^{-1}, serum urea N 133 mg dl^{-1}, serum creatinine 11·3 mg dl^{-1}, and serum uric acid 21·6 mg dl^{-1}. Urine uric acid and creatinine were both 0·5 mg dl^{-1} and there was no erthyrocyturia. Since the urine (urate)/(creatine) ratio was unity, it was believed that this contraindicated urate nephropathy as defined by Kelton et al. (1978). (NB: Fluid balance had been disturbed by lower intestinal haemorrhage.) However, both cases had complicating factors: in Case 1 there was a histopathological diagnosis of acute interstitial nephritis from a percutaneous renal biopsy, and the aetiology of the ARF may have been complex; in the second case there had been a high alcohol intake, which could have contributed to the rhabdomyolysis. PPA-induced ARF may occur in the absence of rhabdomyolysis (Duffy et al., 1981), and it has been suggested that in such cases PPA may cause the liberation of endogenous catecholamines leading to ischaemic renal tubular epithelial necrosis.

A few cases of rhabdomyolysis have been described in association with severe intoxication from the street drug 3,4-methylenedioxyamphetamine (Simpson and Rumack, 1981; Brown and Osterloh, 1987).

Strychnine

Strychnine is a white, bitter tasting alkaloid which is obtained from the seeds of Strychnos nux vomica, a tree native to India. It is rapidly absorbed from the gastrointestinal tract and from subcutaneous or im injection sites. The lethal dose is estimated around 25–100 mg in adults, but in children may be as low as 15 mg (Polson and Tattersall, 1969; Gosselin et al., 1976). Strychnine is readily metabolized by hepatic microsomal enzymes, with about 20% of the unchanged alkaloid being excreted in urine. Strychnine has been incorporated into a number of preparations for the extermination of vermin, and into a variety of tonics, cathartics, analgesics, sedatives and stimulants, for which no pharmacological basis exists (Franz, 1980). However, there is some indication that strychnine may be therapeutically useful in the management of obstructive sleep apnoea and non-ketotic hyperglycinaemia (Nyhan, 1983; Spyker, 1983). Additionally, many 'street drugs' are adulterated with strychnine.

Strychnine causes convulsions as a result of competing with the inhibitory neurotransmittor glycine by blocking central postsynaptic glycine receptors, and possibly also by a more potent presynaptic inhibition of release of glycine. Spyker (1983) has noted that following strychnine poisoning there may be rhabdomyolysis, characterized by increased *s*CPK activity and myoglobinuria. Since strychnine does not produce any direct effect on muscle or neuromuscular junction, it is believed that the rhabdomyolysis is a consequence of the profound muscle contractions during the convulsions.

Boyd et al. (1983) described the case of a 19-year-old male who 'snorted' white powder believed to be cocaine, but it was subsequently determined to be strychnine left over from the cutting of cocaine. He developed myalgia, muscle twitching and extensor spasms within 15 to 30 minutes. This was followed by severe convulsions, hyperthermia (43 °C), marked lactic acidosis, and rhabdomyolysis. Salient admission chemical pathology features were: arterial blood pH 6·55, *s*[lactate] 32 mmol l^{-1}, serum uric acid 32 mg dl^{-1}, *s*CPK 1900 mU ml^{-1} (peaking at 1900 mU ml^{-1} at 2 days), serum creatinine of 186 mmol l^{-1} (peaking at 327 mmol l^{-1} 4 hours postadmission), urea N 4·6 mmol l^{-1}, *s*[K^+] 3·9 mmol l^{-1}, a positive *o*-toluidine test in the absence of erythrocyturia, and a urine myoglobin concentration of 124 mg dl^{-1} (12 hours postadmission). He required intubation, paralysis with pancuronium, artificial ventilation and cooling. Pancuronium was continued for 9 hours and extubation was at 20 hours. Convalescence was complicated by severe muscle weakness, myalgia, myoedema and anterior tibial compartment syndrome. A less severely affected case was also described involving a 26-year-old female who 'snorted' the same powder. She developed myalgia, muscle cramps, nausea, vomiting, sweating and blurred vision. She was given iv diazepam and bicarbonate for management of cramps and acidaemia. There was complete recovery within 4 days.

Major complications of strychnine poisoning, for which intensive management may be required, include rapid onset of marked spasm of the thoracoabdominal muscles leading to a lethal asphyxia. Treatment may include phenobarbital and/or diazepam to suppress convulsions and permit airways management, pancuronium with artificial ventilation, minimization of absorption by gavage (with prior endotracheal intubation), activated charcoal and cathartics. Boyd et al. (1983) note that the currently available evidence suggests that benzodiazepines provide anticonvulsant activity on the basis of gamma-aminobutyric acid (GABA) agonist activity. The anticonvulsant barbiturates provide the same GABA agonist activity as benzodiazepines, and thus probably exhibit the same efficacy in treating strychnine poisoning. Since neither diazepam nor the barbiturates have the same receptor activity as strychnine, neither will likely provide pharmacological reversal in very large strychnine concentrations. Since excess seizure activity may result in neuronal degeneration, cerebral anaesthesia is probably preferable to neuromuscular paralysis when diazepam is ineffective. Boyd et al. (1983) conclude that the use of phenobarbitol is preferable, initially in GABA agonist doses, and then in large doses if anaesthesia is necessary.

Neuroleptics

Various neuroleptics have caused rhabdomyolysis, particularly when given by closely spaced im injections. Additionally, a specific collection of effects, constituting the neuroleptic malignant syndrome (NMS), has been described and confirmed by several investigators. General aspects of neuroleptic-induced rhabdomyolysis and a description of the NMS are presented below.

Neuroleptic-Induced Rhabdomyolysis

Loxapine, a dibenzoxazepine derivative used in the treatment of acute and chronic schizophrenia, may lower the convulsive threshold, especially in those with epilepsy and organic brain disease (Varga and Simpson, 1971). Tam *et al.*, (1980) described the case of a 28-year-old male who overdosed with loxapine succinate and developed *grand mal* seizures; a total of 84×50 mg loxapine succinate had been swallowed. He received sodium phenytoin and subsequently diazepam to control the convulsions. He started to pass dark urine, and chemical pathology was BUN 145 mg dl^{-1}, serum creatinine 22·8 mg dl^{-1}, $s[Ca^{++}]$ 5·5 mmol l^{-1}, and *s*CPK 1500 iu ml^{-1}. The patient became anuric and hypertensive, and was treated initially by peritoneal dialysis and, because of lack of improvement, subsequently by hemodialysis with return to health.

An example of the precipitation of rhabdomyolysis from rapid neuroleptization is provided by the case reported by Thase and Shostak (1984) of a 31-year-old male who developed rhabdomyolysis following 3 injections of loxapine and 1 of benztropine over a 7-hour period.

Several cases of rhabdomyolysis have been associated with the tricyclic antidepressant, amoxapine. Fredin and Swainson (1985) described a 21-year-old who over dosed on 50×50 mg amoxapine tablets with 5 Digesic tablets and 5 naproxene tablets, and who developed acute rhabdomyolysis and ARF, shown to be acute tubular necrosis on renal biopsy. There were characteristic increases in *s*CPK and *s*AST with high creatinine and high *s*[creatine]/[urea] ratio. As the *s*CPK and *s*AST activities decreased, hypercalcaemia developed.

Jenning et al. (1983) described a 27-year-old male who overdosed on amoxapine (1–2 g), having previously taken 100–150 mg day^{-1}. He became drowsy and developed one seizure of 1 to 2 minutes duration. During the subsequent 24 hours, urine output decreased with serum UN increasing to 24 mg dl^{-1} and creatinine to 3–4 mg dl^{-1}. He gradually recovered and did not require haemodialysis. The *s*CPK peaked at 2970 iu l^{-1}, and serum myoglobin was 2500 mg ml^{-1} (normal < 85). They also analyzed 111 cases of amoxapine over-dosage reported to the manufacturers, and found that ARF occurred in 12 patients during the first few days following overdose; 10 of the 12 survived, and 2 died with prolonged status epilepticus. Although 7 of 12 had seizures, myoglobinuria (definitive or presumptive, i.e. positive haemostick but no erythroctyes) occurred in 7 and was not related to the occurrence of convulsions. They recommended rapid hydration with iv saline to reduce the incidence of ARF.

Abreo et al. (1982) also described a case of rhabdomyolysis in a 39-year-old female who ingested about 5 g amoxapine, and had been on 50 mg daily increasing to 300 mg. There was no evidence of trauma, muscle tenderness, or swelling. However, *s*CPK increased to around 50 000 iu l^{-1} on the third day and she developed ARF requiring peritoneal dialysis.

Neuroleptic Malignant Syndrome (NMS)

Myonecrosis, as indicated by serum biochemistry, may occur as part of a specific syndrome caused by neuroleptics, and was first recognized about 1960. NMS is characterized by muscular rigidity, hyperthermia, altered consciousness and autonomic dysfunction, which follows the use of high potency neuroleptics in therapeutic doses, but appears unrelated to duration of treatment. It has been described as a consequence of treatment with phenothiazines, butyrophenones and thioxanthenes, with haloperidol and fluphenazine being most commonly incriminated (Smego and Durak, 1982).

Clinically, signs and symptoms of NMS develop rapidly over 24 to 72 hours, and persist for 5–10 days after cessation of therapy, although this may be longer if long-action depot injections have been used. There is diffuse muscle rigidity and akinesia, which develops concomitantly with, or shortly before, an increase in temperature (up to 42 °C). Extrapyramidal signs may develop or worsen. Autonomic adverse effects include tachycardia, labile BP, diaphoresis and urinary incontinence. There may also be associated sialorrhoea, dyskinesia, dysarthria and dysphagia. There is a progressive alteration in consciousness with varying degrees of unresponsiveness and fluctuations of alertness, and agitation may precede stupor or even coma.

Laboratory findings include marked increase in *s*CPK, *s*AST, *s*ALT, and *s*LDH, reflecting the myonecrotic process. There may be a leucocytosis with a shift-to-the-left.

Fatality from NMS has been estimated at around 20%, resulting from respiratory or renal failure, cardiovascular collapse, or cardiac arrythmias (Smego and Durack, 1982). The clinicopathological features of NMS have been discussed in detail by Caroff (1980) and Smego and Durack (1982).

Although NMS has been compared with the malignant hyperthermia syndrome (Kleinknect et al., 1982), NMS appears to be primarily a central phenomenon rather than a direct muscle response, as is the case with malignant hyperthermia. Thus, muscle relaxation can be achieved with diazepam or pancuronium bromide in NMS, but not in malignant hyperthermia (Smego and Durack, 1982). Also, the pyrexia of NMS is most likely of hypothalamic origin, since induced relaxation of muscle contraction does not abolish pyrexia. NMS has been attributed to a disturbance of the dopaminergic system in the basal ganglia and hypothalamus.

Clinical support for this comes from a report of a 51-year-old male patient with Parkinson's disease who received Sinemet 25 (250 mg tablets) thrice daily, amatadine 100 mg twice daily, and diphenylhydramine 50 mg thrice daily (Hendersen and Wooten, 1981). A 2-week history of agitation and delusion led to the use of haloperidol, 15 mg daily. About 2 weeks later all antiparkinsonian therapy was withdrawn. The following day he began to develop signs of NMS in the form of tremor, rigidity, bradykinesia and pyrexia. After 3 days, pertinent clinical chemistry was BUN 45 mg dl^{-1}, WBC 26 200 mm^{-3}, *s*CPK 6000 iu l^{-1}. Recovery occurred with interim treatment for hyperpyrexia. It would appear that dopamine receptor blockade by haloperidol was potentiated by withdrawal of dopaminergic Sinemet and amantadine. Also, early in a case of NMS with a therapeutic level of haloperidol (6 ng ml^{-1}) it was found that lowered BP was to responsive to iv dopamine, but several days later when haloperidol levels had fallen to lower values (1 ng ml^{-1}) there was cardiovascular responsiveness to dopamine, supporting an association between NMS and dopamine receptor block (Hashimoto et al., 1984).

That the muscle rigidity and hyperpyrexia of NMS can lead to myoglobinuric ARF has been demonstrated by several case reports. Eiser et al. (1982) described 3 patients in whom therapy was as follows: Case 1, haloperidol and amitriptyline; Case 2, haloperidol alone; Case 3, haloperidol, amitriptyline and chlorpromazine. All developed signs typical of NMS, namely hyperpyrexia, lachrymation, diaphoresis together with rhabdomyolysis as indicated by positive serum and urine myoglobin, high serum aldolase, *s*CPK and *s*LDH. All had 2 to 4 weeks of peritoneal dialysis for ARF, but one patient died due to the development of bilaterial bronchopneumonia; at autopsy there was renal tubular necrosis with myoglobin casts and interstitial inflammation. Hashimoto et al. (1984) described a case with rapid onset of NMS and myoglobinuric ARF. The patient, a 29-year-old male paranoid, received 90 mg haloperidol and 100 mg chlorpromazine HC1, and within 24 hours developed NMS characterized by acute pyrexia (41·3 °C), extensive muscle rigidity, autonomic instability (blood pressure effects) and coma. Rhabdomyolysis developed with bilateral tibial compartment syndrome and ARF. Relevant clinical chemistry on admission was *s*$[K^+]$ 7·7 mmol l^{-1}, serum creatinine 3·5 mg dl^{-1}, BUN 44 mg dl^{-1}, prolactin 150 mg ml^{-1} (normal 5–15), *s*ALT 1830 iu l^{-1}, *s*AST 332 iu l^{-1}, *s*CPK 220 000 iu l^{-1}, WBC 15 800 mm^{-3}, with haloperidol 6 mg ml^{-1} and chlorpromazine 230 mg ml^{-1} (i.e. therapeutic range). He was treated by cooling, fluids and dopamine HC1 (unresponsive), and subsequently norepinephrine; anuria was treated by haemodialysis. By the sixth day, the patient was responsive to dopamine infusion (15 μg kg^{-1} min^{-1}) with increased blood pressure and heart rate.

Klemknecht et al. (1982) described rhabdomyolysis with ARF in 6 patients with NMS, one of whom had two episodes of rhabdomyolysis. ARF was prerenal in 5 of the 7 patients, and acute tubular necrosis occurred in 2. Three patients died of cardiorespiratory failure or septicaemia. Most were on multiple therapy, but the drugs involved included benzemide, diazepam, levomepromazine, fluphenazine, chlorpromazine, haloperidol, phenobarbital, nomifensine, amitriptyline, meprobamate, meclofenoxate, sulphiride and cyamemazine.

Surmont et al. (1984) described 3 fatal cases of hyperthermia in the course of neuroleptic drug administration. ARF developed in 3, and 2 had histopathologically diagnosed rhabdomyolysis. One patient receive multiple therapy (including haloperidol, chlorpromazine and diazepam), the second haloperidol and promethazine, and the third amitriptyline, haloperidol and leropromazine.

Anaesthesia-Related Malignant Hyperthermia

This syndrome is found in association with the administration of succinyldicholine and generally consists of pyrexia, intense muscle rigidity, acidosis, hyperkalaemia and high activities in serum for muscle enzymes, and frequently myoglobinuria is present. The incidence is generally stated at 1 in 10 000 general anaesthetic procedures (Britt, 1973), and fatality for the full malignant hyperthermia syndrome is estimated at 70% to 90% (Wilson et al., 1967; Britt and Kalow, 1970; Aldrete et al., 1971).

During the mid-1960s it was observed that administration of suxamethonium to a number of children, instead of causing muscle relaxation, produced muscle spasm and rigidity leading to a difficulty in endotracheal intubation. This was followed by pyrexia (up to 41 °C), muscle weakness, myalgia, myoglobinuria and increases in *s*CPK, serum aldolase, and *s*LDH activities. It is now appreciated that exposure to certain depolarizing muscle relaxants (particularly suxamethonium) and/or gaseous anaesthetic (particularly halothane), can induce a clinical spectrum which varies from slight increase in *s*CPK without clinical manifestations, through muscle weakness, myalgia, slight temperature increase and myoglobinuria with increased serum activities of muscle enzymes, to fulminating hyperpyrexia, severe muscle rigidity and rhabdomyolysis, and marked increases in plasma enzymes. It is the latter condition which constitutes the 'classical' malignant hyperthermia or malignant pyrexia syndrome (Aldrete et al., 1971; Lewandowski et al., 1975; Auerbach et al., 1976). Thus, temperature elevation may be absent, particularly if there is a predisposing factor such as muscular dystrophy or myopathy (Moore et al., 1976; McKishnie et al., 1983). It has therefore been suggested that the term 'anaesthesia-induced rhabdomyolysis' is a more appropriate description for this form of rhabdomyolysis which is devoid of pyrexia. It has been proposed on the one hand that this represents an exaggeration of the normal response to depolarizing neuromuscular blockade (Moore et al., 1976; Schaer et al., 1977; Miller et al., 1978) and on the other hand, it may represent an incomplete form of malignant hyperpyrexia (Bernhardt and Hoerder, 1978; Lewandowski, 1982).

As with other causes of rhabdomyolysis, ARF and/or hypocalcaemia may develop in malignant hyperpyrexia and its clinical variants (Bennike and Jarnum, 1964; McKishnie et al., 1983), and potentially cardioplegic or arrythmogenic hyperkalaemia and/or hypocalcaemia (Schaer et al., 1977; Lewandowski, 1982).

The degree of muscle injury is influenced by several factors; for example, by preceding inhalation induction with halothane, or repeat of intermittent doses of succinylcholine (Tammisto and Airaksinen, 1966; Innes and Stromme, 1973). Complications include cardiac arrest, cardiac arrythmias, hyperkalaemia, and ARF. Early recognition of the developing syndrome is important in aborting the development of the full clinical picture, e.g. strong muscle fasciculations, masseteric spasm, and persistent skeletal muscle hypertonicity in the early phase after suxamethonium (Carballo, 1975).

Management includes continuous monitoring of temperature, serum creatinine, $s[K^+]$, $s[Ca^{++}]$ and sCPK; cooling for pyrexia; fluids and, if necessary, diuretics; iv $NaHCO_3$ for acidosis; and treatment of hyperkalaemia.

A specific therapeutic drug is dantrolene sodium (Bianchine, 1985), with an effective dose being that which produces maximal muscle relaxation, which is about 2·4 mg/kg i.v. (Nelson and Llewellen, 1983). Dantrolene may also be used prophylactically at a dosage of 4 to 8 mg/kg per day for one or two days, with the last dose being administered two hours before anaesthesia (Nelson and Flewellen, 1983). Dantrolene acts directly on skeletal muscle, probably blocking signal transfer from sarcolemmal depolarization to Ca^{++} release from storage sites in the sarcoplasmic reticulum, and inhibiting excitation-contraction coupling. When it is known or suspected that patients are susceptible to malignant hyperthermia, alternatives to halogenated anaesthetics may be employed, and if skeletal muscle paralysis is required the non-depolarizing agent pancuronium is preferred.

The most frequently used and reliable test to determine susceptibility to malignant hyperthermia has been to assess the response of a skeletal muscle biopsy to caffeine and halothane. Muscle from susceptible patients undergoes hypercontraction in response to caffeine, and this is potentiated by halothane (Nelson et al., 1983). More recent studies have suggested that measurement of the effect of anaesthetic challenge on Ca^{++} in blood mononuclear cells may be useful; halothane significantly increases $[Ca^{++}]$ in mononuclear cells in malignant hyperthermia patients, but not in controls (Klip et al., 1987). The authors suggest that this could form the basis for a screening test for malignant hyperthermia. Also, Solomons and Masson (1984) examined the nucleotide profiles of platelets from malignant hyperthermia and control subjects; they chose the platelet because of many chemical similarities with skeletal muscle. There were significant changes in the profiles of platelets from malignant hyperthermia patients in response to halothane challenge, that were not seen in the nucleotide profiles of platelets from controls. Their results showed a complete correlation with the skeletal muscle contraction test. The authors conclude that the platelet-halothane bioassay is highly reproducible and specific for detecting malignant hyperthermia susceptibility, and could form the basis for a diagnostic test.

Aetiology and Pathogenesis

Malignant hyperpyrexia was originally attributed to widespread fasciculations preceding suxamethonium-induced neuromuscular blockade (Meadows, 1971; Rowland and Penn, 1971). However, it now appears that a major factor in the genesis of the syndrome may be an exaggeration of skeletal muscle membrane permeability. Any considerations on the aetiology and pathogenesis of malignant hyperpyrexia require that the following observations be taken into consideration.

Administration of suxamethonium to normal subjects leads to an increase in sCPK without clinical signs (Tammisto and Airaksinen, 1966). sCPK increase is most marked when suxamethonium is given intermittently during general anaesthetic procedures (Airaksienen and Tammisto, 1966; Tammisto et al., 1967). Halothane alone also increases sCPK activity, but to a lesser extent (Pearson et al., 1957). Halothane apparently potentiates the effect of suxamethonium on muscle membrane integrity. Suxamethonium, especially when given during halothane anaesthesia, leads to an increase in 'skeletal muscle characteristic' enzyme activity in serum, in otherwise biochemically normal subjects (Auerbach et al., 1973). Also myoglobinuria may occur following the administration of suxamethonium (McLaren, 1968).

Ryan et al. (1971) found an increased susceptibility of the young during a study on the incidence of myoglobinuria after a single iv dose of succinylcholine in 40 children and 30 adults, using a precipitin technique sensitive to 5 μg myoglobin ml^{-1}. Myoglobin was detected in one adult and 16 children after iv succinylcholine; concentrations at 16 to 60 minutes postinjection ranged 0–85 μm ml^{-1}. Prior administration of drugs which reduce the strength of fasciculations, e.g. thiopentone or d-tubocurarine, impedes the development of malignant hyperpyrexia (Tammisto et al., 1967) and the development of myoglobinuria and increase in *s*CPK (Plotz et al., 1981). On the other hand, halothane anaesthesia appears to potentiate or be a prerequisite for the development of suxamethonium rhabdomyolysis, possibly by increasing fasciculations (Tammisto and Airaksienen, 1966; Baraka, 1968). A detailed study on the development of myoglobinuria in surgical patients receiving succinylcholine during nitrous oxide-oxygen-halothane anaesthesia was conducted by Inagaki et al. (1980) using a radioimmunoassay sensitive to 1·0 ng ml^{-1}. They found that the mean value ($\pm$SEM) for serum myoglobin before pre-anaesthetic medication was 143 $\pm$ 3·8 ng ml^{-1}. Atropine and pentazocine premedication had no effect, but hydroxydine (given im) caused a slight increase in serum myoglobin. With N_2O-O_2-halothane anaesthesia alone, there was no change in serum myoglobin concentration, but iv succinylcholine (1 mg kg^{-1}) with inhalational anaesthesia caused marked increases in serum myoglobin, being significantly greater in children than adults. Thus, the mean ($\pm$SEM) values at 30 minutes postsuccinylcholine were:

Children = 1369 $\pm$ 433 ng ml^{-1} (N = 25)
Adults = 208 $\pm$ 40 ng ml^{-1} (N = 15)

When d-tubocurarine was given iv before succinylcholine, serum myoglobin concentrations remained unchanged. They found abnormal increases in serum myoglobin to concentrations 10 000 ng ml^{-1} in 3 patients who developed masseteric spasm after succinylcholine, and in 2 there was myoglobinuria.

Fasciculations can be attenuated by a prior injection of a small dose of succinylcholine ('self-taming') about 1 minute before the subsequent larger and pharmacologically active dose (Baraka, 1977). However, Plotz and Braun (1982) found that in children scheduled for urological surgery, those who received a 'self-taming' dose of succinylcholine did not have an inhibition of *s*CPK activity rise compared with a control group receiving a single dose of succinylcholine. Although the frequency of visible fasciculations was reduced in the self-taming group, the mean postoperative *s*CPK activity was higher in the self-taming group than in those receiving the single injection of succinylcholine. They suggested that fasciculations are not the basis for muscle cell injury and subsequent altered ionic and enzyme fluxes. Whatever the mechanism for the membrane injury these are abnormal ion fluxes whose magnitude is dependant on the degree of injury, and in particular there is an excessive myoplasmic Ca^{++} influx.

There is a definite susceptibility to malignant hyperpyrexia in those with a pre-existing defined myopathy, and also in certain individuals with a subclinical myopathy. Some cases follow an autosomal dominant inheritance, and are probably a consequence of genetic aberrations of receptor proteins. Particularly susceptible are those with Duchenne muscular dystrophy or those at high genetic risk for latent myopathy (Moore et al., 1976; Miller et al., 1978; Seay et al., 1978; Bolthauser et al., 1980; Lewandowski, 1982; Kelfer et al., 1983; McKishnie et al., 1983; Rosenberg and Heinman-Pathison, 1983; Henderson, 1984). Aldrete et al. (1971), for example, described a case of malignant hyperthermia during anaesthesia of a 17-year-old male who was subsequently shown to have (along with some other family members) increased *s*CPK and pyrophosphate. Moore et al. (1976) described a 13-year-old boy who developed myoglobinuria and muscle weakness after succinylcholine. He and some family members were found to have increased *s*CPK activity with a myopathic EMG, and a diagnosis of 'familial non-progressive muscular dystrophy' was made. Tammisto et al. (1970) and Lewandowski (1982) suggest that strabismus may be a possible sign of latent muscle disease predisposing to suxamethonium-induced myotoxicity. Even in apparently normal individuals who have experienced a malignant hyperpyrexia-like syndrome there may be some evidence of 'muscle membrane' leak. For example, Lewandowski (1981) described the case of a 4-year-old boy who developed muscle rigidity, rhabdomyolysis, myoglobinuria, hyperpyrexia and muscle weakness after receiving halothane anaesthesia and a single iv 25 mg dose of suxamethonium. On the day of the anaesthetic, relevant chemical pathology was as follows: *s*CPK 32 000 iu l^{-1} (normal 0–50), *s*LDU 1,360 iu l^{-1} (normal 0–400), *s*AST 580 iu l^{-1} (normal 0–40), *s*ALT 163 iu l^{-1} (normal 0–4). Although there was rapid clinical improvement, with discharge on the third postoperative day, *s*CPK and *s*LDH remained elevated (being, respectively, 180 and 480 iu l^{-1} at 1 month). There were no neurological abnormalities, and no evidence for muscle disease by histology and EMG. The mother, who was physically normal, also had increased *s*CPK (116 iu l^{-1}) and *s*LDH (750 iu l^{-1}).

All recent studies have indicated that malignant hyperthermia is precipitated by an increase in sarcoplasmic $[Ca^{++}]$. Thus, Lopez et al. (1985) used a Ca^{++} selective microelectrode to measure the free $[Ca^{++}]$ in myoplasm of skeletal muscle from patients who earlier had developed signs of malignant hyperthermia. They found an increased free cytosolic $[Ca^{++}]$; $0{\cdot}39 \pm 0{\cdot}01$ SD μM ($N = 18$) compared with $0.11 \pm 0{\cdot}02$ μM ($N = 10$) in controls. Also, drugs that prevent an increase in myoplasmic $[Ca^{++}]$, such as dantrolene, have a therapeutic or prophylactic effect (Nelson and Flewellen, 1983; Britt, 1984). The Ca^{++}-ion defect may exist in other cell types of patients with malignant hyperthermia. For example, Klip et al. (1987) found that halothane significantly increased $[Ca^{++}]$ in blood mononuclear cells from malignant hyperthermia patients, but not those from normal controls; the increase in cell $[Ca^{++}]$ was highly dependent on the presence of $[Ca^{++}]_e$.

Miscellaneous Therapeutic Agents

The following have been included because isolated cases of rhabdomyolysis have been associated with their use. However, the apparent rarity may, in some cases, be merely a reflection of non-reporting in the readily available medical literature.

Isotretinoin

Isotretinoin (13-cis-retinoic acid) is a synthetic analogue of Vitamin A, used in the treatment of nodulocystic acne and disorders of keratinization. About 15% of patients developed musculoskeletal symptoms and sometimes show increased sCPK activity (Dicken, 1984). Hodak et al. (1986) described 2 patients (16- and 20-year-old males) who received treatment with oral isotretinoin ($0{\cdot}5$ mg kg^{-1}) for severe acne. After a few days they began to complain of muscle weakness and pain, but no history of dark urine. On examination at 4 weeks, muscle tenderness was present. One subject had a normal serum enzyme profile, but the other had sCPK 918 iu l^{-1} (normal 203). Needle EMG showed short duration and low amplitude potentials, mainly in the proximal limb muscles. Improvement occurred following cessation of isotretinoin. Electron microscopic examination of a deltoid muscle biopsy showed the presence of elongated elliptical bodies between the myofibrils.

Diphenhydramine

Hampel et al. (1983) described the case of a 34-year-old male who attempted self-poisoning with diphenhydramine (number of tablets unknown) but did not loose consciousness. Biochemical evidence of rhabdomyolysis was present, as follows: *s*AST (maximum) 540 iu l^{-1} and *s*CPK 30 000 iu l^{-1} (day 2) with serum myoglobin 3550 ng ml^{-1} and urine myoglobin 50 370 ng ml^{-1}. He complained of nausea, weakness and general malaise. The myoglobin and serum enzyme activities steadily declined and the patient slowly recovered.

Amphotericin B

Hypokalaemia is a known potentially serious complication of amphotericin B therapy (McChesney et al., 1964). That this can lead to rhabdomyolysis is suggested by a case reported by Drutz et al. (1970) of a 20-year-old male who was treated with amphotericin B for cryptococcal meningitis. He received 25 mg amphotericin B daily, which maintained therapeutic serum levels of $0{\cdot}39$ to $0{\cdot}78$ μg ml^{-1}. After 40 days, and 985 mg amphotericin B, generalized muscle weakness and aching developed in spite of potassium supplements. The weakness became much more severe over the next 6 days. $s[K^+]$ was in the range $1{\cdot}5$–$2{\cdot}2$ mmol l^{-1}. With aggressive potassium supplementation, muscle strength improved. On the forty-eighth day there was discoloured urine, a positive *o*-toluidine urine test, essentially no erythrocyturia, and colourless serum; there was also increased *s*CPK, *s*ALT and *s*AST. Muscle fibre degeneration was seen in a biopsy from the deltoid muscle.

Drugs of Addiction

A wide variety of central nervous system excitants and depressants are taken in deliberately large and pharmacologically active doses in order to obtain differing and bizarre mental experiences. Many of these drugs are used in clinical practice, including sympathomimetics, opioids, analgaesics and arylcyclohexylamines. The sympathomimetics have been conveniently discussed earlier in the section devoted to CNS stimulants. A variety of adverse effects have been described for drugs of addiction, during both clinical use and addictive abuse; amongst these is rhabdomyolysis.

Although some drugs may be directly myotoxic, in many cases a major or compounding effect resulting in rhabdomyolysis is pressure necrosis occurring after coma, and/or the effects of convulsions. In many instances there may be a complex situation. For example, Penn et al. (1972) found myoglobinuria, raised *s*CPK activity, and ARF in 4 patients after ingestion or injection of a variety of drugs (including barbiturates, methadone, heroin, glutethimide and chlorpromazine). They suggested that myoglobinuria may have been a consequence of several effects, including coma (periods of immobilization estimated at 24–48 hours), direct pressure, ischaemia anoxia, hypotension, hypothermia and acidosis. The role of local muscle pressure in the pathogenesis of rhabdomyolysis in cases associated with drug induced coma has been emphasized by Chaikin (1980), who described the case of a 22-year-old male who had ingested 'mescalin', methadone and alcohol, and developed a swollen left arm and, subsequently, left leg. He became anuric and required several courses of dialysis. Renal function returned to normal, but residual weakness persisted in the left limbs. Chaikin (1980) stresses that radionuclide scanning can play a significant role in determining the extent of soft tissue injury in such cases.

That significant soft tissue pressures may develop from limb compression due to coma is indicated by the experimental findings of Owen et al. (1979), who measured intramuscular pressure using catheters inserted into the volar forearm and anterior tibial compartment of healthy volunteer subjects, who were then instructed to lay in various positions. Compression of the forearm or leg by the subjects own head or torso caused significant increases in intramuscular pressure. Normal osteofascial compartment pressures range 0–8 mm Hg. On hard surfaces, im pressures increased to 20–240 mm Hg, with 80% of values being > 50 mm Hg. The most severe situation was forearm compression by the subjects own rib cage, when pressures increased to 100–225 mm Hg. Owen et al. (1979) estimated that pressure in the range of 30–50 mm Hg can cause muscle ischaemia, and maintenance of such pressures for 4 to 8 hours may cause necrosis. Chaikin (1980) refers to the compartmental syndrome involving local pressure leading to ischaemia and oedema, and resultant increased osteofacial compartment pressure. This may lead to infarction and the systemic manifestations of rhabdomyolysis.

In an attempt to identify factors responsible for the diverse clinical manifestations of drug-associated rhabdomyolysis, Cadnapaphornchai et al. (1980) analyzed their experience with 30 patients who had rhabdomyolysis associated with alcohol, narcotics or sedatives (details not specified). Rhabdomyolysis was diagnosed on the basis of muscle weakness and swelling, myalgia, and *o*-toluidine-positive dark urine in the absence of erythrocyturia, and marked increases in *s*CPK, *s*AST and *s*LDH. Amongst the 30 patients, one-third did not develop ARF, one-third had oliguric ARF, and one-third non-oliguric ARF. For the purpose of identifying factors which could lead to such a diversity with respect to ARF, they also included 51 published drug-related cases of rhabdomyolysis in their analysis. Patients with ARF had a higher incidence of coma, and there were more patients with very high serum enzyme activities than was the case with non-ARF patients. Patients with oliguric ARF were slightly younger, had a higher incidence of muscle swelling, and a higher $s[K^+]$ than those with non-oliguric ARF. Also oliguric ARF was more severe, lasted longer, and required more dialysis than non-oliguric ARF. Hypercalcaemia was present in 22 of 81 patients, but not seen in those without ARF. There were no differences in age, incidence of coma, muscle swelling and serum enzyme activities between those that did and those that did not develop hypercalcaemia. Sixteen patients with nerve entrapment had a higher incidence of coma and muscle swelling than the remainder of the patients.

In some cases, where coma and pressure ischaemia have not occurred, rhabdomyolysis due to direct myotoxicity may be a significant factor. In other cases there may be both direct toxicity and a compounding influence of local muscle pressure. For example, Vissuzine et al. (1976) described a fatal case of rhabdomyolysis from self-poisoning with nitrazepam (200 mg) and Immenoctal (3 g) in a 25-year-old male. There was hypothermia and anuria on admission, and the patient died on the seventh day of hospitalization. There was evidence of necrosis and fragmentation in muscles both subjected to pressure and those not subjected to pressure, as well as in the myocardium. Features of rhabdomyolysis, and its complications, associated with abuse and overdosage from opioids and psychodelics are reviewed below.

Opioids

HEROIN

Neurological complications of heroin addiction include transverse myelitis, acute and chronic polyneuropathy and plexitis (Richter and Rosenberg, 1968; Richter and Baden 1968). Rhabdomyolysis, and ARF, have been described in several cases involving iv heroin, in which loss of consciousness did or did not occur. The first description was apparently by Richter et al. (1971) who observed rhabdomyolysis in 4 males, aged 19–38 years, who had been abusing heroin for between 4 months and 17 years. Before admission all had iv heroin, but there was no history of trauma, convulsions or other toxic exposures. Clinically there was generalized muscle tenderness, oedema and profound weakness. Urinary myoglobin, by a specific immunological method, was present up to $3 \cdot 25$ ng ml^{-1}; serum myoglobin concentration was up to $0 \cdot 31$ ng ml^{-1}; the myoglobin concentrations reduced to zero within 4 to 5 days. Maximum serum enzyme activities were as follows: CKP 14 000 units, LDH 24 600 units, AST 4360 units, and ALT 2500 units. Nerve conduction studies were normal, and the EMG showed myopathic motor unit potentials. Histological examination of muscle biopsies showed acute myolysis; particular features were pale irregular necrotic muscle cells, with type I and II fibres equally involved, and macrophages present in the muscle cells. Renal failure occurred in 2 patients, one of whom died. It was noted that there was recurrence of the effects in one patient following a subsequent heroin injection. Some typical case reports of muscle-related complications of heroin abuse are as follows for different exposure conditions.

Greenwood (1974) described the case of a 22-year-old male who was found unconscious 24 hours after an iv injection of impure heroin. On admission he was unconscious, pyrexial, hypotensive and tachypnoeic. Investigation showed $s[K^+]$ $7 \cdot 5$ mmol l^{-1}, arterial blood pH $7 \cdot 24$, plasma urea 65 mg dl^{-1}, *s*AST 1240 units; he was oliguric, with dark brown benzidine-positive urine in the absence of erythrocytes. Over the next 3 days, plasma urea increased to 250 mg dl^{-1}, and dialysis was given for 7 days with improvement. At 4 weeks there was a normal creatinine clearance. Pain developed in the right leg the day following admission, and the anterior compartment became swollen; there was weakness of the tibialis anterior, extensor hallucis longus, and extensor digitorum longus. EMG, of the tibialis anterior, showed a myopathic pattern, with low amplitude, short duration, polyphasic motor unit potentials.

Nicholls et al. (1982) described two young males who developed ARF after iv street heroin. Chemical pathology in the first case was $s[K^+]$8·2 mmol l^{-1}, *s*ALT 600 units l^{-1} (normal < 65), *s*CPK 1400 units l^{-1} (normal < 130 units l^{-1}), and the urine was positive for myoglobin and contained pigmented casts. Values for the second case were $s[K^+]$ 6·6 mmol l^{-1}, *s*CPK 30 000 units l^{-1}, *s*ALT 2010 units l^{-1}, and a muscle biopsy showed patchy fibre degeneration.

Schwartzfarb et al. (1977) described the case of a 23-year-old heroin abuser who was admitted complaining of a swollen right leg and darkening urine. Admission chemical pathology was blood UN 92 mg dl^{-1}, $s[K^+]$ 6·6 mmol l^{-1} increasing to 8·0 mmol l^{-1}. Peritoneal dialysis was performed. Urine was positive on haemotest in the absence of haemolysis or haemocyturia. Although dialysis successfully lowered blood urea and serum K^+, the patient died on the fourth hospital day. Histology of the right soleus showed extensive necrosis but no thrombosed vessels; the kidney showed acute tubular necrosis; the myocardium showed necrosis and subsarcolemmal proliferation.

D'Agostino and Arnett (1979) described myoglobinuria in a 20-year-old male following snorting of heroin. Additionally, there developed cramping pains in the thighs which increased over the next few days, and the pain spread to involve the calves and upper arms. There was tenderness, but no weakness, of the quadriceps, gastrocnemius and biceps brachii. The BUN was 8 mg dl^{-1}, serum creatinine 1·2 ml dl^{-1}, with (BUN)/(creatinine) ratio of 7, *s*CPK 2665 iu l^{-1} (positive for MM and MB fractions). He was treated with iv fluids and discharged well on the fourth day.

Rhabdomyolysis may also occur in novice (non-addicted) persons. For example, Klock and Sexton (1973) described rhabdomyolysis and ARF in 2 non-addicted subjects who injected heroin iv. One case, a 20-year-old male, gave himself a single injection of heroin and went to sleep for 6 hours, and then awoke with generalized weakness and pain in the right hip and back. He noticed that his urine appeared dark brown. On admission there was muscle tenderness in the thighs, buttock and lower back. Chemical pathology was as follows: *s*CPK 36 000 (day 1), 64 000 (day 2) and 39 000 (day 3), iu l^{-1}, with only the skeletal muscle fraction on isozyme fractionation. Urine was positive for myoglobin. He was oliguric and hyperkalaemic ($s[K^+]$7·0 $mmol^{-1}$), and was treated with insulin, glucose, bicarbonate and oral polystyrene sulphonate, and subsequently mannitol which induced a diuresis. Muscle biopsy showed scattered necrosis and oedema. The patient recovered completely. The second case was that of a 30-year-old male who, two days before hospital admission, injected himself with heroin iv. He developed severe pain in the right arm and shoulder and developed a dark urine. Chemical pathology was as follows: $s[K^+]$ 8·8 mmol l^{-1}, *s*AST 1020 iu, *s*CPK 38 300 iu l^{-1}, *s*LDH 2905 iu l^{-1}. Due to oliguria, the patient received iv fluids, mannitol and furosemide, followed by glucose, insulin, bicarbonate, sodium polystyrene sulphonate and peritoneal dialysis. The development of a neurologic deficit in the right hand required fasciotomy. The patient recovered.

With acute opioid self-overdose in non-addicted subjects, there may be rhabdomyolysis without marked clinical evidence of myopathy. For example, Blain et al. (1985) described 3 patients with opioid self-poisoning (dipipanone, dihydrocodeine, and slow-release morphine) who developed rhabdomyolysis as evidenced by increased *s*AST, *s*CPK and creatinine, with hypocalcaemia, hyperphosphataemia, and the presence of serum myoglobin. One patient developed ARF requiring haemodialysis. Clinical evidence of myopathy was minimal.

The above cases indicate that clinical and biochemical evidence of rhabdomyolysis may occur in the absence of coma or convulsions, suggesting the possibility for a direct myotoxic effect with heroin. However, when there is coma associated with the myotoxic component the pressure ischaemia and necrosis may compound to produce a more severe clinical picture (Rohling et al., 1984).

METHADONE

Several cases of rhabdomyolysis have been described, with and without coma, following self-abuse or self-poisoning with methadone. A typical case, without coma, was reported by Nanji and Filipenko (1983). A 31-year-old male had taken 'a large amount' of methadone orally and had been found vomiting. He did not become comatose or immobilized, and there was no trauma. Laboratory investigations on admission were as follows on arterial blood: pH 7·12, $s[K^+]$ 8·9 mmol l^{-1}, $s[Ca^{++}]$ 7·6 mg dl^{-1}, BUN 24 mg dl^{-1}, serum uric acid 17·5 mg $dl^{<1}$, serum creatinine 2·2 mg dl^{-1}, *s*CPK 7500 iu l^{-1}, *s*LDH 2200 iu l^{-1}, *s*AST 2150 iu l^{-1} phosphate 12·8 mg dl^{-1}. Hyperkalaemia was managed with iv saline, bicarbonate, calcium gluconate and insulin. After 8 hours the level of consciousness decreased, and there was a marked drop in blood pressure (80/0 mm Hg); he was given naloxone and saline and became alert with stabilization of the BP. Peak enzyme activities were measured in serum at 12 hours; CPK 22 900 iu l^{-1}, LDH 14 200 iu l^{-1} and ALT 11 340 iu l^{-1}. Because of progressive oliguria and azotaemia he was treated with haemodialysis, with subsequent improvement of renal function. The conditions of this case suggest a direct myotoxicity of methadone. However, in a case reported by Chaikin (1980) which involved methadone intoxication it is likely that local pressure resulting from coma was the major cause of rhabdomyolysis and associated ARF.

Psychodelics

PHENCYCLIDINE (PCP).

Phencyclidine (phenylcyclohexylpiperidine HCl) is a dissociative anaesthetic which was used in human medicine in the late 1950s, but withdrawn in the mid-1960s because of postanaesthetic excitement, visual delusions and delirium (Burns et al., 1975). It is now used legally only as a tranquillizing agent in veterinary practice, and available as Sernylan. In connection with its illicit use as a street drug a variety of curious and colourful names have been employed, which include: 'Hog', 'PeaCe Pill' (PCP), 'Rocket Fuel', and 'Angel Dust'. In this connection it has been smoked, swallowed, 'snorted', and given iv. It is a major drug of abuse as a psychodelic and hallucinogen (having schizophrenomimetic effects). Some cases showing the severity of the possible presentation and complications are cited below.

Cogen et al (1978) presented the cases of 2 males, 21- and 19-years-old, one of whom self-iv-injected PCP, and the other ingested 21 tablets. One was semi-stuporous and the other lost consciousness, but both had exaggerated and hyperactive movements for which physical restraint was required. In the case involving iv injection of PCP salient findings were: *s*CPK 210 000 iu l^{-1}, *s*AST 2200 iu l^{-1}, *s*LDH 600 iu l^{-1}, urine was *o*-toluidine positive in the absence of erythrocyturia, and myoglobin was demonstrated by a complement fixation technique. A quadriceps muscle biopsy was normal by light microscopy, but electron microscopy showed Z-band smearing and lysosomal swelling. Vigorous diuresis was instituted and ARF did not develop. The patient was discharged on the eighth hospital day. The second case, with peroral PCP, showed *s*CPK of 1900 iu l^{-1}, *s*AST 90 iu l^{-1}, LDH 160 iu l^{-1}, urine was positive by *o*-toluidine test in the absence of erythrocyturia. Due to increasing myotonic activity against restraint and increasing *s*CPK (40 000 iu l^{-1} by the third day), peripheral muscle blockade with pancuronium was instituted to maintain the airway. The *s*CPK activity dropped to 9000 iu l^{-1} within 24 hours of pancuronium-induced paralysis. Renal function remained unaffected, and by the fifteenth day he was alert. Rhabdomyolysis was believed to have been a consequence of the intense muscle activity.

Akmal et al. (1981) analyzed 1000 cases of PCP intoxication and found 25 cases of rhabdomyolysis (2·5% incidence) and 10 of these cases (40%) developed ARF and a further 7 had mild impairment of renal function. Marked hyperuricaemia was present in all 17 cases of renal impairment, and marked hyperphosphataemia with hypocalcaemia was present in the 10 patients with ARF, and 3 of the latter developed hypercalcaemia during the diuretic phase. Pyrexia, tachycardia, and hypertension were found frequently among the rhabdomyolysis patients, and all had leucocytosis (WBC 12 000–24 900 mm^{-3}).

McCarron et al. (1981) analyzed the clinical findings in 1000 cases of acute PCP intoxication, and found a high incidence of violence (35%) and agitation (34%). Motor signs consisted of *grand mal* seizures (3·1%), generalized rigidity (5·2%), localized dystonias (2·4%), catalepsy and athetosis (1·3%). They commonly found increases in *s*CPK, uric acid and transaminases. Thus *s*CPK (normal 25–200 units) was > 300 units in 356 cases (70%), in 22 cases $> 24\,000$ units, and the highest measured value was 423 045 units; CPK isozyme fractionation showed 95–100% of CPK-3 (MM fraction). *s*ALT and *s*AST were normal (40 units) in 50% of subjects tested, and the highest *s*AST was 9760 units and *s*ALT 2630 units. No subject had increased bilirubin. Hyperuricaemia (> 7 mg dl^{-1}) with the serum creatinine of 1·3 mg dl^{-1} or less occurred in 122 cases; in a further 15 patients the serum uric acid ranged 9·4–28·0 mg dl^{-1} with serum creatinine concentrations of 1·4 to 1·5 mg dl^{-1}. All but 24 of the patients with increased serum uric acid had increased *s*CPK, hence there was a relatively high incidence of biochemically-indicated rhabdomyolysis.

Patel and Conner (1985) noted that over a 20-month period, at King-Drew Medical Center, CA, out of 2024 patients who reported to the emergency room with symptoms of PCP intoxication there were 10 cases of rhabdomyolysis complicated by ARF (incidence 0·5%), the total number of cases of rhabdomyolysis could not be determined. During the period 1979–1984 they saw 15 cases of rhabdomyolysis-associated ARF with PCP intoxication, and collected a further 15 cases from the literature. Their general conclusion from analyzing these 30 cases was as follows:

1. *s*CPK: mean 65 028 iu l^{-1} (range 1057–520 000)
   s[creatinine]: mean 9·5 mg dl^{-1} (range 2·3–18·0)
   s[Ca^{++}]: mean 7·1 mg dl^{-1} (range 4·5–9·2)
   s[$PO_4{}^{3-}$]: mean 8·4 mg dl^{-1} (range 4·0–21·0)
   s[uric acid]: mean 21·1 mg dl^{-1} (range 11·9–36·0)
2. Seven of the patients with hypocalcaemia showed transient hypercalcaemia after the onset of diuresis.
3. All patients had a positive urine *o*-toluidine test.
4. PCP was detected in the urine of all patients in whom it was sought.

Special considerations may be necessary with respect to the management of PCP intoxication where rhabdomyolysis may be present. PCP is a lipid soluble weak base (pK_a8·6–9·4) that is readily ionized. Thus, as a generalization, in the treatment of PCP intoxication excretion can be enhanced by acidification measures; ammonium chloride and/or ascorbic acid is a frequently recommended therapy (Aronow and Done, 1978; Gossel and Bricker, 1984), followed by furosemide after urine pH has been reduced to about 5·0. Barton et al. (1980) and Norton (1984) have drawn attention to the fact that this could potentiate the precipitation of myoglobin or uric acid in the renal tubules if there is a coexistent rhabdomyolysis. Thus, it is necessary to determine whether rhabdomyolysis is, or is not, present for the optimum safe treatment of PCP intoxication.

A reasonably large amount of experimental work has been conducted on the toxicity of PCP, which allows conclusions on the probable mechanism of production of rhabdomyolysis in PCP poisoning. It is well known that PCP increases motor activity in free running rats, but under such conditions there is no increase in *s*CPK (Chen et al., 1959; Goode and Meltzer, 1975). However, Kuncl and Meltzer (1974) produced locomotor activity in rats injected with PCP, and found that when restrained there was a marked increase in *s*CPK to about 100 times normal activity. The increase in *s*CPK was highly correlated with isometric muscle tension during restraint. Muscle biopsies from restrained animals showed scattered necrosis of fibres and myofibrillar disruption; denervation essentially abolished this effect. Also, rhabdomyolysis did not occur in restrained untreated animals, or in drug treated and unrestrained animals.

Goode and Meltzer (1975) found that restrained rats given nociceptive stimuli developed both an increase in isometric motor activity and in *s*CPK activity, with a close correlation between the two. These effects were smaller, but qualitatively similar, to the dose-response curves for PCP-induced increased isometric muscle tension and paralleled changes in *s*CPK activity. Since the relationship between isometric activity and *s*CPK activity is qualitatively similar for PCP and nociceptive-stimulated animals, they suggest that the increase in isometric muscle tension during restraint is a major factor in the production of muscle injury and subsequent elevation of *s*CPK activity. Support for this proposal comes from the observation that abolition of motor stress in one of the patients of Cogen et al. (1978) by pancuronium resulted in a decrease in *s*CPK activity.

All the above evidence indicates that PCP-induced rhabdomyolysis is associated with the excess isometric motor activity rather than being due to a direct myotoxicity of PCP. However, in some cases there may, additionally, be a compounding effect from pressure necrosis if consciousness is lost (Akmal et al., 1981).

LYSERGIC ACID DIETHYLAMIDE

Rhabdomyolysis may occur in subjects taking lysergic acid diethylamide (LSD) if they exhibit violent movements. It is probable that, as with PCP, the muscle injury is secondary to the development of high isometric tension during restraint. For example, Mercieca and Brown (1984) described 2 patients who had been placed in strait-jackets after LSD, and subsequently developed rhabdomyolysis and ARF; one of the patients died. The first case, a 19-year-old male, was taken to the hospital in a strait-jacket where he was sedated with chlorpromazine. He became oliguric over the next 4 days, at which time chemical pathology was as follows: *s*CPK 45 000 iu l^{-1} (normal > 90), *s*ALT 1690 iu l^{-1} (normal > 35), *s*[urate] 1155 μmol l^{-1} (normal 100–400). Renal function spontaneously improved. The second case, a 25-year-old male, was restrained in a strait-jacket during transportation to the hospital where he was sedated with iv haloperidol and chlorpromazine, and eventually sodium thiopentone. He was hyperpyrexial (41·6 °C), hypotensive, and passed only a small volume of urine overnight. Chemical pathology (the following morning) was plasma urea 105 mg dl^{-1}, plasma creatinine 5·7 mg dl^{-1}, *s*CPK 13 760 iu l^{-1}, *s*ALT 1100 iu l^{-1}, and *s*AST 1715 iu l^{-1}. He remained hypertensive, had three episodes of cardiac arrest, and died.

COMMERCIAL PRODUCTS

Some materials used in commercially prepared foods, junk foods and beverages which, taken in modest amounts, are apparently devoid of adverse health effects, may cause toxic effects if taken in excess. Two examples of such materials which produce rhabdomyolysis, are liquorice and ethanol. They are discussed below.

Liquorice

Liquorice, in its natural form, is an extract of the root of glycyrrhiza glabra, and contains glycyrrhizin which is a glucuronide of glycyrrhetinic acid and possesses mineralocorticoid activity, leading to Na^+ retention with kaluresis, oedema and hypertension (Koster and David, 1968). Epstein et al. (1977) studied the electrolyte status and renin–angiotensin–aldosterone axis after withdrawal of liquorice in 4 symptomatic females aged 33–55 years, who had long-term liquorice ingestion (25–200 g a day for 6 months to 35 years). During the first few days after withdrawal, excess amounts of K^+ were still excreted in urine, despite a subnormal s[K^+]; presumably this was due to the continued action of the glycyrrhyzinic acid component on renal tubular K^+ secretion. This was followed by a phase of Na^+ loss with K^+ retention (in contrast to the Na^+-K^+ retention seen in Conn's syndrome); they suggested that the naturesis with K^+ retention was related to the effects of extracellular volume expansion and paralysis of the renin–angiotensin–aldosterone system. Subnormal urine and plasma aldosterone levels and subnormal plasma renin activity was measured initially and continued up to the twelfth day of a low NaCl challenge. Plasma aldosterone and angiotensin II, whilst relatively normal under basal conditions, were abnormally low during low salt challenge. Later follow-up (2 to 4 months) showed normal electrolyte and renin–angiotensin–aldosterone axis, indicating that long-term suppression of the axis is uncommon despite prolonged liquorice consumption.

Several cases of hypokalaemic myopathy, with microscopical or biochemical indications of muscle degeneration, have been described. For example, Gross et al. (1966) described the case of a 45-year-old female who for 9 months had consumed 30 to 40 g of liquorice each day. She became lethargic, developed flaccid weakness and hypoactive reflexes. Serum $[K^+]$ was 1·6 mmol l^{-1}, and the urine was dark brown and positive for myoglobin. Muscle water content was normal; $[K^+]$ was reduced to 51·7 mmol kg^{-1} (normal 93) and $[Na^+]$ was increased to 51·9 mmol kg^{-1} (normal 34·7). Muscle biopsy revealed myopathic changes, and electron microscopy showed spherical and concentric lamellar bodies. She improved markedly after potassium supplements.

ARF may occur with liquorice-induced rhabdomyolysis. Mourad et al. (1979), for example, described a 51-year-old male with a history of hypertension, muscle weakness and pain for about 6 months. He was given furosemide and potassium supplements, but an intensification of the muscle pain occurred. It later became known that he consumed about 600 mg a day of glycyrrhyzinic acid. On admission he was oliguric with a BP of 190/110 mm Hg and he had a flaccid quadriparesis. $s[K^+]$ was 1.4 mmol l^{-1}, and the urine was *o*-toluidine positive in the absence of erythrocyturia. Other relevant chemical pathology was: *s*AST 256 mU ml^{-1} (normal 6–11), *s*LDH 1840 mU ml^{-1} (normal 110–180), and *s*CPK 9264 mU ml^{-1} (normal 16–35). He was treated with KCl iv, and in a few hours muscle tone and reflexes reappeared. He was given a 3-week course of peritoneal dialysis. A quadriceps muscle biopsy showed microvacuolor degenerative changes in fibres, necrosis, inflammatory reaction and macrophage infiltration.

That a severe and life-threatening hypokaleamia may occur is illustrated by the case report of Bannister et al. (1977). They described a case of cardiac arrest in a 58-year-old woman due to liquorice-induced hypokalaemia (1·8 kg of liquorice sweets per week). She was admitted to the hospital for increasing fatigue and weakness, and had an admission $s[K^+]$ of 1.3 mmol l^{-1}. Soon after admission she developed ventricular fibrillation, which was treated by external cardiac massage and iv KCl. She was given potassium supplements for 2 days with return of muscle power.

Ethanol

Rhabdomyolysis due to heavy ethanol consumption is not an uncommon cause of rhabdomyolysis and cardiomyopathy. For example, Gabow et al. (1982) studying 87 episodes of rhabdomyolysis in 77 patients found that in this series alcoholism was the commonest aetiological factor (67%). The first recognition of a causative association between alcohol and acute myopathy was apparently by Fahlgren et al. (1957). Clinical presentation may vary considerably and range from chronic myopathy with few symptoms and minor clinical signs, to acute myalgia, muscle tenderness and swelling, cramps, increased serum muscle activities, myoglobinuria and hyperkalaemia (Hed et al. 1962; Perkoff et al., 1967; Lafair and Myerson, 1968; Goertz et al., 1978). Schneider (1970) analyzed the literature to date and stated that the mortality rate for acute alcoholic myopathy was 22%, and in patients presenting with ARF approximately 50%. However, if rhabdomyolysis and ARF are appreciated as complications of heavy alcoholic intoxication, then early diagnosis and treatment should be possible with a consequent reduction in mortality. For example, Haapanen et al. (1984) described 5 cases of severe ARF caused by ethanol-induced rhabdomyolysis of whom 4 required haemodialysis, and one of these required artificial ventilation because of hypoxia due to uraemic lung; all patients recovered. Hypercalcaemia is a frequent feature of ARF in acute alcoholic rhabdomyolysis during the diuretic phase, with an associated hyperparathyrodism (Wu et al., 1972).

The variability in clinical presentation and course is illustrated by the two cases of acute alcoholic myopathy described by Schneider (1970). The first patient, a 36-year-old male, was admitted with a two-day history of painful swelling in both arms and pain in the back and legs. He had dark urine, $s[K^+]$ 7·6 mmol l^{-1}, and *s*CPK > 640 units. He developed acute renal tubular necrosis and severe renal insufficiency which was treated with mannitol and ethacrynic acid iv. A right forearm muscle biopsy showed extensive muscle fibre necrosis, but liver biopsy was normal. The second case, a 38-year-old male, was admitted with pain in the extremities and tenderness, but no swelling, of the muscles. Investigations included: WBC 19 000 mm^{-3}, $s[K^+]$ 6·8 mmol l^{-1}, *s*CPK 7080 units, *s*AST 3170 units, *s*ALT 552 units, and *s*LDH 1750 units; muscle biopsy of the right calf showed severe necrosis with normal vessels. He did not develop ARF, but had evidence of myocardial injury in the form of precordial T-wave inversion, and low R-wave over V_{1-3}. Cardiac involvement has also been described in several other reports. For example, Seneviratne (1975) found acute congestive cardiac failure with disturbances of rhythm and conduction in 3 of 5 alcoholic patients who developed acute rhabdomyolysis; myocardial infarction, thiamine deficiency and cobalt intoxication were excluded. ECG-defined abnormalities were as follows: paroxysmal atrial tachycardia with block, left anterior hemiblock and right bundle branch block, atrioventricular block.

Factors in the aetiology of rhabdomyolysis in the absence of coma and compression have included hypophosphataemia of ATP depletion, and direct myotoxicity. Knochel et al. (1975) demonstrated a relationship between hypophosphataemia and alcoholic myopathy. Thus, when serum phosphate was < 1 mg dl^{-1}, and remained at that concentration for 1 to 2 days, *s*CPK increased sharply (Knochel, 1977). Total muscle phosphorous was markedly subnormal, with an average of 13·2 mmol/100 g (fat free) dry solid (normal 28 mmol/100 g). Also, the resting muscle membrane potential was subnormal at −70·4 mV (normal −86·7 mV). To examine the possibility that phosphate deficiency might cause a myopathy, the effect of phosphate depletion was examined experimentally by Fuller et al. (1976). They found that the resting muscle membrane potential was reduced, the Na^+, Cl^- and H_2O content increased, and the K^+ content decreased; this was reversed when phosphate was replenished. Also, administration of excessive calories to partially starved dogs resulted in a profound hypophosphataemia and sharp increases in *s*CPK with rhabdomyolysis (Knochel et al., 1978).

Evidence for a direct myotoxicity from ethanol comes from the observations of Song and Ruben (1977) who gave ethanol on a daily basis for 28 days to human volunteers at a level of 42% of total calories (225 g ethanol). In all subjects there was a progressive increase in *s*CPK during the period of alcohol consumption, with return to normal within 2 weeks of stopping the consumption of ethanol. Light microscopic examination of deltoid and gastrocnemius muscle biopsies showed no abnormality, but electron microscopy demonstrated intercellular oedema, dilated and vesicular sarcoplasmic reticulum, and irregular mitochondria. However, that fasting may also be a factor in the genesis of acute alcoholic rhabdomyolysis is suggested by the findings of Haller and Drachman (1980) who produced marked increases in *s*CPK and myoglobin in rats by a combination of 2 to 4 weeks of exposure to ethanol and a brief period (1 to 3 days) of food deprivation; blood alcohol levels were maintained at 100–300 mg dl^{-1} by using alcohol vapour chambers. Rhabdomyolysis was confirmed histologically in the ethanol + fast group, but muscle histology was normal in rats exposed to alcohol but not fasted. They propose that the observations suggest that fasting may trigger muscle injury during binge drinking. The authors suggested that the effect of fasting is partly the result of increased blood ethanol due to its decreased clearance, and in part a consequence of fasting-induced potentiation of the toxic effects of high concentrations of ethanol on skeletal muscle. The toxicity of ethanol on muscle cells is indicated by a positive correlation between blood [ethanol] and *s*CPK activity.

Factors influencing the serum and urine myoglobin concentrations in alcoholics was investigated by Hallgren et al. (1980). They studied the following three groups:

- Group A: Chronic alcoholics who had not consumed ethanol for 2 to 4 weeks before investigation. None had increased serum myoglobin, and indeed it was subnormal in 31%.
- Group B: Chronic alcoholics who were serially investigated after a period of heavy alcohol abuse. Five showed an increase in serum myoglobin, with a consistent pattern of decrease and return to normal levels within 4 to 7 days.
- Group C: Ambulatory out-patients with alcoholism of varying duration. Increased serum myoglobin was found in 18%.

There was a significant correlation between *s*[myoglobin] and *s*CPK activity, and decreases in myoglobin concentration and *s*CPK activity generally paralleled each other. No subjects had impaired GFR as judged by *s*[creatinine], and there was no correlation between serum myoglobin on laboratory assessment of hepatic function (*s*AST, *s*ALT, gamma-glutamyl transpeptidase, bilirubin and galactose elimination). A transient, slight increase in the urinary excretion of myoglobin was paralleled by an increased excretion of β_2-microglobulin in two alcoholics, suggesting that myoglobinuria in alcoholics having recent heavy drinking may be due to transient minimal tubular dysfunction.

The above, and other findings, indicate a complex biochemical and physiological situation in the muscle injury associated with alcoholism. Ethanol appears to be myotoxic, but the precipitation of an acute attack of rhabdomyolysis may involve a variety of factors; one of these appears to be abrupt nutritional deficiency. As with other potentially coma-inducing materials, when loss of consciousness occurs then muscle injury secondary to pressure necrosis may develop and compound with that due to ethanol toxicity. The clinical picture may be variable, and ARF can develop.

INDUSTRIAL MATERIALS

Several substances used in industry, and to which overexposure may occur, have been shown to produce rhabdomyolysis and complications thereof. These materials may also find their way into other areas of commerce or the home, where even greater overexposure and a potential for production of adverse health may occur. Because of their circumstances of occurrence, and the unsatisfactory methods available for reporting adverse effects from industrial materials, specific toxic injuries from particular materials are usually not as well documented as is the case for medicinal products. Therefore, the incidence of adverse effects, such as rhabdomyolysis, may well be much greater than is apparent from reviews of readily available literature. Brief summaries of chemicals for which rhabdomyolysis has been reported are given below.

Carbon Monoxide

Several cases of rhabdomyolysis secondary to acute carbon monoxide poisoning have been described and, as indicated in general above, it is believed to be more common than is generally appreciated (Howse and Seddon, 1966). Larrey (1812; cited by Howse and Seddon, 1966) studied troops during the occupation of Berlin by Napoleon in 1806. Soldiers heated their quarters by burning coal in open stoves, which led to cases of carbon monoxide poisoning because of a lack of ventilation. At necropsy he found that there was discolouration and softening of muscles often with necrosis of overlying skin. By 1977, Finley was able to identify 13 case reports of myonecrosis associated with CO poisonings in the English literature; up to that time the majority believed that rhabdomyolysis was a consequence of coma-related pressure necrosis. Tintinalli et al. (1983) lists CO as a cause of rhabdomyolysis and myoglobinuria-associated renal failure. Some typical case reports are given below.

Loughridge et al. (1958) reported the case of a 23-year-old female with CO (coal-gas) poisoning who was found in a coma, but recovered consciousness on admission to the hospital one hour later where she complained of pain in both legs. She became oliguric over the next 24 hours. By the sixth hospital day the right thigh was tender and swollen, the BUN had increased to 325 mg dl^{-1}, $s[K^+]$ was 5·9 mmol l^{-1}, and $s[HCO_3^-]$ was 126·9 mmol l^{-1}. She died on the ninth hospital day. At autopsy the adductor muscles of the thigh were pale and swollen; histologically there was fragmentation, vacuolation, phagocytosis and perivascular cuffing with polymorphs and mononuclear cells. The kidneys were pale and swollen, and distal convoluted tubules and collecting ducts showed benzidine-positive casts. The proximal tubules were normal in some areas, and in other areas there was flattening and the tubules were lined with a degenerating epithelium.

Howse and Seddon (1966) described two cases of ischaemic necrosis of muscles of the upper limbs associated with coma due to CO poisoning, and which lead to ischaemic contractions.

Finley et al. (1977) described two cases of myonecrosis as a complication of CO poisoning. The first case, a 20-year-old male, was believed to have resulted from a leaking heating unit associated with inadequate room ventilation. He was found, after 9 hours, comatose. Shortly after admission he was found to have haemoglobin 25% saturated with CO, and to have a red-brown urine. He developed progressive leg oedema. The *s*CPK was 142 000 iu. Fasciotomy was performed. Myoglobinuria persisted for 4 days. There was some residual muscle injury, requiring the use of a short leg-brace. The second case, a 70-year-old female, was affected by CO leaking from a stove and causing diffuse soreness in both arms and legs, which had been present for one week. On admission, *s*CPK was 29 000 iu, and she was later noted to have amber coloured urine. The *s*CPK rose to 60 000 iu and then decreased promptly. There was transient renal failure from which she recovered.

Durocher et al. (1980) described 3 cases of CO-induced rhabdomyolysis in males aged, respectively, 21, 31 and 32 years. They developed muscle tenderness with increased activities of *s*AST, *s*ALT, *s*LDH and *s*CPK (maximum values were, respectively, 750, 400, 2550 and 22 000 iu). One subject developed oliguria. Coma was present in two, and pressure necrosis may have been a significant factor in producing rhabdomyolysis.

When coma occurs in CO poisoning, then the associated localized pressure necrosis may be a contributing factor. However, the formation of carboxyhaemoglobin may lead to a diffuse myopathy if there is a sufficient degree of hypoxia. The following are relevant in assessing the influence of COHb-related hypoxia in the production of rhabdomyolysis.

1. A reversible decrease in rat myocardial cytochrome c oxidase activity occurs with exposure to CO (Pankow and Ponsold, 1984).
2. Walum et al. (1985) noted that CO caused an inhibition of O_2 uptake by cultured heart cells by as much as 18% under the conditions of the study.
3. Degenerative changes have been demonstrated ultrastructurally in rabbit myocardium following exposure to 100 ppm CO for more than 4 hours; thus 100 ppm for 4 hours was regarded as the threshold for myocardial toxicity, and 180 ppm for 4 hours produced myocardial injury (Thomsen and Kjeldsen, 1974).
4. Brief (2 hours) high concentration (1500 ppm) exposures to CO induced increases in *s*LDH and *s*CPK, returning to control values within a few hours (Penney and Maziarka, 1976).

Toluene

Reisin et al. (1975) described severe myoglobinuria and ARF following acute exposure to toluene in a 49-year-old male. He was found unconscious in an enclosed space following exposure to toluene from a burst hose, 18 hours after the incident. He had burns over the shoulders and arms, and had possibly aspirated toluene. His urine was black and chemical pathology was: blood pH 7·33, BUN 7·6 mmol l^{-1}, *s*[creatinine] 371 μmol l^{-1} (and a urea N/creatinine ratio of 5), *s*[K^+] 7·4 mmol l^{-1}, and the urine gave a 3+ NH_4SO_4 test for myoglobin. Five days after admission the following values were observed: *s*AST 90 units, *s*CPK 53 units, *s*LDH 1196 units, and aldolase 7·2 units. He was given mannitol followed by furosemide to maintain diuresis, but subsequently developed ARF requiring haemodialysis. The relative contribution of rhabdomyolysis to the development of ARF is not clear in this case, since other reports indicate the potential for a direct nephrotoxic effect from toluene. For example, kidney injury has been described in association with solvent abuse by 'sniffing' which produces hallucinations, relaxation and tranquillity of several hours duration (Wyse, 1973); if high concentrations are inhaled this may lead to cardiac arrhythmias, pulmonary and cerebral oedema, hepatic injury and nephrotoxicity (Hayden et al., 1977; Musclow and Awen, 1977).

Patel and Benjamin (1986) described the case of a 32-year-old female who developed severe quadriparesis, hypokalaemia (1·6 mmol l^{-1}) with hyperchloraemic metabolic acidosis, and distal renal tubular acidosis following toluene sniffing for one week. There was no clinical or biochemical evidence of rhabdomyolysis. She was treated with iv normal saline, KCl, $NaHCO_3$, and calcium gluconate for transient tetany with hypocalaemia. There was complete recovery. This case further indicates the nephrotoxicity of toluene.

An association of distal renal tubular acidosis with toluene inhalation has also been described by Streicher et al. (1981), Taher et al. (1974) and Weinstein et al. (1985). Other nephropathies associated with toluene inhalation overexposure include nephrolithiasis (Kroeger et al., 1980; Weinstein et al., 1985), acute renal insufficiency (Will and McLaren, 1981), and abnormal urinalysis in the presence of normal renal function, including haematuria, pyuria and proteinuria (Streicher et al., 1981). Most cases of nephropathy are in patients who have inhaled toluene in high concentrations over short periods. Nephrotoxic inhaled concentrations are difficult to assess, but Nielsen et al., (1985) found that there were no significant changes in the urinary excretion rates of β_2-microglobulin and albumin in 43 male subjects exposed to 382 mg m^{-3} for 6·5 hours under controlled conditions.

The above findings indicate that rhabdomyolysis may occur in toluene intoxication, but apparently only secondary to pressure necrosis of muscle tissue during coma. However, in the more complex situation of paint sniffing (toluene-containing) Steichner et al. (1981) described rhabdomyolysis as a complication in 10 of 25 subjects. In 6, this occurred in the presence of hypokalaemia and hypophosphataemia, but in the remaining 4 these biochemical features were not present. This led the authors to suggest a possible direct myotoxic potential for toluene. Kidney injury in toluene poisoning is usually due to the direct nephrotoxicity of the material, rather than to rhabdomyolysis.

Methanol

Swartz et al. (1981) described increases in *s*CPK in several cases of methanol poisoning, and in one case myoglobinuria was suggested as a possible cause of mild renal insufficiency. Tephly and Martin (1984) note muscle pain as a symptom in some cases of methanol poisoning.

Grufferman et al. (1985) described a case of methanol poisoning with evidence for myoglobinuria and in which ARF developed. A 30-year-old man arrived at the hospital about 90 minutes after ingesting an estimated 700 ml of windshield washer in an attempted suicide. Initial chemical pathology was: normal BUN and creatine, *s*CPK 311 iu l^{-1} (normal 43–235), *s*[methanol] 410 mg dl^{-1}. He was treated with ethanol infusion (10 ml kg^{-1}, as 10% solution) and haemodialysis. On the second day he developed progressive oliguria and reddish-brown discoloured urine which was positive for blood in the absence of erythrocyturia. The urinary [myoglobin] was 600 mg l^{-1} and *s*CPK 435 iu l^{-1}. By the fifth day there was marked oliguria, BUN 56 mg dl^{-1}, and *s*[creatinine] 9·6 mg dl^{-1}; a renal sonogram showed bilateral kidney enlargement. Haemodialysis was then reinstituted. At this stage he discharged himself, but telephone enquiry one month later indicated he was feeling well and urinating normally. In relating the renal failure to rhabdomyolysis, it should be noted that this patient had a brief hypotensive episode because of volume depletion, and at the same time he was mildly hypokalaemic and slightly acidotic (arterial blood pH 7·32).

Methanol-induced rhabdomyolysis is probably rare, since it is not described in several extensive reviews on the clinical toxicology of methanol (e.g. Becker, 1983).

Methylene Chloride

Milles et al (1985) described the case of a 19-year-old male who worked for 2 days in a poorly ventilated room with tile remover containing methylene chloride. He developed nausea, vomiting, anorexia, abdominal pain and oliguria. An intravenous pyelogram showed a dense and prolonged nephrogram, consistent with acute tubular necrosis, which was confirmed by renal biopsy. A technetium Tc 99 m pentetic acid renal flow and scan demonstrated poor visualization of the kidney, and a sodium iodohippurate ^{131}I renogram showed persistent visualization, again consistent with acute tubular necrosis. Peak chemical pathology was *s*ALT 2320 units l^{-1}, *s*CPK 280 units l^{-1}, *s*LDH 3000 units l^{-1}, *s*AST 2500 units l^{-1}, alkaline phosphatase 162 units l^{-1}, total billirubin 2·8 mg dl^{-1}, urine positive for myoglobin. He gradually recovered and was discharged on the fourteenth day. This is a suggestive, but not proven, case of rhabdomyolysis.

p-Phenylenediamine

p-Phenylenediamine (PPDA) is commonly used as a cosmetic hair dye and has a wide range of industrial applications. Its toxicity has been reviewed in detail (Report, 1985).

The occurrence of ARF in acute PPDA poisoning has been described by several authors, but it is not clear if this was due to a direct nephrotoxic effect, secondary to haemolysis and methaemoglobinaemia, or resulted from the muscle injury (Chugh et al., 1982; El-Ansary et al., 1983).

Baud et al. (1983) described 2 cases of accidental ingestion of PPDA which had contaminated hair dye, and in whom rhabdomyolysis and ARF developed. The first case was that of a 50-year-old male who accidentally swallowed PPDA-containing hair dye, and within 3 hours developed epigastric pain and facial oedema. Within 2 hours, he developed severe respiratory failure and the oedema spread to the neck, trunk and arms. Urine became dark brown and ARF developed. Myoglobin (urine) was 45 nmol l^{-1}. Muscle biopsy from the deltoid at 24 hours after admission showed massive muscle necrosis. Maximum enzyme activities were *s*CPK 114 600 iu l^{-1}, *s*AST 5840 iu l^{-1}, *s*LDH 14 100 iu l^{-1}, which began to fall by 7 days and were near normal by 24 days. He developed anuria, requiring haemodialysis, and died on day 25 from sepsis. The second case, a 48-year-old female, drank a significantly lesser amount of the same fluid and developed epigastric pain, but no oedema. There was slight increase in *s*CPK on day 4. Renal function remained normal.

It has been demonstrated experimentally that degenerative changes occur in the muscles of rats given dimethyl-*p*-phenylenediamine by subcutaneous injection (Jasmin and Gareau, 1981). The lesions developed within 24 hours, consisting of swelling and homogenization of muscle fibres followed by fragmentation and coagulation necrosis with a histiocytic reaction and the formation of multinucleated giant cells. There was a significant reduction in succinic dehydrogenase and NADH:tetrazolium reductase activities in the degenerating muscle fibres. Regenerative changes occurred which paralleled the severity of the damage, and by 20 days healing was complete without fibrosis. However, in the myocardium there was a granular degeneration which appeared by the third day, and which became fibrotic. Meijer and Israel (1979) also studied skeletal muscle injury following subcutaneous dimethyl-*p*-phenylenediamine (20 mg kg^{-1}, twice daily on 5 consecutive days). On the fourth day there was coagulation necrosis, fragmentation and disintegration of fibres, with an inflammatory infiltrate between the muscle fibres; this reaction reached a peak at 7 to 9 days and thereafter subsided. Histochemically, the activity of acid phosphatase, β-glucuronidase, and E-600 resistant non-specific esterase was increased in both a granular and diffuse pattern in skeletal muscle; a less marked increase in granular leucine aminopeptidase occurred. The increased activity of acid hydrolases was parallel to the severity of the pathology and was maximum at 7 to 9 days. There was no difference in either the activity or localization of acid hydrolases of Type I and Type II fibres.

Organophosphate Anticholinesterases

As a consequence of their peripheral and central anticholinesterase activities, organophosphates produce a clinical picture of muscarinic and nicotinic cholinergic crisis, some of the major features of which include excess lachrymal, salivary and respiratory tract secretions, miosis, vomiting, muscle weakness progressing to paralysis, respiratory difficulties, bradycardia, muscle twitching, convulsions and coma. As a result of convulsions and coma it might be expected that rhabdomyolysis would be a complication of acute anticholinesterase poisoning; however, this is not frequently seen as a typical clinical finding (Albright, 1984). There is evidence from experimental studies and clinical cases of poisoning that organophosphate anticholinesterases may produce skeletal muscle necrosis. Thus, in the rat it has been shown that cholinesterase inhibition produces a skeletal muscle fibre necrosis (Wecker and Detbarn, 1976; Wecker et al., 1978). Detbarn (1984) found that the organophosphates soman, paroxon and phospholine induced a dose-related necrosis of rat skeletal muscle in concentrations that caused cholinergic effects. The number of fibres affected was greatest with soman. Necrosis healed within a week. Atropine and gentamicin in concentrations not blocking neuromuscular transmission attenuated the necrotic effect of organophosphates by interaction with the presympatic Ca^{++} uptake mechanism.

DeReuck and Willems (1975) reported the case of an individual who died 9 days after ingesting parathion. The diaphragm showed patchy and focal necrosis with some areas having degeneration of muscle fibres. Wecker et al. (1986) reported a 51-year-old male who became contaminated from spraying an organophosphate mixture. On admission he was unconscious, unresponsive and had increased muscle tone and neuromuscular excitability. The serum cholinesterase activity was 0·79 iu l^{-1} (normal 3·42). He subsequently developed cardiac arrest and died on the fourth day. The intercostal muscle showed acetylcholinesterase activity decreased to 53% of control activity, and histologically there were scattered necrotic fibres.

Although rhabdomyolysis-associated ARF has not been reported in acute organophosphate poisoning, renal involvement has been described. Albright et al. (1983) presented the case of a 65-year-old male who developed renal insufficiency with proteinuria 3 weeks after exposure to intense malathion spraying. This resolved without requiring specific treatment. A renal biopsy showed a membranous glomerulonephropathy. This coupled with a marginal decrease in C3 suggested antigenic exposure with subsequent immune complex deposition in the kidney. Wedin et al (1984) described a 26-year-old male who ingested dimpylate and developed decreased urine output and several days of crystalluria. The nature of the crystals was not defined, and the causal relationship between poisoning and crystalluria is questionable. Also, the initial low urine volume was probably a reflection of volume depletion rather than nephrotoxicity.

The available evidence suggests that typical rhabdomyolysis must be rare in cases of organophosphate anticholinesterase poisoning, although massive doses may cause focal myonecrosis. Renal involvement is probably due to toxicity of the parent material and/or metabolite(s).

Lindane

Lindane (gamma-hexachlorocyclohexane; HCH) is a highly liposoluble insecticide, which is rapidly absorbed and distributed. It is a known cause of convulsions, hepatic necrosis, renal failure and aplastic anaemia. Several cases of rhabdomyolysis associated with HCH poisoning have been presented.

Munk and Nantel (1977) described the case of a 35-year-old male who ingested lindane-contaminated food (estimated as approximately 15–30 ml HCH). Within 30 minutes he developed *grand mal* seizures which recurred over a 2-hour period. On admission he was severely acidaemic: arterial blood pH 6·57, $[HCO_3^-]$ 1·7 mmol l^{-1} (normal 24–28), $[Na^+]$ 147 mmol l^{-1}, $[K^+]$ 4·3 mmol l^{-1}, $[Cl^-]$ 106 mmol l^{-1}, *s*ALT 57 iu l^{-1} (normal 5–19), *s*LDH 240 iu l^{-1} (normal 29–92). By the fourth day he had developed muscle weakness and pain (predominantly proximal), myoglobinuria and acute renal failure. On the fifth day the *s*CPK activity was 35 000 iu l^{-1} (normal 0–130). Pancreatitis developed on the fifteenth day of illness. A left deltoid muscle biopsy on the fifteenth day showed widespread necrosis with regeneration. His condition improved and he was discharged on the twenty-fourth day.

Jaeger et al. (1984) reported 6 cases of peroral poisoning with a lindane-solvent mixture in which rhabdomyolysis developed in one subject who ingested 100 g of the mixture. By 90 minutes he was unresponsive, agitated and convulsive. After receiving diazepam, tremor and muscle twitching were still present. He was therefore given suxamethonium, thiopental, and put on assisted ventilation. On admission chemical pathology was; pH 6·72, $s[K^+]$ 7·6 mmol l^{-1}, BUN 21 mg dl^{-1}, and WBC 24 000 mm^{-3}. He was given bicarbonate, and by 8 hours values were, pH 7·35, $s[K^+]$ 2·9 mmol l^{-1}, *s*CPK 832 iu l^{-1}, *s*AST 35 iu l^{-1}, *s*ALT 17 iu l^{-1}, *s*LDH 500 iu l^{-1}. At 3 days there was a peak *s*CPK of 82 500 iu l^{-1} and *s*[myoglobin] was 2292 ng ml^{-1} at 5 days. He subsequently made a recovery without dialysis.

Kurt et al. (1986) described 5 cases of accidental acute HCH ingestion, and in one rhabdomyolysis developed. However, this case was complicated by aspiration during vomiting after ipaecac, seizures and anoxic brain damage.

The case reports would indicate that there may be clinical and biochemical evidence of rhabdomyolysis following acute peroral HCH poisoning, and that this is probably a consequence of associated convulsions.

Triethylene Tetramine

Triethylene tetramine is a copper chelator, and has been used as an alternative in the treatment of Wilson's disease. Epstein and Sherlock (1980) described rhabdomyolysis in a patient in whom triethylene tetramine dihydrochloride (Trien) was used as an alternative to penicillamine in primary biliary cirrhosis. Rhabdomyolysis developed within 48 hours of receiving a 400 mg dose. The patient complained of hand cramps on the day of dosing, and during the second day developed severe muscle pain in both gastrocnemii and lesser pain in the shoulder and pelvic muscle groups. There was associated muscle tenderness and weakness. There was no ARF, but *s*AST increased to 315 iu l^{-1} and *s*CPK to 9100 iu l^{-1}; myoglobinuria was present. Over the ensuing week, without Trien, the weakness and myalgia resolved and *s*CPK and *s*ALT activities decreased to pretreatment levels. Three other patients receiving Trien did not develop rhabdomyolysis, and the fact that the affected patient had a previous history of 'non-specific' myopathy may be relevant in this respect.

Mercuric Chloride

Acute mercuric chloride poisoning is well known to produce direct renal tubular injury (Schreiner and Maher, 1965; Bank et al., 1967). Chugh et al (1978b) presented a case of acute mercuric chloride poisoning in which ARF developed and where rhabdomyolysis may have been a contributing factor. The patient, a 22-year-old male, ingested 2 g of mercuric chloride in a suicide attempt. He vomited, had haematemesis, and developed fluid imbalance. On the third day he was observed to be oliguric. Relevant amongst a series of investigations 8 days after poisoning were: $s[K^+]$ 6·0 mmol l^{-1}, s[phosphate] 4·39 mmol l^{-1}, $s[Ca^{++}]$ 2·13 mmol l^{-1}, *s* aldolase 84 SL units ml^{-1}, *s*LDH 463 iu l^{-1} (normal 70–240), *s*CPK 104 Sigma units ml^{-1} (normal 0–12), serum urea N 43 mmol l^{-1}, and the urine was positive for myoglobin. He was treated with iv fluids (bicarbonate and dextrose), calcium gluconate and insulin, and renal function slowly returned to normal over several days. Left leg muscle biopsy showed a varying degree of 'basiphilic regeneration'.

Potassium Cyanide

Although convulsion is a common clinical feature of severe acute cyanide poisoning, rhabdomyolysis appears not to have been frequently reported (Ballantyne, 1987). However, Brivet et al. (1983) described the case of a 43-year-old male who swallowed a 'capsule' of potassium cyanide and developed signs of severe acute cyanide poisoning, including coma, convulsions, cardiac arrest and lactate acidosis. He was treated symptomatically; O_2, volume expansion, $NaHCO_3^-$ and anticonvulsants. About 20 hours after ingestion of the KCN, he described a pain in the right leg and partial paralysis of the first toe. At this time the *s*CPK was 13 260 iu l^{-1} and *s*AST 519 iu l^{-1}. He was discharged on the third day.

SUMMARY

A variety of therapeutic substances, industrial chemicals and domestically available materials have been shown to be capable of causing rhabdomyolysis. In general, and principally because of the current reporting and documenting procedures, the evidence is most complete and convincing for rhabdomyolysis induced by therapeutic substances. Implied in this is a probability that rhabdomyolysis is more common with industrially and domestically encountered chemicals than is currently appreciated, and it is likely that the incidence is greater with chemicals known to produce rhabdomyolysis and that a greater number of (as yet unknown) chemicals are capable of causing rhabdomyolysis. In view of the potentially life-threatening complications of rhabdomyolysis, and the fact that these may be avoided by the early clinical and biochemical recognition of the disease state, there is adequate justification to plead for reporting of definitive or highly suspect cases.

From a pathogenic viewpoint, rhabdomyolysis may be classified as primary and secondary. Primary rhabdomyolysis is due to a direct effect of the causative agent on muscle leading to membrane leak, abnormal ion and enzyme fluxes, and subsequently degenerative and necrotic changes in the fibre; with such myotoxicity there is usually a clear dose-response relationship. Secondary rhabdomyolysis occurs when the primary effect(s) of a chemical results in a functional or biochemical state which is conducive to the development of ischaemic, degenerative, necrotic or membrane destabilizing changes in muscle, producing the clinical and biochemical features of rhabdomyolysis. Most frequently rhabdomyolysis is secondary to a metabolic derangement, a result of abnormally excessive movement, excessive isometric tension by attempted movement against resistance, or coma leading to increased intramuscular pressure, ischaemia, hypoxia and necrosis. In some circumstances where a material is both myotoxic and a convulsant or narcotic, rhabdomyolysis may be a compounded effect from both primary and secondary mechanisms. In other cases the mechanism by which a particular material produces a well defined rhabdomyolytic response is unknown.

The onset of xenobiotic-induced rhabdomyolysis will depend on the clinical and pharmacological nature of the material, the circumstances of poisoning and the presence of any precipitating factors. The most clearly defined onset-severity relationships, in terms of the magnitude of the absorbed dose, are with primary rhabdomyolytics. However, some of the most severe cases of rhabdomyolysis may be seen where there is a status epilepticus or where the subject has been comatose for several hours and suffered extensive pressure myonecrosis. In many circumstances there are no (obvious) precipitating factors, but in a few cases there may be a suggestion of the rhabdomyolytic process having been precipitated or its development facilitated by exercise or a preceeding subclinical myopathy. In certain circumstances the physician should be aware that there may be a predisposition to the development of rhabdomyolysis and its complications. Clear examples include exercise-induced muscle injury, particularly in hot environments, and malignant hyperthermia (or its variants) in those with clinical, biochemical or genetic evidence for a pre-existing myopathy. Although rhabdomyolysis may be obvious early in cases where a major aetiological factor is hyperkinetic movements or coma, and in some primary rhabdomyolytic processes such as those due to suxamethonium or opioids, in other circumstances there may be a significant delay to the onset of rhabdomyolysis and it may only occur when there have been multiple exposures over a period of many days or weeks; a typical example is that of rhabdomyolysis induced by epsilon-aminocaproic acid. The presentation, and nature and severity of the complications is variable, often depending on the cause of the rhabdomyolysis, the exposure dose (magnitude and frequency), the condition of the patient and circumstances of the poisoning. Some cases, for example one of the variants of alcoholic myopathy, may present with few signs and symptoms as a chronic myopathy. In most cases of xenobiotic-induced rhabdomyolysis, patients present with clinical, biochemical and metabolic features characteristic of the condition, but varying in severity. There will be progressive muscle weakness, tenderness, myalgia and, if injury is sufficient, there will also be obvious swelling due to oedema. The distribution of the muscle effects may vary considerably, depending to a large extent on causation. For example, with primary rhabdomyolytics there may be a diffuse effect, when hyperkinetic movements are present then the limbs will be mainly affected, and when there has been coma the muscular parts of the body subject to compression will be principally involved. As with other cases of rhabdomyolysis, there may be circulatory deficits or peripheral neuropathy due to increased osteofascial compartment pressure. Also, postnecrotic fibrous contractures may occur in the limbs.

The most life-threatening complications are electrolyte disturbances, ARF, cardiac disturbances and respiratory impairment. In most instances, due to K^+ leak from muscle, there will be a moderate to marked hyperkalaemia; the major exception is where rhabdomyolysis is caused by hypokalaemia due to kaluresis.

Phosphorous release produces a hyperphosphataemia, and calcium deposition in muscle leads to hypocalcaemia; during the diuretic phase of rhabdomyolysis-induced ARF there is frequently hypercalcaemia. Some cases may present with significant metabolic acidaemia, and the muscle injury with oedema may lead to a significant hypervolaemia. The cause of ARF in most cases of rhabdomyolysis is unknown, although the increased loads of uric acid and myoglobin may contribute. Factors influencing the probability of acute renal tubular necrosis include the mass of muscle injured, the occurrence of hypotension, and the development of hypovolaemia. The ARF of rhabdomyolysis is potentially reversible, and its anticipation and early diagnosis are important to avoid the development of acute tubular necrosis. Most cardiac effects are a consequence of electrolyte changes and result in atrial and ventricular arrhythmias, conduction delays and bundle branch blocks with non-specific S-T segment and T-wave abnormalities. Potentially cardioplegic hyperkalaemia may develop. A few xenobiotics may produce myocardial injury and the development of signs and symptoms attributable to cardiomyopathy. When there is respiratory muscle involvement in the rhabdomyolytic process there may be difficulty with breathing, ranging from dyspnoea to respiratory paralysis requiring artificial ventilation. In a few cases there may be evidence, often transient, of a disseminated intravascular coagulation syndrome.

The laboratory diagnosis of rhabdomyolysis may be established by measurement of serum enzyme activities and the detection in serum and urine of myoglobin. Serum enzymes which are particularly valuable to establishing a diagnosis are CPK, LDH (with isozyme fractionation), ALT and aldolase. Specific sensitive methods now exist for the quantitative detection of myoglobin in urine and serum. However, in their absence, valuable confirmation of the presence of myoglobin can be obtained by the finding of a positive *o*-toluidine test for haem in the absence of erythrocyturia and when serum is clear and unstained. Serial measurements of enzyme activities and myoglobin concentrations can be used to follow the progression and regression of skeletal muscle injury. Other biochemical features include hyperuricaemia, increased serum creatinine and, in the absence of severe renal failure, a marked decrease in the [BUN]/[creatinine] ratio. Biopsy of clinically affected muscle will show degenerative and necrotic changes with phagocytosis, but no vascular pathology. The EMG generally shows non-specific myopathic effects.

In the management of cases of rhabdomyolysis it is essential to monitor for the degree of muscle involvement and whether it is progressing, and also for the development of complications. In this respect it is important (though by no means exclusive) to monitor the following: serial serum enzyme activities and urine/serum myoglobin, $s[K^+]$, $s[Ca^{++}]$, $s[PO_4^{3-}]$, $s[HCO_3^-]$, blood pH, *s*[urea], *s*[uric acid], urine volume and colour, and ECG. With xenobiotic-induced rhabdomyolysis it is important to recognize and prevent further exposure to the causative drug or chemical. Specific treatment for the xenobiotic involved is required. However, some general principles of antidotal treatment may require to be modified if they are likely to enhance rhabdomyolysis or precipitate any complication, e.g. the avoidance of acidification of urine in PCP intoxication. With respect to the specific treatment of rhabdomyolysis the first important requirement is to rapidly correct any fluid and acid-base derangements. This is an extremely important part of the initial phase of management in order to avoid hypotension and reduce the potential for ARF. Hydration and, in most cases, bicarbonate are essential. The use of mannitol and frusemide, along with fluid replacement and alkalinization of urine, have been found to be useful to increase renal intratubular pressure, flush out debris and minimize the likelihood for development of acute renal tubular necrosis. The correction of hyperkalaemia is important at the earliest opportunity possible, and if there is a severe degree of hyperkalaemia then any associated hypocalcaemia should be treated. Should ARF develop then treatment should be along conventional lines; however, if there has been extensive rhabdomyolysis, then peritoneal dialysis may be inadequate. Also required may be fasciotomy if there are indications that excess osteofascial compartment pressures are developing, and that vascular and neurological complications could develop.

REFERENCES

Abourizk N., Khalil B. A., Bahuth N. et al. (1979) Clofibrate-induced muscular syndrome. *J. Neurol. Sci.* **42**, 1–9.

Abraham A. A., Veronesi B., Alleva F. R. et al. (1986) Ultrastructural changes in skeletal muscles of rats treated neonatally with 6-mercaptopurine. *Toxicol. Ind. Health* **2**, 41–50.

Abreo K., Shelp W. D., Koseff A. et al. (1982). Amoxaphine-associated rhabdomyolysis and acute renal failure: case report. *J. Clin. Psychiatry* **43**, 426–427.

Ahte E. L. and Buncum B. E. G. (1974) Metoclopramide induces catalepsy and increases striatal homovanillic acid content in mice. *Arch. Pharmacol. Toxicol.* **35**, 429–432.

Airaksinen M. M. and Tammisto T. (1966) Myoglobinuria after intermittent administration of succinylcholine during halothane anesthesia. *Clin. Pharmacol. Ther.* **7**, 583–587.

Akmal A. and Massry S. G. (1983) Peripheral nerve damage in patients with non-traumatic rhabdomyolysis. *Arch. Intern. Med.* **143**, 835–836.

Akmal M., Goldstein D. A., Telfer N. et al. (1978) Resolution of muscle calcification in rhabdomyolysis and acute renal failure. *Ann. Intern. Med.* **89**, 928–930.

Akmal M., Valdin J. R., McCarron M. M. et al. (1981) Rhabdomyolysis with and without acute renal failure in patients with phencyclidine intoxication. *Am. J. Nephrol.* **1**, 91–96.

Albright R. K. (1984) Letter to Editor. *JAMA* **252**, 1408.

Albright R. K., Kram B. W. and White R. P. (1983) Malathion exposure associated with acute renal failure. *JAMA* **250**, 2469.

Aldrete J. A., Padfield A., Solomon C. C. et al (1971) Possible predictive test for malignant hyperpyrexia during anesthesia. *JAMA* **215**, 1465.

Alleva F. R., Haberman, B. H., Slaughter L. J. et al. (1981) Muscular degeneration in rats after postnatal treatment with 6-mercaptopurine. *Drug Chem. Toxicol.* **4**, 133–146.

Allera F. R., Slaughter L. J., Abraham A. A. et al. (1986) Toxicological studies with 6-mercaptopurine in neonates. *Toxicol. Ind. Health* **2**, 11–23.

Andersson O., Berglund G. and Hansson L. (1976) Anti-hypertensive action, time of onset and effects on carbohydrate metabolism of labetol. *Br. J. Clin. Pharmacol. Suppl.* **3**, 757–761.

Anderson R., Cohen M., Haller R. et al. (1980) Skeletal muscle phosphorus and magnesium deficiency in alcoholic myopathy. *Mineral Electrolyte Metab.* **4**, 106–112.

Anderson R. J., Reed G. and Knochel J. (1983) Heatstroke. *Adv. Intern. Med.* **28**, 115–140.

Aronow R. and Done A. K. (1978) Phencyclidine overdose: An emergency concept of management. *J. Am. Coll. Emerg. Phys.* **7**, 56–59.

Auerbach V. H., DiGeorge A. M., Mayer B. W. et al. (1973) Rhabdomyolysis and hyperpyrexia in children after administration of succinylcholine. In: *International Symposium on Malignant Hyperthermia*, 30. Illinois: Thomas.

Ayer G., Grandchamp A. and Truniger B. (1971). Intrarenal hemodynamics in glycerol-induced myochemoglobinuric acute renal failure in the rat. *Circ. Res.* **29**, 128–135.

Balducci L., Collier B., Markov A. et al. (1986) Skeletal muscle changes during chronic doxorubicin administration. *J. Exptl. Clin. Cancer Res.* **5**, 155–164.

Ballantyne B. (1987) Toxicology of Cyanides. In: Ballantyne B. and Marrs T. C. (ed.) *Clinical and Experimental Toxicology of Cyanides*. 41–126. Bristol: Wright.

Bank N., Mutz B. F. and Aynedjion N. H. S. (1967) The role of leakage of tubular fluid in anuria due to mercury poisoning. *J. Clin. Invest.* **46**, 695.

Bank W. J., DiMauro S., Bonella E. et al. (1975) A disorder of muscle lipid metabolism and myoglobinuria. Absence of carnitine palmityltransferase. *N. Engl. J. Med.* **292**, 443–449.

Bannister B., Ginsburg R. and Shneerson J. (1977) Cardiac arrest due to liquorice-induced hypokalaemia. *Br. Med. J.* **2**, 738–739.

Baraka A. (1968) Effect of halothane on tubocurarine and suxamethonium block in man. *Br. J. Anaesth.* **40**, 602.

Baraka A. (1977). Self-taming of succinylcholine-induced fasculations. *Anesthesiology* **46**, 292–293.

Barnes P. C. and Leonard J. H. C. (1971) Hypokalemic myopathy and myoglobinuria due to carbenoxolone sodium. *Postgrad. Med. J.* **47**, 813–814.

Barton C. H., Sterling M. L. and Vaziri N. D. (1980) Rhabdomyolysis and acute renal failure associated with phencyclidine intoxication. *Arch. Intern. Med.* **140**, 568–569.

Bateman D. N. and Gokal R. (1980) Metoclopramide in renal failure. *Lancet* **1**, 982.

Baud F., Bismuth Ch., Galliot M. et al. (1983) Rhabdomyolysis in para-phenylenediamine intoxication. *Lancet* **ii**, 514.

Becker C. E. (1983) Methanol poisoning. *J. Emerg. Med.* **1**, 51–58.

Bennett J. R. (1972). Myopathy from E-aminocaproic acid: a second case. *Postgrad. Med. J.* **48**, 440–442.

Bennett H. S., Spiro A. J., Pollack M. A. et al. (1982) Ipecac-induced myopathy simulating dermatomyositis. *Neurology* **32**, 91–94.

Bennike K. A. and Jarnum S. (1964) Myoglobinuria with acute renal failure possibly induced by suxamethonium. A case report. *Br. J. Anaesth.* **36**, 730–736.

Bergin J. J. (1966) The complications of therapy with epsilon-aminocaproic acid. *Med. Clin. North Am.* **50**, 1669–1678.

Berman P. H., Nigro M. A. and Harris M. B. (1973) Activation of fibrinolysis in muscular dystrophy. *Arch. Neurol.* **29**, 65–66.

Bernhardt D. and Hoerder M. H. (1978) Anesthesia-induced myoglobinuria without hyperpyrexia—an abortive form of malignant hyperthermia? In: Aldrete J. A. and Britt B. A. (ed.) *Malignant Hyperthermia*, 419–425. New York: Grune and Stratton.

Best M. M. and Duncan C. H. (1966) Effect of clofibrate and dextrothyroxine singly and in combination on serum lipids. *Arch. Intern. Med.* **118**, 97–102.

Bianchine J. R. (1985) Drugs for Parkinson's disease, spasticity, and acute muscle spasms. In: *Goodman and Gilman's The Pharmacological Basis of Therapeutics*. Ed. Gilman A. G., Goodman L. S. and Ralland T. W., Murad F. pp. 487–488. New York, Macmillan.

Bichet D. G., Levi M. and Schrier R. W. (1985) Polyuria, dehydration, and overhydration. In: Seldin D. N. and Giebisch G. (ed.) *The Kidney, Physiology and Pathophysiology*, 851–894. New York: Raven Press.

Bindoff L. and Cullen M. J. (1978) Experimental (-) emetine myopathy. Ultrastructural and morphometric observations. *J. Neurol. Sci.* **39**, 1–15.

Biswas C. K., Reid Milligan D. A., Agte S. D. et al. (1980) Acute renal failure and myopathy after treatment with aminocaproic acid. *Br. Med. J.* **281**, 115–116.

Black W. D. and Murphy W. M. (1984) Nontraumatic rhabdomyolysis and acute renal failure associated with oral phenmetrazine hydrochloride. *J. Tennessee Med. Assoc.* **77**, 80–81.

Blain P. G., Lane R. J. M., Bateman D. N. et al. (1985) Opiate-induced rhabdomyolysis. *Human Toxicol.* **4**, 71–74.

Blessing W. and Walsh J. C. (1977) Myotonia precipitated by propanolol therapy. *Lancet* **1**, 73–74.

Blick K. E. and Liles S. M. (1985) *Principles of Clinical Chemistry*. New York: Wiley.

Bolli P. and Wool-Manning H. J. (1977) Treatment of hypertension with labetol. *NZ. Med. J.* **86**, 557–563.

Bolthauser E., Steinmann B., Meyer A. et al. (1980) Anaesthesia-induced rhabdomyolysis in Duchenne muscular dystrophy. *Br. J. Anaesth.* **52**, 559.

Bon C. and Jeng T.-W. (1979) Crotoxin: a possible mechanism of action. In: Ceccarelli B. and Clementi F. (ed.) *Avances in Cytopharmacology*, Vol. 3, 231. New York: Raven Press.

Bonnici F. (1973) Antidiuretic effect of clofibrate and carbamazepine in diabetes insipidus—studies on free water clearance and response to water load. *Clin. Endocrinol.* **2**, 265–267.

Bowden D. H., Frazer D. and Jackson S. H. (1956) Acute recurrent rhabdomyolysis (paroxysmal myoglobinuria). *Medicine* **35**, 335–353.

Boyd J. F. (1987) Fatal rhabdomyolysis in marathon runner. *Lancet* **1**, 1089.

Boyd R. E., Brennan P. T., Deng J. F. et al (1983) Strychnine poisoning. Recovery from profound lactic acidosis, hyperthermia, and rhabdomyolysis. *Am. J. Med.* **74**, 507–512.

Bradley W. S., Fewings J. D., Harris J. B. et al. (1976) Emetine myopathy in the rat. *Br. J. Pharmacol.* **57**, 29–41.

Braun S. R. (1970) Evaluation of the renal toxicity of heme proteins and their derivatives: A role in the genesis of acute tubule necrosis. *J. Exp. Med.* **131**, 443–460.

Bridgman C. J. F., Rosen S. M. and Thorp J. M. (1972) Complications during clofibrate treatment of nephrotic-syndrome hyperlipoproteinaemia. *Lancet*, **11**, 506–509.

Britt B. A. (1973) Prevention of malignant hyperthermia. In: Gordon R. A., Britt B. A. and Kalow W. (ed.) *International Symposium on Malignant Hyperthermia*. Springfield, Ill: Thomas.

Britt B. A. (1984) Dantrolene—a review. *Can. Anaesth. Soc. J.* **31**, 61–75.

Britt B. A. and Kalow W. (1970) Malignant hyperthermia: a statistical review. *Can. Anaesth. Soc. J.* **17**, 293–315.

Britt C. W., Light R. L., Peters B. H. et al. (1980) Rhabdomyolysis during treatment with epsilon-aminocaproic acid. *Neurology* **37**, 187–188.

Brivet F., Delfraissy J. F., Duche M. et al. (1983) Acute cyanide poisoning: recovery with non-specific supportive therapy.l *Intensive Care Med.* **9**, 33–35.

Brodkin H. M. (1980) Myoglobinuria following epsilon-aminocaproic acid (EACA) therapy. *J. Neurosurg.* **53**, 690–692.

Brotman M. C., Forbath N., Garfinkel P. E. et al. (1981) Myopathy due to ipecac syrup poisoning in a patient with anorexia nervosa. *Can. Med. Assoc. J.* **125**, 453–454.

Brown C. and Osterloh J. (1987) Multiple severe complications from recreational ingestion of MDMA ('Ectasy'). *JAMA* **258**, 780–781.

Brown J. A., Wollmann R. L. and Mullan S. (1982) Myopathy induced by epsilon-aminocaproic acid. Case report. *J. Neurosurg.* **57**, 130–134.

Browne P. M. (1979). Rhabdomyolysis and myoglobinuria associated with acute water intoxication. *West J. Med.* **130**, **459.**

Buckle R. M. (1965) Exceptional (march) haemoglobinuria: reduction of haemolytic episodes by the use of sorbo-rubber soles. *Lancet* **1**, 1136–1138.

Burns R. S., Lerner S. E., Corrado R. J. James S. H. et al. Phencyclidine—states of acute irritation and fatalities. *West. J. Med.* **123**, 345.

Butikofer E. and Molleyeres J. (1968). Akute ischamische Muskelnekrosen revisible Muskelverbalkungen and sekundare Hypercaliamie bei akuter Anurie. *Schweiz. Med. Wochenschr.* **98**, 961–965.

Bywaters E. G. L. (1944) Ischemic muscle necrosis. *JAMA* **124**, 1103–1109.

Bywaters E. G. L. and Beall D. (1941) Crush injuries with impairment of renal functions. *Br. Med. J.* **1**, 427–432.

Bywaters E. G. L., Delroy G. E., Remington C. et al. (1941) Myohaemoglobin in urine of air raid casualties with crushing injuries. *Biochem.* J. **35**, 1164–1168.

Cadnapaphornchai P., Taher S. and McDonald F. D. (1980) Acute drug-associated rhabdomyolysis: an examination of its diverse renal manifestations and complications. *Am. J. Med. Sci.* **280**, 66–72.

Campion D. S., Arias J. M. and Carter N. W. (1972) Rhabdomyolysis and myoglobinuria. Association with hypokalemia of renal tubular acidosis. *JAMA* **220**, 967–969.

Carballo A. S. (1975) Aborted malignant hyperthermia: case report. *Can. Anaesth. Soc. J.* **22**, 227–231.

Caroff S. N. (1980) The neuroleptic malignant syndrome. *J. Clin. Psychiatry* **41**, 79–83.

Carter S. K. (1975) Adriamycin—a review. *J. Natl Canc. Inst.* **55**, 1265–1274.

Chaikin H. L. (1980) Rhabdomyolysis secondary to drug overdose and prolonged coma. *South. Med. J.* **73**, 990–994.

Chang C. C. and Lee J. D. (1977) Crotoxin, the neurotoxin of South American rattlesnake venom, is a presynaptic toxin acting like B-bungarotoxin. Nzunyn-Scheidebergs *Arch. Pharmacol.* **296**, 159.

Chen G., Ensor R., Russell D. et al. (1959). The pharmacology of 1,(1-phenylcyclohexyl)piperidine HCl. *J. Pharmacol. Exper. Therap.* **127**, 241–250.

Chowdhury U. M., Carey P. C. and Hussein M. M. (1979) Prevention of early recurrence of spontaneous subarachnoid hemorrhage by E Amino-caproic acid. *Lancet*, **1**, 741–743.

Chugh K. S., Malik G. M. and Singhal P. C. (1982) Acute renal failure following para-phenylene diamine (hair dye) poisoning. Report of two cases. *J. Med.* **13**, 131–137.

Chugh K. S., Singhal P. C. and Khatri G. K. (1978a) Rhabdomyolysis and renal failure following status asthmaticus. *Chest* **73**, 879.

Chugh K. S., Singhal P. C., Nath I. V. S. et al. (1979) Acute renal failure due to non-traumatic rhabdomyolysis. *Postgrad. Med. J.* **55**, 386–392.
Chug K. S., Singhal P. C. and Uberoi H. S. (1978b) Rhabdomyolysis and renal failure in acute mercuric chloride poisoning. *Med. J. Aust.* **2**, 125–126.
Clark J. G. and Sumerling M. D. (1966) Muscle necrosis and calcification in acute renal failure due to barbiturate intoxication. *Br. Med. J.* **2**, 214–215.
Clarkson A. R., MacDonald M. K., Fuster V. et al. (1970) Glomerular coagulation in acute ischaemic renal failure. *Q. J. Med.* **39**, 585–598.
Cogen F. L., Rigg G., Simmons J. L. et al. (1978) Phencyclidine-associated acute rhabdomyolysis. *Ann. Intern. Med.* **88**, 210–212.
Cumming W. J. K., Hardy M., Hudgson P. et al. (1976) Carnitine–parmityl–transferase deficiency. *J. Neurol. Sci.* **30**, 247–258.
Cunningham E., Kohli R. and Venuto R. C. (1979). Influenza-associated myoglobinuric renal failure. *JAMA* **242**, 2428.
D'Agostino R. S. and Arnette E. N. (1979) Acute myoglobinuria and heroin snorting. *JAMA* **24**, 277.
Demos M. A., Gitin E. L. and Kagen L. J. (1974) Exercise myoglobinemia and acute external rhabdomyolysis. *Arch. Intern. Med.* **134**, 669–673.
DeRuck J. and Willems J. (1975) Acute parathion poisoning: myopathic changes in the diaphragm. *J. Neurol.* **208**, 309–314.
Descamps C, Vandenbroucke J. M. and Ypersele de Strihou C. van (1977) Rhabdomyolysis and acute tubular necrosis associated with carbenoxolone and diuretic treatment. *Br. Med. J.* **1**, 272.
Dettbarn W-D. (1984). Pesticide induced muscle necrosis: mechanism and prevention. *Fund. Appl. Tox.* **4**, S18–S26.
Devereux S. and Knowles J. M. (1985) Rhabdomyolysis and acute renal failure in sickle-cell anaemia. *Br. Med. J.* **290**, 1707.
Dicken C. H. (1984) Retinoids: A review. *J. Am. Acad. Dermatol.* **11**, 541–552.
DiMauro S. and Melis-DiMauro P. M. (1973) Muscle carnitine palmityltransferase and myoglobinuria. *Science* **182**, 929–931.
Doroshow J. H. (1983) Effects of anthracycline antibiotics on oxygen radical formation in rat heart. *Cancer Res.* **43**, 460–472.
Doroshow J. H., Locker G. Y., Ifrim I. et al. (1981) Prevention of doxorubicin cardiac toxicity in the mouse by N-acetylcysteine. *J. Clin. Invest.* **68**, 1053–1064.
Doroshow J. H., Tallent C. and Schechter J. E. (1985) Ultrastructural features of adriamycin-induced skeletal and cardiac muscle toxicity. *Am. J. Pathol.* **118**, 288–297.
Drutz D. J., Fan J. H., Tai T. Y. et al. (1970) Hypokalemic rhabdomyolysis and myoglobinuria following amphotericin B Therapy. *JAMA* **211**, 824–826.
Duane D. D. and Engel A. G. (1970) Emetine myopathy. *Neurology* **20**, 733–738.
Duffy W. B., Senekjian H. O., Knight T. E. et al. (1981) Acute renal failure due to phenylpropanolamine. *South. Med. J.* **74**, 1548–1549.
Dukes M. N. G. (1980) Drugs affecting lipid metabolism. In: Dukes M. N. G. (ed.) *Meyler's Side Effects of Drugs*, 9th ed., 728–732. Amsterdam: Excerpta Medica.
Durocher A., Chopin C., Gosselin B. et al. (1980) Toxic and drug-induced rhabdomyolysis. *Rev. Med. Interne.* **1**. 223–226.
Eiser A. R., Neff M. S. and Slifkin R. F. (1982) Acute myoglobinuric renal failure. A consequence of the neuroleptic malignant syndrome. *Arch. Intern. Med.* **142**, 601–603.
El-Ansary E. H., Ahmed M. E. K. and Clague H. W. (1983) Systemic toxicity of paraphenylenediamine. *Lancet* **i**, 1341.
Elion G. B. (1986) Historical background of 6-mercaptopurine. *Toxicol. Ind. Health.* **2**, 1–9.
Foley R. J., Kapatikin K., Verani R. et al. (1984) Amphetamine-induced acute renal failure. *South. Med. J.* **77**, 258–259.
Forfar J. C., Brown G. J. and Cull R. E. (1979) Proximal myopathy during beta-blockage. *Br. Med. J.* **2**, 1331–1332.
Franz D. N. (1980) Central nervous system stimulants. In: Gilman A. H., Goodman L. S. and Gilman A. (ed.) *Goodman and Gilman's The Pharmacological Basis of Therapeutics*, 6th ed., 585–591. New York: Macmillan.
Fraser W. D., Gardner M. D. and Dryburgh F. J. (1986) Acute renal failure induced by rhabdomyolysis. *Br. Med. J.* **292**, 410.
Frendin T. J. and Swainson C. P. (1985) Acute renal failure secondary to non-traumatic rhabdomyolysis following amoxapine overdose. *N.Z. Med. J.* August, 690–691.

Friedman E. J. (1984) Death from ipecac intoxication in a patient with anorexia nervosa. *Am. J. Psychiatry* **141**, 702–703.
Fuller T. J., Carter N. W., Barcenas C. et al. (1976) Reversible experimental myopathy associated with phosphorus depletion. *J. Clin. Invest.* **57**, 1019.
Gabow P. A., Kaehny W. D. and Kelleher S. P. (1982) The spectrum of rhabdomyolysis. *Medicine* **61**, 141–152.
Geltner D., Shapiro M. and Chaco M. (1975) Reversible myopathy induced by clofibrate. *Postgrad. Med. J.* **51**, 184–185.
George C., Brun-Bruisson C., Amamon M. et al. (1979) Acute renal failure due to rhabdomyolysis in sickle-cell trait. *Intensive Care Med.* **2**, 204–205.
Geronemus R., Herz D. A. and Shulman K. (1974) Streptokinase clot lysis time in patients with ruptured intracranial aneurysms. *J. Neurosurg.* **40**, 499–503.
Gloetzner F. L., Planner M. and Gaab M. (1979) Creatine kinase in serum after *grand mal* seizures. *Europ. Neurol.* **18**, 399–404.
Goertz B., Kunst H. and Heitmann R. (1978). Toxische Rhabdomyolyse nach alkohol—und Medikametenvergiflungen. *Dtsch. Med. Wochemschr.* **103**, 121–123.
Good D. J. and Meltzer H. Y. (1975) The role of isometric muscle tension in the production of muscle toxicity by phencyclidine and restraint stress. *Psychopharmacologia* **42**, 105–108.
Gopalakrishnakone P., Dempster D., Hawgood B. et al. (1984) Cellular and mitochondrial changes induced in the structure of murine skeletal muscle by crotoxin, a neurtoxic phospholipase A_2 complex. *Toxicon* **2**, 85.
Gossel T. A. and Bricker J. D. (1984) *Principles of Clinical Toxicology*, 316–317. New York: Raven Press.
Gosselin R. E., Hodge H. C. and Smith R. P. (1976) *Clinical Toxicology of Commercial Products*, 4th ed., 303–307. Baltimore: Williams and Wilkins.
Green K. G. and Margetts G. (1967) Long-term follow-up of multicentre trial of ethyl-α-p-chlorophenoxyisobutyrate (clofibrate, Atromid S) and clofibrate plus androsterone ('Atromid'). In: Kritchevsky D., Paoletti R. and Steinberg D. (ed.) *Progress in Biochemical Pharmacology, Vol. 2.*, 378–392. Basel: Karger.
Greenberg J. and Arneson L. (1967) Exertional rhabdomyolysis with myoglobinuria in a large group of military trainees. *Neurology* **17**, 216–222.
Greenwood R. J. (1974) Lumbar plexitis and rhabdomyolysis following abuse of heroin. *Postgrad Med. J.* **50**, 772–773.
Gross E. G., Dexter J. D. and Roth R. G. (1966) Hypokalemic myopathy with myoglobinuria associated with licorice ingestion. *N. Engl. J. Med.* **274**, 602–606.
Grossman H. H. and Large H. (1968) Hypercalcemia in acute renal failure. *Ann. Intern. Med.* **69**, 1332.
Grossman R. A., Hamilton R. W., Morse B. M. et al. (1974) Non-traumatic rhabdomyolysis and acute renal failure. *New Engl. J. Med.* **291**, 807–811.
Grufferman S., Morris D. and Alvarez J. (1985) Methanol poisoning complicated by myoglobinuric failure. *Am. J. Emerg. Med.* **3**, 24–26.
Gutman R. A. (1986) Acute renal failure. In: Rakel R. L. (ed.) *Conn's Current Therapy*, 555–558. Philadelphia: Saunders.
Haapanen E., Pellinen T. J. and Bartanen J. (1984) Acute renal failure caused by alcohol-induced rhabdomyolysis. *Nephron* **36**, 191–193.
Haller R. G. and Drachman D. B. (1980) Alcoholic rhabdomyolysis: an experimental model in the rat. *Science* **208**, 412–414.
Hallgren R., Lundin L., Roxin L-E. et al. (1980) Serum and urinary myoglobin in alcoholics. *Acta Med. Scand.* **208**, 33–39.
Hampel G., Horstkotte H. and Rumpf K. W. (1983) Myoglobinuric renal failure due to drug induced rhabdomyolysis. *Human Toxicol.* **2**, 197–203.
Hart G. R., Anderson R. J., Crumpler C. P. et al. (1982) Epidemic classical heatstroke: Clinical characteristics and course of 28 patients. *Medicine* **61**, 189.
Harvey, S. C. (1980). Gastric antacids and digestants. In: Gilman A. G., Goodman L. S. and Gilman A. (ed.) *Goodman and Gilman's The Pharmacological Basis of Therapeutics*, 6th ed., 997. New York: Macmillan.
Harwood S. J., Cartou P. G. and Cole G. W. (1978) Creatine phosphokinase isoenzyme fractions in the serum of a patient struck by lightning. *Ann. Intern. Med.* **138**, 645–646.
Hashimoto F., Sherman C. B. and Jeffrey W. H. (1984) Neuroleptic malignant syndrome and dopaminergic blockade. *Arch. Intern. Med.* **144**, 629–630.

Hayden J. W., Peterson R. G. and Bruckner J. V. (1977) Toxicology of toluene (methylbenzene): review of current literature. *Clin. Toxicol.* **11**, 549–552.

Hed R., Lundmark C., Fahlgren H. et al. (1962) Acute muscular syndrome in chronic alcoholism. *Acta Med. Scand.* **171**, 585–599.

Henderson W. A. V. (1984) Succinylcholine-induced cardiac arrest in unsuspected Duchenne muscular dystrophy. *Can. Anesth. Soc. J.* **31**, 444–446.

Henderson V. W. and Wooten G. F. (1981) Neuroleptic malignant syndrome: a pathogenetic role for dopamine receptor blockade? *Neurology* **31**, 132–137.

Henrich W. L., Prophet D. and Knochel J. P. (1980) Rhabdomyolysis associated with *Escherichia coli* septicaemia. *South. Med. J.* **73**, 936–937.

Hodak E., Gadoth N., David M. et al. (1986) Muscle damage induced by isotretinon. *Br. Med. J.* **293**, 425–426.

Howell R. R. and Williams J. C. (1983). The glycogen storage diseases. In: Stanbury J. B., Wyngaarden J. B., Fredrickson, D. S. Goldstein J. L. and Brown M. S. (ed.) *The Metabolic Basis of Inherited Disease*, 5th ed., 141–166. New York: McGraw-Hill.

Howse A. J. G. and Seddon H. (1966) Ischaemic contracture of muscle associated with carbon monoxide and barbiturate poisoning. *Br. Med. J.* **1**, 192–195.

Hwang K. M., Yang L. C., Carrico C. K. et al. (1974) Production of membrane whorls in rat liver by some inhibitors of protein synthesis. *J. Cell. Biol.* **62**, 20–31.

Hyser C. L. and Drake M. E. Jr (1983) Myoclonus induced by metoclopramide therapy. *Arch. Intern. Med.* **143**, 2201–2202.

Iannaccone S. T. and Griggs R. C. (1981) Animal model for EACA-induced myopathy. *Muscle Nerve* **4**, 176.

Inagaki M., Koyama A., Sakata S. et al (1980) Changes in serum myoglobin levels due to succinylcholine administration during GOF (nitrous oxide-oxygen-halothane) anaesthesia. *Masui* **29**, 1476–1482.

Indo T. and Ando K. (1982) Metoclopramide-induced parkinsonism: clinical characteristics in ten cases. *Arch. Neurol.* **39**, 494–496.

Innes R. and Stromme J. (1973) Rise in serum creatinine phosphokinase associated with agents used in anaesthesia. *Br. J. Anaesth.* **45**, 185–190.

Jaeger V., Podczeck A., Haubenstock A. et al. (1984) Acute oral poisoning with lindane-solvent mixture. *Vet. Hum. Toxicol.* **26**, 11–14.

Jaenke R. S. (1974) An anthracycline antibiotic-induced cardiomyopathy in rabbits. *Lab. Invest.* **30**, 292–304.

Jasmin G. and Gareau R. (1961). Histopathological study of muscle lesions produced by para-phenylenediamine in rats. *Br. J. Exper. Path.* **42**, 592–596.

Jaweed M. M., Alleva F. R., Herbison G. J. et al. (1986b) Muscle atrophy and histopathology of the solcus in 6 mercaptopurine-treated rats. *Toxicol. Ind. Health* **2**, 31–40.

Jaweed M. M., Ferraro T. N., Allevo F. R. et al (1986a) Methylhistidine changes in tibialis anterior muscles of 6-mercaptopurine-treated rats. *Toxicol. Ind. Health* **2**, 69–77.

Jehn A. E., and Fink M. K. (1980) Myositis, myoglobinemia, and myoglobinuria associated with enterovirus Echo 9 infection. *Arch. Neurol.* **37**, 457–458.

Jendrzejewski J. W., Jones S. R. and Newcombe R., L. (1978) Non-traumatic clostridial myonecrosis. *Am. J. Med.* **65**, 542–546.

Jenning A. E., Levey A. S. and Harrington J. T. (1983) Amoxaphine-associated acute renal failure. *Arch. Intern. Med.* **143**, 1525–1527.

Jensen O. B., Mosdal C. and Reske-Nielson E. (1977) Hypokalemic myopathy during treatment with diuretics. *Acta Neurol. Scand.* **55**, 465–482.

Kagen L. J. (1972) Myoglobinuric syndromes. *Am. J. Med. Sci.* **264**, 141–142.

Kaiser A. B., Rieves D., Price A. H. et al. (1985) Tularemia and rhabdomyolysis. *JAMA* **253**, 241–243.

Kalish S. B., Tallman M. S., Cook F. V. et al. (1982) Polymicrobial septicemia associated with rhabdomyolysis, myoglobinuria, and acute renal failure. *Arch. Intern. Med.* **142**, 133–134.

Kantor R. J., Norden C. W. and Wein T. P. (1978) Infectious mononucleus is associated with rhabdomyolysis and renal failure. *South Med. J.* **71**, 346.

Kelfer H. M., Singler W. D., and Reynolds R. N. (1983) Malignant hyperthermia in a child with Duchenne muscular dystrophy. *Pediatrics* **71**, 118–119.

Kelton J., Kelly, W. N. and Holmes E. W. (1978) A rapid method for the diagnosis of acute uric acid nephropathy. *Arch. Intern. Med.* **138**, 612–615.

Kendrick W. C., Hull A. R. and Knochell J. P. (1977) Rhabdomyolysis and shock after intravenous amphetamine administration. *Ann. Intern. Med.* **86**, 381–387.
Kennard C., Swash M. and Henson R. A. (1980) Myopathy due to epsilon-aminocaproic acid. *Muscle Nerve*, **3**, 202–206.
Klip A., Britt B. A., Elliott M. E. et al. (1987) Anaesthetic-induced increase in ionised calcium in blood mononuclear cells from malignant hyperthermia patients. *Lancet* **1**, 463–466.
Klock J. C. and Sexton M. J. (1973) Rhabdomyolysis and acute myoglobinuric renal failure following heroin abuse. *Calif. Med.* **119**, 5–8.
Kleinknecht D., Parent A., Blot P. et al (1982) Rhabdomyolysis with acute renal failure and the malignant neuroleptic syndrome. *Ann. Med. Interene.* **133**, 549–552.
Klinenberg J. R., Kippen L. and Bluestone R. (1975) Hyperuricemic nephropathy: pathologic features and factors influencing waste deposition. *Nephron* **14**, 88–98.
Knochel J. P. (1976) Renal injury in muscle disease. In: Suki W. and Eknoyan G. (ed.) *The Kidney in Systemic Disease*, 129–140. New York: John Wiley.
Knochel J. P. (1976) Rhabdomyolysis. *West J. Med.* **125**, 312–314.
Knochel J. P. (1977) The pathophysiology and clinical characteristics of severe hypophosphatemia. *Arch. Ind. Med.* **137**, 203–220.
Knochel J. P. (1985) Deranged phosphorus metabolism. In: Seldin D. W. and Giebisch G. (ed.) *The Kidney: Physiology and Pathophysiology*, 1397–1416. New York: Raven Press.
Knochel J. P. (1982) Rhabdomyolysis and myoglobinuria. *Ann. Rev. Med.* **33**, 435–443.
Knochel J. P., Barcenas C., Cotton R. J. et al. (1978) Hypophosphatemia and rhabdomyolysis. *J. Clin. Invest.* **62**, 1240–1246.
Knochel J. P., Bilbrey G. L., Fuller T. J. et al. (1975) The muscle cell in chronic alcoholism: The possible role of phosphate depletion in alcoholic myopathy. *Ann. NY Acad. Sci.* **252**, 274–286.
Knochel J. P. and Carter N. W. (1976) The role of muscle cell injury in the pathogenesis of acute renal failure after exercise. *Kidney Int.* **10**, S.58–S.64.
Knochel J. P., Dotin L. N. and Hamburger R. J. (1974) Heat stress, exercise and muscle injury: Effects on waste metabolism and renal function. *Ann. Intern. Med.* **81**, 321–328.
Knochel J. P. and Schlein E. M. (1972) On the mechanism of rhabdomyolysis in potassium depletion. *J. Clin. Invest.* **51**, 1750–1758.
Knolph R. D. (1969) Mechanics for inefficient peritoneal dialysis in acute renal failure associated with heat stress and exercise. *Am. J. Int. Med.* **71**, 317–326.
Koeffler H. P. and Haskell C. M. (1978) Rhabdomyolysis as a complication of 5-azacytidone. *Cancer Treat. Rep.* **62**, 573–574.
Koffler A., Friedler R. M. and Massry S. G. (1976) Acute renal failure due to non-traumatic rhabdomyolysis. *Ann. Intern. Med.* **85**, 23–28.
Konttinen A., Martel G. and Louhija A. (1970) Multiple serum enzyme analyses in chronic alcoholics. *Acta Med. Scand.* **188**, 257.
Kouyoumdjian J. A., Harris J. B. and Johnson M. A. (1986) Muscle necrosis caused by the sub-units of crotoxin. *Toxicon* **6**, 575–583.
Korsan-Bengtsen K., Ysander L., Blohme G. et al. (1969) Extensive muscle necrosis after long-term treatment with aminocaproic acid (EACA) in a case of hereditary periodic edema. *Acta Med. Scand.* **185**, 341–346.
Koster M. and David G. K. (1968) Reversible severe hyptertension due to licorice ingestion. *N. Engl. J. Med.* **278**, 1381–1383.
Kroeger R. M., Moore R. J., Lehman T. H. et al. (1980) Recurrent urinary calculi associated with toluene sniffing. *J. Urol.* **123**, 89–91.
Kuncl R. W. and Meltzer H. Y. (1974) Pathologic effect of phencyclidine and restraint on rat skeletal muscle: prevention by prior denervation. *Exper. Neurol.* **45**, 387–402.
Kurt T. L., Bost R., Gilliland M. et al. (1986) Accidental Kwell (lindane) ingestions. *Vet. Hum. Toxicol.* **28**, 479.
Kwiechinski H. (1978) Myotonia induced with clofibrate in rats. *J. Neurol.* **219**, 107–116.
Lafair J. S. and Myerson R. M. (1968) Alcoholic myopathy with special reference to the significance of creatine phosphokinase. *Arch. Intern. Med.* **122**, 417.
Laggner A. N., Kaik S., Lenz K. et al. (1984) Treatment of severe poisoning with slow release theophylline. *Br. Med. J.* **288**, 1497.
Lancet (1982). Editorial. Phenylpropanolamine over the counter. *Lancet* **i**, 839.
Lane, R. J. M., McLelland N. J., Martin A. M. et al. (1979) Epsilon-aminocaproic acid (EACA) myopathy. *Postgrad. Med. J.* **55**, 282–285.

Langer T. and Levy R. I. (1968) Acute muscular syndrome associated with administration of clofibrate. *N. Engl. J. Med.* **279**, 856–858.

Langman M. J. S. (1980) Gastrointestinal drugs. In: Dukes M. N. G. (ed.) *Meyler's Side Effects of Drugs*, 9th edn., 619–620. Amsterdam: Excerpta Medica.

Layzer R. B., Rowland L. P. and Ranney H. M. (1967) Muscle phosphofructokinase deficiency. *Arch. Neurol.* **17**, 512.

Leaf A. (1970) Regulation of intracellular fluid volume and disease. *Am. J. Med.* **49**, 291–295.

Lenaz L. and Page J. A. (1976) Cardiotoxicity of adriamycin and related anthracyclines. *Cancer Treat. Rev.* **3**, 111–120.

Leonard C. D. and Eichner E. R. (1970) Acute renal failure and transient hypercalcemia in idiopathic rhabdomyolysis. *JAMA* **211**, 1539–1540.

Lewandowski K. (1981) Rhabdomyolysis, myoglobinuria and hyperpyrexia caused by suxamethonium in a child with increased serum creatine kinase concentration. *Br. J. Anaesth.* **53**, 981–984.

Lewandowski K. B. (1982) Strabismus as a possible sign of subclinical muscular dystrophy predisposing to rhabdomyolysis and myoglobinuria: a study of an affected family. *Can. Anesth. Soc. J.* **29**, 372–376.

Lewandowski K. B., Hollmen A. and Reunanen M. (1975) Malignant hyperpyrexia. A study of an affected family. *Ann. Chir. Gynecol. Fenn.* **64**, 112.

Lewin P. K. (1985) Rhabdomyolysis and acute failure in sickle-cell anaemia. *Br. Med. J.* **291**, 413.

Lewis R. V. and McDevitt D. G. (1986) Adverse reactions and interactions with β-adrenoceptor blocking drugs. *Med. Toxicol.* **1**, 343–361.

Lietman P. S. (1971) Mitochondrial protein synthesis: inhibition by emetine hydrochloride. *Molec. Pharmacol.* **7**, 122–128.

Llach F., Felsenfeld A. J. and Haussler M. R. (1981) The pathophysiology of altered calcium metabolism in rhabdomyolysis-induced acute renal failure. *N. Engl. J. Med.* **305**, 117–123.

Logan J. L. and Ogden D. A. (1985) Rhabdomyolysis and acute renal failure following the bite of the giant desert centipede Scolopendra heros. *West. J. Med.* **142**, 549–550.

Lonka L. and Pdersen R. S. (1987) Fatal rhbdomyolysis in marathon runner. *Lancet* **1**, 857–858.

Lopez J. R., Alamo L., Caputo C. et al. (1985). Intracellular ionized calcium concentration in muscles from humans with malignant hyperthermia. *Muscle Nerve* **8**, 355–358.

Loughridge L. W., Leader L. P. and Bowen D. A. L. (1958) Acute renal failure due to muscle necrosis in carbon monoxide poisoning. *Lancet* **ii**, 349–351.

Louw A. and Nielsen H. E. (1944) Paroxysmal paralytic hemoglobinuria. *Act Med. Scand.* **117**, 424–436.

Lulich K. M., Goldie R. G., Ryan G. et al. (1986) Adverse reactions to β_2-agonist bronchodilators. *Med. Toxicol.* **1**, 286–299.

MacDonald J. B., Jones H. M. and Cowan R. A. (1985). Rhabdomyolysis and acute renal failure after theophylline overdose. *Lancet* **i**, 932–933.

MacKay A. R., Sang V. H. and Weinstein P. R. (1978) Myopathy associated with epsilon-aminocaproic acid (EACA) therapy. Report of two cases *J. Neurosurg.* **49**, 587–601.

McArdle B. (1951) Myopathy due to a defect in muscle glycogen breakdown. *Clin. Sci.* **10**, 13–51.

McCarron M. M., Schulze B. W., Thompson G. J. et al. (1981) Acute phencyclidine intoxication: incidence of clinical findings in 1000 cases. *Ann. Emerg. Med.* **10**, 237–242.

McChesney J. A., and Marquardt J. F. (1964) Hypokalaemic paralysis induced by amphotericin B. *JAMA* **189**, 1029–1031.

McClaren C. A. B. (1968) Myoglobinuria following the use of suxamethonium chloride. *Br. J. Anaesth.* **40**, 901–902.

McKishnie J. D., Muir J. M. and Girvan D. P. (1983) Anaesthesia induced rhabdomyolysis. A case report. *Can. Anaesth. Soc. J.* **30**, 295–298.

Manno B. R. and Manno J. E. (1977) Toxicology of ipecac: a review. *Clin. Toxicol.* **10**, 221–242.

Martindale (1977) In: Wade A. (ed.) *The Extra Pharmacopoeia.* London: The Pharmaceutical Press.

Massry S. C., Dua S., Garty J. et al. (1978) Role of uremia in the skeletal resistance to the calcemic action of parathyroid hormone. *Mineral Electrolyte Metab.* **1**, 172–180.

Mateer J. E., Farrell B. J., Chon S. S. M. et al. (1985) Reversible ipecac myopathy. *Arch. Neurol.* **42**, 188–190.

Meadows J. C. (1971) Fasciculation caused by suxamethonium and other cholinergic drugs. *Acta Neurol. Scand.* **47**, 381–391.

Medical Staff Conference (1976). Rhabdomyolysis. *West J. Med.* **125**, 298–304.

Meijer A. E. F. H. and Israel D. E. (1979) The increase in activity of acid hydrolases in muscles of rats after subcutaneous administration of dimethyl-para-phenylene diamine. A combined histochemical and biochemical investigation. *Histochemistry* **61**, 81–91.

Meltzer H. (1971) Possible mechanism of increased intravascular coagulation in malignant hyperpyrexia. *Lancet* **1**, 918–919.

Meltzer H. Y., Mrozak S. and Boyer M. (1970) Effect of intramuscular injections on serum creatine phosphokinase activity. *Am. J. Med. Sci.* **259**, 42–48.

Mercieca J. and Brown E. A. (1984) Acute renal failure due to rhabdomyolysis associated with use of a strait-jacket in lysergide intoxication. *Br. Med. J.* **288**, 1949–1950.

Meroney W. H., Arney G. K., Segar W. E. et al. (1957) The acute calcification of traumatized muscle with particular reference to acute post-traumatic renal insufficiency. *J. Clin. Invest.* **36**, 825–832.

Meyer-Betz F. (1911). Beobachtungen an einem ugenartigen mit muskellahmungen verbundemen Fall von Hamoglobinurie. *Dtsch. Arch. Klin. Med.* **101**, 85–127.

Miller E. D., Sanders D. B., Rowlingson J. C. et al. (1978) Anesthesia induced rhabdomyolysis in a patient with Duchenne's muscular dystrophy. *Anesthesiology* **48**, 146–148.

Miller L., Pateras V., Friederici H. et al. (1985) Acute tubular necrosis after inhalation exposure to methylene chloride. Report of a case. *Arch. Intern. Med.* **145**, 145–146.

Minow R. A., Gorbach S., Johnson B. L. Jr et al. (1974) Myoglobinuria associated with influenza A infection. *Ann. Intern. Med.* **80**, 359–361.

Modi K. B., Horn E. H. and Bryson S. M. (1985) Theophylline poisoning and rhabdomyolysis. *Lancet* **ii**, 160–161.

Mohamed S. D., Chapman R. S. and Crooks J. (1966) Hypokalemia, flaccid quadriparesis, and myoglobinuria with carbenoxolone (Biogastrone). *Br. Med. J.* **1**, 1581–1582.

Moore W. E., Watson R. L. and Summary J. J. (1976) Massive myoglobinuria precipitated by halothane and succinylcholine in a member of a family with elevation of serum creatine phosphokinase. *Anesth., Anal.* **55**, 680–682.

Morris C. D. W., Jacobs P., Berman P. A. et al. (1983) Epsilon-aminocaproic acid-induced myopathy. A case report. *S. Afr. Med. J.* **64**, 363–366.

Morris R. C. (1981) Renal failure, myoglobinuria, and hemoglobinuria. *JAMA* **246**, 685.

Morton A. R. and Waldek S. (1985) Myoglobinuric renal failure after prolonged sponsored activity. *Br. Med. J.* **291**, 1767.

Mourad G., Gallay P., Oules R. et al. (1979) Rhabdomyolyse et insuffisance reinale aigue. Role d'une déplétion potassique induite par une intoxication à la réglisse. *J. Urol. Nephrol.* (Paris) **85**, 315–319.

Munk Z. M. and Nantel A. (1977) Acute lindane poisoning with development of muscle necrosis. *Canad. Med. Assoc. J.* **117**, 1050–1054.

Musclow C. E. and Awen C. F. (1977) Glue sniffing: report of fatal case. *Canad. Med. Assoc. J.* **104**, 315–319.

Nanji A. A. and Filipenko J. D. (1983) Rhabdomyolysis and acute myoglobinuric renal failure associated with methadone intoxication. *J. Toxicol., Clin. Toxicol.* **20**, 353–360.

Nelson T. E. and Flewellen E. H. (1983) The malignant hyperthermia syndrome. *N. Engl. J. Med.* **309**, 416–518.

Nelson T. E., Flewellen E. H. and Gloyna D. F. (1983) Spectrum of susceptibility to malignant hyperthermia: diagnostic dilemma. *Anesth. Analg.* **62**, 545–552.

Nibblelink D. W., Torner J. C. and Henderson W. G. (1975) Intracranial aneurysms and subarachnoid hemorrhage: a comparative study—antifibrinolytic therapy in recent onset subarachnoid hemorrhage. *Stroke* **6**, 622–629.

Nicholls K., Niall J. F. and Moran J. E. (1982) Rhabdomyolysis and renal failure. Complications of narcotic abuse. *Med. J. Australia* Oct., 387–889.

Nielson H. K., Krusell L., Baelum J. et al. (1985) Renal effects of acute exposure to toluene. *Acta Med. Scand.* **218**, 317–321.

Norton R. L. (1984) Phencyclidine-management of acute intoxication. In: Bayer M. J., Rumack B. H. and Wanke L. A. (ed.) *Toxicologic Emergencies*, 191–197. Buvie, Maryland: Brady.

Nygren A. (1966) Serum creatine phosphokinase activity in chronic alcoholism in connection with acute alcohol intoxication. *Acta Med. Scand.* **179**, 623.

Nyhan W. L. (1983). Nonketotic hyperglycinemia. In: Stranburg J. B., Wyngaarden J. B., Frederickson D. S. et al. (ed.) *The Metabolic Basis of Inherited Disease*, 5th edn. 561–569. New York: McGraw-Hill.

Olerud J. E., Homer L. D. and Carroll H. W. (1976) Incidence of acute exertional rhabdomyolysis. *Arch. Intern. Med.* **136**, 692–697.

Olson K. R., Benowitz N. L., Woo O. F. et al. (1985) Theophylline overdose: acute single ingestion versus chronic repeated over medication. *Am. J. Emerg. Med.* **3**, 386–394.

Ono I. (1953) Studies on myoglobinuria. *Tohoku J. Exp. Med.* **57**, 273–281.

Orgain E. S.,, Bogdonoff M. D. and Cain C. (1967) Clofibrate and androsterone effect on serum lipids. *Arch. Intern. Med.* **119**, 80–85.

Owen C. A., Mubarak S. J. and Hargens A. R. (1979) Intramuscular pressures with limb compression. *N. Engl. J. Med.* **300**, 1169–1172.

Palmer E. P. and Guay A. T. (1985) Reversible myopathy secondary to abuse of ipecac in patients with major eating disorders. *N. Engl. J. Med.* **313**, 1457–1459.

Pankow P. and Ponsold W. (1984) Effect of carbon monoxide exposure on heart cytochrome c oxidase activity of rats. *Biomed. Biochim. Acta* **10**, 1185–1189.

Patel R. and Benjamin J. Jr (1986) Renal disease associated with toluene inhalation. *Clin. Toxicol.* **24**, 213–223.

Patel R. and Connor G. (1985) A review of thirty cases of rhabdomyolysis-associated acute renal failure among phencyclidine users. *Clin. Toxicol.* **23**, 547–556.

Patten B. M., Wood J. M., Harati Y. et al. (1979) Familial recurrent rhabdomyolysis due to carnitine–palmityl–transferase deficiency. *Am. J. Med.* **67**, 167–171.

Patten B. R., Pearn J. H., DeBuse P. et al. (1985) Prolonged intensive therapy after snake bite. *Med. J. Aust.* **142**, 467–469.

Pearce M. B., Bullock R. T. and Murphy M. L. (1971) Selective damage of myocardial mitochondria due to emetine hydrochloride. *Arch. Pathol.* **91**, 8–81.

Pearson C. M., Beck W. S. and Bladh W. H. (1957) Idiopathic paroxysmal myoglobinuria. *Arch. Intern. Med.* **99**, 376.

Pearson C. M. and Kalyanaraman K. (1983) Familial periodic paralysis. In: Stanbury J. B., Wyngaarden J. B., Fredrickson D. J., Goldstein J. L. and Brown M. S. (ed.) *The Metabolic Basis of Inherited Disease*, 5th ed., 1496. New York: McGraw-Hill.

Penn A. S., Rowland L. P. and Fraser D. W. (1972) Drugs, coma, and myoglobinuria. *Arch. Neurol.* **26**, 336–343.

Penney D. and Maziarka T. (1976) Effect of acute carbon monoxide poisoning on serum lactate dehydrogenase and creatine phosphokinase. *J. Toxicol. Environ. Health* **1**, 1017–1021.

Perkoff G., Dioso M. M., Bleisch V. et al. (1967) A spectrum of myopathy associated with alcoholism. I. Clinical and laboratory findings. *Ann. Intern. Med.* **67**, 481–482.

Perkoff G. T. and Tyler F. H. (1958) Estimation and physical properties of myoglobin in various species. *Metabolism* **7**, 751.

Pierides A. M., Alvarez-Ude F., Kerr D. N. S. et al. (1975) Clofibrate-induced muscle damage in patients with chronic renal failure. *Lancet* **ii**, 1279–1282.

Plotz J. and Braun J. (1982). Failure of 'self-taming' doses of succinylcholine to inhibit increases in postoperative serum creatine kinase activity in children. *Anesthesiology*, **56**, 207–209

Plotz J., Braun J. and Stallenberger R. (1981) The inhibitory effect of dantrolene on the rise of serum creatine kinase activity after combined use of halothane and suxamethonium in man. *Anesthesiology* **30**, 338–342.

Podgorny G. (1983) Venomous reptiles and arthropods of the United States and Canada. In: Hadded L. M. and Winchester J. F. (ed.) *Clinical Management of Poisoning and Drug Overdose*, 275–294. Philadelphia: Saunders.

Polson C. J. and Tattersall R. N. (1969) *Clinical Toxicology*, 2nd ed., 558–568. Philadelphia: Lippincott.

Porter G. A. and Bennett W. M. (1981) Toxic nephropathies. In: Brenner B. M. and Rector F. C. (ed.) *The Kidney*. Philadelphia: Saunders.

Posner M. R., Caudill M. A., Brass R. et al. (1980) Legionnaires' disease associated with rhabdomyolysis and myoglobinuria. *Arch. Intern. Med.* **140**, 848–850.

Publicover S. F., Duncan C. J. and Smith J. L. (1978) The use of A23187 to demonstrate the role of intracellular calcium in causing ultrastructural damage in mammalian cells. *J. Neuropath. Exper. Neurol.* **37**, S554–557.

Quintanilla A. P. (1982) Pigment nephropathy. In Earle D. P. (ed.) *Manual of Clinical Nephrology*, 269–276. Philadelphia: Saunders.

Raifman R. A., Berant B. and Lenarsky C. (1978) Cold weather and rhabdomyolysis. *J. Pediatr.* **93**, 970–971.

Rainey R. L., Estes P. W., Neely C. L. et al. (1963) Myoglobinuria following diabetic acidosis. With electromyographic evaluation. *Arch. Intern. Med.* **111**, 564.

Ratnesar V. C. and Pobee J. (1962) Emetine toxicity with predominant neuromuscular manifestations. *Postgrad. Med. J.* **38**, 586–588.

Reisin E., Teichner A., Jaffe R. et al. (1975) Myoglobinuria and renal failure in toluene poisoning. *Br. J. Ind. Med.* **32**, 163–168.

Relman A. S. (1972) Metabolic consequences of acid–base disorders. *Kidney Int.* **1**, 347–359.

Report (1985). Final report on the safety assessment of *p*-phenylenediamine. Expert Scientific Panel, Cosmetic and Toilet Fragrancy Association. *J. Am. Coll. Toxicol.* **4**, 203–266.

Revis N. and Marusic N. (1979) Sequestration of $^{45}Ca^{2+}$ by mitochondria from rabbit heart, liver, and kidney after doxorubicin or digoxin/doxorubicin treatment. *Exper. Molec. Path* **31**, 440–451.

Rheingold A. J., Greenwald R. A. and Hayes P. J. (1977) Myoglobinuria and renal failure associated with typhoid fever. *JAMA* **238**, 341.

Richter R. W. and Baden M. M. (1969) Neurological complications of heroin addiction. *Trans. Am. Neurol. Assoc.* **94**, 330–332.

Richter R. W., Challenor Y. B., Pearson J. B. et al. (1971) Acute myoglobinuria associated with heroin addiction. *JAMA* **216**, 1172–1176.

Richter R. W. and Rosenberg R. N. (1968). Transverse myelitis associated with heroin addiction. *JAMA* **206**, 1255–1257.

Rizza R. A., Sclonick S. and Conley C. L. (1976) Myoglobinuria following aminocaproic acid administration. *JAMA* **236**, 1845–1846.

Robinson D. C. (1984) Renal disease. In: Herfindal E. T. and Hirschman J. L. (ed.) *Clinical Pharmacy and Therapeutics*, 629–645. Baltimore: Williams and Wilkins.

Robinson O. P. W. (1973) Metoclopramide: its side effects and safety. *Postgrad. Med. J.* **49**, *Suppl.* **4**, 77–80.

Rodriguez E. E., Woods K. L., Deno R. E. et al. (1983) Rhabdomyolysis-induced acute renal failure in Legionnaires' disease. *South. Med. J.* **76**, 1328–1329.

Rohling T., Hecking E. and Weihrauch T. (1984) Heroin-induzierte Rhabdomyolyse mit ukutem Nier enversagen. *Med. Klin.* **79**, 616–618.

Rollo I. M. (1980) Drugs used in the chemotherapy of amebiasis. In: Gilman A. G., Goodman L. S. and Gilman A. (ed.) *The Pharmacological Basis of Therapeutics*, 1065–1067. New York: Macmillan.

Rosenberg H. and Heiman-Patterson T. (1983) Duchennes's muscular dystrophy and malignant hyperpyrexia: another warning. *Anesthesiology* **59**, 362.

Ross J. H., Attwood E. C. and Atkin G. E. (1986) Acute renal failure induced by rhabdomyolysis. *Br. Med. J.* **292**, 694.

Ross J. H., Attwood E. C., Atkin G. E. et al. (1983) A study on the effects of severe exercise on serum myoglobin. creatinine kinase, transaminases, and lactate dehydrogenase. *Q. J. Med.* **52**, 268–279.

Rowland L. P. and Penn A. S. (1972) Myoglobinuria. *Med. Clin N. Am.* **56**, 1233–1256.

Ruiz-Guinazu A., Coelho J. B. and Paz R. A. (1967) Methemoglobin-induced acute renal failure in the rat. *In vivo* observations, histology and micropuncture measurements of intratubular and postglomerular vascular pressures. *Nephron* **4**, 257–275.

Rumpf K. W., Kaiser H. F., Horstkotte H. et al. (1983) Rhabdomyolysis after ingestion of an appetite suppresant. *JAMA* **250**, 2112.

Rumpf K. W., Wagner H., Criee C-P. et al. (1985). Rhabdomyolysis after theophylline overdose. *Lancet* **i**, 1451–1452.

Ryan J. F., Kagen L. J. and Hyman A. I. (1971) Myoglobinemia after a single dose of succinylcholine. *N. Engl. J. Med.* **285**, 824–827.

Salako L. A. (1970) Effects of emetine on neuromuscular transmission. *Europ. J. Pharmac.* **11**, 342–348.

Schaer H., Steinmann B., Jerusalem S. et al. (1977) Rhabdomyolysis induced by anaesthesia with intra-operative cardiac arrest. *Br. J. Anaesth.* **49**, 495–499.

Scheulen J. J. and Munster A. M. (1983) The lightning injury. *J. Burn Care Rehab.* **4**, 101–105.

Schiff H. B., MacSearraigh E. T. M. and Kallmeyer J. C. (1978) Myoglobinuria, rhabdomyolysis and marathon running. *Q. J. Med.* **47**, 463–472.

Schlesinger J. J., Gandara D. and Bensch K. G. (1978). Myoglobinuria associated with herpes-group viral infections. *Arch. Intern. Med.* **138**, 422–424.

Schneider R. (1970). Acute alcoholic myopathy with myoglobinuria. *South. Med. J.* **63**, 485–489.

Schofield P. M., Beath S. V., Mant T. G. K. et al. (1985) Recovery after severe oxprenolol overdose complicated by rhabdomyolysis. *Human Toxicol.* **4**, 57–60.

Schreiner G. E. and Maher J. F. (1965) Toxic nephropathy. *Am. J. Med.* **38**, 409.

Schrier R. W., Henderson H. S., Tischer C. C. et al. (1967) Nephropathy associated with heat stress and exercise. *Ann. Intern. Med.* **67**, 356–376.
Schulze-Delrieu K. (1961) Metoclopramide. *N. Engl. J. Med.* **305**, 28–33.
Schwartzfarb L., Singh G. and Marcus D. (1977) Heroin-associated rhabdomyolysis with cardiac involvement. *Arch. Intern. Med.* **137**, 1255–1257.
Seay A. R., Ziter F. A. and Thompson J. A. (1978) Cardiac arrest during anaesthesia in Duchenne muscular dystrophy. *J. Pediatr.* **93**, 88.
Segal A. J., Miller M. and Moses A. M. (1968) Hypercalcemia during the diuretic phase of acute renal failure. *Ann. Intern. Med.* **68**, 1066–1068.
Seneviratne B. I. (1975) Acute cardiomyopathy with rhabdomyolysis in chronic alcoholism. *Br. Med. J.* **4**, 378–380.
Simpson D. L. and Rumack B. H. (1981) Methylenedioxyamphetamine: clinical description of overdose, death, and review of pharmacology. *Arch. Int. Med.* **141**, 1507–1509.
Slaughter L. J., Alleva F. C. and Balazs T. (1986) 6-Mercaptopurine-induced muscular lesions in rats: gross and light microscopic pathology. *Toxicol. Ind. Health* **2**, 25–29.
Smalls A. G. M., Bess L. V. A. M. and Kloppenborg P. W. C. (1978) Clofibrate-induced muscle damage with myoglobinuria and cardiomyopathy. *N. Engl. J. Med.* **299**, 942.
Smego R. A. and Durack D. T. (1982) The neuroleptic malignant syndrome. *Arch. Intern. Med.* **42**, 1183–1185.
Smit A. J., Mulder P. O. M., deJong P. E. and van der Hem G. K. (1986) Acute renal failure after overdose of labetol. *Br. Med. J.* **293**, 1142–1143.
Smith S. G., Black-Schaffer B. and Lasater T. E. (1950) Potassium deficiency syndrome in the rat and the dog. *Arch. Pathol.* **49**, 185–199.
Solomons C. C. and Masson N. C. (1984) Platelet model for halothane-induced effects on nucleotide metabolism applied to malignant hyperthermia. *Acta Anaesthiol. Scand.* **28**, 185–190.
Somers J. E. and Winer N. (1966) Reversible myopathy and myotonia following administration of a hypocholesterolemic agent. *Neurology* **16**, 761–765.
Somerville P. J. and Kaye A. M. (1978) Resistance to parathyroid hormone in renal failure: role of vitamin D metabolites. *Kidney Int.* **14**, 245–254.
Somerville P. J. and Kaye A. M. (1979) Evidence that resistance to the hypercalcaemic action of parathyroid hormone in rats with uremia is caused by phosphate retention. *Kidney Int.* **16**, 552–560.
Song S. K. and Rubin E. (1972) Ethanol produces muscle damage in human volunteers. *Science* **175**, 327–328.
Sonntag V. K. H. and Stein B. M. (1974) Arteriopathic complications during treatment of subarachnoid haemorrhage with epsilon-aminocaproic acid. *J. Neurosurg.* **40**, 480–485.
Soule T. I. and Cunningham G. R. (1973) Herbicopi lathyri septicemia, myoglobinuria, and acute renal failure. *JAMA* **223**, 1265–1266.
Spyker D. A. (1983) Strychnine. In: Haddad L. M. and Winchester J. F. (ed.) *Clinical Management of Poisoning and Drug Overdose*, 728–729. Philadelphia: Saunders.
Statham H. E., Duncan C. J. and Smith J. L. (1976) The effect of the ionophore A23187 on the ultrastructure and electrophysiological properties of frog skeletal muscle. *Cell Tissue Res.* **173**, 193–207.
Steel T. H. and Rieslebach R. E. (1975) Renal urate excretion in normal man. *Nephron* **14**, 21–32.
Streeton J. A. (1967) Traumatic haemoglobinuria caused by karate exercises. *Lancet* **2**, 191–192.
Streicher H. Z., Gabow P. A., Moss A. H. et al. (1981) Syndromes of toluene sniffing in adults. *Ann. Intern. Med.* **94**, 758–762.
Stryer L. (1981) *Biochemistry*, 2nd ed., 43–64. New York: Freeman.
Surmont D. W. A., Colardyn F. and de Reuck J. (1984) Fatal complications of neuroleptic drugs. A clinico-pathological study of three cases. *Acta Neurol. Belg.* **84**, 75–83.
Swartz R. D. Millman R. P. Billi J. E. et al. (1981) Epidemic methanol poisoning: clinical and biochemical analysis of a recent episode. *Medicine* **60**, 373–382.
Swenson R. D., Golper T. A. and Bennett W. M. (1982) Acute renal failure and rhabdomyolysis after ingestion of phenylpropanolamine-containing diet pills. *JAMA* **248**, 1216.
Taher S. M., Anderson R. J. McCartney M. et al. (1974) Renal tubular acidosis associated with toluene sniffing. *N. Engl. J. Med.* **290**, 765–768.
Tam C. W., Olin B. R. and Ruiz A. E. (1980) Loxapine-associated rhabdomyolysis and acute renal failure. *Arch. Intern. Med.* **140**, 975–976.
Tammisto T. and Airaksinen M. (1966) Increase of creatine kinase activity in serum as a sign of

muscular injury caused by intermittently administered suxamethonium during halothane anaesthesia. *Br. J. Anaesth.* **38**, 510–515.

Tammisto T., Leikkonen P. and Airaksinen M. (1967) The inhibitory effects of d-tubocurarine on the increase of creatinine kinase activity produced by intermittent suxamethonium administration during halothane anaesthesia. *Acta Anaesthiol. Scand.* **11**, 333–340.

Tammisto T., Brander P., Airaksinen M. M. et al. (1970) Strabismus as a possible sign of latent muscular disease predisposing to suxamethonium-induced muscular injury. *Ann. Clin. Res.* **2**, 126–130.

Tang T. T., Sedmak G. V. and Siegesmund K. A. (1975). Chronic myopathy associated with coxsackie virus type A9: A combined electron microscopical and viral isolation study. *N. Engl. J. Med.* **292**, 608–611.

Tarui S., Okuno G., Ikura Y. et al. (1965) Phosphofructokinase deficiency in skeletal muscle: A new type of glycogenolysis. *Biochem. Biophys. Res. Commun.* **34**, 77–83.

Tavill A. S., Evanson J. M., Baker S. B. et al. (1964) Idiopathic paroxysmal myoglobinuria with acute renal failure and hypocalcaemia. *N. Engl. J. Med.* **271**, 283–287.

Teicher A., Rosenthal T., Kissin E. et al. (1981) Labetol-induced toxic myopathy. *Br. Med. J.* **282**, 1824–1825.

Tephly T. R. and Martin R. E. (1984) Methanol metabolism and toxicity. *Food Sci. Technol.* **12**, 111–140.

Thase M. E. and Shostak M. (1984) Rhabdomyolysis complicating intramuscular neuroleptization. *J. Clin. Psychopharmacol.* **4**, 46–48.

Thayer W. S. (1977) Adriamycin stimulated superoxide formation in submitochondrial particles. *Chem. Biol. Interact.* **19**, 265–278.

Thomsen H. K. and Kjeldsen K. (1974) Threshold limit for carbon monoxide-induced myocardial damage. *Arch. Environ. Health* **29**, 73–78.

Tintinalli J. E., Rominger M. and Kittleson K. (1983) Carbon Monoxide. In: Haddad L. M. and Winchester J. F. (ed.) *Clinical Management of Poisoning and Drug Overdose*, 748–753. Philadelphia: Saunders.

de Torrente A., Berl T., Cohn P. D. et al. (1976) Hypercalcaemia of acute renal failure. *Am. J. Med.* **61**, 119–123.

Tribble C. J., Persing J. A., Morgan R. F. et al. (1985) Lightning injuries. *Compr. Ther.* **11**, 32–40.

Tsung J. S. and Tsung S. S. (1986) Creatine kinase isoenzymes in extracts of various human skeletal muscles. *Clin. Chem.* **38**, 1568–1570.

Ulvila J. M. and Nessan V. J. (1973) Hypernatremia with rhabdomyolysis. *Am. J. Med. Sci.* **265**, 79.

Van Horn G., Drori J. B. and Schuartz F. D. (1970) Hypokalemic myopathy and elevation of serum enzymes. *Arch. Neurol.* **22**, 335–341.

Varga E. and Simpson G. M. (1971) Loxapine succinate in the treatment of uncontrollable destructive behaviour. *Curr. Therap. Res.* **13**, 737–742.

Vissuzaine C., Coste F. and Bocqnet L. (1976) Rhabdomyolyse cardique et squelettique au cours d'un coma par intoxication médicamenteuse. *Couer Med. Int.* **15**, 615–623.

Walton K. W., Scott P. J., Verrier Jones J. et al. (1963) Symposium on atromid. *J. Atheroscl. Res.* **3**, 396–414.

Walum E., Varnbo I. and Peterson A. (1985) Effects of dissolved carbon monoxide on the respiratory activity of perfused neuronal and muscle cell cultures. *Clin. Toxicol.* **23**, 299–308.

Wardle E. N. and Wright N. A. (1973) Intravascular coagulation and glycerin hemoglobinuric acute renal failure. *Arch. Pathol.* **95**, 271–275.

Warren D. J., Leitch A. C. and Leggett R. J. E. (1975) Hyperuricaemic acute renal failure after epileptic seizures. *Lancet* **ii**, 385–387.

Wecker L. and Dettbarn W-D. (1976) Paraoxon-induced myopathy: muscle specificity and acetylcholine involvement. *Exp. Neurol.* **51**, 281–291.

Wecker L., Kiauta T. and Dettbarn W-D. (1978) Relationship between acetylcholinesterase inhibition and the development of a myopathy. *J. Pharmacol. Exp. Ther.* **206**, 97–104.

Wecker L., Mrack R. E. and Dettbarn W-D. (1986) Evidence of necrosis in human intercostal muscle following inhalation of organophosphate insecticide. *Fund. Appl. Toxicol.* **6**, 172–174.

Wedin G. P., Pennente C. M. and Sachder S. S. (1984). Renal involvement in organophosphate poisoning. *JAMA* **252**, 1408.

Weinstein S., Scottolini A. G. and Bhagran A. V. (1985) Low neutrophil alkaline phosphatase in renal tubular acidosis with hypophosphatemia after toluene sniffing. *Clin. Chem.* **31**, 330–331.

Welt L. G., Hollander W. Jr and Blythe W. B. (1960) The consequences of potassium depletion. *J. Chronic Dis.* **11**, 213–254.

Will A. M. and McClaren E. H. (1981) Reversible renal damage due to glue sniffing. *Br. Med. J.* **2**, 163–164.

Wilson D. R., Thiel G., Arce M. L. et al. (1967) Glycerol induced hemoglobinuric acid renal failure in the rat. III. Microfunctional studies of the effects of mannitol and isotonic saline on individual nephron function. *Nephron* **4**, 337–355.

Wilson D. R., Dent T. E. and Traber D. L. (1967) Malignant hyperpyrexia with anesthesia. *JAMA* **202**, 183–186.

Woolfe G. (1965) Chemotherapy of amoebiasis. *Progr. Drug. Res.* **8**, 11–52.

Wright J., Coucitonnai G. and Hodges G. R. (1979) Adenovirus type 21 infection: Occurrence with pneumonia, rhabdomyolysis, and myoglobinuria in an adult. *JAMA* **241**, 2420–2421.

Wright J. P., Laurence S., Holt S. et al. (1987) Rhabdomyolysis with hyperkalaemia after aminophylline overdose. *Med. Sci. Law* **27**, 103–105.

Wu B. C., Pillay V. K. G., Hawker C. D. et al. (1972) Hypercalcaemia in acute renal failure of acute alcoholic rhabdomyolysis. *S. Afr. Med. J.* **46**, 1631–1633.

Wyse D. G. (1973) Deliberate inhalation of volatile hydrocarbon. A review. *Can. Med. Assoc. J.* **108**, 71–74.

Yander G. and Haji H. (1984) Investigating the myopathic effects of 6-mercaptopurine on developing skeletal muscle *in vitro*. *Drug Chem. Toxicol.* **7**, 177–192.

Yander G., Jaweed M. M. and Kaji H. (1986) Effects of 6-mercaptopurine on developing muscle cells *in vitro*. *Toxicol. Ind. Health.* **2**, 51–56.

Yang W. C. T. and Dubick M. (1980) Mechanism of emetine cardiotoxicity. *Pharmacol. Ther.* **10**, 15–26.

Yost J. W. and Holmes F. F. (1974) Myoglobinuria following lightning stroke. *JAMA* **228**, 1147–1148.

Chapter 5

Drug-induced Oesophagitis

David B. Doman

Drug-induced oesophagitis is an underdiagnosed entity. Many patients have primary structural or motility disorders that not only predispose the oesophagus to prolonged mucosal contact with injurious agents, but are often blamed for oesophagitis so that the possibility of reversible drug-induced injury is overlooked. Furthermore, many cases of atypical chest pain and dyspepsia can, in retrospect, be related to drug injury.

The pathogenesis of drug-oesophagitis appears to be a local mucosal inflammatory effect unrelated to systemic pharmacology of the medication (Oakes and Sherck, 1985). Of note, a recently published animal study (Carlbourg and Densert, 1980) suggests that the mucosal pressure alone will not produce oesophageal ulcerations. Five hours of mucosal contact with chemically inert tablets such as barium sulphate or calcium lactate does not cause oesophageal injury. By contrast, lesions are seen regularly after similar application of more caustic chemical compounds such as ferrosuccinate, ferrous sulphate, doxycycline, propranolol, alprenolol, emepronium, acetylsalicylic acid, potassium chloride, and ascorbic acid.

Symptoms of drug-induced oesophagitis are usually acute and follow closely on the ingestion of the causative agent. However, they may have an insidious onset, particularly if there is an underlying oesophageal disorder. The pain is retrosternal, may be continuous or intermittent, and is usually aggravated by swallowing. Pathologically, the oesophageal lesions may be present as diffuse inflammation, or less commonly, as focal ulceration. In more severe cases, stricture formation with resultant dysphagia, perforation and haemorrhage have all been reported as complications. These complications may be life-threatening; in one series of forty-one cases of drug-induced oesophagitis, there were nine deaths from haemorrhage or perforation (Collins et al., 1974).

Drug-induced oesophagitis occurs in three patient categories:

1. Patients with underlying oesophageal structural abnormalities impeding tablet-passage, e.g. abnormalities that may be intrinsic (e.g. peptic stricture, neoplasm or hiatal hernia), or extrinsic (e.g. oesophageal compression by a hypertrophied left atrium or great vessels).
2. The second category is those with motility disturbances, i.e. individuals at risk include those with increased lower oesophageal sphincter pressure (e.g. achalasia, hypertensive lower oesophageal sphincter), which fails to relax

completely upon swallowing, or those with abnormal peristalsis (e.g. scleroderma, diffuse oesophageal spasm). The patients with structural or peristaltic disorders are particularly difficult to manage because it is all too easy for the physician to overlook medication the patient is taking, and to attribute symptoms to the underlying disease process.

3. Perhaps the most common group is those patients with a normal oesophagus who take medication in a recumbent position, or drink inadequate amounts of liquid, or both. The significance of gravity in promoting the passage of pills or capsules down the oesophagus is not widely appreciated. Similarly, the need for an adequate liquid bolus swallowed with the medication has never been stressed enough. Such a bolus makes swallowing easier by promoting oesophageal peristalsis and by initiating tablet dissolution.

Since drug-induced oesophagitis was first described, it has been intuitively obvious that swallowing time of the medication must play an intrinsic role. It was not until recently, however, that data was published to evaluate objectively this aspect of the phenomenon. Evans and Roberts (1976) used tablets of barium sulphate identical in size and shape to commercial aspirin to study the dynamics of swallowing in 98 consecutive patients with and without oesophageal pathology. After swallowing two tablets with approximately 15 ml of water, the patients immediately lay down. Of 57 patients, tablets were retained within the oesophagus for more than five minutes; in 14 of these, retention exceeded ten minutes. Delay was extremely common in patients with anatomic or functional oesophageal abnormalities: 21 of 29 such patients demonstrated retention. It is even more noteworthy that under these conditions tablet retention was documented in 30 of 69 individuals with a normal oesophagus (52%).

Applegate et al. (1979) used a scintigraphic method to quantitate oesophageal emptying of liquids, solids and capsules. A review of their data includes the following points:

1. There are significant differences between oesophageal emptying of water, capsules and liver cubes.
2. Oesophageal emptying of capsules was altered significantly by body position and ingestion of a chaser.
3. In some subjects, capsules may remain in a distal oesophagus for a prolonged period despite repeated swallows.

The authors concluded that if capsules are administered, the patient should be sitting upright and should swallow at least 15 ml of liquid as a chaser.

Over a dozen agents (*Table* 5.1) have been implicated in the pathogenesis of drug-induced oesophagitis. A recent review (Oakes and Sherck, 1985) described that 83% of such cases were due to tetracycline, potassium chloride and emepronium bromide.

Several antibiotics, including tetracycline and doxycycline, have been noted to cause discrete ulcers (Stillman and Martin, 1979; Bohey and Hugh, 1975). It is of note that most of the reported antibiotic cases occurred in patients who swallowed inadequate liquids, or swallowed in a recumbent position, or both. One paper (Crowson et al., 1976) evaluated the potential hazard as it relates to tetracycline. The authors reported that when the antibiotic was dissolved in 2 to 3

Oakes D. D. and Sherck J. D. (1985) Drug-induced esophagitis. In: DeMeester T. R. and Skinner D. B. (ed.) *Esophageal Disorders Pathophysiology and Therapy*, 241. New York: Raven Press.
O'Meara T. F. (1980) A new endoscopic finding of tetracycline-induced esophageal ulcers. *Gastrointest. Endosc.* **26**(3), 106–107.
Pannuti F. (1973) Oesophageal injury caused by fluorouracil. *Gazzeta Medica Italiana* **132**, 303.
Stillman A. E. and Martin R. J. (1979) Tetracycline-induced esophageal ulcerations. *Arch. Dermatol.* **115**, 1105.
Teplick J. G., Teplick S. K., Ominsky S. H. et al. (1980) Esophagitis caused by oral medication. *Diagn. Radiol.* January, 23–25.
Walta D. C., Giddens J. D., Johnson L. F., et al. (1976) Localized proximal esophagitis secondary to ascorbic acid ingestion and esophageal motor disorder. *Gastroenterology* **70**, 766–769.

Chapter 6

Review of Recent Advances in the Development and Application of the Micronucleus Test System

R. S. Slesinski and P. J. Guzzie

INTRODUCTION

Short-term genotoxicity tests have become routine procedures for evaluating xenobiotics for mutagenic and carcinogenic potential. Agents which cause damage to the genome may produce gene mutations and/or chromosomal abnormalities which are possible initiating events in carcinogenesis, or which can result in hereditable genetic disorders. Increases in chromosome damage have particular relevance to humans because a significant fraction of human genetic diseases are related to abnormalities in the structure or number of the chromosomes (Yunis, 1977; Riccardi, 1977; Sperling, 1984). Also, most tumours are characterised by alterations in chromosome structure or number which suggests a direct or indirect involvement in abnormal growth patterns of tumour cells (Berger, 1981; Yunis, 1983). The high degree of correlation between chromosome breaking (clastogenic) potential and carcinogenic activity (Radman et al., 1982) suggests a valuable role for clastogen screening tests in short-term testing programmes to identify potential carcinogens. Thus, a concerted effort has been devoted to develop and improve test systems which can rapidly and reliably detect agents with clastogenic ability.

The need to evaluate potential genetic hazards of a large number of chemicals prompted the rapid development of a diverse number of test systems. Cytogenetic analyses of chromosomes from bone marrow cells or lymphocytes from blood samples are relatively well-established procedures, but they are time consuming and require highly trained observers. The micronucleus test developed by Schmid (1973, 1975, 1976, 1977) and by Heddle (1973) is an appealing method for determining potential clastogenicity because the test is relatively rapid and inexpensive, and it can be performed with a modest degree of training and experience. However, the test has been criticized by cytogeneticists because it is an indirect method for evaluating chromosome breakage, and the results do not provide mechanistic data, nor supply information on reciprocal exchanges or alterations in chromosome number. Despite these limitations, the advantages of the micronucleus test may outweigh the criticisms. Genotoxicity screening tests are not intended primarily as mechanistic studies, and with the development of simpler procedures a greater number of agents can be tested more rapidly. Modifications and improvements in the micronucleus test, its extension to animal and human tissues, and tests with transplacentally active agents are some of the recent examples for a useful role for this test system in genotoxicity screening programmes.

Numerous excellent and complete reviews on the history, development, validation and performance of this test procedure are available (Schmid, 1976, 1977; Heddle and Salamone, 1981; Jenssen, 1982; Heddle et al., 1983, 1984) and these details will not be repeated in this report. The purpose of this chapter will be to review the recent developments and applications of the micronucleus test procedure and to evaluate the rapid advances made in extending the use of this method to diverse areas of cytogenetic testing with mammalian systems.

BACKGROUND AND PRINCIPLE OF THE METHOD

Micronuclei were observed first by Howell (1891) as distinct cellular inclusions in red blood cells from anaemic cats. Jolly (1905) later confirmed the existence of micronuclei during studies of erythrocyte development with mouse and rat embryos. In medicine, presence of Howell–Jolly bodies (micronuclei) in erythrocytes is diagnostic for various anaemias (Miale, 1982). Presence of micronuclei in blood cells can also indicate dysfunction of the spleen that should under normal conditions act to remove abnormal erythrocytes (Miale, 1982). Micronuclei appear as round, membrane-bound cellular inclusions which vary from 1 to 4 micrometres in size and contain deoxyribonucleic acid (DNA) (Schmid, 1973, 1975, 1977; Heddle, 1973; Heddle and Carrano, 1977). Micronuclei are believed to form as a result of damage to chromosomes or to the mitotic apparatus, resulting in acentric chromosomal fragments or in abnormal mitotic segregation. The fragments, 'lagging' chromosomes or chromosomes with multiple centromeres, form small nuclei ('micronuclei') which are distinct from the cell nucleus, but which stain similarly because of their DNA content. *Fig*. 6.1 shows typical micronuclei in mouse bone marrow cells and in cells from peripheral blood.

Heddle and Carrano (1977) quantified the DNA content of micronuclei from mouse bone marrow cells and concluded that the amount of DNA was in agreement with the hypothesis that micronuclei arise from chromosomal fragments. Hayashi et al. (1984a) also found the same agreement between distributions for the DNA content of micronuclei and the lengths of acentric fragments in mouse bone marrow cells. Other evidence suggest that the sizes of micronuclei may indicate the mechanism of chromosome damage. Yamamoto and Kikuchi (1980) observed that micronuclei produced by clastogens were smaller than those produced by spindle inhibitors such as vincristine. This finding indicates that the size of micronuclei can discriminate between agents which operate by different cytogenetic mechanisms. Högstedt and Karlsson (1985) independently verified the findings of Yamamoto and Kikuchi (1980), and also showed that agents which produce chromosome fragments (X-rays and mitomycin C) had smaller sized micronuclei than agents which affect chromosomes and the mitotic spindle (colcemid and vincristine). Thus, the micronucleus test can discriminate between different clastogenic mechanisms in addition to its role as a biological monitor of potential chromosome damage.

A number of test systems have been developed in which micronuclei are used as indicators of chromosome damage in plants (Ma, 1979), animals (von Lebedur and Schmid, 1973; Schmid, 1973, 1975, 1976, 1977; Matter and Grauwiler, 1974) and in mammalian cell cultures (Obe et al., 1975; Countryman and Heddle, 1976; Lasne et al., 1984). In animals, micronuclei are most easily discernible in polychromatic erythrocytes (PCEs) which are anucleated cells whose relative age can be determined by staining differences. PCEs contain residual RNA which results in a pale-bluish staining of the cytoplasm by Giemsa stains (Schmid, 1973). PCEs are a relatively late stage in the erythrocyte maturation process, and they exist in the mouse bone marrow and peripheral blood for 24 to 30 hours prior to maturation into normochromatic erythrocytes (NCEs). Schmid (1973) recognized that restricting studies of micronuclei to observations with PCEs would increase the sensitivity of detecting clastogenic effects because the young target cells, which developed during the exposure period to the test material, could be distinguished. Other advantages of evaluating PCEs for clastogenic effects are the large number of cells available for examination, and eliminating the requirement for obtaining mitotic cells necessary for classic metaphase chromosome procedures.

Although technically less demanding than examination of chromosome aberrations, the micronucleus test still requires a moderate degree of experience for accurate identification of micronuclei, and to avoid technical artefacts. As stated more directly by Schmid (1975), 'the micronucleus test is a relatively simple method but it was not designed for evaluation by fools'. Aminoacridines are apparently one group of chemicals which present difficulties for evaluation in this system. Several aminoacridines, which did not increase chromosome aberrations in metaphase analyses of mouse bone marrow cells, produced significant increases in what appeared to be micronuclei in mouse erythrocytes (Jenssen et al., 1974). Further work showed that the 'micronuclei' were artefacts because they were Feulgen-negative, they were neither membrane-bound nor spherical (like true micronuclei), and they contained RNA rather than DNA (Maier and Schmid, 1975; Jenssen, 1982). However, the artefacts caused by aminoacridines may not represent a common problem. Jenssen (1982) cited preliminary data suggesting that aminoacridines interact with microtubules, and they may alter the nucleolar organizers resulting in fragmented nucleoli which were mistaken for micronuclei. The number of chemicals which specifically affect nucleoli is apparently very low because other chemically produced artefacts, like those found for the aminoacridine example, are not common.

Methods to avoid technical artefacts in identifying micronuclei are now available. Two reports by Hayashi et al. (1983) and by MacGregor et al. (1983a) describe fluorescent staining procedures that discriminate between RNA and DNA, and thus provide a more definitive identification of micronuclei. Hayashi et al. (1983) stained bone marrow smears using 0·24 mM acridine orange in 1/15 M Sorensen's buffer (pH 6·8) for 3 minutes followed by 3 rinses in buffer. Under fluorescence illumination, the micronuclei emitted bright green fluorescence and were easily distinguished from granules and contaminants which fluoresced red. MacGregor et al. (1983a) used a double dye procedure using Hoechst 33258, which binds to DNA and emits blue fluorescence, and pyronin Y, which stains

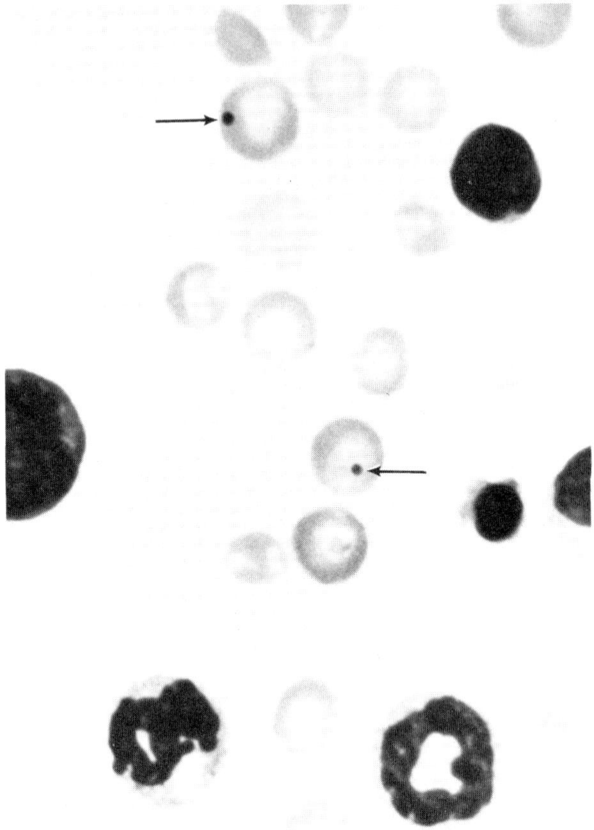

a

Fig. 6.1. Micronuclei in mouse bone marrow (*a*) and

both DNA and RNA and emits red-orange fluorescence. The advantages of this procedure included differentiation of micronuclei from basophilic granules, selective identification of DNA-containing objects, and a reduction in the number of staining manipulations. Fluorescence methods are significant advancements for studies of micronuclei because they open up possibilities both for application of flow cytometry and image analysis methods in quantifying micronuclei in cells (MacGregor et al., 1983b).

Pascoe and Gatehouse (1986) recently developed a haematoxylin-eosin staining procedure which differentiates micronuclei from cellular inclusions and produces permanent staining, in contrast to fluorescence procedures. The haematoxylin-eosin procedure stains micronuclei blue-black but does not stain micronuclei-like inclusions, such as mast cell granules which are numerous in rat bone marrow preparations. Other micronuclei-like artefacts produced by acridine dyes (e.g. quinacrine) (Maier and Schmid, 1975) also stain with haematoxylin-eosin dye, but with much less intensity than micronuclei so that they can be discriminated and avoided.

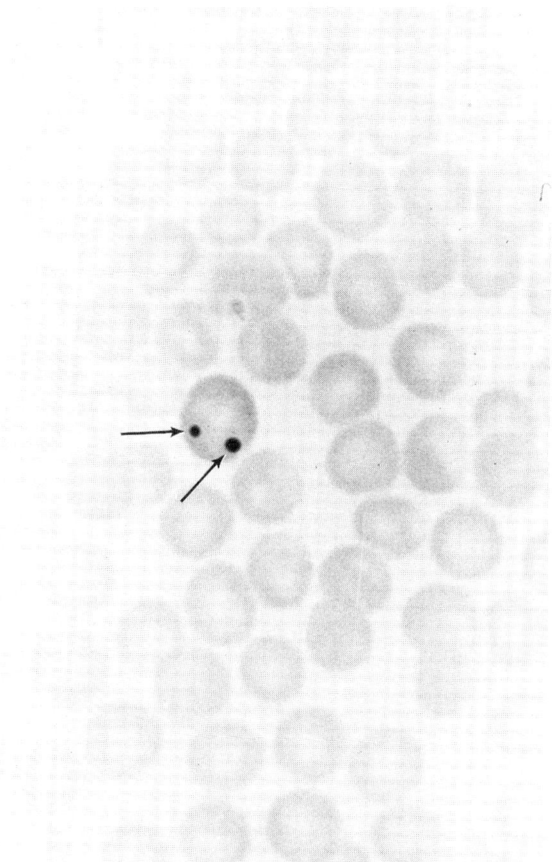

b

peripheral blood polychromatic erythrocytes (*b*).

FACTORS AFFECTING THE SENSITIVITY OF THE TEST SYSTEM

Reliability of the micronucleus test for detecting the clastogenic potential of chemicals has been criticized because the test is an indirect measurement of only a portion of the possible types of chromosomal damage. In order for a test system to be useful as a screen for potential clastogens, it should detect activity of a variety of agents which act by different mechanisms, and the test must be reproducible in multiple laboratories. Experiments to validate genetic screening tests are necessary for assessing both the sensitivity and, of equal importance, the limitations of the test system. Several of the studies to be discussed in the following section are directed at comparing results obtained using the micronucleus test to those using 'classical' cytogenetic metaphase analysis. Other examples compare the effects of modifying various parameters of the testing protocol in order to increase the sensitivity of the assay. In typical comparative studies, modification of test parameters involved varying the time between dosing and tissue sampling, studying the effects of multiple injections of a fractionated dose as compared to a single dose, and quantifying the micronucleus response in different tissues.

Comparison of the Micronucleus Test to Classical Cytogenetics Methods

The classical method of cytogenetic analysis involves the laborious and skilled task of observing large numbers of metaphase cells for anomalies of chromosome number and structure. Detailed information can be obtained from a cytogenetic study regarding the nature of the chromosomal lesions and the mechanisms of interaction with the genome. A major advantage of metaphase analysis is the ability to detect numerical additions and deletions of chromosomes and translocation of chromosomal segments. However, the direct method of chromosome evaluation is extremely time consuming, and this limits both the number of possible tests and the speed of obtaining final results. The informational advantages of metaphase analyses are not particularly relevant to routine screening tests, which are intended primarily to identify genotoxic potential rather than to be mechanistic studies.

A break in the chromosome or chromatid is the primary lesion induced by most clastogens. Since a break in the chromatid material, if not repaired, produces an acentric fragment, breakage can be detected and quantified by counting micronuclei which form from chromosomal fragments. Thus, the major concern for micronucleus testing is whether clastogenic effects can be detected with the same agents and dose levels as those detected by metaphase analysis. Because clastogens produce a spectrum of lesions, some of which are not associated with chromosomal breakage, a larger number of cells is required for evaluation in the micronucleus test to achieve comparable sensitivity to metaphase analyses. However, 1000 or more exposed cells can be observed easily with the micronucleus test in a fraction of the time required to evaluate the 50 to 100 metaphase cells generally evaluated in metaphase test protocols.

In early studies, Goetz et al. (1975) compared the clastogenic response induced by cyclophosphamide using bone marrow metaphase analysis and the micronucleus test in mice, rats and Chinese hamsters. Cyclophosphamide is an indirect clastogen that requires biotransformation to produce an active metabolite. In all three species, the proportion of PCEs with micronuclei correlated well with the percentage of cells with aberrations detected by metaphase analyses. Although positive increases of chromosome damage were detected similarly by both methods, the slope of the dose-response curve for chromosome breaks was steeper than the curve for the percent of PCEs with micronuclei. The peak response for micronuclei was six times higher than the control values. However, the maximum response using cytogenetic evaluation was approximately 62 times greater than the control. Although both methods demonstrated unequivocal dose-related effects, the use of classical metaphase analysis appeared to be more sensitive than micronucleus analysis with the limited number of cells sampled.

In later studies, Frank et al. (1978) compared activity of cyclophosphamide in both the micronucleus test and a bone marrow cytogenetics assay using four routes of administration: intravenous, intraperitoneal, subcutaneous and peroral. The micronucleus test detected chromosome damage in the PCEs of bone marrow cells at the lowest dose level of cyclophosphamide tested (5 mg/kg) by each route of dosage administration. Although the micronucleus test required evaluation of more cells, a positive dose-related effect could be obtained in most cases in less than half the time required using metaphase analysis.

In a similar study, Kliesch et al. (1981) compared the sensitivities of the micronucleus test and bone marrow cytogenetic analysis after treatment of mice with methyl methanesulphonate, mitomycin C and procarbazine. Both methods showed comparable positive responses at the same dose level after exposure to mitomycin C and procarbazine. However, in order to detect a significant response to methyl methanesulphonate, a short-lived and highly reactive alkylating agent, the micronucleus test required a dose level two times higher than that employed with animals evaluated by metaphase analysis. This result indicates that selection of the dosing interval may be a critical factor for attaining adequate sensitivity of the micronucleus test. Also, for some highly reactive chemicals, a larger sample of cells may be required to detect a positive micronucleus response in the bone marrow.

Tsuchimoto and Matter (1979) compared results from the micronucleus test to those obtained using chromosome metaphase analysis and sister chromatid exchange (SCE) evaluations with Chinese hamsters. Triethylenemelamine (TEM) is a bifunctional alkylating agent and a potent inducer of chromosome aberrations. Significant and dose-related increases were induced by TEM in all three test systems. SCE analysis was the most sensitive indicator of chromosome damage, and a statistically significant response was obtained with a dose of 0·032 mg/kg. A positive response was detectable at the next higher dose of 0·062 mg/kg by metaphase analyses, and at 0·125 mg/kg in the micronucleus test. Azathioprine, another recognized clastogen, produced significant increases only at the maximum dose tested (500 mg/kg) with either the micronucleus test or by metaphase analysis. No significant response was observed in the SCE test. The results demonstrate the variation in sensitivity between the various test systems for detecting activity of specific agents; however, the study supports the comparability of the micronucleus results to those obtained by metaphase analyses.

The micronucleus test has an additional advantage in that it can detect spindle poisons. Spindle poisons such as colchicine and vincristine have been shown to affect the microtubules involved in chromosome movement, and this may result in errors in the segregation of the chromosomes at mitosis (mitotic non-disjunction). Segregation errors produce 'lagging' chromosomes that are not integrated with the other chromosomes into the two newly formed cellular nuclei at cell division. These isolated (lagging) chromosomes are usually incorporated into membranous vesicles to form micronuclei. Experiments with colchicine by Tsuchimoto and Matter (1979) showed positive results in the micronucleus test using mice, but only weak effects in the test with Chinese hamsters. Mice may, thus, be a more sensitive species for detecting non-disjunctional events.

Although all three test systems can detect effects on the chromosome level, the molecular mechanisms which lead to the various endpoints differ both for the individual assays and for different chemicals. Therefore, each test has unique value in a test battery to reveal possible differences in mutagenic mechanisms for various agents. A large number of chemicals have been tested and compared using these approaches. In most studies with known clastogens, micronucleus testing alone is sufficient to detect a positive response. However, the limitations of this test system must be considered when evaluating negative test data from studies on chemicals with unknown genetic specificity. Many modifications of the basic test system have been shown to increase the sensitivity and reproducibility of the micronucleus test (Heddle et al., 1983), and these improvements should be incorporated into current testing protocols. Factors such as multiple sampling times, fractionated dose administration, use of adequate positive and negative controls, and appropriate dose selection have all been found to affect the sensitivity of the micronucleus test. The following sections will summarize some of the principal factors found to affect performance and reliability of this test system.

Determination of Optimum Numbers of Exposures and Sampling Intervals

Bone-Marrow Kinetics of Micronucleus Formation:

Detection of genotoxic agents with 'weak' levels of effect in the test system necessitates sampling the target cells at a period of maximum response. In order to determine the optimum time period to detect peak responses in the micronucleus test, it is first necessary to understand the kinetics of erythrocyte maturation in the bone marrow. Cole et al. (1979, 1981) described the effect of the cell-cycle kinetics of the adult bone marrow erythroblast (*Fig.* 6.2) upon the time of appearance of micronuclei. Each erythroblast was shown to undergo 6 to 7 divisions in the bone marrow, and each of the last two divisions required

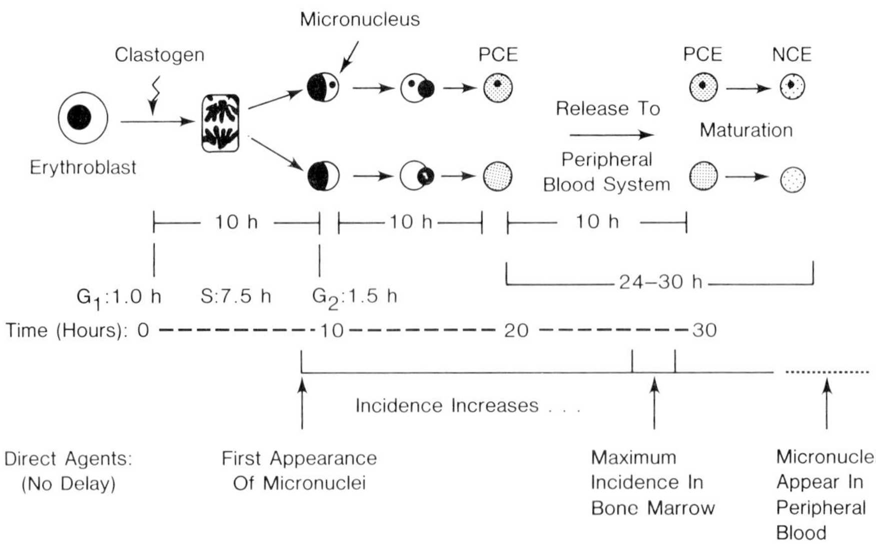

Fig. 6.2. Timing of micronucleus formation during erythroblast differentiation in adult mouse bone marrow cells (Cole et al., 1979, 1981).

approximately 10 hours for completion: 1.0 hour for G_1, 7.5 hours for DNA synthesis (S-phase), and 1.5 hours for G_2. After mitosis, the cells matured in the bone marrow for 10 hours before the nucleus was extruded. On the basis of these times, it was not considered to be useful to sample bone marrow for treatment-induced micronuclei earlier than 10 hours after dosing. Following nuclear expulsion, the resulting anucleated polychromatic erythrocytes, rich in ribosomal material, remain in the bone marrow an additional 10 hours before release into the peripheral circulation. Some agents, because of their cytotoxic properties, also cause delays at various points of the cell cycle, and this can produce a further delay in the time interval for observing maximal responses. Therefore, when screening agents with unknown metabolic requirements and undefined bone-marrow cytotoxicity, it is extremely important to sample the bone marrow at several time intervals after treatment.

Jenssen and Ramel (1978) confirmed the results of Cole et al. (1979) by using autoradiography of [^{3}H]thymidine-labelled nuclei to measure the time required to expel the nucleus after the S-phase of mitosis is complete. These tests indicated that the time interval between the end of S-phase in bone marrow erythroblasts until nuclear expulsion was approximately 12 hours. Their results showed that micronuclei were produced by X-rays both in G_2- and S-phases of the cell cycle but MMS, in contrast, produced micronuclei predominantly in S-phase.

Hart and Hartly-Asp (1983) recently demonstrated increases in micronuclei in bone marrow erythrocytes significantly earlier than 10 hours after treatment. The authors suggested a revised model of cell-cycle timing where the final mitosis occurs only 5 hours before the expulsion of the nucleus, in contrast to the 10 hours originally determined by Cole et al. (1979). Results from tests with the spindle poison vincristine, and with X-rays which do not produce delays in cell division, indicated that there was a 5 hour interval for expulsion of the nucleus following the final mitosis in the bone marrow. The 9 to 12 hour interval determined by Jenssen and Ramel (1978) using X-rays was explained on the basis that [^{3}H]thymidine itself caused a delay in cell division (Morimoto and Wolff, 1980), and this delay may have affected the results of their studies. Agents such as cyclophosphamide, which are known to produce delays in cell division, required 9 to 10 hours to elicit a positive increase of micronuclei in bone-marrow erythrocytes. Thus, although the 10 hour cell division time proposed by Cole et al. (1979) was supported by this study, the nuclear extrusion phase was shown to require only 5 hours with the agents employed.

A summary of the results from the various studies discussed in this section reveals some general areas of agreement and a few discordant findings. In the studies cited, the time interval between the final erythroblast division until enucluation varies from 5 to 12 hours; with the greatest agreement for a 5 to 8 hour time interval (Jenssen and Ramel, 1978; Hart and Hartley-Asp, 1983; Hayashi et al., 1984a). The estimated time interval that PCEs remain in the bone marrow also ranges from 10 hours (Cole et al., 1979; Hart and Hartley-Asp, 1983) to 24 hours; with the greatest agreement for an 18 to 24 hour residence interval (Jenssen and Ramel, 1978; Heddle et al., 1984; Hayashi et al., 1984a). In general terms, therefore, the predominant evidence suggests that sampling bone marrow for micronuclei prior to 6 hours would be of little or no value, and that 15 to 36 hour samples generally will provide maximum responses for direct-acting agents (Heddle et al., 1984).

Numbers of Doses and Sampling Times:

In the original test protocol proposed by Schmid (1975), dosing was performed twice, at 24 hour intervals, and bone marrow was sampled once at 30 hours. Salamone et al. (1980) studied the influence of multiple injections and multiple sample times with three different classes of compounds. After a single injection, each chemical produced a different pattern of micronucleus responses over time. Mitomycin C produced the earliest increase of micronuclei which attained maximal values at 36 hours. Cyclophosphamide produced a maximum number of micronuclei between 42 and 48 hours, and the micronucleus response to 9,10-dimethyl-2,3-benzanthracene (DMBA) did not attain values maximum until 72 hours. A significant increase in the incidence of micronuclei was detected by 24 hours after injection of mitomycin C and cyclophosphamide, but effects of DMBA were not evident until the 36 hour sample. Thus, a single sample at 30 hours would not detect a delayed micronuclear response for agents which act like DMBA. For all three chemicals, the incidence of micronuclei returned to baseline level by 96 hours. Return to control levels would be expected at 96 hours because by this time all of the bone marrow erythrocytes from the exposed population at risk would have been released into the peripheral circulation. Thus, sampling at 96 hours or later would not generally be recommended or useful for this test in bone marrow.

In the same study, Salamone et al. (1980) compared the time-response curve after a single injection at 0 hours and double injection regime at 0 and 24 hours. For all three agents, two injections with a single 48 hour sample time produced similar total numbers of micronuclei as obtained following a single injection and summing the individual values for the 24 hour and 48 hour evaluations. With the double injection protocol, the peak incidence of micronuclei produced by mitomycin C and cyclophosphamide was delayed for 12 hours, but the peak in the time-response curve for DMBA was similar with either single or double injections. Although two injections at 0 and 24 hours generally produced additive micronucleus values, more than two injections produced excessive cytotoxicity and decreased the total numbers of micronuclei and the sensitivity of the test system. The authors concluded that a double treatment protocol, with a single 30 hour sample of bone marrow (as recommended by Schmid, 1975), does not eliminate the need for multiple sampling times. Also, the excessive cytotoxicity noted by a decrease in PCEs following more than two injections indicates that subchronic administration would not be appropriate for routine testing.

In contrast to the results of Salamone et al. (1980), Kliesch et al. (1981) observed lower numbers of micronuclei in mouse bone marrow PCEs when the same total dose was administered in two injections rather than one. The incidence of micronuclei at 30 and 48 hour sampling times was lower for three clastogens when tested in the double versus single injection schedule. Kliesch et al. (1982) discussed the possibility that the sensitivity of the micronucleus test could be reduced by multiple exposures because of induced changes in cell-cycle kinetics and erythroid-cell maturation. Also, each exposure produces cell damage leading to death, and thus reduces the relative number of affected cells in the sample. For routine genotoxicity screening studies, the use of a single injection schedule may be preferable for agents with undefined bone marrow cytotoxicity, metabolism and pharmacokinetics. A double injection schedule may serve to increase test sensitivity for chemicals which possess a short biological half-life, and which do not adversely affect frequency of bone marrow PCEs.

In addition to the single injection and double injection protocols, several investigators have studied the effects of a 5-daily injection schedule using fractionated doses. Yamamoto and Kikuchi (1981) employed a repeat-dosing protocol in the study discussed previously and found that the 5-treatment schedule produced micronuclei responses which were similar to those obtained with a single injection of the five alkylating agents. However, with antimetabolites, the 5-injection protocol increased the sensitivity for detecting positive effects. With all agents, multiple injections at high dose levels produced bone marrow cytotoxicity and decreased the incidence of micronuclei in PCEs. Thus, a lower total dose is required when a multiple injection protocol is used. The value of a multiple dosing regime for micronucleus evaluations in bone marrow is apparently limited to only a few specific agents (eg. antimetabolites). Because bone marrow micronuclei do not reveal cumulative effects in a consistent fashion, similar results can generally be obtained with one or, at most, two injections of the test material.

Yamamoto and Kikuchi (1981) studied the effects of sequential sampling of mouse bone marrow erythrocytes on the sensitivity of detecting increases in numbers of micronuclei. Several of the alkylating agents that were tested with a single dose produced peak frequencies of micronuclei at 24 hours following injection. With 6-mercaptopurine, an antimetabolite of nucleic acid synthesis, although no response was observed at 24 hours, the incidence of micronuclei peaked sharply at 30 hours. Vincristine, a spindle poison, produced a highly significant increase in numbers of micronuclei at the 24 hour sample, values then peaked at the 30 hour sample, and only a marginal elevation in numbers of micronuclei was observed after 48 hours. Therefore, for a single dose administration, the optimal time to sample bone marrow for these agents was apparently 30 hours posttreatment.

Multiple sampling times are particularly important for increasing the sensitivity and reliability of the test system. Some chemicals require varying time intervals for biotransformation and transport of active metabolites to the bone marrow. Treatment-related effects are detected only if different sampling intervals are employed. Several testing protocols reviewed in this section show that various agents produce a different pattern of response which necessitates multiple doses or samplings. Although there is no single protocol that will produce optimal results for all test agents, the US EPA Gene-Tox Program (Heddle et al., 1983) recommended that a single treatment with multiple posttreatment sampling times was a preferable protocol when testing agents of unknown activity.

Selection of Appropriate Dose Ranges

As with most biological assays, testing over an effective range of concentrations is a crucial factor that affects both the sensitivity of the test system and relevance of the results. Some agents are clastogenic within a relatively narrow range of cytotoxicity, whereas others may be effective at low, non-cytotoxic levels. Several chemicals, particularly alkylating agents, produce damage to chromosomes at dose levels that correlate directly with cytotoxic effects. However, excessive cytotoxicity can decrease the yield of micronuclei because damaged cells may be selectively eliminated in the surviving population. The relative degree of bone marrow cytotoxicity in the micronucleus test system can be assessed by evaluating the proportion of PCEs relative to the total population of NCEs. However, Kliesch et al. (1982) found decreases in the incidence of both micronuclei and

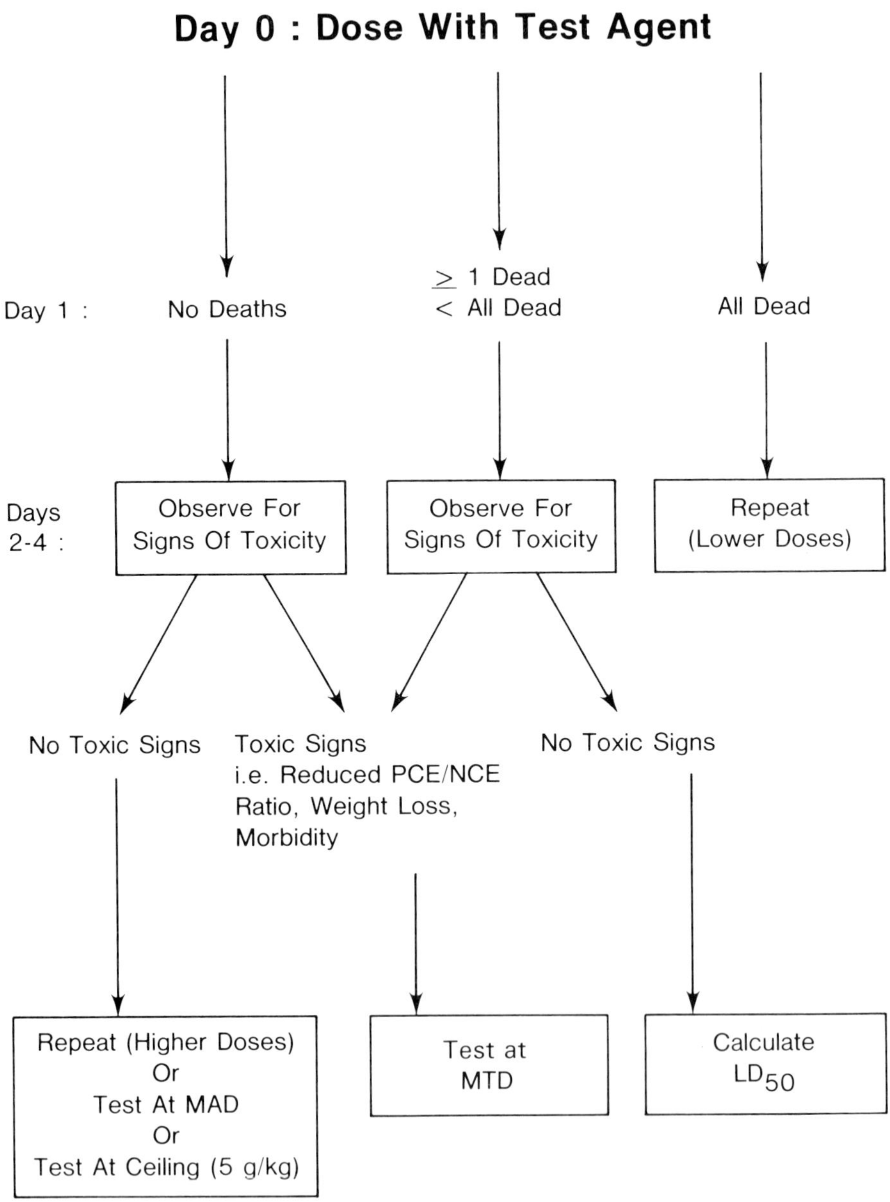

Fig. 6.3. Flow diagram of preliminary tests suitable for identifying appropriate dose ranges for micronucleus testing.

chromosome aberrations at high dose levels of benzo[*a*]pyrene even when there was no indication of either a reduced PCE:NCE ratio or reduction of the mitotic index.

Hayashi et al. (1984b) recognized the need for a standard procedure to identify appropriate dose ranges for the micronucleus test, and they have proposed a preliminary test protocol to determine suitable dosage ranges and sampling times. With their approach, 4 different dose levels were administered ip to 2 male mice (or 1 male and 1 female), and bone marrows were sampled at 18, 24, 30, 48 and 72 hours after injection. Following staining, the PCE:NCE ratio of 200 erythrocytes and the incidence of micronuclei in 1000 PCEs were scored. The maximum dose level for the preliminary test was chosen as twice the published LD_{50} value when available, otherwise, 5 g/kg was used arbitrarily. Subsequent dose levels were 50%, 25% and 12·5% of the maximum selected dose. Appropriate experimental parameters for the definitive test were determined from the preliminary data by the sampling time and dose which gave maximum numbers of micronuclei in PCEs when data were arranged two-dimensionally. For chemicals which did not produce significant increases of micronuclei, the maximum dose would be the highest dose which produced no deaths.

The US EPA Gene-Tox Program (Heddle et al., 1983) recommended that a minimum of three dose levels be tested over a reasonably wide range. In general, the highest dose level should be either the maximum tolerated dose (MTD) or approximately 80% of the LD_{50}. For agents of undetermined toxicity, a 4-day LD_{50} was considered adequate to determine the maximum dose for short-term testing. Preliminary assessment of the PCE:NCE ratio after exposure to several dose levels can be used for some agents to assess cytotoxicity to bone marrow erythrocytes and to detect delays in the cell cycle by multiple sampling at 24 hour intervals. The MTD may be determined as the highest dose that does not produce excessive signs of toxicity, which can be defined as significant weight losses, behavioural effects, or depression of the PCE:NCE ratio by more than 50 to 75% of control values. In the case of non-cytotoxic test agents, the maximum attainable dose level (MAD) should be administered as the highest dose level using 5 g/kg as a reasonable maximum dose ('limit test'). Additional dose levels are typically set at 50%, 25%, and 12.5% of the LD_{50}, MTD or MAD as appropriate to the test agent. *Fig.* 6.3 presents a flow diagram that illustrates one possible scheme for preliminary determination of appropriate test doses as discussed in this section. In practice, dosages which depress the PCE:NCE ratio below 5 per 1000 are extremely difficult to evaluate properly, and should be considered as excessively cytotoxic.

Scoring and Evaluation of Micronucleus Data

Evaluation of incidences of micronuclei for significant differences from concurrent vehicle control values typically relies upon some statistical procedure to analyze the data. The value of statistical analyses and the power of various tests to reveal actual differences is affected by the group size, the sample size/animal and the variability between animals. Typically, a group size of 5 males and females per dose level and 1000 PCEs per animal are recommended minimal sample sizes by various guidelines for this test (Heddle et al., 1983; EPA, 1985;

OECD, 1987). Schmid (1973) originally recommended that 'per animal a total of 2000 to 5000 erythrocytes are examined for presence of micronuclei. The findings grouped in (a) polychromatic erythrocytes with one or several micronuclei, and (b) other erythrocytes with micronuclei.' This recommendation was misquoted by Ashby and Mohammed (1986) who stated that 'Schmid (1973) originally recommended that between 2000 to 5000 polychromatic erythrocytes should be assessed per slide' in their recent proposal that evaluation of at least 2000 PCEs/animal would be a prudent sample size to reduce variability of bone marrow evaluations. In fact, Schmid (1973) apparently grouped both polychromatic and normochromatic erythrocytes in his recommendation, and because NCEs are present in much greater numbers than PCEs, current guidelines for this test of 1000 PCE (minimum) actually *exceed* rather than ignore Schmid's recommendation. However, for statistical analyses, apparently 2000 cells/animal is preferable to reduce frequency of zeros in the data for mathematical transformations of the data prior to statistical analyses (Mitchell and Brice, 1986).

Ashby and Mohammed (1986) made several excellent and pertinent observations and recommendations concerning evaluation of the adequacy of spontaneous micronucleus values and evaluation of results. They stressed the importance of adequate historical negative control data for each testing facility which show that the spontaneous variation is within a reasonably expected range of (approximately) 0–4 mPCE/1000 PCE. If the spontaneous incidence is outside this range, then problems in slide preparation or errors in scoring micronuclei should be suspected. Interestingly, Ashby and Mohammed (1986) concluded that they have yet to find a consistent method to prepare homogeneous slides which would reduce counting variability for the bone marrow procedure. Apparently, with the typical methods used to disperse bone marrow preparations, using smear or paintbrush techniques, they found that certain areas of the slide can contain higher/lower numbers of mPCE. These authors stressed the importance of using a standardized method of slide reading to reduce variability caused by these 'runs' of specific cells. In subsequent sections of this chapter, the problem of non-homogeneity of bone marrow and subsequent slide reading problems may be circumvented by scoring PCEs in blood samples from dosed animals either instead of using bone marrow or to provide additional data. Blood is presumably a more homogeneous tissue than bone marrow and less variability would be expected in slide preparation. Also, repetitive sampling from the same animal reduces animal usage and lowers variability since animal to animal variations constitute the principal source of variance. Interesting comparisons and complementary data could be obtained from blood PCEs with no more effort than by the suggested doubling of cells from 1000 to 2000 in evaluation of bone marrow slides (Ashby and Mohammed, 1986).

Tissue Differences

As mentioned in previous sections, some agents are tissue specific and affect only one or a few tissues. Tissue specificity may depend on the route of dose administration, biotransformation, the tissue distribution of either the parent compound or active metabolites, the rate of transport and concentration of the active agent in a given tissue, and the rate of elimination. Thus, sampling only one tissue, such as bone marrow, following dose administration by a single route will not always effectively detect all potential clastogens. A number of micronucleus procedures which use specific cells or tissues have been developed to overcome the limitations of the bone marrow procedure, and some of these methods are presented in the following sections.

Goldberg et al. (1983) examined epithelial cells from the colon following dissection of the colon, fixation with buffered formalin, and preparation of histological sections in paraffin. Sections were stained with Feulgen-Fast Green Stain and the cells in each of 10 crypts were scored for presence of micronuclei. Bone marrow PCEs and colon epithelial cells were compared for ability to detect the effects of 1,2-dimethylhydrazine (DMH) and cyclophosphamide. DMH, a specific colon carcinogen, induced an approximate incidence of 5% of colon cells with micronuclei. However, in the bone marrow of the same animals, there was no increase in the incidence of micronuclei, even at the highest dose levels. In contrast, cyclophosphamide affected primarily the bone marrow erythrocytes with little increase of micronuclei in the colon. The tissue-specific effects of DMH were not believed to be caused by preferential distribution because studies by Rublo et al. (1980) showed that the agent and its metabolites can reach the colon through the blood stream. Therefore, the specificity of this agent may be due either to selective metabolism by specific enzymes in the colon (Grab and Zedeck, 1977) or to other undefined mechanisms.

Shindo et al. (1983) compared the incidence of micronuclei from the spleen to those from PCEs in the bone marrow using the same mouse. Unlike rats and man, haematopoiesis is active in both the spleen and bone marrow of the adult mouse (Loem et al., 1978). Spleens were removed 30 hours after treatment, and the spleen cells were rinsed, suspended in foetal calf serum, and dissociated by forcing the tissue through a syringe. The cells were centrifuged and resuspended in a small volume of calf serum, and slides were then prepared and stained using routine bone marrow techniques. PCEs were found in the spleen cells at a frequency of 9%, a value that is similar to the 13% typically seen in the bone marrow. For mitomycin C, cyclophosphamide and fosfomycin, evaluations of micronuclei in the spleen and the bone marrow produced similar conclusions. A significant increase in the incidence of micronuclei was observed in animals treated with either mitomycin C or cyclophosphamide. However, numbers of micronuclei were slightly higher in the bone marrow PCEs than in those from the spleen. Fosfomycin, a broad-spectrum antibiotic, did not increase the incidence of micronuclei in either spleen or bone marrow cells. Use of spleen cells may have value for confirming effects found in bone marrow PCEs, or to provide an alternate tissue with comparable sensitivity when bone marrow is needed for other studies such as cytogenetic analyses or for pathology preparations.

Liver is not a typical tissue used for the micronucleus test because it is composed principally of non-dividing cells, and at least one cell division following genetic damage is necessary for production of micronuclei. Tates and den Engelse (1982) circumvented this problem by stimulating cell division in the liver by partial hepatectomy. Following a single ip injection of DMN, DEN or EMS, rats were partially hepatectomized at 1, 6 and 28 days following injection of EMS , and at an additional time of 56 days following administration of DMN or DEN. DMN was shown to induce statistically significant increases in the incidence of micronuclei in hepatocytes isolated from livers of treated animals as long as 28 days after injection of the test chemicals. The incidence of micronuclei in hepatocytes tested with DEN was significantly elevated at all four time intervals tested. However, EMS did not produce a significant increase in the frequency of micronuclei in the hepatocytes at any sampling time. The hepatocyte method appears to be a sensitive and useful method for evaluating agents which are activated in the liver. However, for direct alkylating agents such as EMS, the test either lacks adequate sensitivity or, more likely, additional sampling at earlier time periods is necessary to detect treatment-related effects.

Human lymphocytes offer another potential source of readily available cells amenable to micronucleus analyses (Countryman and Heddle, 1976; Hartley-Asp, 1979). However, the lymphocyte, unlike the erythrocyte, is a nucleated cell with only a small amount of cytoplasm. These two characteristics lead to significant problems in identifying and counting micronuclei. Högstedt (1984) developed a modified method for studying micronuclei in lymphocytes in which the cytoplasm of the cell is preserved by elimination of the typical hypotonic-fixation steps. Human whole blood was cultured for 72 to 96 hours in McCoy's 5A medium supplemented with calf serum and with the mitogen phytohaemagglutinin (PHA). After incubation, the cells were centrifuged, medium was removed and slides were prepared by smearing cells resuspended in a small amount of medium across each slide. With styrene, lymphocyte cultures of blood from 38 exposed workers showed a weak but statistically significant correlation between increases in numbers of micronuclei and increases in numerical chromosome aberrations. For human monitoring, evaluation of clastogenic effects using the lymphocyte micronucleus procedure appears to provide similar data to the more laborious metaphase evaluations. However, recent studies by Fenech and Morley (1985a) show that endogenous levels of micronuclei in human lymphocytes increase with increasing age of the donor, and responses to clastogenic agents increase in an inverse relation to age. Thus, additional studies appear to be necessary to verify the application of this procedure for routine use.

Vehicle Effects

Several vehicles have been shown to affect the results and apparent sensitivity of the micronucleus test. Raj and Katz (1984) demonstrated that corn oil and/or its constituents inhibited the induction of micronuclei and chromosome aberrations by DMBA. Corn oil is a widely used vehicle for agents that are mixed in the diet, applied topically, or for those which are not water soluble. The fats, oils and lipids contained in corn oil are essential for the optimal function of some microsomal enzymes. The cytochrome P450 mixed function oxidase system acts in the biotransformation of a large number of xenobiotics to either more or less biologically active forms, and rats fed diets supplemented with corn oil have increased levels of cytochrome P450 (Norred and Wade, 1972; Marshall and McLean, 1971). Because of these possible effects upon metabolism, use of corn oil as a vehicle should be considered in interpreting results of genotoxicity tests. Wade et al. (1978) observed that corn oil increased the metabolic conversion of DMN and decreased the mutagenic activity of the agent. However, in other studies, rats fed diets enriched with polyunsaturated fatty acids were more susceptible to tumour induction by other carcinogens. There may be quite distinct differences in assessing genotoxicity and carcinogenicity, but the added role of the vehicle in affecting these endpoints should not be forgotten.

Dimethylsulphoxide (DMSO) is a solvent that is commonly used for agents that are not water soluble. When DMSO was administered by ip injection in our laboratory, we found that DMSO was lethal to weanling Swiss-Webster mice at 10 ml/kg (Guzzie and Slesinski, unpublished results). Mice administered 5 ml/kg of DMSO were lethargic and their fur appeared unkempt within one day after injection. No adverse clinical signs were noted at dose levels between 2 to 3 ml/kg. Salamone (1981) also reported that DMSO was toxic to mice at 9–11 ml/kg, ip. In addition, there are reports that DMSO may potentiate the toxicity of some substances, possibly by increasing the rate of distribution of the agent to the target tissue. Salamone (1981) speculated that the toxicity of cyclophosphamide was increased slightly when DMSO was used as the vehicle in comparison to saline (424 *v.* 584 mg/kg, respectively). Finally, there is one report that DMSO was clastogenic following ip dosing of rats (Kapp and Eventhoff, 1980).

Caution should be employed when using ethanol as a vehicle in micronucleus studies. We observed (unpublished data) that absolute ethanol was lethal when administered ip to Swiss-Webster mice at the relatively low level of 0·05 ml to a 30 g mouse (1·67 ml/kg).Administration of a 50% solution of ethanol in water and a 0·05 ml injection volume produced transient sedation but no deaths. In addition to toxicity, ethanol has also been shown to be a clastogenic agent in human studies on alcoholics (Obe and Herha, 1975). Other studies also indicate that ethanol can induce the formation of ring and dicentric chromosomes (Obe et al., 1979). In studies in our laboratory, we have not observed significant effects of ethanol upon the spontaneous aberration values in either *in vitro* tests with CHO cells or in mouse peripheral blood micronucleus tests using a 50% ethanol vehicle (1·0 g/kg). Korte et al. (1979) also found no effect of ethanol administered in drinking water upon chromosome aberrations in bone marrow; and ethanol did not alter the clastogenic effects of cyclophosphamide or aflaxtoxin B1. However, chromosome damage produced by patulin, which is a direct-acting mutagen, were suppressed by ethanol to 50% below control values.

The adverse experiences noted for both DMSO and ethanol in the preceeding examples suggest that organic solvents should only be employed in this system if there is no other suitable vehicle.

Sex and Species Differences in Sensitivity

Detection of clastogenic activity of some chemicals can be affected significantly by metabolic or hormonal difference in the test animals. Henry et al. (1980) observed repeatable sex-related differences in the micronucleus response of male and female mice to EMS, a direct-acting alkylating agent. In their study, females had greater numbers of micronuclei in PCEs than males, and similar differences in cytotoxicity were also apparent by lower numbers of PCEs in the females. Although the observed sex-related differences were unexplainable, and were only obtained with EMS, Henry et al. (1980) speculated that other chemicals may be encountered with similar specific effects.

In contrast to the increased response of females to EMS, a direct-acting, alkylating agent (Henry, 1980), Madle et al. (1986) reported that male rats and mice were clearly more responsive than females to aflatoxin B1 which requires metabolic conversion for activation. However, they speculated that the differences in sensitivity were more closely related to hormonal effects upon metabolic inactivation of the reactive metabolite, than to differences in mixed function oxidases between sexes. Rabello-Gay et al. (1985) reported essentially identical increased sensitivity of male mice to activation-dependent cyclophosphamide and they noted that a greater number of micronuclei were produced in older vs. younger males, but no age-related differences were apparent with females.

Benzene is a clastogenic chemical for which sex-related differences are also apparently related to hormonal factors. Siou et al. (1981) administered benzene orally to mice and Chinese hamsters, and determined clastogenic effects by both micronucleus and metaphase analyses. In male and female mice, chromosomal aberrations and the increase in numbers of micronuclei were greater in males than in females. The existence of sex-related differences in clastogenicity of benzene also applies to long-term exposures as evident in micronucleus studies on blood samples from carcinogenesis studies on mice (Choy et al., 1985). In earlier studies conducted by Siou et al. in 1980, as cited by Siou et al. (1981), no sex-related differences could be demonstrated with castrated or immature males. However, when castrated males were administered testosterone, they regained the greater degree of sensitivity to benzene which confirmed the probable hormonal mechanism for the sex-related differences. In the same study, Siou et al. reported that benzene produced only small and inconclusive effects upon both chromosome aberrations and the incidence of micronuclei in Chinese hamsters. The mechanism for different sensitivity in the response to benzene by mice and hamsters was not studied, but differences in pharmacokinetics or metabolism were suggested as likely possibilities.

Similar findings of lower responses of hamsters to clastogens were reported by Madle et al. (1986) and aflatoxin B1 produced clearly positive micronucleus increases in bone marrow of rats but no significant increases in hamsters. These authors speculated that the species differences may be due to differences in the ability to inactivate the reactive epoxide metabolite of the aflatoxin B1 molecule, and mice and rats, for example, differ significantly in this regard. In contrast to metabolic-activation-dependent clastogens, Aeschbacher (1986) reported that, except for inbred strain MS/Ae, no significant differences in production of micronuclei were observed with three inbred mouse strains AKR, BALB/c and C57 BR, or in outbred strains OF1 and NMRI.

The studies on EMS and benzene discussed in this section serve as illustrations of the possible chemical-specific effects which cannot be anticipated in routine screening programmes. In the case of EMS, females were more sensitive and had greater clastogenic responses than males. With benzene, and other metabolic-activation dependent clastogens, the opposite sex-relationship was found. Although differences between species and sexes should not be surprising in toxicological studies on chemicals which have diverse metabolic activation requirements, the possible existence of such differences must be considered during statistical comparisons and for study interpretation.

DETERMINATION OF MICRONUCLEI IN CIRCULATING ERYTHROCYTES

A significant advance in simplifying the performance of the micronucleus test originated from the finding that micronuclei persisted in polychromatic erythrocytes in the blood stream following release from the bone marrow. MacGregor et al. (1980) were the first to demonstrate conclusively that clastogen-induced increases in the incidence of micronuclei in peripheral polychromatic erythrocytes from blood and bone marrow of mice followed a similar dose-effect relationship after administration of cyclophosphamide (25 mg/kg), nitrogen mustard (2.5 mg/kg), or 7,12-dimethylbenz[*a*]anthracene (40 mg/kg). Their method employed air-dried blood smears which were fixed with absolute methanol, and the cells were then stained with Wright-Giemsa stain to distinguish PCEs and micronuclei. Selected slides were stained with Feulgen and DNA-specific stains to assure correct identification of cellular inclusions and micronuclei.

MacGregor's finding of increases of PCEs in peripheral erythrocytes contradicted earlier studies by von Lebedur and Schmid (1973), who concluded that peripheral blood from mice was not an appropriate tissue for quantifying micronuclei. MacGregor et al. (1980) speculated that the differences in the data between the two groups were probably attributable to experimental variations, in that von Lebedur and Schmid (1973) used highly cytotoxic doses and evaluated lower numbers of cells. These are reasonable explanations because the destruction of nucleated bone marrow cells was evident in the study of von Lebedur and Schmid (1973); a finding which is indicative of excessive cytotoxicity. High levels of cytotoxicity, at a minimum, would cause a lengthy delay in the entry of new PCEs into the bloodstream, and positive effects upon the incidence of micronuclei would not be detected without extending the sampling period.

Examination of micronuclei using blood smears has considerable advantages over bone marrow studies, but some differences in the methods must be considered. A minor, but noteworthy, difference between the bone marrow and peripheral blood methods is that there is a difference in the sampling interval required to attain maximum numbers of micronuclei. Although dependent to some extent upon the specific test chemical, micronucleated PCEs in blood attain maximum values about 24 hours later than PCEs in the bone marrow. This additional time is required for the release of PCEs from bone marrow and for their appearance in the bloodstream (Russel and Bernstein, 1966). Thus, a 24 hour sampling time, which is appropriate for bone marrow, is not likely to reveal treatment-related effects in peripheral blood PCEs for most agents which act during or prior to S-phase of mitosis.

Assessments of micronuclei with peripheral blood are particularly advantageous because only a small drop of blood is required for the evaluation and the same animal(s) can be sampled repeatedly. Consecutive sampling from the same animal(s) increases the uniformity of the test results, reduces the number of animals required and eliminates variability encountered in typical group comparison experiments. Finally, the peripheral blood method allows a better estimation of the cellular kinetics of clastogenic effects because consecutive samples can be obtained using the same dosed animals.

A question of obvious concern is whether the evaluation of micronuclei in peripheral PCEs is as sensitive as the examination of micronuclei in bone marrow PCEs. MacGregor et al. (1980) observed equal to two-fold greater numbers of micronuclei/1000 PCEs using blood smears in comparisons to the incidence in bone marrow cells from the same mice. This finding was consistent with the three clastogens they evaluated, and the results indicated that evaluation of peripheral blood PCEs provided comparable or greater sensitivity to micronucleus evaluations with bone marrow cells. Styles et al. (1983) compared the micronucleus response of three strains of mice (C_{57}B1/6J; hybrid C_3H/C_{57}; and hybrid BALBc/CBA) following administration of two doses of cyclophosphamide (75 mg/kg) or hexamethylphosphoramide (1.28 ml/kg), and sampling bone marrow at 48 and 72 hours. They concluded that there were significant increases in numbers of micronuclei in both bone marrow PCEs and 'mature erythrocytes' from peripheral blood for all but the CBA hybrid, which showed a positive micronucleus response only with bone marrow PCEs. The critical point to realize in the study by Styles et al. (1973) is that they compared PCEs in bone marrow with 'mature erythrocytes' in the bloodstream, rather than with the younger PCEs evaluated by MacGregor et al. (1980). Quantitative comparisons between the different cells examined were likely to be affected significantly by the cellular dynamics of the bone marrow. Thus, the comparison does not serve to evaluate possible differences in sensitivity for blood and bone marrow cells as target tissues in the micronucleus test. Although Styles et al. (1973) found that the number of micronuclei/1000 cells was lower in normochromatic erythrocytes (mature cells) than in PCEs, this result would be expected in this test because of simple dilution of the micronucleated (target) cells with the anucleated normochromatic cells already present in the peripheral blood.

Steinheider et al. (1985) reported that similar numbers of micronuclei were produced by cyclophosphamide treatment in bone marrow and peripheral blood PCEs. They concluded that the peripheral blood micronucleus test was as sensitive as evaluations with bone marrow in three strains of mice used for these comparisons (BALB/c, DBA/2 and NMRI).

Schlegel and MacGregor (1982) reported that evaluation of micronucleated NCEs could provide a useful method to determine cumulative chromosome damage when mice are exposed to multiple doses of clastogenic agents. After 8 ip injections of 0.2 mg/kg of triethylenemelamine over a 17 day period, they observed progressive increases in micronucleated NCEs/1000 cells. Significant increases of micronuclei were observed beginning on the fifteenth day after 5 injections, and significant differences from control values persisted for approximately 21 days after treatment was stopped. The level of micronucleated NCEs did not return to control levels until approximately 30 days after the last injection, a total time period which approximates the calculated 45 day lifespan of erythrocytes.

Schlegel and MacGregor (1983) extended their observation of cumulative micronucleus effects in mice to propose a rapid screening test employing mice administered 5 daily injections of the test materials. They found that weaning mice were preferable for these studies, rather than older animals, because they had a greater percentage of PCEs in the peripheral blood which then produced higher numbers of micronucleated NCEs. Apparently with weaning mice, there was a more rapid release and accumulation of erythrocytes exposed to the test material during the erythroblast stage in the bone marrow. The advantage of this repeated dosing protocol over acute exposures (Schlegel and MacGregor, 1983) was the possibility of increasing the sensitivity of the test for weak clastogens. With repeated dosing, the critical time for sampling was eliminated, because appearance of micronucleated NCEs was found to be a cumulative process. For example, following repeated doses of nitrogen mustard, Schlegel and MacGregor (1983) observed a progressive increase in micronucleated NCEs, and the incidence of micronuclei attained a steady-state value after 5 weeks of exposures. Steinheider et al. (1985) were in agreement with these conclusions, and they also found that NCEs were sensitive and appropriate cells for detecting clastogenic effects in both acute and chronic exposure studies with mice.

The observation of cumulative increases in numbers of micronuclei was an exciting finding because, for subchronic toxicology studies employing mice, a blood smear prepared for haematological evaluation could now additionally be used to score for micronucleated NCEs as an inexpensive screen for potential clastogens. This same speculation prompted us (unpublished data), as well as Schlegel and MacGregor (1984), to attempt the same approach with rats, a species more commonly employed in routine toxicology testing programmes. Unfortunately, these efforts were fruitless, and only showed that the accumulation of micronucleated NCEs does not occur in rats. The same result is likely to be true in other species with efficient spleens which remove these abnormal micronucleated erythrocytes (e.g. humans). Thus, for a time, it appeared that the peripheral blood micronucleus test could only be performed with mice.

Using a clever modification, Schlegel and MacGregor (1984) discovered that splenectomy of rats can be employed to circumvent the removal of micronucleated NCEs by the spleen, thus allowing the application of the peripheral blood micronucleus test to rats. When these authors administered 11 daily injections of 0·2 mg triethylenemelamine/kg to splenectomized rats, the incidence of micronucleated NCEs rose to approximately 9 times the baseline level, and the increase persisted for 50 to 55 days. Although splenectomy provides one approach for the extension of their method, it still does not permit the concomitant application of the peripheral blood micronucleus test to routine toxicology screening studies with normal, non-splenectomized, rats ... or to humans.

Choy and MacGregor (1984) developed a novel procedure employing density enrichment techniques which may yet permit application of the peripheral blood micronucleus procedure to studies of rats and other species. Using Percoll density gradients, more than 75% of the PCEs could be separated from blood samples of mice. The incidence of micronucleated PCEs, following single injections of cyclophosphamide (25 mg/kg) or triethylenemelamine (0·5 mg/kg) were essentially the same for PCEs evaluated with whole blood smears or with the fractionated cells. The ability to concentrate PCEs may ultimately allow the extension of this test to rats or other animals in toxicology studies and perhaps to monitoring human exposures as well.

A further note of caution concerning the interpretation of results from the peripheral blood micronucleus test stems from findings of Steinheider et al. (1985), which show that excessive blood loss, haemolysis or toxicity to the spleen can cause transient but measurable increases in the micronucleus frequency. Slight increases in mPCEs after the first bleeding interval can be verified as a treatment-related effect by using animals sampled only at this particular interval in an independent test.

TRANSPLACENTAL MICRONUCLEUS TEST

The placenta, although a protective barrier to many agents, allows a variety of both hydrophilic and hydrophobic agents to cross from mother to foetus. The foetus is not only susceptible to direct acting agents, but also to indirect agents that require metabolic activation. The active metabolites of indirect agents may be produced in the maternal liver, and these are usually short-lived and tissue specific. However, the foetus also has the capability of biotransforming agents to active metabolites. Both foetal liver and the placenta of humans and other animals have been shown to be capable of mixed function oxidase metabolism (Yaffe et al., 1970; Sehgal and Hutton, 1977). Russell and Bernstein (1966) showed that erythropoiesis occurs exclusively in the liver of the foetal mouse between day 12 and 16 of gestation. Thus, for chemicals that require metabolic activation by the liver, the ultimate metabolite would be produced in close proximity to the cells undergoing erythropoiesis.

Rapid DNA synthesis during foetal development, and a quantitative and qualitative lack of repair enzymes, are two factors that contribute to the increased susceptibility of the foetus to damage produced by occupational and environmental exposures to genotoxic agents. Deficient repair and excretory mechanisms may increase the levels of genotoxins in foetal cells (Klinger et al., 1981), and these factors could enhance the probability of genetic damage. In addition, foetal cells during organogenesis are in a rapid state of DNA replication and cell division, and both of these factors increase the risk of clonal expansion of the altered genotype. Genetic alterations to somatic stem cells and germ cells during foetal development may be of consequence during the lifetime of the organism, and they could also result in hereditable changes which increase genetic risk for subsequent generations. Foetal exposures to dangerous xenobiotics have been correlated with early foetal death, malformations at birth (teratogenesis) and childhood cancers (transplacental carcinogenesis). A fraction of these agents are also clastogenic and produce damage to the chromosomes. The transplacental micronucleus test can reveal clastogenic damage, and it may be useful for evaluating chemicals which could pose potential genetic risks to the foetuses of exposed pregnant females.

The Sensitivity of the Transplacental Test System

Cole et al. (1979) compared the micronucleus response in PCEs from maternal bone marrow, foetal liver and foetal peripheral blood after treatment with mitomycin C and procarbazine. Both agents were found to produce significant increases in numbers of micronuclei in PCEs from all three tissues. In tests with mitomycin C, the maximum increase in numbers of micronuclei was higher in the maternal PCEs than in foetal PCEs. However, with procarbazine, the incidence of micronuclei in foetal cells was significantly higher than the incidence in maternal bone marrow PCEs. Thus, for some agents, the determination of micronuclei in foetal cells may provide a more sensitive indicator both for potential foetal genotoxicity and for assessing agents difficult to detect with adult tissues.

In preliminary studies, King and Wild (1979) found that the cellular composition of the foetal mouse blood is highly amenable for the evaluation of micronuclei. Foetal blood contains a high percentage of PCEs, ranging from 45 to 49%, which compares to the maternal bone marrow PCE frequency of approximately 16%. In addition, the foetal blood cells were predominantly

(98%) anucleated on days 16 and 17 compared to approximately 30% in the maternal bone marrow. However, Cole et al. (1981) suggested that foetal liver was preferable and more sensitive than foetal blood for micronucleus testing. The life-span of the peripheral blood PCE is considerably longer than PCEs in the liver, and fewer target cells at risk to the test agent would be assessed in blood as compared to liver. In addition, micronucleated PCEs that enter the peripheral circulation from bone marrow are mixed and diluted with pre-existing PCEs, and this dilution would result in a lower incidence of micronuclei/PCE.

An important asset of transplacental micronucleus testing is that the foetal cells and maternal bone marrow cells can be assessed from the same chemically exposed dam. However, Cole et al. (1979, 1981) showed that foetal cell division and maturation of PCEs each require approximately 6 hours, in contrast to 10 hours in the adult mouse. These differences in division time must be considered when comparing the micronucleus response from maternal and foetal cells sampled at the same time. The cellular kinetics illustrated in *Fig.* 6.4 indicate that the optimal sampling time for foetal liver PCEs is 12 to 18 hours after chemical administration. However, the optimal sampling time for foetal peripheral blood PCEs would be approximately 30 hours, which is similar to an appropriate sampling time of adult bone marrow PCEs.

King and Wild (1979) tested cyclophosphamide, procarbazine, trenimon and mitomycin C for the induction of micronuclei in foetal mouse peripheral blood PCEs. Procarbazine, trenimon and mitomycin C were shown to induce significantly higher incidences of micronuclei in foetal blood PCEs than in maternal bone marrow PCEs. Mitomycin C induced comparable numbers of micronuclei in the foetal blood PCEs; however, at the lowest dose level the incidence in the foetus was only 30% of that observed in the mothers. All four test agents induced a significant, dose-related increase in the incidence of micronuclei in the foetal blood PCEs. The direct relationship obtained in this study for known clastogens supports the applicability of transplacental micronucleus testing for assessing potential *in utero* genetic effects.

Several studies have confirmed that the transplacental micronucleus test is particularly sensitive for detecting clastogenic effects produced by agents that are biotransformed to the active metabolite by the liver. These agents are difficult

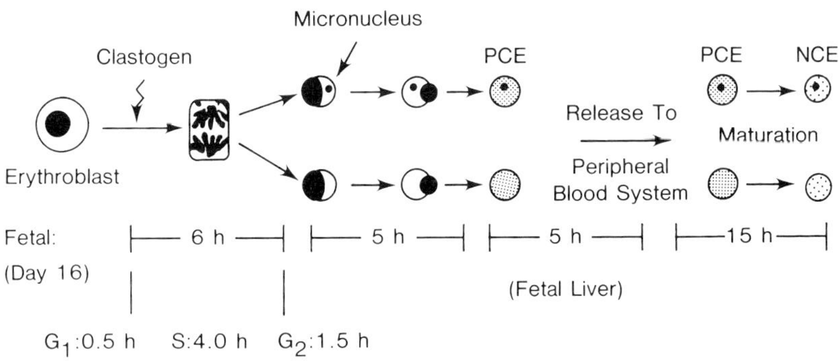

Fig. 6.4. Kinetics of the formation of micronuclei in fetal liver cells during erythrocyte maturation.

to detect in cytogenetic assays that employ adult animals because the active metabolite is often short-lived and it fails to reach the bone marrow in sufficient quantities to produce significant increases in clastogenic damage. In addition, the foetal liver has greater metabolic activity than the adult liver and it is more active in biotransformation(s).

Adult bone marrow cells that are primarily used for micronucleus testing are incapable of transforming nitrosamines to the active electrophiles. Electrophiles formed by biotransformation in the liver react quickly with biological nucleophiles and often fail to reach the bone marrow (Margison and O'Connor, 1979). Diethylnitrosamine (DEN) was shown by Cole et al. (1982a) to induce small but significant increases in the incidence of micronuclei in PCEs from liver of foetal mice exposed on either day 15 or day 17 of gestation, whereas maternal bone marrow cells did not show an increased response. N-methyl-N′-nitro-N-nitrosoguanidine (MNNG) is known to be carcinogenic to mice, but it has not yet been found to be active *in vivo* with mammalian mutagenicity test systems in adult animals. MNNG is thiocatalysed to diazomethane, which is the biologically active form (Frei and Lawley, 1976). Diazomethane is also a very reactive alkylating agent and, like the active metabolite of DEN, it reacts very rapidly in biological systems. Yamamoto and Kikuchi (1984) were able to demonstrate positive increases in numbers of micronuclei in foetal mouse liver PCEs following *in utero* exposure to MNNG. In a similar study, Stoyel and Clark (1980) tested the alkaloid lasiocarpine in the transplacental micronucleus test and compared the maternal and foetal response. Lasiocarpine also requires biotransformation to produce a highly reactive and short-lived metabolite. Similar to results obtained with DEN and MNNG, lasiocarpine did not increase the incidence of micronuclei in the maternal bone marrow PCEs, but it was active in examinations of foetal liver PCEs. Thus, foetal liver appears to be an excellent tissue for detecting genetic effects of genotoxins which require metabolic activation.

A multiple-dose testing regime was studied by Cole et al. (1982) as a means of increasing the sensitivity of the transplacental micronucleus test. Methyl methanesulphonate (MMS), a relatively short-lived alkylating agent, was administered ip to pregnant mice once, twice or three times at six hour intervals. Two injections produced a directly additive response in foetal mouse liver PCEs, and the response to three injections was more than additive. The data suggested that multiple injections increased the sensitivity of the test system. However, as in the adult, a protocol employing a single fixed sample time for the exposed foetuses may not necessarily detect an optimal response for all agents. On the basis of the cell kinetics of the foetal erythrocyte, Cole et al. (1982b) recommended that cells be sampled from the foetal liver or peripheral blood at multiple harvest times, commencing 12–15 hours or 24–30 hours after the last injection, respectively.

Determination of SCEs has been shown to be a sensitive indicator of genotoxic damage, and in most cases determination of SCE effects is more sensitive than classical cytogenetic techniques. However, not all agents that induce chromosomal aberrations also increase the frequency of SCEs; and likewise, not all agents that induce SCEs are clastogenic. Kram et al. (1979) have demonstrated the applicability of transplacental SCE testing for detecting genetic damage induced *in utero*. Thus, *in utero* studies may provide complementary data from both SCE and cytogenetic endpoints.

In comparative studies, Cole et al. (1983) evaluated the transplacental micronucleus test and *in vivo/in vitro* determinations of SCEs in foetal liver erythrocytes. After *in vivo* exposure to the test agent, foetal erythroblasts were cultured for two cell cycles in media containing erythropoietin, needed for promoting cell division, and bromodeoxyuridine, required for SCE differentiation. Results for six chemicals administered to pregnant mice on gestation day 15 showed that, with the exception of procarbazine, the lowest effective dose of all 5 test chemicals produced similar increases in both the SCE and micronucleus test systems. Procarbazine is recognized to be an ineffective inducer of SCEs; thus the increase in SCEs did not parallel the steep dose-response curve obtained for production of micronuclei.

Henderson et al. (1984) compared foetal and maternal responses to three carcinogens which differed in requirements for metabolic activation. Cyclophosphamide and procarbazine produced similar SCE responses in cells derived from foetal liver and maternal bone marrow. When chromosome damage was assessed, however, cyclophosphamide and procarbazine produced significantly greater numbers of micronuclei in foetal liver PCEs than in maternal bone marrow cells. In contrast, mitomycin C produced slightly greater increases in SCEs and numbers of micronuclei in maternal bone marrow rather than in foetal liver cells. These comparative data illustrate the differences which can be encountered in tissue sensitivities and metabolic capabilities for different chemicals. Also, the greater sensitivity of the transplacental test employing foetal tissues appears to be a valuable adjunct to clastogen screening programmes.

Gestational age at exposure is apparently an important variable that can produce differences in the maternal and foetal response as well as affect test sensitivity to particular agents (e.g. for carcinogens that require metabolic activation). The enzyme and metabolic systems required for biotransformation, DNA repair, detoxification and elimination are in a constant state of change throughout gestation. Although several metabolic pathways are not fully functional until after birth, Galloway et al. (1980) demonstrated that the enzyme systems capable of activating aromatic hydrocarbons are present early in embryogenesis. Likewise, the activity of enzymes that biotransform nitrosamines were shown to exceed adult values by the fifteenth to sixteenth day of gestation (Rao and Vesselinovitch, 1973). As another example, cyclophosphamide (CP) is biotransformed by the cytochrome P-450 mixed function oxidase system into a variety of products that each differs in potential to produce increases of SCEs and chromosome aberrations, depending upon the time of administration during gestation (Au et al., 1980). Kram et al. (1980) tested cyclophosphamide *in utero* and found an elevated foetal SCE response when the dam was treated on day 11 of gestation. However, on the fifteenth day of gestation, the SCE response was only 50% of the response observed at day 11, and SCE values had decreased to those found in maternal bone marrow. The differences in metabolic activity throughout gestation must be considered as an important variable when designing dosing and sampling protocols for *in utero* test systems.

Several other variables can effect the response of transplacental micronucleus induction, including factors such as excessive chemical toxicity and delays in cell division. The foetal cell cycle time is significantly faster than the adult cycle, and the cell division time interval changes throughout gestation. Thus, when designing test protocols, cell harvest times must be coordinated to consider variations in both cell cycle time and changes in metabolic activation during development.

Intralitter variation appears to be another factor which alters the micronucleus response when the dose is administered ip. Yamamoto and Kikuchi (1984) observed that foetuses located closest to the site of MNNG injection had a higher incidence of micronuclei than foetuses further from the injection site. This variation may be attributable either to accidental injection into the uterine horn or to a direct diffusion of the test agent into the horn proximal to the injection site. Intralitter variation can be circumvented in several ways, such as by selectively evaluating foetuses located on the uterine horn opposite that from the injection site (Stoyel and Clark, 1980), by pooling data from all foetuses, or by randomly sampling from both uterine horns.

In conclusion, the transplacental micronucleus test appears to be a promising test system with some advantages over micronucleus tests using adults. Chemicals which produce short-lived, clastogenic metabolites are likely to be detected with greater success with the *in utero* procedure, especially when foetal liver is employed for the determinations. Thus, even for general screening, where *in utero* effects are not of principal concern, the transplacental methods may be a preferable protocol for xenobiotics which require metabolic activation.

APPLICATION TO HUMAN MONITORING

Genetic screening tests attain particular relevance to humans when the method can also be employed for monitoring individual or population exposures. In medicine, observation of micronuclei (Howell–Jolly bodies) in blood smears is an established diagnostic sign for abnormalities in the function of the spleen (Miale, 1982). Hyposplenism and asplenia are serious human disorders associated with increases in micronuclei in peripheral erythrocytes. Hyposplenism apparently occurs spontaneously in a number of disease states including coeliac disease and ulcerative colitis (Ryan et al., 1978). Asplenia is a congenital condition resulting in severe cardiovascular and pulmonary anomalies, and is a cause of unexpected, sudden infant death (Roguin et al., 1979; Katcher, 1980). Increases in micronuclei observed in haematological preparations provide a useful monitor which can confirm the diagnosis of both of these serious conditions.

In patients undergoing radio- or chemotherapy, determination of micronuclei in bone marrow cells has been employed for dosimetry of potential genetic effects of the treatments. In chemotherapy studies with trimethoprimsulphamethoxazole, Sorensen and Krogh Jensen (1981) reported that the incidence of micronuclei in bone marrow cells was a more sensitive indicator of chromosome damage than was metaphase analyses of aberrations. In an earlier study on patients with pernicious anaemia, Krogh Jensen (1977) also concluded that the micronucleus method was more sensitive than metaphase analyses. Although both of these studies were too limited to provide definitive proof for differences in sensitivity, the comparative data suggest that determinations of micronuclei provide comparable data to the more time-consuming metaphase studies. In partial support of this conclusion, the data of Krogh Jensen et al. (1979) and Hartley-Asp (1979) showed that there were similar increases in both micronuclei and chromosome aberrations for patients undergoing therapy with penicillamine and metronidizole, respectively. Krogh Jensen and Nyfors (1979) reported similar agreement and greater sensitivity for human bone marrow micronucleus determinations in comparisons with data from metaphase evaluations of patients treated with methotrexate. Additional work will be needed to validate the micronucleus system in multiple laboratories, and to prove whether it provides comparable or greater sensitivity than classic cytogenetic procedures employed for human monitoring.

Because of obvious difficulties encountered in obtaining human bone marrow samples, blood lymphocytes were proposed as an alternative source of cells for human studies. Huber et al. (1983) concluded that micronucleus studies with lymphocytes lacked suitable sensitivity because of inherent problems in manipulating these cells. Unlike studies with PCEs, young target lymphocytes were not distinguishable by staining procedures, and these authors could not identify an optimum cell-culture interval for attaining maximum responses to clastogenic agents. Krogh Jensen and Nyfors (1979b) agreed that lymphocytes were not sufficiently sensitive in detecting clastogenic effects of methotrexate in human studies on bone marrow cells and cultured lymphocytes. In contrast to these two negative reports, Högstedt (1984) found that preservation of the cytoplasm of human lymphocytes, by eliminating the hypotonic swelling and fixation steps, resulted in greater precision for identification of micronuclei and provided greater sensitivity than attainable by the typical hypotonic cell-preparation procedures as employed by Huber et al. (1983). Recent studies by Högstedt and Karlsson (1985), using human lymphocytes with preserved cytoplasm, showed that X-rays and mitomycin C produced micronuclei which were significantly smaller than micronuclei produced by vincristine and colcemid. This finding showed that the micronucleus procedure is capable of differentiating between agents which cause chromosomal fragments, versus those affecting the mitotic spindle and producing whole-chromosome changes (i.e. colcemid and vincristine).

The application of the lymphocyte method to human monitoring requires further validation, and it is still premature to speculate whether it will prove to be a sensitive biological monitor. However, a recent report by Pincu et al. (1984) suggests that there is still good reason not to rule out the use of lymphocytes in human micronuclei studies. By culturing human lymphocytes with 4×10^{-4} M bromodeoxyuridine in the cell-culture medium, followed by staining by the FPG method (Perry and Wolff, 1974), both the nuclei and micronuclei in proliferating lymphocytes were stained blue, while non-proliferating cells had nuclei that were stained red. Fenech and Morley (1985b) used cytochalasin B to block lymphocytes in mitosis *in vitro*, and the proliferating cells could be easily recognized by their binucleate appearance. Ability to recognize dividing lymphocytes is a significant advance, because evaluations can be restricted to cells which would have divided at least once—a necessary condition for production of micronuclei—and non-dividing cells incapable of forming micronuclei would be excluded. Pincu et al. (1984), employing lymphocytes exposed to ^{60}Co, achieved a significant increase in sensitivity of the test by counting micronuclei only in the blue (i.e. dividing) cells, and noted that the evaluations were faster, less variable, and the method permitted a positive identification of micronuclei.

Hans Stich and co-workers (1982a,b,c, 1983, 1984) were pioneers in the use of the micronucleus test method for assessing clastogenic effects of chemical, food and tobacco products in humans. They recognized that chromosomal damage to epithelial cells could be observed and quantified in exfoliated cells from various mucosal tissues such as buccal or bronchial mucosa, urinary bladder, ureter, cervix and oesophagus. Cell samples could be obtained readily for micronucleus studies from centrifuged urine samples, scrapings of the oral cavity, and from sputum or cervical smears. Elegant studies performed by this group involved quantifying of micronuclei in human buccal (oral) mucosa cells exposed to putative mutagens or carcinogens. In a study on 27 tobacco chewers in India (Stich et al., 1982a,c), significant increases in numbers of micronuclei in buccal cells were found in all of the individuals examined. The presence of clastogenic agents in Indian tobacco was then confirmed *in vitro* with both Chinese hamster ovary and human cells. Similar positive associations between betel nut chewing and clastogenic effects were obtained in parallel studies (Stich et al., 1982b,c).

Stich and Rosin (1983) did not find a significant increase in micronuclei of oral mucosa cells from either tobacco smokers or users of alcohol when each agent was ingested alone. However, significant increases in the incidence of micronuclei were observed for smokers who also drank alcohol. An increase of four-fold above respective control values was found for persons who ingested at least 150 ml of ethanol and who also smoked one or two packs of cigarettes/day. For drinkers who smoked three or more packs/day, the incidence of micronuclei in oral mucosal cells was almost eight-fold greater than for drinkers who did not smoke.

The use of the micronucleus assay as a dosimeter for human exposure to food and environmental agents provides a high degree of ease and relevance unmatched by other available short-term clastogenicity test systems. An excellent review of the possible uses of this monitoring approach is available in a recent article by Stich and Rosin (1984).

APPLICATION OF THE MICRONUCLEUS TEST TO SCREENING POTENTIAL CARCINOGENS

Although the major value of the micronucleus test is its ability to simplify detection of clastogenic agents, several of the developers of the method proposed that the test could also serve to detect carcinogens. This screening role appeared reasonable because many, if not all, proven clastogens are also animal carcinogens (Radman et al., 1982). The Gene-Tox Program of the Environmental Protection Agency (Preston et al., 1981) reported that there was a striking positive correlation of 94% (17 of 18 cases) between carcinogenic and clastogenic activity when there was agreement in at least two cytogenetic test systems. Although the sample size in this study was limited, these data are highly suggestive of a direct relationship between clastogenic activity and carcinogenic potential. At the molecular-genetic level, there is growing evidence that oncogenes present in the mammalian genome may become derepressed and 'activated' by positional changes caused by chromosomal damage and rearrangement (Gilbert, 1983). Derepression of oncogenes is one of the current and appealing hypotheses on possible mechanisms for initiating cellular neoplasia. Lastly, evidence for a direct relationship between chromosomal changes and carcinogenesis increases the relevance of clastogenicity test results for humans.

Various attempts to validate the accuracy of the micronucleus method as a predictive test for carcinogens have produced mixed results. Trzos et al. (1978) and Jenssen and Ramel (1980) concluded that the micronucleus test did not possess appropriate sensitivity in a predictive role for identifying carcinogens. Wild (1978) used a different group of chemicals and concluded that the correlation between carcinogenic potential and positive micronucleus effects suggested a useful role for the test in a screening battery. The Gene-Tox program (Heddle et al., 1983) evaluated published micronucleus studies and found a 50% accuracy in predicting carcinogenic potential. These authors speculated that this relatively low value would be greater with more rigorous protocols and testing procedures and they recommended several changes which are very likely to improve the degree of detection of potential carcinogens in the future.

The value of the micronucleus test should not be judged solely upon the prediction of carcinogenic potential for two reasons. First, the degree of correlation is greatly influenced by the percentage of carcinogens in the group of chemicals evaluated. Secondly, the degree of correlation will be additionally affected by the percentage of clastogens within the group of carcinogens in the panel of chemicals. It is unrealistic to expect the micronucleus test to predict carcinogenic potential for all carcinogens, simplistically because not all carcinogens are clastogens. Some carcinogens cause gene mutations but not chromosome damage (de Serres and Ashby, 1981), while other carcinogens may act by extragenetic mechanisms which are not detectable in routine genotoxicity assays.

A reasonable application of the micronucleus test in carcinogen screening programmes would be its use as an *in vivo* confirmation of clastogenic activity detected *in vitro* or in other cytogenetic assays. In this role, the micronucleus test has the apparent advantage of a low 'false positive' rate (Heddle et al., 1983) which is a desirable characteristic for confirmatory test systems. Once again, as discussed in previous sections, the sensitivity and accuracy of the test as a confirmatory procedure becomes a significant issue. Heddle et al. (1983) indicated that when appropriately high doses and sufficient numbers of cells are evaluated, as in currently acceptable protocols, a negative result in the micronucleus test may be considered to be a definitive result. This statement contained the caveat that a negative result does not prove non-clastogenicity, which, however, is an equally true statement for metaphase analyses or for other tests which cannot be used to 'prove' non-mutagenicity or non-carcinogenicity. When a negative result is obtained in the micronucleus test in the presence of other positive clastogenicity data, further work would be necessary to determine whether the test agent reaches the bone marrow, or whether tissue-specific metabolism is required for activation. The finding of disagreement between positive *in vitro* results and negative results *in vivo* is becoming more common as chemicals appear which can be inactivated *in vivo*, or with chemicals which show effects only in artificial *in vitro* conditions aimed at providing a maximum exposure condition.

MONITORING CHROMOSOMAL DAMAGE IN GERM CELLS

Evaluation of chromosomal damage in meiotic cells involves both laborious and technically complex procedures. For these reasons, progress in applying meiotic screening tests of genotoxicity has proceeded at a steady but relatively slow pace. Determination of micronuclei in meiotic cells offers a simplified approach for monitoring clastogenic effects in germ cells, and evidence is accumulating that this procedure provides comparable sensitivity to other more complex methods.

In one example of an indirect application of the micronucleus method to determination of potential germ cell effects, Oud and Peters (1978) compared six different *in vivo* methods for detecting clastogenic effects of the potent alkylating agent triaziquone. Positive increases in chromosome damage were found at comparable doses in a bone marrow cytogenetics test, a bone marrow micronucleus test, and in both a mouse dominant lethal test and F_1 translocation test. No significant increases were observed directly in mouse meiotic cells, either in the spermatogonial metaphase test, or by the evaluation of spermatocyte translocations using identical doses. This study showed that the evaluation of micronuclei in somatic cells provided greater sensitivity and ease in scoring than the latter two meiotic clastogenicity tests. Also, the spermatogonial metaphase test and evaluations of spermatocyte translocations did not detect the known clastogenic effects of triaziquone, possibly because of cytotoxicity or insufficient sample size.

Lähdetie and Parvinen (1981) were first to study clastogenic effects directly in mammalian germ cells by determining the incidence of micronuclei. They isolated spermatids from seminiferous tubules of Sprague-Dawley rats by applying gentle pressure to the tubules isolated by dissection. Micronuclei were observed by phase-contrast microscopy using a transillumination procedure. In parallel studies, the identification of micronuclei was verified using Hoechst 33258 dye and fluorescence microscopy to assure the presence of DNA. In studies of X-ray exposures, they observed linear increases in the frequency of spermatid micronuclei. The sensitivity of the micronucleus determinations following low X-ray doses (0–600 rads) was comparable to analyses of spermatocyte chromosomes reported by others employing similar exposure doses. These workers concluded that evaluation of meiotic micronuclei was faster and required less specific skills than time-consuming analyses of complex meiotic chromosome preparations.

In more recent work, Lähdetie (1983a,b) extended the application of the meiotic micronucleus method to evaluate other agents, including adriamycin, ethyl methanesulphonate, cyclophosphamide and dimethylbenzanthracene. Sampling spermatocytes from animals at different time intervals after dosing revealed that S-phase dependent mutagens (cyclophosphamide and dimethylbenzanthracene) predominantly increased numbers of micronuclei in preleptotene stage spermatocytes. Significant increases in numbers of micronuclei were detected only after a relatively lengthy interval of 17 days after injection. Ethyl methanesulphonate, an S-phase independent mutagen, produced increases of micronuclei only at 1 day following injection, indicating that with this agent, spermatocytes at the diplotene-diakinesis stage of division were the most sensitive cell stage.

Before the meiotic micronucleus method attains increased acceptance and application, additional work will be necessary to evaluate the relative sensitivity and reproducibility of the test among different research groups. Tates et al. (1983) developed an enzymatic digestion method for isolating spermatids from seminiferous tubules, which should simplify the further application of this test. The enzymatic method provides a means for preparing spermatids reproducibly from a number of different species, and it allows application of routine staining procedures for identifying micronuclei. Tates and de Boer (1984) used this procedure to study whether lagging chromosomes produced by non-disjunction during meiotic reduction divisions contributed to micronucleus formation in early spermatids. In three strains of mice with known abnormal chromosome configurations and a high frequency of spontaneous non-disjunction, no remarkable increases in numbers of micronuclei were found in comparisons with normal mouse strains. This result indicated that micronuclei resulting from whole chromosomes do not seem to occur in second division spermatocytes, and it implies that the spermatid micronucleus assay would be insensitive to agents which increase non-disjunction.

Simplification of the meiotic micronucleus method should foster increased effort in this relatively complex segment of chromosome research. Evaluations of meiotic tissues should continue to be an exciting area of clastogenicity research for the future.

APPLICATION TO BIOLOGICAL DOSIMETRY

The micronucleus test has found growing acceptance as a biological dosimeter for radiation exposure, and as a monitor for genetic effects of various workplace chemicals and environmental pollutants. In this role, the sensitivity of the test to low-level exposures and the linearity of the dose-effect curves are significant and controversial questions.

Appelgren et al. (1978) studied effects of ethylene oxide exposures of rats and mice with the bone marrow micronucleus method. An iv dose of 0.1 g/kg (approximately $\frac{1}{3}$ of LD_{50}), a concentration which did not produce positive effects in their earlier mouse dominant lethal study, produced significant increases in micronuclei in bone marrow PCEs from both rats and mice. This study showed that the micronucleus test had greater sensitivity than the dominant lethal procedure for detecting clastogenic damage.

Clastogenic potential of benzene was evaluated following subcutaneous injection by Diaz et al. (1980), and by oral intubation by Hite et al. (1980). Both groups noted significant, dose-related increases in numbers of bone marrow micronuclei as a result of exposure to benzene. The latter group observed significant increases of micronuclei as late as 5 days following two treatments with 0.125 ml/kg, but micronucleus values were similar in treated groups and controls after 9 and 16 days. Siou et al. (1981) confirmed the clastogenic activity of benzene in mice and Chinese hamsters, and they found agreement in data from both metaphase and micronucleus evaluation. The clastogenic activity of benzene determined by micronucleus evaluations was further supported in retrospective examinations of blood smears from a National Toxicology Program long-term carcinogenicity bioassay (Choy et al., 1985). This latter study indicated that the sensitivity of the micronucleus procedure is sufficient to be used as a measure of genotoxicity as part of routine bioassays of carcinogenicity. Blood smears prepared for haematology can be used to obtain further information on genotoxicity.

Dosimetry studies of low-level radiation exposures using the micronucleus test system have been appealing as a possible method for monitoring biological and genetic effects. With standard bone marrow procedures, Garriott and Grahn (1982) observed significant increases of micronuclei in bone marrow PCEs of mice, even with the lowest exposures to neutrons (range 10–120 rads) or X-rays (range 50–600 rads). The range of exposures employed in each case was stated to be comparable to values which caused positive effects in dominant lethal tests and in reciprocal translocations in the same strain of mouse.

In other radiation dosimetry studies, attempts to use a lymphocyte micronucleus detection system have produced mixed results. A lymphocyte micronucleus procedure has obvious relevance to humans because of the greater ease in sampling blood as compared to obtaining bone marrow cells. Countryman and Heddle (1976) were the first to use phytohaemagglutinin (PHA)-stimulated, human whole-blood cultures to quantify micronuclei following X-ray irradiation *in vitro*. Later studies with X-rays by Huber et al. (1983) concluded that PHA-stimulated, human lymphocyte cultures presented multiple problems during interpretation of results, and that this procedure '. .. is not sensitive enough to detect a significant increase in the incidence of micronuclei after exposure to low doses (< 0·3 Gy)'. The major problems they identified were: a high spontaneous micronucleus frequency in control cultures—leading to low test sensitivity; the inability to identify cells in the first mitotic division following treatment; and the lack of a standard time interval necessary to identify maximal responses.

Boyes and Koval (1983) arrived at a different conclusion about the possible monitoring value of the human lymphocyte micronucleus test in studies on interactions of X-rays, caffeine and cell-culture timing intervals. These authors observed that when human blood cultures were stimulated with PHA 48 hours prior to X-irradiation instead of immediately prior to treatment, according to usual procedures, the magnitude of the micronucleus response was significantly enhanced. Also, when 1 mM caffeine was added to the cultures following irradiation, sensitivity of the micronucleus response was enhanced further. With cultures stimulated with PHA and then irradiated immediately, only a marginal increase in numbers of micronuclei was observed in the absence of caffeine, and a decrease in numbers of micronuclei was observed when caffeine was present. These results suggested that the micronucleus response was significantly affected by cell cycle events, and that enhancement of sensitivity by caffeine was obtained only with growing (stimulated) lymphocyte cultures. The absence of effects of caffeine in earlier micronucleus studies on X-rays by Jenssen and Ramel (1978) may be explainable by the potentiation of cell-lethal damage by caffeine when bone marrow erythrocytes are sampled shortly after exposure (Boyes and Koval, 1983).

Biological monitoring of environmental pollutants appears to be another prospective area of practical application of the micronucleus test method. Siboulet et al. (1984) studied the use of the newt, *Pleurodeles waltl*, for monitoring clastogenic pollutants in aquatic environments. Larvae of the newt was reared in water containing various test substances, and micronuclei were examined in blood samples obtained by intracardiac puncture. Significant dose-effect increases in numbers of micronuclei were obtained for X-rays and for 5 of 6 of the known clastogens tested by this procedure, although effects of formaldehyde were not evident in this study.

Wantabe et al. (1982) studied the clastogenic effects of combinations of chemical carcinogens and environmental pollutants using bone marrow PCEs from strain ddY mice. Their results indicated the possibility of synergistic positive effects for some combinations of clastogenic agents. Cadmium, for example, which was inactive alone in producing increases in micronuclei, produced an enhanced positive response to dimethylnitrosamine. However, no synergistic effects of DMN and polychlorinated biphenyls were observed in this same study. Synergistic responses are serious concerns for complex environmental pollutants, and the data of Watanabe et al. (1982) show the possible role of the micronucleus method for detection of synergism for clastogenic chemicals.

The application of the micronucleus method in monitoring environmental agents and pollutants will likely increase as new procedures are developed and verified. The relevance of these data for assessment of biological risks will require additional study before they can be applied in a routine fashion. The primary role of this test in detecting clastogens should not be forgotten in applications to environmental monitoring. A negative result in this test indicates only the absence of agents which damage chromosomes and does not imply the absence of mutagens or carcinogens which act by different mechanisms. Thus, the micronucleus method may find a useful role in environmental monitoring and biological dosimetry if the purpose and limitations of the test are kept in proper perspective.

SUMMARY

The goal of this chapter was to review the recent advances in the development and application of the micronucleus test method and to credit the efforts of the principal scientists who have fostered this procedure through periods of criticism and doubt. Although this test is an indirect cytogenetic method, it has proven to be useful in various areas of biological investigation, medicine and genetic toxicology, and for human and environmental monitoring. Significant scientific advances are readily apparent in the extension of this test to monitoring of peripheral blood cells, germ cells, exfoliated human epithelial cells and transplacental clastogens. A number of improvements in procedures and protocols are now available for increasing the sensitivity and reproducibility of this test system. The relative simplicity and rapidity of micronucleus determinations will likely spur continued improvements and applications of this method to areas of increasing relevance to humans and the environment.

ACKNOWLEDGEMENTS

The authors are grateful to Drs E. R. Homan, R. H. Garman and C. M. Troup for helpful comments and review of the manuscript. Special thanks are due to Mrs V. L. Trout for typing the manuscript and its several revisions.

REFERENCES

Aeschbacher H. U. (1986) Rates of micronuclei induction in different mouse strains. *Mutat. Res.* **164**, 109–115.

Appelgren L-E., Eneroth G., Grant C. et al. (1978) Testing of ethylene oxide for mutagenicity using the micronucleus test in mice and rats. *Acta Pharmacol. Toxicol.* **43**, 69–71.

Ashby J. and Mohammed R. (1986) Slide preparation and sampling as major sources of variability in the mouse micronucleus assay. *Mutat. Res.* **164**, 217–235.

Au W., Sokova O.I., Koprin B. et al. (1980) Cytogenetic toxicity of cyclophosphamide and its metabolites *in vitro*. *Cytogenet. Cell Genet.* **26**, 108–116.
Berger F. (1981) The chromosomes in haematology. *Cancer Genet. Cytogen.* **4**, 69–88.
Boyes B. G. and Koval J. J. (1983) Clastogenic interactions of γ-radiation and caffeine in human peripheral blood cultures. *Mutat. Res.* **108**, 239–249.
Choy W. N. and MacGregor J. T. (1984) Density-gradient enrichment of newly-formed mouse erythrocytes. Application to the micronucleus test. *Mutat. Res.* **130**, 159–164.
Choy W. N., MacGregor J. T., Shelby M. D. et al. (1985) Induction of micronuclei by benzene in $B6C3F_1$ mice: Retrospective analysis of peripheral blood smears from the NTP carcinogenesis bioassay. *Mutat. Res.* **143**, 55–59.
Cole R. J., Taylor N. A., Cole J. et al. (1979) Transplacental effects of chemical mutagens detected by the micronucleus test. *Nature* (London) **277**, 317–318.
Cole R., Taylor N. A., Cole J. et al. (1981) Short-term tests for transplacentally active carcinogens. I. Micronucleus formation in fetal and maternal mouse erythroblasts. *Mutat. Res.* **80**, 141–157.
Cole R. J., Taylor N., Cole J. et al. (1982a) Short-term tests for transplacentally active carcinogens. Sensitivity of the transplacental micronucleus test to diethylnitrosamine. *Mutat. Res.* **104**, 165–171.
Cole R. J., Aghamohammadi Z., Cole J. et al. (1982b) Short-term tests for transplacentally active carcinogens. Multiple-dose regimes in the transplacental micronucleus test. *Mutat. Res.* **105**, 115–120.
Cole R. J., Cole J., Henderson L. et al. (1983) A comparison of sister-chromatid exchange and the micronucleus test in mouse foetal liver erythroblasts. *Mutat. Res.* **113**, 61–75.
Countryman I. and Heddle J. A. (1976) The production of micronuclei from chromosome aberrations in irradiated cultures of human lymphocytes. *Mutat. Res.* **41**, 321–332.
de Serres F. J. and Ashby J. (1981) Evaluation of short-term tests for carcinogens. Report of the International Collaborative Program. *Progress in Mutation Research. Vol. I.* New York: Elsevier/North-Holland, Inc.
Diaz M., Reiser A., Braier L. et al. (1980) Studies on benzene mutagenesis. I. The micronucleus test. *Experientia* **36**, 297–299.
Environmental Protection Agency (EPA; 1985) Toxic Substances Control Act Test Guidelines. Part 798. Health Effect Testing Guidelines. Subpart F. Genetic Toxicity, *Federal Register* **50**, 39435–39458.
Fenech M. and Morley A. A. (1985a) The effect of donor age on the spontaneous and induced micronuclei. *Mutat. Res.* **148**, 99–105.
Fenech M. and Morley A. A. (1985b) Measurement of micronuclei in lymphocytes. *Mutat.Res.* **147**, 29–36.
Frank D. W., Trzos R. J. and Good P. I. (1978) A comparison of two methods for evaluating drug-induced chromosome alterations. *Mutat. Res.* **56**, 311–317.
Frei J. V. and Lawley P. D. (1976) Tissue distribution and mode of DNA methylation in mice by methyl methanesulfonate and N-methyl-N′-nitro-N-nitroso-guanidine: lack of thymic lymphoma induction and low extent of methylation of target tissue DNA at 0–6 of guanine. *Chem. Biol. Interact.* **13**, 215-222.
Garriott M. L. and Grahn D. (1982) Neutron and γ-ray effects measured by the micronucleus test. *Mutat. Res.* **105**, 157–162.
Galloway S. M., Perry P. E., Meneses J. et al. (1980) Cultured mouse embryos metabolise benzo[*a*]pyrene during early gestation: Genetic differences detectable by sister chromatid exchanges. *Proc. Natl Acad. Sci. USA* **77**, 3524–3528.
Gilbert F. (1983) Chromosome aberrations and oncogenes. *Science* **303**, 475.
Goetz P., Sram R. J. and Dohnalova J. (1975) Relationship between experimental results in mammals and man. 1. Cytogenetic analysis of bone marrow injury induced by a single dose of cyclophosphamide. *Mutat. Res.* **31**, 247–254.
Goldberg M. T., Blakey D. H. and Bruce W. R. (1983) Comparison of the effects of 1,2-dimethylhydrazine and cyclophosphamide on micronucleus incidence in bone marrow and colon. *Mutat. Res.* **109**, 91–98.
Grab D. J. and Zedeck M. S. (1977) Organ-specific effects of the carcinogen methylazoxymethanol related to metabolism by nicotinamide adenine dinucleotide-dependent dehydrogenases. *Cancer Res.* **37**, 4182–4189.
Hart J. W. and Hartley-Asp B. (1983) Induction of micronuclei in the mouse. Revised timing of the final stage of erythropoiesis. *Mutat. Res.* **120**, 127–132.

Hartley-Asp B. (1979) Metronidazole exhibits no cytogenetic effect in the micronucleus test in mice or on human lymphocytes *in vitro*. *Mutat. Res.* **67**, 193–196.
Hayashi M., Sofuni T. and Ishidate M. Jr. (1983) An application of acridine orange fluorescent staining to the micronucleus test. *Mutat. Res.* **120**, 241–247.
Hayashi M., Sofuni T. and Ishidate M. Jr. (1984a) Kinetics of micronucleus formation in relation to chromosomal aberrations in mouse bone marrow. *Mutat. Res.* **127**, 129–137.
Hayashi M., Sofuni T. and Ishidate M. Jr (1984b) A pilot experiment for the micronucleus test. The multi-sampling at multi-dose levels method. *Mutat. Res.* **141**, 165–169.
Heddle J. A. (1973) A rapid *in vitro* test for chromosome damage. *Mutat. Res.* **18**, 187–190.
Heddle J. A. and Carrano A. V. (1977) The DNA content of micronuclei induced in mouse bone marrow by γ-radiation: evidence that micronuclei arise from acentric chromosomal fragments. *Mutat. Res.* **44**, 63–69.
Heddle J. A. and Salamone M. F. (1981) The micronucleus assay. I. *In vivo*. In: Stich H. F. and San R. H. C. (ed.) *Short-Term Tests for Chemical Carcinogens*, 243–249. New York: Springer-Verlag.
Heddle J. A., Hite M., Kirkhart B. et al (1983) The induction of micronuclei as a measure of genotoxicity. A report of the US Environmental Protection Agency Gene-Tox Program. *Mutat. Res.* **123**, 61-118.
Heddle J. A., Stuart E. and Salamone M. F. (1984) The bone marrow micronucleus test. In: Kilby B. J., Legator M., Nichols W. and Ramel C. (ed.) *Handbook of Mutagenicity Test Procedures* 2nd edn., 441–457. New York: Elsevier.
Henderson L., Cole R., Cole J., et al. Sister-chromatid exchange and micronucleus induction as indicators of genetic damage in maternal and foetal cells. *Mutat. Res.* **126**, 47–52.
Henry M., Lupo S. and Szabo K. T. (1980) Sex differences in sensitivity to the cytogenetic effects of ethyl methanesulfonate in mice demonstrated by the micronucleus test. *Mutat. Res.* **69**, 385–387.
Hite M., Pecharo M., Smith I. et al. (1980) The effect of benzene in the micronucleus test. *Mutat. Res.* **77**, 149–155.
Högstedt B. (1984) Micronuclei in lymphocytes with preserved cytoplasm. A method for assessment of cytogenetic damage in man. *Mutat. Res.* **130**, 63–72.
Högstedt B. and Karlsson A. (1985) The size of micronuclei in human lymphocytes varies according to the inducing agent used. *Mutat. Res.* **156**, 229–232.
Howell W. H. (1891) The life history of the formed elements of the blood, especially of the red corpuscles. *J. Morphol.* 4, 57–116.
Huber R., Streng S. and Bauchinger M. (1983) The suitability of the human lymphocyte micronucleus assay system for biological dosimetry. *Mutat. Res.* **111**, 185–193.
Jenssen D., Ramel C. and Gothe R. (1974) The induction of micronuclei by frameshift mutagens at the time of nucleus expulsion in mouse erythroblasts. *Mutat. Res.* **26**, 553–555.
Jenssen D. and Ramel C. (1978) Factors affecting the induction of micronuclei at low doses of X-rays, MMS and dimethylnitrosamine in mouse erythroblasts. *Mutat. Res.* **58**, 51–65.
Jenssen D. and Ramel C. (1980) The micronucleus test as part of a short-term mutagenicity test program for the prediction of carcinogenicity evaluated by 143 agents tested. *Mutat. Res.* **75**, 191–202.
Jenssen D. (1982) The induction of micronuclei. In: Sandberg A. A. (ed.) *Sister Chromatid Exchange*, 47–63. New York: Alan R. Liss, Inc.
Jolly M. J. (1905) Sur l'évolution des globules rouges dans le sang des embryons de mammifères. *C. R. Soc. Biol.* (Paris) **58**, 593–595.
Kapp Jr. R. W. and Eventhoff B. E. (1980) Mutagenicity of dimethylsulfoxide (DMSO). *Teratogenisis Carcinog. Mutagen.* **1**, 141–145.
Katcher A. L. (1980) Familial asplenia, other malformations, and sudden death. *Pediatrics*, **65**, 633–635.
King M-T. and Wild D. (1970) Transplacental mutagenesis: The micronucleus test on fetal mouse blood. *Human Genet.* **51**, 183–194.
Kliesch U., Danford N. and Adler I-D. (1981) Micronucleus test and bone-marrow chromosome analysis. A comparison of 2 methods *in vivo* for evaluating chemically induced chromosomal alterations. *Mutat. Res.* **80**, 321–332.
Kliesch U., Roupova I. and Adler I-D. (1982) Induction of chromosome damage in mouse bone marrow by benzo[a]pyrene. *Mutat. Res.* **102**, 265–273.
Klinger W., Muller D., Kleeberg U. et al. (1981) Peri- and postnatal development of phase I reactions. In: Kimmel C. A. and Buelkesam J. (ed.) *Developmental Toxicology*. New York: Raven Press.
Korte A., Slacik-Erben R. and Obe G. (1979) The influence of ethanol treatment on cytogenetic

effects in bone marrow cells of Chinese hamsters by cyclophosphamide, aflatoxin B1 and patulin. *Toxicology* **12**, 53–61.

Kram D., Bynum G. D., Senula G. C. et al. (1979) *In utero* sister chromatid exchange analysis for detection of transplacental mutagens. *Nature* **279**, 531.

Kram D., Bynum G. D., Senula G. C. et al (1980) *In utero* analysis of sister chromatid exchange: Alterations in susceptibility to mutagenic damage as a function of fetal cell type and gestational age. *Proc. Natl Acad. Sci. USA* **77**, 4784–4787.

Krogh Jensen M. (1977) Cytogenetic findings in pernicious anaemia. Comparison between results obtained with chromosome studies and the micronucleus test. *Mutat. Res.* **45**, 249–252.

Krogh Jensen M., Gorm Rasmussen G. and Ingeberg S. (1979) Cytogenetic studies in patients treated with penicillamine. *Mutat. Res.* **67**, 357–359.

Krogh Jensen M. and Nyfors A. (1979) Cytogenetic effect of methotrexate on human cells *in vivo*. Comparison between results obtained by chromosome studies on bone-marrow cells and blood lymphocytes by the micronucleus test. *Mutat. Res.* **64**, 339–343.

Lähdetie J. and Parvinen M. (1981) Meiotic micronuclei induced by X-rays in early spermatids of the rat. *Mutat. Res.* **81**, 103–115.

Lähdetie J. (1983a) Meiotic micronuclei induced by adriamycin in male rats. *Mutat. Res.* **119**, 79–82.

Lähdetie J. (1983b) Micronuclei induced during meiosis by ethyl methanesulfonate, cyclophosphamide and dimethylbenzanthracene in male rats. *Mutat. Res.* **120**, 257–260.

Lasne C., Gu Z. W., Venegas W. et al (1984) The *in vitro* micronucleus assay for detection of cytogenetic effects induced by mutagen-carcinogens: comparison with *in vitro* sister-chromatid exchange assay. *Mutat. Res.* **130**, 273–282.

Loem W. F., Bannerman R. M., Rininger B. F. et al. (1978) Hematologic disorders. In: Benirschke K., Garner F. M. and Jones T. C. (ed.) *Pathology of Laboratory Animals*, 889–1032. New York: Springer-Verlag.

Ma T-H. (1979) Micronuclei induced by X-rays and chemical mutagens in meiotic pollen mother cells of *Tradescantia*. A promising mutagen test system. *Mutat. Res.* **64**, 307–313.

Madle E., Korte A. and Beek B. (1986) Species differences in mutagenicity testing: I, Micronucleus and SCE tests in rats, mice, and Chinese hamsters with aflatoxin B1. *Teratogen., Carcinog. Mutagen.* **6**, 1–13.

Maier P. and Schmid W. (1975) The non-induction of micronuclei by quinacrine. *Mutat. Res.* **30**, 299–302.

MacGregor J. T., Wehr C. M. and Gould D. H. (1980) Clastogen-induced micronuclei in peripheral blood erythrocytes: the basis of an improved micronucleus test. *Environ. Mutagen.* **2**, 509–514.

MacGregor J. T., Wehr C. M. and Langlois R. G. (1983a) A simple fluorescent staining procedure for micronuclei and RNA in erythrocytes using Hoechst 33258 and pyronin Y. *Mutat. Res.* **120**, 269–275.

MacGregor J. T., Schlegel R., Choy W. N. et al. (1983b) Micronuclei in circulating erythrocytes: A rapid screen for chromosomal damage during routine toxicity testing in mice. In: Hayes A. W., Schnell R. C. and Miya T. S. (ed.) *Developments in the Science and Practice of Toxicology*, 555–558. New York: Elsevier.

Margison G. P. and O'Connor P. J. (1979) Nucleic acid modification by N-nitroso compounds. In: Grover P. J. (ed.) *Chemical Carcinogens and DNA*, 111–160. Boca Raton: CRC Press.

Marshall W. J. and McLean A. E. M. (1971) A requirement for dietary lipids for induction of cytochrome P-450 by phenobarbitone in rat liver microsomal fraction. *Biochem. J.* **122**, 569–573.

Matter B. E. and Grauwiler J. (1974) Micronuclei in mouse bone-marrow cells. A simple *in vivo* model for the evaluation of drug-induced chromosomal aberrations. *Mutat. Res.* **23**, 239–249.

Miale J. B. (1982) *Laboratory Medicine Hematology*, 6th ed. St Louis: C. V. Mosby Co.

Mitchell I. deG. and Brice A. J. (1986) Investigations into parametric analysis of data from in vivo micronucleus assays by comparison with non-parametric methods. *Mutat. Res.* **159**, 139–146.

Morimoto K. and Wolff S. (1980) Cell kinetics in human lymphocyte cultures. *Nature* **288**, 604–606.

Norred W. P. and Wade A. E. (1972) Dietary fatty acids—induced alterations of hepatic microsomal drug metabolism. *Biochem. Pharmacol.* **21**, 2887–2897.

Obe G., Beek B. and Vaidya V. G. (1975) III. Premature chromosome condensation from chemically and X-ray induced in micronuclei. *Mutat. Res.* **27**, 89–101.

Obe G. and Herha J. (1975) Chromosomal damage in chronic alcohol users. *Humangenetik* **29**, 191–200.

Obe G., Natarajan A. T., Meyers M. and den Hertog A. (1979) Induction of chromosomal aberrations in peripheral lymphocytes of human blood *in vitro*, and of SCEs in bone-marrow cells of mice *in vivo* by ethanol and its metabolite acetaldehyde. *Mutat. Res.* **68**, 291–294.

Organization for Economic Cooperation and Development (OECD; 1987) Genetic Toxicology: Micronucleus Test *Guidelines for Testing of Chemicals*. Guideline 474 (adopted 1985).

Oud J. L. and Peters P. W. J. (1978) A sequential screening of the cytogenetic damage induced by triaziquone. *Mutat. Res.* **54**, 175–184.

Pascoe S. and Gatehouse D. (1986) The use of a simple haematoxylin and eosin staining procedure to demonstrate micronuclei within rodent bone marrow. *Mutat. Res.* **164**, 237–243.

Perry P. and Wolff S. (1974) New Giemsa method for differential staining of sister chromatids. *Nature* **252**, 156–158.

Pincu M., Bass D. and Norman A. (1984) An improved micronuclear assay in lymphocytes. *Mutat. Res.* **139**, 61–65.

Preston R. J., Au W., Bender M. A. et al. (1981) Mammalian *in vivo* and *in vitro* cytogenetics assays: A report of the US EPA's Gene-Tox Program. *Mutat. Res.* **87**, 143–188.

Rabello-Gay M. N., Carvalho M. I. deO., Otto P. A. et al. (1985) The effects of age, sex and diet on the clastogenic action of cyclophosphamide in mouse bone marrow. *Mutat. Res.* **158**, 181–188.

Radman M., Jeggo P. and Wagner R. (1982) Chromosomal rearrangement and carcinogenesis. *Mutat. Res.* **98**, 249–264.

Rao K. V. N. and Vesselinovitch S. D. (1973) Age and sex-associated diethylnitrosamine dealkylation activity of the mouse liver and hepatocarcinogenesis. *Cancer Res.* **33**, 1625–1627.

Raj A. S. and Katz M. (1984) Corn oil and its minor constituents as inhibitors of DMBA-induced chromosomal breaks *in vivo*. *Mutat. Res.* **136**, 247–253.

Riccardi V. M. (1977) *The Genetic Approach to Human Disease*. New York: Oxford University Press.

Roguin N., Auslander L., Zeltzer M. et al. (1979) Asplenia syndrome: Report of two cases. *Isr. J. Med. Sci.* **15**, 451–453.

Rublo C. A., Nylander G. and Santos M. (1980) Experimental colon cancer in the absence of intestinal contents in Sprague-Dawley rats. *J. Natl Cancer Inst.* **64**, 569–572.

Russell E. S. and Bernstein S. E. (1966) Blood and blood formation. In: Green E. L. (ed.) *Biology of the Laboratory Mouse*, 351–372. New York: Dover Press.

Ryan F. P., Smart R. C., Holdsworth C. D. et al. (1978) Hyposplenism in inflammatory bowel disease. *Gut* **19**, 50–54.

Salamone M. F. (1981) Toxicity of 41 carcinogens and noncarcinogenic analogs. In: de Serres F. J. and Ashby J. (ed.) *Evaluation of Short-Term Tests for Carcinogens, Report of the International Collaborative Program—Progress in Mutation Research. Vol I*, 682–685. New York: Elsevier-/North Holland, Inc.

Salamone M., Heddle J., Stuart E. et al. (1980) Towards an improved micronucleus test. Studies on 3 model agents: mitomycin C, cyclophosphamide and dimethylbenzanthracene. *Mutat. Res.* **74**, 347–356.

Schmid W. (1973) Chemical mutagen testing on *in vivo* somatic mammalian cells. *Agents Actions*, **3**, 77–85.

Schmid W. (1975) The micronucleus test. *Mutat. Res.* **31**, 9–15.

Schmid W. (1976) The micronucleus test for cytogenetic analysis. In: Hollaender A. (ed.) *Chemical Mutagens: Principles and Methods for their Detection. Vol. 4*, 31–53. New York: Plenum Press.

Schmid W. (1977) The micronucleus test. In Kilbey B. J., Legator M., Nichols W. and Ramel C. (ed.) *Handbook of Mutagenicity Test Procedures*, 235–242. Amsterdam: Elsevier.

Schlegel R. and MacGregor J. T. (1982) The persistence of micronuclei in peripheral blood erythrocytes: detection of chronic chromosome breakage in mice. *Mutat. Res.* **104**, 367–369.

Schlegel R. and MacGregor J. T. (1983) A rapid screen for cumulative chromosomal damage in mice. Accumulation of circulating micronucleated erythrocytes. *Mutat. Res.* **113**, 481–487.

Schlegel R. and MacGregor J. T. (1984) The persistence of micronucleated erythrocytes in the peripheral circulation of normal and splenectomized Fischer 344 rats: Implications for cytogenetic screening. *Mutat. Res.* **127**, 169–174.

Sehgal C. B. and Hutton J. J. (1977) Homogenates of pregnant rat and foetal tissues metabolize carcinogens to mutagens detected by *Salmonella typhimurium* TA98 and TA100. *Mutat. Res.* **46**, 325–344.

Shindo Y., Hirano F., Maeda H. et al. (1983) The micronucleus test with mouse spleen cells. *Mutat. Res.* **121**, 53–57.

Siboulet R., Grinfeld S., Deparis P. et al. (1984) Micronuclei in red blood cells of the newt *Pleurodeles waltl* Michah: induction with X-rays and chemicals. *Mutat. Res.* **125**, 275–281.

Siou G., Conan L. and el Haitem M. (1981) Evaluation of the clastogenic action of benzene by oral administration with 2 cytogenetic techniques in mouse and Chinese hamster. *Mutat. Res.* **90**, 273–278.

Sorensen per J. and Krogh Jensen M. (1981) Cytogenetic studies in patients treated with trimethoprim-sulfamethoxazole. *Mutat. Res.* **89**, 91–94.

Sperling K. (1984) Frequency and origin of chromosome abnormalities in man. In: Obe G. (ed.) *Mutations in Man*, 128–146. Berlin: Springer-Verlag.

Steinheider G., Neth R. and Marquardt H. (1985) Evaluation of non-genotoxic and genotoxic factors modulating frequency of micronucleated erythrocytes in the peripheral blood of mice. *Cell Biol. Toxicol.* **1**, 197–211.

Stich H., Curtis J. R. and Parida B. B. (1982a) Application of the micronucleus test to exfoliated cells of high cancer risk groups: tobacco chewers. *Int. J. Cancer* **30**, 553–559.

Stich H., Stich W. and Parida B. B. (1982b) Elevated frequency of micronucleated cells in the buccal mucosa of individuals at high risk for oral cancer: betel quid chewers. *Cancer Lett.* **17**, 125–134.

Stich H. F. and Stich W. (1982c) Chromosome-damaging activity of saliva of betel nut and tobacco chewers. *Cancer Lett.* **15**, 193–202.

Stich H. F. and Rosin M. P. (1983) Quantitating the synergistic effect of smoking and alcohol consumption with the micronucleus test on human buccal mucosa cells. *Int. J. Cancer* **31**, 305–308.

Stich H. F. and Rosin M. P. (1984) Micronuclei in exfoliated human cells as a tool for studies in cancer risk and cancer intervention. *Cancer Lett.* **22**, 241–253.

Stoyel C. and Clark A. (1980) The transplacental micronucleus test. *Mutat. Res.* **74**, 393–398.

Styles J. A., Richardson C. R. and Burlinson B. (1983) A comparison of the incidence of micronuclei in blood and bone marrow in 3 strains of mouse dosed with cyclophosphamide or hexylmethylphosphoramide (HMPA). *Mutat. Res.* **122**, 143–147.

Tates A. D. and den Engelse L. (1982) Time dependent induction of chromosome damage in rat hepatocytes in relation to alkylation damage of DNA. In: Natarajan A. T., Obe G. and Altman H. (ed.) *DNA Repair, Chromosome Alterations and Chromatin Structure. Progress in Mutation Research. Vol. 4*, 267–278. New York: Elsevier.

Tates A. D., Dietrich A. J. J., de Vogel N. et al. (1983) A micronucleus method for detection of meiotic micronuclei in male germ cells of mammals. *Mutat. Res.* **121**, 131–138.

Tates A. D. and de Boer P. (1984) Further evaluation of a micronucleus method for detection of meiotic micronuclei in male germ cells of mammals. *Mutat. Res.* **140**, 187–191.

Trzos R. J., Petzold G. L., Brunden M. N. et al. (1978) The evaluation of sixteen carcinogens in the rat using the micronucleus test. *Mutat. Res.* **58**, 79–86.

Tsuchimoto T. and Matter B. E. (1979) *In vivo* cytogenetic screening methods for mutagens, with special reference to the micronucleus test. *Arch. Toxicol.* **42**, 239–248.

von Ledebur M. and Schmid W. (1973) The micronucleus test. Methodological aspects. *Mutat. Res.* **19**, 109–117.

Wade A. E., Norred W. P. and Evans J. S. (1978) Lipids in drug detoxification. In: Hathcock J. N. and Coon J. (ed.) *Nutrition and Drug Interrelations*, 475–503. New York: Academic Press.

Watanabe M., Honda S., Hayashi M. and Matsuda T. (1982) Mutagenic effects of combinations of chemical carcinogens and environmental pollutants in mice as shown by the micronucleus test. *Mutat. Res.* **97**, 43–48.

Wild D. (1978) Cytogenetic effects in the mouse of 17 chemical mutagens and carcinogens evaluated by the micronucleus test. *Mutat. Res.* **56**, 319–327.

Yaffe S. J., Rane A., Sjoqvist F. et al. (1970) The presence of a mono-oxygenase system in human fetal liver microsomes. *Life Sci.* **9**, 1189–1200.

Yamamoto K. I. and Kikuchi Y. (1980) A comparison of diameters of micronuclei induced by clastogens and by spindle poisons. *Mutat. Res.* **71**, 127–131.

Yamamoto K. I. and Kikuchi Y. (1981) Studies on micronuclei time response and on the effects of multiple treatments of mutagens on induction of micronuclei. *Mutat. Res.* **90**, 163–173.

Yamamoto K. I. and Kikuchi Y. (1984) Induction of micronuclei in mouse fetal liver after exposure *in utero* to N-methyl-N′-nitro-N-nitrosoguanidine. *Mutat. Res.* **128**, 173–179.

Yunis J. J. (1977) *New Chromosomal Syndromes*. New York: Academic Press.

Yunis J. J. (1983) The chromosomal basis of human neoplasia. *Science* **221**, 227–236.

Chapter 7

Chemical Induction of Dominant Lethal Mutations in Mammals

A. Philip Leber

A first step in the discussion of the topic of dominant lethal mutations is to define the components of the term. In reverse order, a mutation is a sudden variation in some heritable characteristic of an individual. Lethal is a factor or influence which induces death. Dominant is that which controls with superior power over lesser influences. Taken together, a dominant lethal mutation is a controlling influence which leads to death as an inherited variation in a biological species. For the purposes of this chapter, a chemical which has been administered to a parental animal prior to conception is subsequently considered a dominant lethal mutagen if there is a demonstration of induction of death in the fertilized egg or developing embryo as an apparent result of chromosomal aberration(s).

The phenomenon of dominant lethal mutagenesis is self-limiting in that it is expressed as a terminal event *in utero*, and therefore there is no opportunity for this form of chemically induced mutation to perpetuate itself. Its natural history extends from exposure and genetic alteration of germ cells of one of the sexually paired individuals, and ends with the death of the resulting gamete or embryo.

The evaluation of chemicals for their potential as mutagens is well founded. Ionizing radiation has long been known as an agent capable of inducing teratogenesis, carcinogenesis and mutagenesis (Miller, 1978). It was subsequently discovered that various chemicals also had the capacity to induce one or more of these biological anomalies. As with radiation, the threat of excessive exposures of humans to chemicals became evident as various occupational and therapeutic incidents later demonstrated. Genetic anomalies are implicated in human disease by virtue of (1) the presence of chromosomal abnormalities in individuals who are affected with various clinical disorders (often hereditable) including spontaneous abortions (Brusick, 1980); and (2) findings that agents, including chemicals which are capable of inducing chromosomal or gene changes, also produce deleterious health effects in experimental test species, including mammals.

Estimates of dominant non-lethal disorders in humans suggest that the frequency is approximately 9 per 100 live births (Carter, 1980). These conditions include various diseases of the nervous system, kidneys, skeleton, blood and other organs. Most frequently these conditions do not obviate reproductive function in affected individuals, but allow perpetuation of genetically related aberrations in subsequent generations. However, estimating dominant lethal mutation frequencies in humans is more difficult. As pointed out by Wilcox (1983), determinations of spontaneous abortion rates as defined by pregnancy loss before 20 to 28 weeks of gestation is most difficult, although 15% appears to be a reasonable estimate. This pregnancy loss encompasses dominant lethal events in humans, although it is emphasized that spontaneous abortions do not result solely from dominant mutations. However, it is reported that 50% of spontaneous abortuses display chromosomal anomalies (Barlow and Sullivan, 1982), demonstrating that this genetic condition appears to be related to embryonic death.

It is this array of observations in humans that drive efforts to evaluate chemicals according to test procedures which assess an agent's potential to induce dominant lethality. The remainder of this chapter will describe some of the experimental and practical aspects of this undertaking.

EXPERIMENTAL METHODS

Various tests have been developed to detect chemical induction of dominant lethality in mammalian test species. It has mainly been the rat and mouse which have been used in this testing. The sex targeted for evaluation has been primarily the male. The rodents have been chosen as models as a result of their extensive use in other toxicity testing, their well-defined germ cell development, and the relative low costs in testing these species. The choice of the male for most dominant lethal assessments stems from the fact that spermatogenesis is a continuous occurrence in adults. At any time point there is a population of cells at each stage of sperm development, beginning with stem cells and terminating with mature spermatozoa. It is these various male cell populations which are then subjected *in vivo* to chemical exposures and potentially mutagenic changes.

According to Brusick (1980), three general types of protocols have been used to assess dominant lethal mutations in rodents. The most commonly used procedure employs 10 or more males per dose group, preferably using individuals which are proven breeders. These males are then treated with test chemical on five consecutive days at levels ranging from zero (controls) up to a level considered to be a maximal tolerated dose. Each male is then housed with separate pairs of virgin females for five day intervals, with two day's rest between breeding periods. These mating periods number seven to ten to ensure encompassing the majority of, or the entire spermatogenic cycle.

The following schematic depicts how this chemical dosing schedule frequently allows designation of the spermatogenic stage during the chemical-chromosomal events. If, for example, a chemical mutagen is given 6 weeks prior to mating, the sperm affected would have been at the spermatocyte stage in their development when the genetic damage was incurred.

SPERMATOGONIA SPERMATOCYTE SPERMATID SPERMATOZOA

−9 −7 −5 −3 −1 Mating

Time of chemical exposure (week) prior to mating

Females are considered to have been inseminated by the appearance of a vaginal plug during their caging with the male. At days 13 to 17 of gestation, the females are sacrificed, and the uterine contents examined for:

1. Verification of pregnancy.
2. Total number of implantation sites in the uterus.
3. Numbers of dead and live foetal implants.

From these data, various calculations can be made which lead to a characterization of the reproductive toxicity and mutagenic activity of the test compound administered to the male animals. Preimplantation losses are reflected by a decrease in total number of implantation sites per pregnant female relative to control values. Alternatively, where ovarian corpora lutea counts are included in the test protocol (which indicate number of ova released for potential fertilization), preimplantation loss can be expressed in terms of a decrease in the ratio of implantation sites per corpora lutea in pregnant females. Post implantation loss is the incidence of dead implants per pregnant female.

These values provide a basis for estimating a chemical's potential to cause dominant lethal mutations in mammals. In addition, because of the serial mating of the test males to individual pairs of females, the susceptible cellular stage(s) for the test chemical's dominant lethal mutagenicity within the spermatogenesis chain can be determined.

Several indices are used to describe dominant lethal mutagenicity. One is the postimplantation index, which is dead implants per dam divided by the total implants per dam as described by Haseman and Soares (1976). This value is increased in animal test groups treated with dominant lethal mutagens relative to values for controls. Another approach is the calculation of per cent dominant lethals by the formula:

$$\left[1 - \frac{\text{Average number of live foetuses (test)}}{\text{Average number of live foetuses (control)}}\right] \times 100$$

This incorporates into one number the dominant lethal activity of the test compound (Generosa, 1984). As the latter author suggests, chemical mutagenic activity can be deduced after observing the trends of increased frequency of dead implantations, increased number of females with one or more dead implants, reduction in numbers of living embryos, reduction in numbers of implantations, and reductions in fertile matings. The latter two criteria are seen only when mutagenic activity towards the sperm is very high.

Various conditions contribute to accomplishing a satisfactory evaluation for dominant lethal mutagenicity in this bioassay:

1. The chemical must be administered by a route, and at a dose level, that will allow *in vivo* exposure of the gonads to the test substance in the targeted sex. The probability for this occurring is optimized by the administration of doses up to those causing a demonstrable clinical effect, such as depression in body weight gains or food intake.
2. The chemical must be administered at times in which the germ cells are sensitive or vulnerable to chromosomal attack by the test compound. Since the window of vulnerability is not known a priori, a test protocol must therefore accommodate by allowing chemical exposures to occur over the entire life cycle of the targeted germ cells.

3. Excessive toxicity in the treated rodents may compromise sexual performance or result in depressed sperm counts. These outcomes would lower the number of pregnancies occurring, making it more unlikely that sufficient conceptions would have occurred to measure dominant lethal mutations.
4. Since the spontaneous rates for pre- and post-implantation losses are relatively high in rodents, adequate numbers of test animals must be used to achieve the sensitivity required. Concomitantly, statistical analyses must be made which take into account unequal variances between test groups. Therefore, non-parametric analysis appears to be most appropriate on data such as dead implants per female (or per total implants) for postimplantation mutagenesis measurements (Haseman and Soares, 1976; Schreiner and Steelman, 1977).
5. Other tests which assess chemical induction of chromosomal aberrations, either *in vitro* or *in vivo*, may be used to support the results of dominant lethal results. Consistency between the outcomes of these tests would substantially increase the confidence that the rodent results assess true dominant lethality.

USE OF THE DOMINANT LETHAL ASSAY

During the development of toxicity information on a chemical, considerations must be given to what tests are needed for providing adequate assessment of potential mutagenic activity. The dominant lethal assay is not routinely performed as a first tier test in mutagenicity assessments, but is a useful follow-up to short-term *in vivo* or *in vitro* assays which indicate that a chemical is capable of inducing chromosomal aberrations. It is not justified to expect that agents which produce chromosomal damage in non-germ cells (somatic cells such as lymphocytes) will automatically cause germ cell mutagenic damage. As suggested by van Buul (1982) in discussing radiation risks, only observations made on primates and/or human germ cells (and not blood lymphocytes) can be expected to estimate human genetic risks arising from structural chromosomal aberrations.

Conceptually, the use of the dominant lethal mutation assay has a strong appeal for the following reasons:

1. It is one of very few mutagenicity endpoints that can be detected in intact animals. Implicit in this is the opportunity to evaluate activities following chemical administration via different exposure routes. Administered test compounds in this assay are subjected to possible metabolic transformation (activation or de-activation in a mutagenic sense), distribution and elimination processes in the animal, which must all be accounted for before any toxic endpoint takes on practical significance.
2. There is a high degree of relevance of the endpoint of the assay (embryonic-foetal lethality) to human reproductive health. This is an outcome of the assay's focus on the mammalian gonads and germ cells as target organs.
3. Many of the compounds which are positive in the dominant lethal mutation test are known to produce chromosomal changes and adverse reproductive outcomes in humans, e.g. cancer therapeutic agents.
4. Finally, dominant lethal mutations have been shown to be related to various chromosomal changes. A positive response may therefore suggest that the

chemical induces certain non-lethal, but potentially harmful, chromosomal changes, as well as lethal types.

Overall, the consensus of scientific opinion on this test is that if a compound gives positive results in the mouse or rat, the material should be used cautiously, because the assumption is that at some exposure level, the chemical has the potential to cause mutagenic injury in humans. However, the test can not be relied upon as a screening technique since the assay, as performed, is relatively insensitive towards compounds with weak activity. This property appears to result from the high and variable background incidences observed in control rodents. The fact that other assays for chromosomal aberrations (e.g. bone marrow cytogenetics, heritable translocation or *in vitro* studies) appear quite sensitive contributes to the dominant lethal test's diminished reputation in this regard.

MODE OF ACTION

The mechanism by which chemicals cause dominant lethal mutations is thought to be related to damage induced in chromosomes of germ cells characterized as structural or numeric changes. This has been established by the non-routine procedure of performing cytogenetic analysis on preimplanted fertilized eggs taken from Fallopian tubes and uteri of rodents. Generosa et al. (1978) describe findings which indicate that alkylating agents which are active towards male germ cells in inducing chromosome breakage in postmeiotic stages (spermatids or spermatozoa) also induced dominant lethality, which further supports its linkage with chromosomal breaks. They also showed that mouse differentiating spermatogonia and early meiotic germ cell stages can be subject to dominant lethal mutagenic attack and chromosomal breakage when treated with the non-alkylating agent 6-mercaptopurine. These latter observations contrast with previously held perceptions that (1) only alkylating agents cause chromosomal breakage, and (2) only postmeiotic germ cells are sensitive to dominant lethal mutagenicity induction by chemicals.

CHEMICAL EXAMPLE

A chemical which has been extensively scrutinized with respect to its genetic toxicity is ethylene oxide (EO). This material derives its qualities as a chemical intermediate and biomedical sterilant from the alkylating properties of its epoxide group. It is this characteristic which also contributes to its mutagenic and toxicological profile.

EO has been described as being active in a wide variety of non-mammalian test systems (Embree et al., 1977; Generosa et al., 1980), inducing gene mutations and chromosomal aberrations (also seen in mammalian somatic cells). A dominant lethal study in rodents was first reported by Embree et al. (1977). After an inhalation exposure of 4 hours to 1000 ppm of EO, male rats were mated with groups of females from week 1 to week 10 posttreatment. Dominant lethality was clearly demonstrated, as numbers of dead implants per total implants were substantially increased over control values (2 to 4 times) in females mated 2 or 3 weeks following EO exposures. This corresponds to late spermatid/early spermatozoa attack by EO in the treated males. Additional data supporting the dominant lethality of EO following inhalation exposures to rats were developed by Snellings (1984).

A mouse study was conducted (Generosa, 1980) in which males were administered one intraperitoneal injection of EO in aqueous solution at a dose of 150 mg/kg. Matings were then conducted in pairs of females up to 21 days after treatment. Percentages of implants found dead were elevated when mating occurred up to 13 days after dosing, indicating that EO has dominant lethal effects in exposed spermatozoa and late spermatids (postmeiotic cells).

A study later conducted by Generosa et al. (1985) was to produce not only further evidence regarding the dominant lethal properties of EO in mice, but important information relative to dose-response and dose-rate-response relationships. In the first experiment, mice were exposed by inhalation to 300, 400 or 500 ppm EO in the air for 6 hours a day for 4 days. The highest incidence of induced dominant lethal mutations occurred when mating was 4·5 to 7·5 days following final EO exposures. With increasing dose levels, the percentage of dead implants at this time interval were 9, 30 and 53, with an average control rate of 3%, clearly demonstrating that the dominant lethal effect is related to the dose administered. However, extrapolation shows that the curve does not extend through zero, indicating that the dose-response is a threshold phenomenon.

The second phase of the experiment examined dose rate effects for EO. Three groups of mice were exposed to equal total doses of EO (1800 ppm hours/day for 4 days), but at the daily schedules of (1) 300 ppm for 6 hours, (2) 600 ppm for 3 hours, or (3) 1200 ppm for 1·5 hours, with matings within the same time interval as the first experiment. Percentages of dead implants were 17, 33 and 56 under exposure conditions 1, 2 and 3, respectively, with a control rate of 3%. This experiment dramatically demonstrates that for the dominant lethality of EO, greater risks are incurred by shorter exposures to high levels of compound, as opposed to longer exposures at low concentrations. Mechanistically, it appears that the former exposure condition either induces greater genetic damage initially, or in some manner inhibits repair mechanisms within the genetic apparatus. In any event, these observations have important implications in terms of the establishment of allowable occupational exposures to mutagens, both for long-term time-weighted averages, and short-term maximal exposures. As discussed by the investigators, further elaboration of factors relevant to human risks may derive from the study of covalent binding of mutagenic adducts to germ cell chromosomes.

Finally, publications on the dominant lethal mutagenicity of 140 chemicals have been reviewed, with results tabulated employing several criteria for acceptability of data (Green et al., 1985). This review is helpful as a compendium of dominant lethal results presented in published literature.

REFERENCES

Barlow S. M. and Sullivan F. M. (1982) *Reproductive Hazards of Industrial Chemicals*, **29**, London: Academic Press.

Brusick D. (1980) *Principles of Genetic Toxicology*, Chapter 3. New York: Plenum Press.

Carter C. O. (1980) Presentation at *International Symposium of Chemical Mutagenesis, Human Population Monitoring and Genetic Risk Assessment*. Ottawa, Ontario, October 14–16.

Embree J. W., Lyon J. P. and Hine C. H. (1977) The mutagenic potential of ethylene oxide using the dominant-lethal assay in rats. *Toxicol. Appl. Pharmacol.* **40**, 261–267.

Generosa W. M. (1984) Dominant-lethal mutations and heritable translocations in mice. In: Chu E. H. Y. and Generosa W. M. (ed.) *Mutation, Cancer, and Malformation*, 369–388. New York: Plenum.

Generosa W. M., Cain K. T., Huff S. W. et al. (1978) Inducibility by chemical mutagens of heritable translocations in male and female germ cells of mice. In: Flamm W. G. and Mehlman M. A. (ed.) *Mutagenesis*, Chapter 6. Washington DC: Hemisphere Publishing Corp.

Generosa W. M., Cain K. T., Hughes L. A. et al. (1986) Ethylene oxide dose and dose-rate effects in the mouse dominant-lethal test. *Environ. Mutagen.* **8**, 1 7.

Generosa W. M., Cain K. T., Krishna M. et al. (1980) Heritable translocation and dominant lethal mutation induction with ethylene oxide in mice. *Mutat. Res.* **73**, 133–142.

Green S., Auletta A., Fabricant J. et al. (1985) Current status of bioassays in genetic toxicology—the dominant lethal assay. A report of the US Environmental Protection Agency Gene-Tox Program. *Mutat. Res.* **154**, 49–67.

Haseman J. K. and Soares E. R. (1976) The distribution of fetal death in control mice and its implication on statistical tests for dominant lethal effects. *Mutat. Res.* **41**, 277–288.

Miller R. W. (1978) The discovery of human teratogens, carcinogens, and mutagens: lessons for the future. In: Hollaender A. and de Serres F. J. (ed.) *Chemical Mutagens—Principles and Methods for Their Detection. Vol. 5*, 101–126. New York: Plenum.

Schreiner C. A. and Steelman J. R. (1977) Oral triethylenemelamine: effects in the dominant lethal assay for mutagenicity. *Toxicol. Appl. Pharmacol.* **42**, 487–495.

Snellings W. M. (1984) Ethylene oxide dominant lethal mutagenicity inhalation study on rats. *Final report to the Ethylene Oxide Producers*. Chemical Manufacturers Association, Washington D.C.

Soares E. R. (1979) Genetic aspects of short-term testing and an appraisal of some *in vivo* mammalian test systems. In: Butterworth B. E. (ed.) *Strategies for Short-Term Testing for Mutagens/Carcinogens*, 67–76. West Palm Beach, Florida: CRC Press.

van Buul P. P. W. (1982) Absence of correlation between the chromosomal radiosensitivity of peripheral blood lymphocytes and stem-cell spermatogonia in mammals. *Mutat. Res.* **95**, 69–77.

Wilcox A. J. (1983) Surveillance of pregnancy loss in human populations. *Am. J. Ind. Med.* **4**, 285–291.

Chapter 8

Developmental Toxicity in Toxicologic Research and Testing

Rochelle W. Tyl

INTRODUCTION AND BACKGROUND

Standard reference texts define toxicity simply as 'the state of being toxic or poisonous', and toxic as 'relating to, or caused by poison or toxin'. Therefore, in order to provide a more meaningful beginning to this discussion of developmental toxicity, the following expanded definition of toxicity is proffered: any structural or functional alteration or perturbation, caused by environmental insult, reversible or irreversible, which interferes with homeostasis, normal growth, differentiation, development and/or behaviour. These alterations, by definition, exceed the limits of tolerance by the system under scrutiny. 'Developmental toxicity' may then be defined as toxicity to the conceptus occurring and expressed pre- or postnatally. Developmental toxicity includes insult to (1) the fertilized egg or zygote prior to implantation, or prior to the formation of the three primary germ layers (ectoderm, endoderm and mesoderm); (2) the embryo during the period of organogenesis, terminating with the closure of the secondary palate; (3) the foetus, in the postembryonic or histogenetic period of gestation; and (4) the neonate and postnatal offspring, occurring or expressed from parturition through the postnatal period until sexual maturity. Developmental toxicity encompasses a spectrum of possible effects which includes death, malformation, functional deficits and developmental delays (Wilson, 1973; Johnson and Christian, 1984), in order from most to least severe.

Death, which represents the ultimate expression of toxicity, may be manifested as preimplantation loss, resorptions, dead foetuses, or spontaneous abortions in test animals, and spontaneous miscarriages or stillbirths in humans, depending on the stage of development at the time of death. Preimplantation loss (fractional loss, commonly expressed as a percentage and calculated as the number of ovarian corpora lutea minus the number of uterine implantation sites divided by the number of corpora lutea), measures the disparity between ovulated eggs (the corpus luteum forming from the follicle after ovulation) and implanted zygotes, and indicates pre-embryonic death. Resorptions include implantation sites (uterine decidual reactions) discernible only after staining apparently non-gravid uteri with ammonium or sodium sulphide (on fresh preparations; Salewski, 1964), or with potassium ferricyanide (on formalin-fixed preparations), or macroscopically visible placental remnants with or without foetal tissue, including dead foetuses without discernible digits. Resorptions indicate death of the conceptus during the embryonic period or early in the foetal period. These uterine site designations may be further subdivided into 'empty' implantation sites (visualized by staining), early resorptions (placental remnants only), middle resorptions (placental remnants with foetal tissue but no discernible limb buds), and late resorptions (placental remnant with foetuses with discernible limb buds but no discernible digits). Dead foetuses indicate death late in the foetal period and are designated (depending on the laboratory) based on a certain minimum body weight, a complete secondary palate, and/or the presence of discernible digits. The time of death may be more or less precisely determined employing external morphological criteria, e.g. those of Rugh (1968) for the mouse. These foetuses may appear pale, autolyzed or macerated to a greater or lesser degree.

Structural malformations are detected in late gestational (term) foetuses or in neonates, presenting as external, visceral (including the craniofacial soft tissue) and/or skeletal lesions, and are expressions of frank teratogenicity resulting from dysmorphogenesis. The criterion of dysmorphogenesis is important since it indicates a diversion from the normal course of development and not a delay in an essentially normal process. Malformations are typically considered incompatible with, or severely detrimental to postnatal survival, and are essentially irreversible without intervention. Parenthetically, there is evidence that some lesions can be repaired prenatally, e.g. cleft palate in rats (Schuepbach and Schroeder, 1984), egg cylinder (early embryonic stage, gestational day 6 to 8) lesions in mice (Hamburgh et al., 1984), and ventricular septal defect in non-human primates (Hendrickx et al., 1983); or postnatally, e.g. wavy ribs in rats (Nishimura et al., 1982), and certain types of ventricular septal defect in children (Bankl,1977). Malformations may involve replication, absence or extensive reduction of essential structure(s) or organs. They may result from cell damage or cell death (cytotoxicity) at a critical location and phase of differentiation or growth. They may also result from partial or complete interference with morphogenetic cell movements, or interference with critical inductions between adjacent tissues to initiate new structures.

The category of malformations may also include syndromes or clusters of otherwise minor anomalies. Aberrations such as deviations or variations (Khera, 1981), for example, include those findings which could be upgraded to malformations depending on severity of expression, and which are not considered, by themselves, lethal or detrimental to postnatal survival. Deviations frequently may involve slight to major reduction or absence of non-essential structures, may be reversible or irreversible, and may be observed with measurable frequency in normal populations (i.e. there may be a predisposition in the specific species or strain examined, a confounding factor which will be discussed later). In term foetuses, an increased incidence in skeletal variations such as extra rib or wavy rib may be indicative of toxicity and not considered a malformation (Kimmel and Wilson, 1973; Khera, 1981). In this category of variations may also be placed findings of reduced skeletal ossification, especially in those skeletal districts or regions indicative of toxicity (Aliverti et al., 1979), if the delayed/retarded/reduced ossification occurs in a normal developmental pattern. To classify the finding as a variation, the diminished ossification observed should occur in those elements which ossify last, so that the normal pattern of cephalocaudal and proximodistal ossification is maintained. However, reduced skeletal ossification is usually considered evidence for developmental delay or growth retardation (*see below*).

Functional deficits or derangements (with presumed underlying microstructural and /or biochemical lesions), detected as altered enzymatic activities or abnormal organ function tests, are demonstrated in foetuses, in neonates, or in older postnatal animals. These alterations may be accompanied by changes in organ-to-body weight ratios and/or histopathologic changes in the affected organ(s). Behavioural development may be altered as detected by the evaluation in older postnatal offspring of such behaviours as open field activity, nestbox emergence, locomotor activity, diurnal activity, passive or active avoidance, operant discrimination, maze learning and swimming activity.

Developmental delay or growth retardation is detected by reduced foetal or neonatal body weights, reduced absolute and relative organ weights, reduced crown-rump length, and reduced ossification of skeletal elements in the term foetus, especially in those skeletal districts which ossify last and are therefore sensitive to insult (Aliverti et al., 1979). The assumption inherent in identifying these skeletal findings as variations is that what is observed is a reduced level of ossification at the particular point in time at which it is conventionally evaluated (gestational day 20 or 21 in rats, gestation day 17 or 18 in mice, gestation day 29 or 30 in rabbits), reflecting a lower rate of ossification which would have proceeded, if the animals had not been sacrificed for examination, to form essentially normal bony structures, and not a premature termination of ossification which would produce an abnormal (missing, short, incomplete) bony structure. This latter situation would result in a malformation if other criteria for the designation were satisfied. To distinguish between a slower rate of ossification and a prematurely terminated ossification sequence, the foetal preparations may be doubly stained with alizarin red S specific for bone and with alcian blue specific for cartilage (Inouye, 1976; Kimmel and Trammel, 1981). This double stain would allow identification of cartilaginous precursors not yet ossified versus the absence of the cartilaginous precursor (anlage). The presumption is that the presence of cartilaginous anlage(n) implies the capability for ossification so that the finding is classified as retarded ossification. The absence of such a precursor is interpreted as a missing bone (or portion of bone) which would not subsequently ossify, hence a malformation. This double staining technique would be useful only for cartilage-replacement bones found in the axial and appendicular skeleton, and not for membranous bones found in the skull plates which do not form initially as cartilage. Developmental delays in postnatal offspring may be indicated by reduced body weight or weight gain, considered a sensitive and consistent measure of developmental effect (Lochry et al., 1984). Altered time courses for acquisition of developmental landmarks may also indicate delays. Landmarks evaluated may include surface righting reflex, pinna detachment, visible pilation (secondary hair growth), cliff avoidance, incisor eruption, wire grasping, auditory startle reflex, eye opening, midair righting reflex, negative geotaxis, testis descent, vaginal patency, etc. These effects may be transient if exposure has ceased, or even in the event of continued exposure. Delays may also be indicated in the time course of more sophisticated behaviours, as outlined previously under functional defects.

The effects described may represent pleiotropic responses to the toxic stimulus, separate, distinct and independent in their development, or they may represent points on a single continuum beginning with growth retardation on a cellular, organ or systemic level, through malformations or functional deficits, and terminating in the death of the conceptus.

The developing conceptus is considered preferentially vulnerable to environmental insult because of qualitative and/or quantitative differences from adults. These differences include the following:

1. *Small cell numbers.* Initially the cells of the conceptus, through morula, blastula and early gastrula stage, are totipotent. If relatively few cells are irreparably damaged or lost, the remaining cells are capable of repair, regulation, or replacement, and the conceptus will appear unharmed, or exhibit intrauterine growth retardation without abnormalities (Fabro et al., 1984) at term. This organismic plasticity is found in the pre-embryonic or predifferentiation stage of development, and is lost with the transition from presumptive to determined cell status. This same transition is found as each tissue and organ becomes biochemically committed by the derepression of structural genes coding for specific cell products characteristic of the tissue or organ. This initial induction occurs in a roughly cephalocaudal sequence in the embryonic period of development as cells commit, and is expressed as recognizable cell and tissue proteins and structures in the histogenetic or foetal period.
2. *Rapid rates of proliferation.* The initial rapid cell divisions with minimal time between each cytokinesis (i.e. a very short G_1 period) require rapid synthesis of energy sources such as ATP and GTP, nucleic acid precursors, chemical messengers such as cyclic AMP, contractile proteins and cell and nuclear membrane components. Interference with this process, even in the absence of microscopically visible cell damage or death, may preclude normal differentiation and growth, and may translate into growth retardation or malformations.
3. *Large proportion of undifferentiated cells.* This pool of totipotent cells (see discussion under (1) above) may confer a regulatory ability on the conceptus, but these cells may lack sophisticated biochemical defence capabilities characteristic of more mature differentiated cells (see (5) and (6) below).
4. *Requirement for precise temporal and spatial localization of cells and cell products.* In the formation of various structures, specific cells (specific for both number and type) and cell products must be present at the appropriate place and time for normal differentiation. This precision is important for morphogenetic movements, programmed cell death and developmental inductions.

   Large scale morphogenetic movements include migration, aggregation, cavitation, delamination, folding, closure and fusion. Migration is critical for the movement of germ cells from the extraembryonic yolk sac to the embryonic germinal ridge, site of the future gonad; neural crest cells move from the lateral edge of the developing neural tube to form axons, ganglia, melanocytes, etc. Masses of cells assemble (or replicate) to form various solid organs. Cavitation occurs in the formation of the coelomic cavity in early embryos. Delamination of early cardiac cells gives rise to the papillary muscles, chordae tendineae and valvular flaps within the heart. Folding, closure and fusion are essential for the formation of the neural tube and palate. Movements of a few or single cells are involved in the organization of the neurones of the central and peripheral nervous system.

Programmed cell death plays an indispensible role in embryonic development. 'Phylogenetic death' eliminates vestiges of evolutionary anlagen; 'histogenetic death' remodels cartilage and bone; 'morphogenetic death' accompanies the formation of folds and the confluence of anlagen (Saunders, 1966). This process is essential for the ontogeny of the higher vertebrate foetal kidney, and for shaping the vertebrate limb. Higher vertebrates elaborate, and then destroy the pronephros and mesonephros as prelude for the formation of the metanephric kidney. Interference with this process precludes formation of the terrestrial vertebrate kidney (Balinsky, 1975). Non-programmed damage to the posterior necrotic zone (PNZ) alters the development of the bones of the limb; excessive damage to the apical ectodermal ridge (AER) of the limb bud results in reduction (oligodactyly) or loss of digits (adactyly). The lack of programmed cell death in the PNZ prevents the sculpting of the appropriate limb bones; this lack in the AER results in the formation of excess digits (polydactyly).

Induction is a major mechanism for formation of a number of organs, e.g. the optic lobes of the diencephalon must grow out and appose the head ectoderm to induce lens formation; the mesoderm at gastrula stage must underlay the dorsal ectoderm to induce formation of neural plate; the mesonephric ducts of the kidney must approximate the metanephrogenic tissue to induce the metanephric kidney (Balinsky, 1975). This need for critical and specific mass in certain tissues or regions at specific times confers unique specific sensitivity upon those tissues or regions. This sensitivity is lost once the critical period has past.

5. *Limited metabolic capability*. The ability of cells (and organisms) to recover from environmental insult depends on the functioning of inducible and/or constitutive enzymes involved in metabolism. These enzymes are responsible for inadvertently activating xenobiotics to toxic metabolites or for detoxifying xenobiotics, again inadvertently, as they are modified, to enhance solubility in water. These enzymes include the mixed function oxidases, cytochrome P_{450} and P_{448}, which are ubiquitous, as well as enzymes specific for certain molecules or classes of molecules and specific as to location. Molecular repair (e.g. unscheduled DNA synthesis), derepression of certain genetic loci, and repression of others for differentiation, regulation or replacement of cells, and higher level repair (tissue, organ, etc.) are also critical for recovery. It has been accepted as dogma that the conceptus has little or no metabolic capability until late in the foetal period when the liver and kidney are functional (Wilson, 1973). The developing conceptus has therefore been viewed as the passive receptacle for parent compound or metabolites produced by the maternal organism and/or the placenta. However, preliminary data by Filler (1982) indicates that the preimplantation (gestational day 3·5) mouse morula has demonstrable inducible enzymatic activity for metabolism of xenobiotics, under appropriate strain-specific genetic control. The metabolic products are present in femtomole quantities, but if additional research confirms Filler's findings, then the

conceptus is at least somewhat capable of generating potentially toxic metabolites, or of detoxifying toxic chemicals throughout the gestational period.

6. *Immaturity of immunosurveillance systems.* The ability to distinguish between 'self' and 'non-self', or between cells with the normal surface markers and transformed cells with altered surface markers is acquired in the postnatal period. This lack of recognition capability implies that the conceptus cannot identify and thus destroy altered cells produced from environmental insult (or from internal genetic error). This lack is of special concern for the induction of transplacental carcinogenesis, documented for diethylstilbestrol (DES) in humans where *in utero* exposure results in clear cell vaginal carcinoma in adolescent women. In animals, many chemicals produce system-specific tumours in adults after exposure in the foetal period (Rice, 1976). The immunosurveillance system itself is also sensitive to environmental insult, expressed in the young adult (Chapman and Roberts, 1984) or the older animal (Spyker and Fernandes, 1973).

Many of the above differences may be invoked to explain the greater sensitivity of developing (or regenerating) organs to insult relative to mature organs.

The conceptus exhibits differing susceptibilities throughout its development. These differences may be qualitative or quantitative in response to the same insult.

The conceptus is considered relatively refractory to the production of terata from environmental insult in the pre-embryonic stage of development, which begins with fertilization and ends at implantation, and lasts approximately 5 to 8 days in most mammals. This resistance is thought to be due to the totipotent cells which comprise the conceptus at this time, and which are capable of regulation and replacement. It may also be due to the isolated status of the conceptus, floating in the uterine lumen, nourished by uterine secretions and not in contact with the maternal blood supply. If the damage to the conceptus at this stage is too severe for repair, the conceptus may die and the insult is detected as preimplantation loss. If regulation is not completely successful, the conceptus at term may be small but structurally normal. The resistance of the pre-embryonic conceptus is not total; hypoxia, hypothermia and actinomycin D do cause malformations if administered at this stage. The embryonic or organogenesis period begins with implantation and formation of the primary germ layers (beginning on gestational days 5 to 6 in conventional test animals, day 8 for humans) and extends until closure of the secondary palate (which occurs on gestational days 15 to 17 in rodents, days 18 to 19 in lagamorphs such as rabbits, and days 58 to 60 in the human). In this period, the conceptus, now termed an embryo, is at maximum susceptibility for induction of structural malformations and also death (detected as resorptions at term in animal models or as miscarriages or spontaneous abortions in humans). In the foetal or histogenetic period, which begins at the closure of the secondary palate and ends at birth, the susceptibility is expressed as functional deficits, since the organ systems present from the embryonic period are now differentiating in terms of intra- and intercellular products. Exposure to certain agents during this period (but not before) may also result in system-specific tumours in the mature postnatal animal (Rice, 1976). The development of many systems is not complete by parturition, but continues into the neonatal or postnatal period, e.g. the central and peripheral nervous system, respiratory system, urogenital system, endocrine system, digestive system, and the cellular and humoral immune system. Insults to these systems from *in utero* exposure would not necessarily be detectable until the systems were called upon to function or were under stress, because of functional reserve capacity, so that the latency from exposure until expression and detection of the lesion could be up to ten years of age or beyond for most human anomalies (including neurofunctional deficits detectable in school children, and reproductive dysfunctions), and until sexual maturity in test animals. However, premature loss of function in a mature or ageing individual may also be caused by *in utero* insult, e.g. methyl mercury exposure and premature senescence of the immune system in mice (Spyker and Fernandes, 1973); hence the need for continued surveillance. In addition, the time to onset of tumours from *in utero* insult (transplacental carcinogenesis—*see above*) may be 12 to 24 months in rodents or 15 to 30 years in humans.

GOVERNMENTAL TEST RULES AND GUIDELINES

The history of governmental regulatory rules and guidelines for evaluation of reproductive and developmental toxicity in test animals began with the recognition, in the early 1960s, that the testing methods then in use worldwide would not have detected, and did not detect, the teratogenic risk to humans of thalidomide; over 8000 children in 28 countries were malformed from maternal use of the drug in the first trimester of pregnancy. A discussion of the deficiencies in testing at this time and the sequence of events which led to governmental intervention has been presented by Wilson (1979). The first formal action by a governmental agency was a letter from the Chief of the Drug Review Branch, US Food and Drug Administration (FDA), sent on March 1, 1966, to all corporate medical directors (Goldenthal, 1966), establishing Guidelines for Reproductive Studies for Safety Evaluation of Drugs for Human Use. These guidelines were promulgated 'as a routine screen for the appraisal of safety of new drugs for use during pregnancy and in women of childbearing potential'. Phase I (or Segment I), designated as the Study of Fertility and General Reproductive Performance, involved exposure of the males for 10 weeks prior to mating to include exposure during all phases of spermatogenesis, estimated as 8 or 9 weeks duration in rats and 5 weeks in mice, and of the females for 2 weeks to include ovulation, a 4 to 5 day cycle in rodents. Exposure was continued for the females through pregnancy, parturition and lactation. One-half the dams were sacrificed on gestational day 13 for examination of number and distribution of live embryos in uterine horns, implantation sites and resorptions. The dams allowed to litter were examined for litter size, stillborn and live births. Dead pups were examined for skeletal anomalies. Live pups were examined for gross anomalies and individually weighed at delivery, postnatal day 4 and 21. This segment would provide information on breeding, fertility, implantation, parturition and lactation in the parental generation and on neonatal effects in the offspring (F_1), but would not detect effects on reproduction in the F_1 generation. FDA subsequently suggested a three-generation reproduction protocol to evaluate long-term effects on reproduction and fertility, beginning with a prebreeding exposure in the P_0 (parental) generation and including effects on the germinal cell line developing *in utero* during exposure to the test material in the F_1 and F_2 generations. Two litters per breeding pair were obtained in each generation, one litter sacrificed at weaning, one litter selected for mating to produce the next generation. Both F_3 litters were sacrificed at weaning, one litter destined for histopathologic examination (FDA, 1970).

Phase II (or Segment II) as originally proposed by the FDA (Goldenthal, 1966), entitled Teratological Study, involved exposure during organogenesis, gestational days 6 through 15 (rodents) or 6 through 18 or 19 (rabbits). Testing in two species was called for, one rodent and one non-rodent. The basis for the two species requirement presumably was to distinguish between an agent uniquely teratogenic to a rodent and one positive in two species, with implications that it may be positive in all mammals (including humans). Dams were sacrificed 1 to 2 days before the anticipated date of parturition and foetuses were delivered by Caesarean section. Data to be collected included number of ovarian corpora lutea and status of uterine implantation sites: live and dead foetuses, and early and late resorptions. Live foetuses were to be weighed and examined for external malformations. In rodents, one-third to one-half of each litter were to be examined for soft tissue deficits by visceral dissection of fresh tissue (Staples, 1974), or by serial freehand cross sectioning of fixed material (Wilson, 1965, 1973). The remaining foetuses were cleared and stained for examination for skeletal anomalies. Rabbit foetuses were to be incubated for 24 hours to assess viability, then all foetuses were examined for external, visceral and skeletal anomalies.

Phase III (or Segment III), entitled Perinatal and Postnatal study, involved exposure of the dam during the final one-third of gestation and continuing through parturition and lactation to weaning. This segment 'should delineate effects of the drug on late fetal development, labor and delivery, lactation, neonatal viability, and growth of the newborn' (Goldenthal, 1966). Cross-fostering was suggested for this phase if survival of pups were impaired. Rearing of pups from this Phase and Phase I to evaluate reproductive and fertility performance in these F_1 animals was also suggested as a possibility.

FDA established good laboratory practice regulations for laboratories involved in toxicology testing (FDA, 1978), including teratogenicity evaluations. The Environmental Protection Agency (EPA) proposed guidelines for hazard evaluation, including teratogenicity and reproductive evaluations (EPA, 1978). These guidelines were basically those of the FDA. In addition, EPA suggested a modified Segment III, with exposures during the last third of pregnancy and observation of the postnatal animals to sexual maturity, with evaluation of central nervous system function. EPA recommended a two-generation reproductive evaluation with one litter per generation, in lieu of the FDA suggestion of three generations and two litters per generation. EPA also deleted the mid-pregnancy sacrifice for one-half of the females in the Segment I reproductive toxicity testing. The explanation was that evaluation for genetic damage, detected in the FDA three-generation study (with the midgestational sacrifice to detect non-viable implants), would better (cheaper, faster, more precisely) be detected in mutagenicity test batteries, including dominant lethal tests, and that, if parental animals were bred when they were mature, the variability commonly associated with first litters in young animals (hence one of the rationales for two litters per generation) would be minimized. These guidelines became EPA proposed test standards for chemicals under the Toxic Substances Control Act (TSCA) in 1979 (EPA, 1979), and final rules in 1983 (EPA, 1983a); the practice standards for chemicals covered by the Federal Insecticide Fungicide and Rodenticide Act (FIFRA) became rules in 1983 (EPA, 1983b) with an effective date of May 2, 1984 (EPA, 1984a). The Interagency Regulatory Liaison Group (IRLG), during this period of rapid regulatory evolution, also proposed draft guidelines for selected studies, including developmental toxicity evaluations (Morgenroth, 1979), and planned to create test standards for all toxicity tests which would satisfy all concerned US Agencies (IRLG, 1980), but was disbanded before it could complete this task. In an attempt to unify test standards internationally (a critical need for companies attempting to satisfy regulatory requirements prior to registering compounds in different countries), the Organization for Economic Cooperation and Development (OECD) developed guidelines for testing of chemicals, including reproductive and developmental toxicity testing (OECD, 1981, 1983), which closely resembled the EPA guidelines and rules. The hope was that member countries could accept these compromise guidelines, and that testing requirements could be made uniform worldwide.

Examination of the current guidelines and rules from FDA, EPA(TSCA), EPA(FIFRA), OECD, Canada, the United Kingdom and Japan (for drugs and agricultural chemicals) with respect to Segment II (teratogenicity) testing indicates very similar protocols and requirements, essentially the same as the initial FDA protocol (Goldenthal, 1966). The differences which do exist are: (1) in the number of pregnant rodents per treatment group—all current groups require 20, except Japan which requires 30 because of the requirement for one-third of the animals in each group to be allowed to litter, and for postnatal examination of the litters, including evaluation of behavioural development; (2) in the number of pregnant rabbits per treatment group—US agencies require 12, Japan requires 10 (drugs) or 8 (agrichemicals); (3) in the onset of dosing, which varies one or two days around gestational day 6; (4) in the percentage of each rodent litter to be evaluated viscerally and skeletally; and (5) in the requirement by Japan (agrichemicals) for histopathologic examination of reproductive organs.

Examination of the guidelines from the same sources for Segment I (Multigeneration Reproduction) testing again indicates very similar requirements. All of the current guidelines suggest rats as the species of choice, and require exposure of the initial animals on study (termed P_0, P_1 or F_0) to begin as weanlings, and to continue for at least the length of one spermatogenesis cycle (minimum 8 weeks) for both sexes (even though ovulation in female rodents is a 4 to 5 day cycle). They also require continued exposure through the breeding period (usually 20 days), pregnancy period (approximately 20 to 22 days), and lactational period (21 days in mice and most rat strains, 28 days in the Fischer 344 rat (Charles River, 1982)). The parental animals are necropsied after the weaning of the F_1 (males may be necropsied after the breeding period is complete unless a second litter is called for). The F_1 weanlings selected to produce the F_2 generation are continually exposed through their growth to adulthood for at least 8 weeks (the weanlings not selected may be necropsied or sacrificed and discarded), and then bred as described above with exposure continuing. The parental F_1 animals are sacrificed after weaning of their litters. If three generations are called for, the F_2 weanlings are similarly selected, exposed and bred. The final generation (F_2 or F_3, depending on the protocol) is sacrificed at weaning and may or may not be examined histopathologically. The guidelines from the various agencies differ in (1) the age of the animals at study onset (5 to 9 weeks of age); (2) the number of animals per sex per dose group (20 to 30); (3) the duration of the prebreeding exposure in F_0 and subsequent generations (8 weeks to 100 days for F_0, 8 weeks to 120 days for F_1 animals; (4) the number of litters per generation (Canada and Japan are the only countries which currently require two litters per generation for preregistration testing of certain classes of chemicals, but this requirement is currently being discussed for possible deletion); (5) the organs selected for histopathologic examinations (FDA and EPA require testes, epididymides, prostate, seminal vesicles, ovaries, uterus, vagina and gross lesions or tumours; OECD requires these plus cervix, coagulating glands and pituitary); and in (6) the requirement by EPA to examine parental animals which failed to mate for determination of the cause of the infertility, which may include histopathology of reproductive organs.

The EPA recently released a draft document detailing current thinking by the Agency on tentative guidelines for developmental toxicity testing (EPA, 1984b). The document presents a balanced, reasonable statement of current methodologies and risk assessment strategies. Given the current developmental toxicity protocols (Segment II studies mandated by the various governmental guidelines and rules), a list of maternal and embryo/foetal endpoints of toxicity can be derived from the data collected. The toxicity endpoints listed by EPA (1984) for Segment II (developmental toxicity) studies, slightly modified for clarity and completeness, are presented in *Table* 8.1 for maternal endpoints, and *Table* 8.2 for reproductive and embryo/foetal endpoints. The embryo/foetal endpoints listed in *Table* 8.2 are litter-based, and are not based on the total number of conceptuses in each dose group, since the dam (or the litter) is the appropriate unit of analysis (Weil, 1970). Embryo/fetotoxicity is calculated in a number of ways to maximize the amount of information obtained. The number (and percentage) of resorptions (early, middle and late) and foetal deaths per litter is determined separately and then pooled under the number (and percentage) of 'non-live' per litter; the percentage is based on the number of total implantations per litter. Similarly, the number (and percentage) of foetuses per litter with individual external, visceral and/or skeletal malformations is determined separately and then pooled initially by category (external, visceral and skeletal), and finally under the number (and percentage) of malformed foetuses per litter; the percentage is based on the number of live foetuses per litter since only live foetuses are conventionally examined for malformations and variations. Since the frequencies of non-live implantations and malformed foetuses are calculated on different bases, implantations for the former and live foetuses for the latter, they cannot be directly summed. However, these two aspects of developmental toxicity, non-live and malformed, can be further pooled as the number (and percentage) of 'affected' implantations per litter; the percentage is based on the number of total implantations per litter. The frequency of affected implants represents the incidence of total developmental toxicity or total embryotoxicity. The use of these pooled 'umbrella' terms allows detection of a toxic effect by the agent on the conceptus, which is expressed with various degrees of penetrance in different foetuses within a litter and in different litters, which might not be detected as exhibiting a significant change when calculated separately.

A similar list of parental and offspring endpoints of toxicity from Segment I

Table 8.1. Maternal endpoints of toxicity in Segment II developmental toxicity studies[a].

Mortality[b]
Number. aborted (rabbits)
Number delivered early
Number (%) pregnant at sacrifice (includes all dams with implants)
Number (%) with live litters[c]
Number with totally non-live litters[d]
Body weight:
Gestational day (gd) 0
First treatment day
Mid treatment day
Last treatment day
Sacrifice day
Corrected (absolute) body weight (body weight at sacrifice minus gravid uterine weight)
Body weight change:
Throughout gestation (gd 0 through sacrifice)
Pre-exposure period (gd 0 to exposure onset)
Exposure period
Postexposure period (end of exposure through sacrifice)
Corrected (absolute) maternal (body weight change throughout gestation minus gravid uterine weight)
Food and water consumption (g/dam/day and/or g/kg/day)[e]
Clinical signs (from gd 0 through sacrifice):
Incidence of clinical signs by dam, by gestational day and by dose group
Observations at scheduled sacrifice
Gravid uterine weight at sacrifice (includes all with implants)
Organ weights at sacrifice (e.g. liver, kidneys, spleen, etc.):
Absolute
Relative to corrected body weight and/or to brain weight

[a] Table modified from EPA draft document (EPA, 1984b).
[b] Number of pregnant females dead/number of pregnant females on study; data from non-pregnant females should not be included in data analyses.
[c] Number of dams with one or more live foetuses at scheduled sacrifice.
[d] Litters with all implantations present as resorptions (early, middle and/or late) and/or dead foetuses at scheduled sacrifice.
[e] If the administration of test chemical is by dosed feed or dosed water, then the amount of chemical consumed may be determined, in mg/kg/day.

(reproductive toxicity) studies can be derived from the data collected from protocols designed to satisfy current rules and guidelines (*Table* 8.3 and 8.4, respectively).

Agencies within the NTP are currently evaluating two new protocols, one possibly to replace multigeneration reproductive toxicity testing, termed 'Fertility Assessment by Continuous Breeding' (Reel et al,. 1985) under the sponsorship of the National Institute of Environmental Health Sciences (NIEHS), and one to screen and prioritize agents for subsequent developmental toxicity testing, called the 'Chernoff Assay', developed by EPA researchers Chernoff and Kavlock (1980, 1982), and now under the sponsorship of the National Institute of Occupational Safety and Health (NIOSH).

The current protocol for fertility assessment by continuous breeding (Reel

Table 8.2. Reproductive and embryo/foetal endpoints of toxicity in Segment II developmental toxicity studies[a].

a. All litters:

Number of ovarian corpora lutea (CL)/dam

Number of uterine implantation sites/dam

% Preimplantation loss $\left[\frac{\text{CL} - \text{implantations}}{\text{CL}}\right] \times 100$

Number of (%) resorptions/litter (early, mid and late, separated and pooled)

Number of (%) litters with resorptions

Number of (%) foetal deaths/litter

Number of (%) non-live (foetal deaths plus resorptions) implants/litter

Number of (%) litters with non-live implants

% Postimplantation loss $\left[\frac{\text{Implantations} - \text{live foetuses}}{\text{Implantations}}\right] \times 100$

Number of (%) affected (non-live plus malformed[b]) implants/litter

Number of (%) litters with affected implants

b. Litters with live foetuses:

Number of Litters with live foetuses

Number of live foetuses/litter

Number of males/litter

Number of females/litter

Sex ratio (% males)

Foetal body weight/litter (all foetuses, males, females)

Foetal crown–rump length/litter (all foetuses, males, females)

Externally malformed foetuses/litter

Viscerally malformed foetuses/litter (including craniofacial malformations)

Skeletally malformed foetuses/litter

Number of (%) malformed foetuses/litter[b]

Number of (%) litters with malformed foetuses[b]

Number of (%) malformed males/litter[b]

Number of (%) malformed females/litter[b]

Incidence of individual malformations[c] (by foetuses, by litters and by dose)

Incidence of individual variations[c] (by foetuses, by litters and by dose)

Individual foetuses and their malformations and variations

[a] Table modified from EPA draft document (EPA, 1984b).

[b] Malformed includes foetuses with one or more malformations (external, visceral and/or skeletal).

[c] A foetus may be represented more than once if it exhibited more than one category of malformations and/or variations.

et al., 1985) consists of five tasks in outbred albino CD-1 mice, not all of which are necessarily performed for a given compound. Task 1 is a 14 day repeated dose or continuous administration range-finding study for 8 animals per sex per dose, for 5 dose groups plus vehicle control. Task 2 is the continuous breeding phase with 20 animals per sex for each of 3 chemical-exposed groups, and 40 per sex for controls, consisting of a 7 day premating exposure, 98 day cohabitation period, and a 21 day segregation period with exposure throughout. During the 98 day cohabitation, any litters born are examined externally, counted, sexed, weighed and discarded at birth. Any litters born during the 21 day segregation period are retained for possible use in Task 4. Task 3 is performed if significant effects of fertility and reproduction are noted in Task 2. Task 3 utilizes the control and high dose parental mice from Task 2 in a crossover breeding design (high dose

Table 8.3. Parental endpoints of toxicity in Segment I reproductive toxicity studies[a].

General:
Mortality
Body weights
Body weight change
Food and water consumption (g/animal/day or g/kg/day)[b]
Clinical signs of toxicity
Histopathology of target organs (all doses or high plus controls)
Reproductive:

Mating index: $\dfrac{\text{Number of females impregnated}^{c}}{\text{Number of females paired}}$; $\dfrac{\text{Number of males impregnating}^{c}}{\text{Number of males paired}}$

Fertility index: $\dfrac{\text{Number of females pregnant}^{d}}{\text{Number of females impregnated}^{c}}$

Gestational length in days
Clinical signs in females during pregnancy, at parturition (e.g. dystocia), and during lactational period
Abnormal nesting and/or nursing behaviour in dams

Prenatal loss: $\dfrac{\text{Number of implantations}^{e} - \text{Number of pups born}}{\text{Number of implantations}^{e}}$

[a] Parents include initial animals on study (variously designated as P_0, P_1 or F_0) and subsequent animals bred (e.g. F_1 and F_2 animals).
[b] If the chemical is administered by dosed feed or dosed water, then the amount of chemical consumed may be determined in mg/kg/day.
[c] Impregnation indicated by vaginal plug or vaginal sperm.
[d] Pregnancy status determined at parturition or by examination of uteri of females not littering.
[e] Number of implantations can be determined at scheduled necropsy by examination of the uterus in females bearing only one litter; these sites are visible at least through postnatal day 42 (Tyl, unpublished observations).

males × control females, high dose females × control males, control males × control females; hence the original requirements in Task 2 for 40 breeding pairs in controls) in order to determine the affected sex(es). If reproductive effects are not observed in Task 2, Task 4 is conducted. Task 4 evaluates reproductive performance in the offspring from the final Task 2 litters (born during the 21 day segregation period) of the control and high dose groups (bred within dose groups), with exposure continuing from birth to adulthood and breeding period. If effects are found in the offspring, these animals may be examined in Task 3 to determine the affected sex. At the conclusion of Task 3 or 4, gross necropsy may be performed on one or both sexes. Blood is collected for hormone assay and the liver, brain, pituitary, female reproductive tract (ovaries, oviducts, uterus, cervix and vagina), testes, epididymides, prostate and seminal vesicles with coagulating glands are weighed. The reproductive organs are fixed for subsequent histopathologic evaluation. If the male is affected by treatment, sperm analysis (number, motility and morphology) also is performed at necropsy. Task 5 evaluates reproductive hormone patterns in plasma samples obtained at necropsy from the affected sex(es). Toxicity data generated from this protocol are presented in *Table* 8.5.

The Chernoff Assay (Chernoff and Kavlock, 1980, 1982) also employs CD-1 mice in a two-phase design. As currently performed, Phase 1 is a dose range-finding study employing 10 non-pregnant females per dose, five doses and

Table 8.4. Offspring endpoints of toxicity in Segment I reproductive toxicity studies.

General:
Number of total pups delivered
Number of (%) live pups at birth
Number of (%) dead ups at birth (stillbirths)
Sex ratio at birth

Postnatal:
External abnormalities at birth
Periodic viability counts[a]
Periodic body weights on individual pups (reported by sex by litter)[b]
Periodic weight gains (reported by sex by litter)[b]
Clinical signs of toxicity
Acquisition of developmental landmarks (see text)
Evaluation of various behaviours (see text)

Survival indices:

$$\text{At birth: } \frac{\text{Number of live pups delivered}}{\text{Number of total pups delivered}}$$

$$\text{4-day: } \frac{\text{Number of live pups on postnatal day } 4^{a} \text{ (precull)}}{\text{Number of live pups at birth}}$$

$$\text{7-day: } \frac{\text{Number of pups on postnatal day 7}}{\text{Number of live pups on postnatal day } 4^{a}}$$

$$\text{14-day: } \frac{\text{Number of live pups on postnatal day 14}}{\text{Number of live pups on postnatal day 4 or 7}}$$

$$\text{21-day: } \frac{\text{Number of live pups on postnatal day 21}}{\text{Number of live pups on postnatal day 4 or 14 (postcull)}}$$

$$\text{Lactational index: } \frac{\text{Number of live pups on postnatal day } 21^{c}}{\text{Number of live pups on postnatal day 4}}$$

Histopathology:
Weanlings (F_1 and F_2) not selected as parents for the next generation (target organs, reproductive systems or complete work up)
Weanlings (F_3) at terminal sacrifice (target organs, reproductive systems or complete work up)
Adults (see *Table* 8.3 for parental animals)

[a] Culling of litters to fixed number (to 8 or 10 depending on strain and guidelines, with an equal number of each sex if possible), if performed, is usually done on postnatal day 4 so subsequent viability counts and survival indices are based on the litter number on postnatal day 4.
[b] Pups may be individually identified, usually on postnatal day 4, by tattooing the dorsal surface of the paws.
[c] Weaning is done on postnatal day 21 for mice and most rat strains; however, the Fischer rat is weaned on postnatal day 28 (Charles River, 1982), so the lactational index for this strain would consider survival to postnatal day 28.

control, with dosing for 5 consecutive days to establish a minimally toxic dose (MTD). The MTD is defined as the dose resulting in significant weight reduction during the treatment period, mortality, or other signs of toxicity. The definitive study employs a block design with 24 to 50 timed-pregnant females at the MTD for each of one to four chemicals, plus a concurrent control (24 to 50 females). Animals are dosed (by gavage or intraperitoneal injection) on gestational days 8 to 12. Maternal weight change for the treatment period is calculated and females are allowed to litter. The litters are counted, sexed, weighed and examined

Table 8.5. Endpoints of toxicity in fertility assessment by continuous breeding studies.

General (all tasks);
Mortality
Body weights
Body weight change
Organ weights (absolute and relative to body weight)
Food and water consumption (g/animal/day or g/kg/day)[a]
Clinical signs of toxicity
Reproductive:
Fertility index: $\frac{\text{Number of fertile}^{b}}{\text{Number of cohabited}}$ (Tasks 2,3,4)
Cumulative days to delivery of litters (each litter in Task 2)
Litters per mating pair (Task 2)
Live pups per litter (males, females, total) (Tasks 2,3,4)
Proportion of pups born live (males, females, total) (Tasks 2,3,4)
Live pup weight per litter (males, females, total)[c] (Tasks 2,3,4)
Reproductive organ weights (absolute and relative to body weight)
Histopathology of reproductive organs (male and female)
Sperm analysis (number, motility and morphology)
Plasma hormone levels[d] (Task 5)

[a] If the chemical is administered by dosed feed or dosed water, then the amount of chemical may be determined in mg/kg/day.
[b] By definition, breeding pairs were classified as fertile if they produced at least one pup (dead or alive).
[c] Absolute pup weight may be adjusted for litter size (by analysis of covariance).
[d] Radioimmunoassays for follicle stimulating hormone (FSH), luteinizing hormone (LH), testosterone (male), estradiol-17β (female), progesterone (female).

externally on postnatal day 1 (defined as gestational day 20—see footnotes to *Table* 8.6) and day 3, and then discarded. Dams not delivering by postnatal day 3 are sacrificed and their uteri examined for implantation sites. The toxicity endpoints available from this assay are listed in *Table* 8.6.

The primary function of this *in vivo* screen (according to Chernoff and Kavlock) 'should be the assignment of priorities to compounds whose developmental toxicity is unknown for subsequent in-depth testing by standard procedures' (Chernoff and Kavlock, 1982, p. 547). They suggest prioritization by assigning compounds into three categories: '(i) those that induce perinatal death should be tested as rapidly as possible, (2) those that induce only perinatal weight changes would be given a lower testing priority, and (3) those producing no effect would be given the lowest priority' (Chernoff and Kavlock, 1982, p. 548). This assay is not designed as a definitive test to replace conventional evaluations, but may be a useful tool for ordering chemicals for subsequent testing, as well as a method for comparing chemicals at a comparable dose (the MTD) to assess structure-activity relationships. This assay does not require the intensive labour or training required in a standard developmental toxicity protocol, and allows the pups to provide their own evaluation, i.e. if they survive and thrive then whatever alterations they carry are not critical. However, if the chemical under scrutiny must have developmental toxicity testing for possible commercial application,

Table 8.6. Endpoints of toxicity in Chernoff Assay.

Adult (non-pregnant in Phase 1, pregnant in Phase 2):
Mortality (Phases 1 and 2)
Body weight (Phases 1 and 2)
Body weight changes (Phases 1 and 2)
Clinical signs of toxicity (Phases 1 and 2)
Minimally toxic dose (MTD, Phase 1)

Reproductive (Phase 2):
Number (%) pregnant[a]
Number (%) with one or more live pups at birth
(or number (%) with totally non-live (resorbed plus dead) litters)
Number of (%) pups with external anomalies
Gestational length in days
Number of total, live, dead pups (postnatal day 1[b])
Sex ratio (live pups postnatal days 1 and 3)
Pup body weight gain (postnatal days 1 and 3)
No. live/dead pups (postnatal day 3)

$$\text{Survival index:} = \frac{\text{Number of live pups on postnatal day 3}}{\text{Number of live pups on postnatal day 1}}$$

$$\text{Prenatal loss} = \frac{\text{Number of implants}^{c} - \text{number of live pups at birth}^{b}}{\text{Number of implants}^{c}}$$

$$\text{Postnatal loss} = \frac{\text{Number of live pups at birth}^{b} - \text{number of live pups on postnatal day 3}}{\text{Number of live pups at birth}}$$

[a]Number pregnant = Number of females producing at least one pup (live or dead).
[b]Postnatal day 1 is defined by Chernoff and Kavlock (1980) as the day of delivery (gestational day 20 since mice in their facility normally delivered on the evening of gestational day 19)
[c]Implantation scars can be visualized in uniparous females until at least postnatal day 42 (Tyl, unpublished observations), so the number of implanted conceptuses may be determined and compared with the number of pups delivered, or used to determine pregnancy status in females which did not deliver.

this assay would not be relevant. This screen has been extensively evaluated and modifications and refinements suggested (Hardin, 1987).

A thoughtful discussion of the FDA's multifaceted approach to reduce risks to the unborn, using animal testing, clinical trials, epidemiology, surveillance, research and education has been presented (Kelsey, 1982).

INTERACTIONS AND IMPLICATIONS

One of the most important determinants of teratogenic (and developmental toxicity) susceptibility is the genotype of the conceptus. The current view is that all observed indications of the developmental toxicity are due to the interaction of the genotype of the conceptus (confounded by maternal genotype if different from that of the conceptus—*see below*) and its environment. There are apparently no 'new' malformations due to exposure to a xenobiotic, just an increase above the spontaneous background incidence of that malformation, due to the interaction of the test chemical (and/or metabolites) with susceptible genetic loci. Landauer (1960) was the first to recognize the production of 'phenocopies', environmentally induced imitations of genetic anomalies. Positive interactions have been demonstrated between teratogens and single genes in test animals in the cases of nicotine and crooked-neck dwarf in chicks (Landauer, 1960), 5-fluorouracil and the luxoid and luxate genes in mice (Dagg, 1967), actinomycin D and the Brachyury gene in mice (Winfield and Bennett, 1971), insulin and the genes rib fusion and crooked in mice (Cole and Trasler, 1980), and retinoic acid and the Splotch gene in mice (Kapon-Bras and Trasler, 1984). In addition, animal strains differ markedly in their response to environmental insult, resulting (presumably) from the interaction between the xenobiotic and a number of genetic loci, many yet unidentified. For example, inbred mouse strains differ in the incidence of cortisone-induced cleft palate (Kalter, 1954), and in the incidence of cadmium-induced testicular and embryonic toxicity (Wolkowski, 1974; Wolkowski-Tyl, 1978; Wolkowski-Tyl and Preston, 1979).

All of the currently used strains of rats, rabbits and mice have demonstrable incidences of spontaneous malformations, a finding which has been interpreted to mean that the strain has a predisposition based on genotype for the specific malformation(s) or variation(s). The best documented historical data bases are for the Charles River CD® rat (Banerjee and Durloo, 1973; Perraud, 1976; Woo and Hoar, 1979) and the New Zealand white rabbit (Cozens, 1967; Fritz et al., 1978; Palmer, 1972, 1978; Woo and Hoar, 1982; Stadler et al., 1983), but a number of smaller studies have documented spontaneous malformation incidence and frequency in the CD-1 mouse (Palmer, 1972; Perraud, 1976; Fritz et al., 1978). The Fischer 344 rat has been, and continues to be employed extensively in toxicity evaluations by the National Cancer Institute (NCI), and now the National Toxicology Program (NTP) and by industry. This strain is being used more extensively in developmental toxicity evaluations in order to compare different toxicity endpoints in the same strain. The Fischer 344 rat does not have a published data base for spontaneous malformations. However, as the number of developmental toxicity studies employing this rat strain increases and is reported in the literature, a growing body of background information is becoming available (e.g. Snellings et al., 1979; Bus et al., 1979; John et al., 1981; DePass and Weaver, 1982; Wolkowski-Tyl et al., 1983a; Tyl et al., 1984; Price et al., 1985). The B6C3F1 mouse hybrid, resulting from the cross C57BL/6 female × C3H male, has also been the strain of choice for lifetime carcinogenicity studies by the NCI and NTP. Its use in developmental toxicity studies is confounded by the problem that if the F_1 parents are B6C3F1 × B6C3F1, then the conceptuses are of varying genotypes (segregating F_2 genotypes and phenotypes) with concomitant varying genetic susceptibilities; if the parents are C57BL/6 × C3H to produce B6C3F1 conceptuses, then the exposure is to the C57BL/6 dams in a developmental toxicity evaluation, and to C57BL/6 females and C3H males in a reproductive toxicity study. The susceptibilities of the parental strains may vary from those of the conceptuses. However, developmental toxicity studies have been performed evaluating the B6C3F1 conceptus (Wolkowski-Tyl et al., 1982a,b).

Other determining factors of susceptibility include the gestational stage at exposure, the specificity of the agent, the doses, the route and duration of exposure, the disposition of the agent, metabolism, transport (especially transplacental), and excretion, as well as maternal status (e.g. age, health, other exposures). The factors of gestational age, dose and route have been adequately reviewed previously (e.g. Wilson, 1965, 1973; Wolkowski-Tyl, 1981). Suffice it to say that although there is some specificity of effect based on the chemical, the kind of response observed depends to a great extent on the stage of development of the conceptus at exposure, with the organs most vulnerable being those which are going through the biochemical transition from presumptive to determined status, commencing prior to any overt indication of organ formation.

The repertoire of enzymes, cofactors, carriers, etc., available to the exposed individual is under genetic control. Therefore, the individual's ability to manipulate a xenobiotic, i.e. by absorption, distribution, equilibrium, metabolism and excretion (collectively defined as toxicokinetics when expressed quantitatively), is a reflection of his/her genotype. However, this aspect of the response to exposure warrants discussion distinct from that of genotype.

Information on the toxicokinetics of the test chemical in the test animal system, which includes maternal, placental and embryo/foetal compartments, is critical for the interpretation of the parental and embryo/foetal/neonatal response in that animal system. It is also critical for the decision as to the 'extrapolability' of the data from that animal to other test animals and to humans. Ethical and technical considerations may limit or preclude evaluation of the toxicokinetics of a given toxicant in humans, but information gleaned from test animals can define the identity and relative quantities of the parent compound and/or metabolite(s) in the maternal blood supply available to the conceptus, as well as the identity and amounts of chemical present in the foetal circulation in test animals, and can provide inferences for humans.

The rate of entry into the maternal (and foetal) blood, time to steady state (or equilibrium), and the elimination half-life ($t_{\frac{1}{2}}$) from the blood can also be determined following various routes of exposure, including the routes most likely for human exposure. Maintenance of the animals in metabolic cages can provide information on the identity, quantity and time-course of eliminated chemical and/or metabolite(s) in the urine, faeces and expired air. These data allow the investigator to conclude that, given the particular dose, by the specific route, with the identified metabolites, and measured maternal and/or foetal blood levels in the animal under test, administration of the test chemical results in the specified maternal and embryo/foetal toxicity (including teratogenicity). These data can also be utilized to infer limits within which the concentrations of the parent compound and/or metabolites are likely to occur in human maternal and embryo/foetal compartments.

The Interagency Regulatory Liaison Group (IRLG) convened a workshop on Reproductive Toxicity Risk Assessment at FDA headquarters in Rockville, Maryland, in 1981. One of the workshops, in which this author participated, dealt with 'The Role of Pharmacokinetics in Reproductive and Developmental Toxicological Research'. In the discussion and published report from those deliberations (Kimmel and Kimmel, 1986), seven general concepts emerged.

1. If the test chemical is transferred to the conceptus by simple diffusion across the placenta, is not metabolized significantly by the placenta or conceptus, and is not excreted by the foetal kidney (into the amniotic fluid), then the toxicokinetic parameters measured or calculated and the concentrations of unbound (available) chemical in maternal blood are useful in predicting the upper limits of unbound chemical in the conceptus of any species. If the chemical is slowly diffusible, the maximum concentrations of chemical in maternal blood occur earlier than that in the conceptus, but maternal blood

levels may still be used to predict the area under the curve (AUC), and thus the average concentration of unbound chemical in the conceptus. The maternal blood level would provide an upper limit to the concentration in the conceptus. If the chemical is metabolized rapidly by the conceptus or placenta relative to the rate of diffusion across the placenta, or if there is active transport of the chemical into or out of the conceptus, then it is not possible to predict chemical concentration in the conceptus solely from maternal blood levels (Gillette, 1979). Blood levels in the test animal conceptus may be measured directly relatively late in gestation, when there is adequate volume of blood available for assay. This might or might not be relevant to significant concentrations at an earlier critical phase because of the evolving status of metabolic capabilities in the conceptus.

2. Not all toxic effects on the conceptus are caused solely by a test chemical and/or its metabolites within the conceptus. Some (or all) of the effects from exposure to a xenobiotic may be mediated at locations external to the conceptus, e.g. alterations in the placenta or in the maternal organism. If the dam is affected such that she does not transport appropriate nutrients, hormones, etc., or transports inappropriate concentrations of these materials, the conceptus can be affected, resulting in any of the four manifestations of developmental toxicity (*see* Section I). To this extent, information on the chemical levels in the conceptus would be irrelevant.
3. Toxicokinetic data from the entire dose range employed in animal studies facilitates interpretation and use of dose-response curves generated from the toxicological data, and provides one basis for a proposed mechanism of action. Knowledge of toxicokinetic parameters in more than one test species facilitates selection of dosage regimens for the evaluation of the susceptibility of another species at equivalent exposure if the parameters are similar. If the parameters differ among test species, then the appropriate animal model to provide information relevant to the human can be selected if the human parameters for that chemical are known.
4. The toxicokinetics of single-dose and repeated-dose exposure regimens may be very different. Single-dose kinetics are more dependent on the structure of the placenta, since diffusional rate constants are more important in limiting the concentration of the chemical within the conceptus after a single dose than after multiple doses. As long as the test chemical is not actively transported and the transfer is pH independent, the maximum concentration of unbound chemical in foetal blood after one dose is no higher than the maximum concentration of unbound chemical in maternal blood. When repeated doses are administered to steady state, the average concentration of unbound chemical in foetal blood is likely to be essentially independent of the diffusion rate across the placenta, again if the compound is not metabolized by the conceptus and not excreted by the foetal kidneys. The average concentration of unbound chemical in the foetal blood will be less than its concentration in maternal blood if its metabolism occurs within the placenta or conceptus, or if it is excreted by the foetal kidney. The magnitude of the difference between foetal and maternal blood depends on the rates of metabolism and excretion relative to the diffusional rate across the placenta.
5. Toxicokinetic data are useful (if not critical) for the elucidation of the

mechanism of reproductive or developmental toxicity, and for the establishment of appropriate parameters for inter-species comparisons. These data can be used to determine whether the toxicity is due to the parent compound or a metabolite. If the former (toxicity due to parent compound), then toxicokinetics in one species can suggest dosage levels to be employed to maintain equivalent blood levels of parent compound in a second species, or to define blood levels at which the particular toxic response from the parent compound could be expected. The relative susceptibility of two species to a test chemical may also be assessed. Evaluation of the toxicokinetic profile in two species can determine whether a toxic response is to be expected at all, e.g. if in one species the test chemical is rapidly metabolized, then toxicity may not occur, as opposed to one case of a species in which the parent compound persists. Alternatively, if a metabolite is responsible for the toxic response in one species, then determination as to whether a second species produces this metabolite, and the extent to which it is produced, may provide information as to the risk of a toxic response in the second species. These data can be used, if the toxicokinetic information is available in humans, to select for each chemical an appropriate test species in which to evaluate the potential for reproductive and/or developmental toxicity. These data can also provide information as to the appropriate route of administration, dose levels, vehicle and dosing schedule.

6. One ideal element of information from any toxicity evaluation is the determination of the relationship between the exposure at the molecular target and the type and time to onset of the lesion. At this time and at this stage in the science, it is not possible to measure directly the concentration of the toxicant at the molecular target; it is not possible in most cases to ascertain the molecular target! But workers in the field are getting closer, and are obtaining indirect estimates by measuring concentrations in target organs or tissues, in foetal blood, in the whole embryo of foetus, or less directly, by utilizing toxicokinetic data in the maternal organism to establish boundaries of the expected concentration in the conceptus. In a few instances, e.g. the developing palate (Zimmerman, 1984), molecular mechanisms of teratogens are being evaluated. These types of measurements can provide a more precise 'dose-response' curve by relating the incidence or severity of the toxic response to the dose administered to the dam (mother), and to the measured or estimated dose to the whole foetus or foetal target organ or tissue. These data are also useful in determining or predicting thresholds (*see below*). If the dose-response is known in one species, i.e. the relationship between maternal and foetal toxicokinetics and the toxic response, then knowledge of the toxicokinetic profile in the mother in another species (including humans) permits an approximation of the toxicokinetics in the conceptus of this second species, and of the relative risk of a toxic response.

The determination of dose and target organ(s) is complicated in a developing system since the target organ(s) may vary depending on the time of exposure (relative to the gestational age), and the doses evoking a response may also differ depending on the gestational age at exposure. These differences may be qualitative: different target organs at different gestational times of exposure, and sensitivity at one time and apparent insensitivity at others; and/or quantitative: differing severity of response in the same target organ(s) with exposure at different gestational stages. This concept has been explored by Wilson and others, and is discussed by Wilson (1965, 1973) and Wolkowski-Tyl (1981).

7. The concept of a threshold, defined as a dose below which an adverse effect does not occur, is relevant to developmental toxicity studies and strongly supported by published data (Wilson, 1973), although its existence is under question in carcinogenicity studies. The assumption of a threshold in developing systems is predicted on the assumption, or biological rationale, that the conceptus is capable of repair after insult (*see above*) and that most malformations and other indications of developmental toxicity are probably multifactorial in nature (EPA, 1984b). There are actually three kinds of thresholds: metabolic, experimental and 'real'. The metabolic threshold is the concentration of agent at which there is a change in the toxicokinetic parameters, e.g. above a given concentration the metabolic profile changes and toxic effects occur presumably from saturation of a given metabolic pathway (enzymes, cofactors, carriers, binding sites), or from exceeding the molecular repair capabilities of the test system. The experimental threshold is the dose below which no statistically significant adverse effects were observed in a given study; this parameter is dependent upon the conditions of the experimental protocol, especially sample size. The real threshold, the dose below which the toxic event would not occur, cannot currently be determined, since the molecular mechanism of action of any developmental toxicant is currently not known. If the mechanism were known, then it might be possible to predict whether a 'real' threshold exists and, with appropriate toxicokinetic data, to predict what it is. Toxicokinetic data, then, can define the metabolic threshold, predict the experimental threshold if toxicity data are available, and provide information as to the 'real' threshold in one test system, with the possibility of extrapolation to other test animals (or exposed humans). The assumption of a threshold in developmental toxicology is really the basis for assigning 'no observable effect levels' (NOELs) from animal study data and safety factors for use in extrapolating animal data to acceptable exposure concentrations and risk assessment in humans (EPA, 1984b).

The above discussion of the role of genotype and toxicokinetics in reproductive and toxicity study design, results, and interpretations has been extensive since these factors confound the toxic response of the parental animals, and therefore of the conceptus, and toxicokinetic information on the dam and conceptus is not routinely collected.

However, information is accumulating on the maternal/foetal toxicokinetics of chemicals evaluated for developmental toxicity, e.g. Greenaway et al. (1984) on biotransformation of salicylates, Bus et al. (1979) on metabolism of *n*-hexane, Nau et at. (1984) on disposition of valproic acid, Slikker et al. (1982a,b) on transplacental pharmacokinetics of oestrogen derivatives, and Juchau (1981) on bioactivation and inactivation of teratogens.

Ideally, this information on toxicokinetics should be available prior to any developmental or reproductive toxicity testing, at least in order to select the appropriate test species and the appropriate doses and route of administration.

The response of the parental animal, primarily, but not exclusively, the mother, in turn also confounds the detection of response to environmental insult in the conceptus.

According to Staples and Wilson (1975): 'A test agent is not usually classified as a teratogen if the dose required to produce the adverse effect in the embryo or foetus is overtly toxic to the mother because the induced stress in the mother may itself be teratogenic or otherwise toxic to the young of many species of animals.' (Staples and Wilson, 1975, p. 26). There are two aspects to this pragmatic definition which deserve consideration. The first is the aspect of 'overt maternal toxicity'. Current governmental rules and guidelines require or suggest collection of maternal data for a limited number of endpoints of toxicity (*see* Section II and *Tables* 8.1, 8.3, 8.5 and 8.6). These data include (1) mortality information; (2) confirmed pregnancy status, i.e. number (%) pregnant/non-pregnant; and (3) percent preimplantation loss, especially important if exposure begins prior to the completion of implantation as it does in the rat (exposure usually begins on gestational day 6 when implantation is not yet complete). Preimplantation loss (death of the preimplantation zygote) may be treatment related. Information on (4), postimplantation loss, is also critical to evaluate embryonic death (resorptions) and foetal death to ascertain if treatment affects the intrauterine environment to preclude maintenance of the pregnancy to term. This information is also important since embryonic or foetal death may mask malformations, i.e. if the conceptus is so severely affected that it dies *in utero*, then the endpoint is embryonic or foetal toxicity, not teratogenicity, although the proximate cause of death may be from malformations. Although both responses, death and malformation, are considered indications of developmental toxicity, the test article is categorized differently (perhaps erroneously (Johnson and Christian, 1984)), with implications for commercial use, product labelling, risk assessment and liability considerations. Also typically evaluated are: (5) periodic maternal body weights and weight gain, (6) periodic food and water consumption, and (7) absolute organ weights and organ-to-body weight or brain weight ratios at sacrifice.

Corrected maternal body weight at term, or corrected maternal weight gain during gestation (maternal body weight at sacrifice or maternal weight gain during gestation minus the gravid uterine weight) are useful parameters to distinguish between effects on the dam as distinct from effects on the conceptuses when effects from the test agent are observed for maternal weight(s) or weight gain. All of these endpoints are relatively crude. More subtle endpoints, but perhaps of equal or more importance, are currently not evaluated routinely. These last evaluations must be selected on a chemical-by-chemical basis based on information on target organ(s) and mechanism of action, if known. These endpoints may include evidence of a metabolic threshold and other information from toxicokinetics in the pregnant animal (dam, placenta, conceptus), histopathology of target organ(s), organ function tests, and haematological evaluation to ascertain if the oxygen-carrying capacity of the mother is impaired, with implications for normal growth and development of the conceptus. Pregnancy *per se* is associated with a 30 to 40% increase in blood volume, a 33% decrease in erythrocytes, a 20 to 30% increase in maternal oxygen consumption, and a greater oxygen debt after exercise and physical activity (Warshaw, 1977). Data from women who smoke during pregnancy support the concept that restricted blood flow to the conceptus results in reduced birth weight and elevated risks in the neonatal period. The developing central nervous system may be especially vulnerable to oxygen deprivation because of its high and continuous oxygen requirement. Damage to haematopoietic organs such as liver, spleen and bone marrow would also impact on the well-being of the mother and therefore her conceptus, or on the conceptus directly if its blood-forming organs (including the yolk sac in early embryos) are affected. For example, Clark et al. (1984) have concluded that chemical-induced maternal anaemia (and not the presence of the chemical) produced malformations in rabbits exposed to diflunisal. Toxicokinetic data can determine maternal blood levels of the test chemical and/or metabolites, and half-life, and if the test article passes into the conceptus, in what form (parent compound, metabolites), in what quantity (blood levels), and localized concentrations in foetal organs. These data can determine if there is a metabolic threshold, with implications for a qualitative or quantitative shift in the toxic response (*see above*). All of these suggested evaluations can result in the determination of legitimate endpoints of toxicity for both the mother and conceptus. These endpoints may be observed at doses (well) below those at which maternal weight or foetal survival is affected. This information may result in a lower maternal NOEL such that embryo/foetal effects observed at this level may, in fact, be due in large part or entirely to the compromised status of the mother. This information is also important since the lower dose now designated as a NOEL may be closer to that at which humans may be exposed, and information will then be available as to possible human toxic responses in the absence of more obvious signs of toxicity. This lower effect level will also impact on the so-called A/D ratio, defined as the ratio of the dose at which the adult exhibits a toxic response, the 'A', to the dose at which the developing organism exhibits a toxic response, the 'D'. This ratio is viewed as an increasingly important parameter in risk assessment (Fabro et al., 1982; Johnson and Gabel, 1983; EPA, 1984b; Johnson, 1984).

The evaluations suggested above, such as toxicokinetics, organ function tests and haematological profile, ought to be performed, not only at the time of scheduled sacrifice just prior to parturition, long after exposure has ceased in a Segment II study, but also at the time of exposure when toxic effects are most likely to be manifested. Evaluation at these two time points will enable detection of an effect and provide evidence for persistence of, or recovery from, the toxic effects. This kind of observation is available for body weight and food and water consumption data if the times for these evaluations are chosen appropriately. Data for these parameters commonly indicate transient effects. The functional evaluations can be done by adding additional adult animals to each treatment group (or only to the control and high dose groups), treating them exactly the same as the other animals in the group, and sacrificing them immediately after the last exposure for evaluation; remaining animals in each group are then sacrificed at term for the typical morphological endpoint evaluations. The plea has been made (Rogers, 1987; Schwetz and Tyl, 1987) to collect, report and publish as complete maternal toxicity profile as is possible in developmental toxicity studies.

The second aspect in the Staples and Wilson (1975) definition is the concept that adverse effects, including malformations observed at maternally toxic doses, are due in whole or in part to maternal toxicity. There is strong support from the literature for this view. Maternal stress in mice, e.g. transportation (Brown et al., 1972), water deprivation and low humidity (Brown et al., 1974), food and water deprivation (Rosenzweig and Blaustein, 1970), or food restriction (Hemm et al., 1977), can, by itself, produce cleft palate in the offspring. This induction of cleft palate is presumably due to elevated endogenous corticosteroids in the mother from stress (Hemm et al., 1977); exogenous steroids produce cleft palate in susceptible strains of mice (Kalter, 1954). On a cellular level, maternal exposure to cold stress, or injection of synthetic glucocorticoid, results in altered development of retinal neurones in the foetal rat (Puro, 1984). Parenthetically, restricted diet *per se* produces a decrease in sperm number and an increase in the number of abnormal sperm in mice (Anderson et al., 1984). These results may be due to stress and may have a bearing on fertility and pregnancy outcome. Maternal diet can also interact with administration of known teratogens to alter the incidence of induced malformations (Miller, 1977; Goad et al., 1984). Kalter (1965) has shown in mice that the spontaneous incidence of cleft palate decreased with increasing parity (number of litters), increasing maternal age and increased maternal weight. It is clear that any major perturbation in maternal homeostasis during pregnancy is liable to influence the development of the conceptus. In humans, malformations are associated with maternal disorders such as diabetes, phenylketonuria, vaginal bleeding and hyperthermia (Kalter and Warkany, 1983). Khera (1983, 1984, 1985) has addressed the issue of the role of maternal toxicity in causing congenital malformations. He initially reviewed the published literature on teratogenicity evaluations performed with diverse mouse strains, to ascertain '...whether any association exists between the type of foetal malformations and maternal toxicity in mice' (Khera, 1984, p. 411). Such an association would suggest that maternal toxicity, regardless of the cause, is a more important factor in the induction of foetal malformation than the test agent itself. Of the 85 studies examined, 13 were performed at dose levels which did not produce maternal toxicity, and 33 had insufficient data on maternal toxicity. Of the remaining 39 studies, 19 produced foetal defects occurring in a characteristic pattern, 9 produced diverse malformations with no specific pattern, and 11 produced maternal toxicity with no foetal malformations. The defects which were produced in a consistent pattern included exencephaly, open eyes, hemivertebrae, fused arches or centra of lumbar or thoracic vertebrae, fused, missing or supernumerary ribs, and fused or scrambled sternebrae (Khera, 1984). The reviewer (Khera, 1984) felt that these defects were induced in a consistent pattern since they did not occur at dose levels which were not maternally toxic, and that the incidence and severity of the foetal defects were positively correlated with the degree and severity of the maternal toxicity exhibited. Embryo/foetal toxicity was also present in many of these mouse studies at maternally toxic dose levels, as indicated by the presence of increased embryonic deaths, resorptions, and foetal deaths, and of reduced foetal body weight, and reduced foetal crown–rump length. Khera (1985) subsequently reviewed data from teratology studies performed on hamsters, rats and rabbits. He found a strong correlation with maternal toxicity and embryo/foetal deaths (nearly all manifested as resorptions) in all three species. The concurrent occurrence of both maternal toxicity and embryo/foetal mortality was observed in all four species in 133 of 177 studies (75%). There was no apparent direct correlation between embryo/foetal mortality and foetal malformation incidence. He also found, as in the mice, that maternal toxicity was associated with consistent patterns of foetal malformations, the latter occurring at low incidence and without a clear dose-response relationship for each individual malformation. Foetal malformations associated with maternal toxicity in hamsters included fused ribs, exencephaly, encephalocele (cranial blister), and micro- or anophthalmia. Omphalocele, shortened or crooked tail, cleft lip, and ectro- or syndactyly were less frequently reported. In rats and rabbits the following malformations were frequently reported in association with maternal toxicity: fused, extra, missing or wavy ribs, fused, retarded, missing or split (bipartite) vertebrae and missing, fused or non-aligned sternebrae. Less frequently reported malformations included ex-, an- or microphthalmia, cleft palate, umbilical hernia, shortened or bent long bones of the limb, ectro- or syndactyly, and crooked, short or absent tail (Khera, 1985). Khera concluded that 'presumptive evidence indicates that embryo-foetal deaths, and the above-mentioned foetal malformations in experimental animals, which in published literature are presently attributed to chemical induction for a large number of chemicals, may be a consequence of maternal toxicity per se' (Khera, 1985, p. 129).

However, the view that any and all adverse effects (including malformations) to the conceptus, observed at dose(s) of an agent which produced maternal toxicity, are due in part or *in toto* to the compromised status of the dam (Staples and Wilson, 1975), may, in some cases, be too categorical and overly simplistic. The conclusion that such an agent which produced malformations should not be termed a teratogen (Staples and Wilson, 1975) may also be erroneous. The EPA (1984b, p. 14) indicates that '...when fairly specific types or syndromes of effects are produced at maternally toxic doses by agents to which adult human exposure may occur at toxic levels (e.g. smoking, alcohol, solvents), these developmental effects should not be ignored'.

The EPA caveat appears concerned with developmental effects observed at maternally toxic doses only for chemicals to which humans may be exposed at toxic levels, e.g. from 'recreational' or emergency exposures. The concern should be broadened to include those foetal defects, observed at maternally toxic dose levels, which are not typical of the background incidence of the species and strain under test (*see above*). In other words, foetal malformations (and other developmental defects) may be due to maternal toxicity, or they may be due to direct intervention by the test agent, even in the presence of maternal toxicity. The fact that the incidence and severity of the observed defects parallel the degree and severity of maternal toxicity, a point which Khera (1984) makes in support of his view of the role of maternal toxicity, does not prove causality; both findings may be coincidental independent responses to the increasing dose levels. One would expect a dose-response relationship for malformations as well as for maternal toxicity if they were both due to the test agent. The absence of foetal defects in the absence of observed maternal toxicity may also be due to similar but independent thresholds of response. The presence of foetal defects in the absence of maternal toxicity implies different thresholds, i.e. an A/D ratio of greater than 1 (dependent in large part on the extent to which parameters of maternal toxicity were evaluated), and a differential risk to the conceptus. The converse situation, where there is maternal toxicity but no foetal defects again implied differing threshold ($A/D < 1$), and relatively less risk to the conceptus (protecting the mother will protect the conceptus). If the substance is equally injurious, in terms of dose levels, to adults and embryos ($A/D = 1$), this does not necessarily imply that there is no developmental risk, e.g. ethanol can cause permanent damage to the conceptus at doses which cause somewhat reparable toxicity to the adult (Johnson and Christian, 1984).

Khera's review of the mouse (Khera, 1983, 1984), rat and rabbit (Khera, 1985) teratology literature to identify categories of foetal responses associated with maternal toxicity represents a laudable beginning. What is needed is a concerted effort to identify, in current test animals, those malformations observed in historical controls specific for species and strain (e.g. Woo and Hoar, 1970, for the CD® rat; Woo and Hoar, 1982, for the New Zealand white rabbit; and others discussed previously), especially those malformations commonly associated with maternal toxicity irrespective of the cause, versus those unique malformations observed in the presence or absence of maternal toxicity which are not observed with measurable frequency in historical controls. Laboratories with an adequate database should be encouraged to publish their information in the open literature (e.g. Kimmel et al., 1985). The consensus may ultimately be that an increased incidence of certain (but not all) malformations may be indicative of maternal and foetal toxicity and not of the teratogenic potential of the test agent, and that the presence of other specific malformations does, in fact, indicate teratogenic potential.

A similar consensual attitude is developing for the interpretation of an increased incidence of foetal variations, especially skeletal, after exposure to a xenobiotic. In 1981, Khera suggested that anatomic alterations in term foetuses after exposure to a test agent may be categorized into malformations and aberrations. He considered aberrations as minor structural changes, distinct from malformations, and subdivided the former into retardations, variations and deviations. Retardations were defined as provisional delays in growth or morphogenesis, localized or generalized, including reduced ossification, especially in sternebrae, vertebrae and skull plates (also targeted and ascribed to toxicity by Aliverti et al., 1979), delayed development such as dilated renal pelvis which has been termed hydronephrosis (identified by Woo and Hoa, 1972, as a normal developmental stage in late gestational CD® rat foetuses), and slower migration of certain organs such as delayed testis descent from the abdomen to the scrotum. Variations are viewed by Khera (1981) as having a genetic basis influenced by environment, such as variations in the vertebral column and number of ribs. Deviations, minor changes from alterations in differentiation, are transitory or permanent but relatively innocuous, resulting in no observable alterations in external morphology, functional activity or survival, such as wavy rib. Khera (1981) concluded that aberrations occur commonly with variable incidence and morphology. If they are associated with malformations, then malformations should provide the basis for risk assessment; if they occur alone, they may suggest 'pathological significance' or they 'may not warrant serious attention' (Khera, 1981, p. 6).

Kimmel and Wilson (1973) observed a number of skeletal variants in rats after exposure to known teratogens, e.g. rudimentary, extra, supernumerary ribs, and variable sternebral centra. They believe that 'none of these skeletal variants should in themselves be considered as malformations' (Kimmel and Wilson, 1973, p. 309), and that these changes may be interpreted as indications of embryotoxicity. Kenel et al. (1984) also interpreted skeletal changes, such as bent ribs in rats, changes in the number of presacral vertebrae and extra ribs in rabbits, and reduced ossification in various skeletal districts as indicators of maternal and foetotoxicity. In contrast, Yasuda and Maeda (1973) have stated that when a dose-response relationship exists between the incidence of lumbar ribs (a common variation) and the dose level of the drug, this finding constitutes a meaningful index of teratogenicity.

Even the vehicle control chosen affects a number of maternal and foetal parameters in rats and mice. In a retrospective study of control animals from many tests (Kimmel et al., 1985), corn oil vehicle *per se* caused reduced maternal gestational weight gain, reduced maternal body weight at sacrifice, and reduced foetal body weight per litter relative to distilled water vehicle in CD® rats, but not in CD® -1 mice. In both species, corn oil as vehicle caused an increase in the percentage of foetuses malformed per litter and in the number of defects (malformations and variations) per foetus per litter relative to distilled water (Kimmel et al., 1985).

In addition to maternal toxicity and foetal aberrations discussed above, four important factors which confound the detection of a developmental toxicity response to a test agent are foetal body weight, litter size, sex and uterine location. Ariyuki et al. (1980, 1982) have examined the relationship between foetal body weight and extent of ossification in the foetal skeleton. They indicate that decreased foetal body weight *per se* is positively correlated with decreased ossification, that is, the lighter the foetus, the less ossified the skeleton. The pattern of ossification, especially in skeletal regions identified as susceptible, has not been systematically evaluated. The pattern in those regions which did ossify (not the extent of ossification) may be different in exposed foetuses from that observed in lighter weight foetuses of the same age (or from that seen in younger foetuses). These differences may be very subtle, based on preliminary observations in this author's laboratory, such as differences in the texture of the ossified elements and in the pattern of bone ray development in the skull plates. Two parameters which affect the body weight are the litter size and the sex of the foetus. Foetal weight is usually inversely correlated with litter size, and the average body weight of male foetuses is greater than that for female foetuses in laboratory animals. These last two truisms have not been previously documented in the literature but are generally accepted (e.g. EPA, 1984). Selected data from the author's laboratory to document these views are presented in *Table* 8.7 which examines litter size and foetal weight, and in *Table* 8.8 which evaluates body weight by sex for the most commonly used rat and rabbit strains. It is clear from these data that litter size and foetal body weight are inversely correlated in rats and rabbits, and that female rat foetuses, but apparently not female rabbits, are lighter than males. A number of considerations follow from these observations. If the litter size is large, then the weight of each individual foetus in that litter is usually less, with concomitant reduction in skeletal ossification, relative to foetal weight and ossification in a litter with fewer foetuses, irrespective of treatment. In addition, if there is embryonic or foetal lethality from a test agent such that the litter size is reduced, then the foetal body weight of remaining live foetuses may be increased relative to a litter with the full complement of foetuses, and an effect from the agent on foetal weight and/or ossification may be obscured. The production of specific malformations is also confounded by foetal weight (and litter size). Kalter (1965) has shown an inverse relationship in mice between the frequency of cortisone-induced cleft palate and mean foetal weight; the lighter weight foetus is more likely to exhibit cleft palate, or perhaps the foetus with cleft palate is more likely to be lighter in weight, than its normal littermate. He (Kalter, 1965) has also reported a positive association between the number of live young per uterine horn (hence litter size) and the incidence of cleft palate, but this is obviously confounded by foetal weight. If there is a skewed sex ratio in a given litter (which occurs commonly, although the average sex ratio for a large number of litters is usually close to 1:1), then the average foetal weight for that litter may be increased (if predominantly males) or decreased (if predominantly females) relative to a litter with an approximately equal number of males and females, again irrespective of treatment. The sex distribution *per se* may also impact on the apparent susceptibility of that litter. Male and female conceptuses have a differing susceptibility to induction of certain malformations (e.g. Scott et al., 1972; Wolkowski-Tyl et al., 1983b) and to toxicity (e.g. Fink et al., 1967) from exposure to a test agent. Male and female conceptuses of laboratory animals may also have a differential susceptibility to spontaneously occurring malformations, variations and foetal wastage, since this phenomenon is known in humans, i.e. preferential loss of males during gestation (Niswander et al., 1974; Bear, 1978) and differential rate of spontaneous malformations presumably due to environmental factors (Rogers and Morris, 1973; Janerich, 1975; Bear, 1978; James, 1979; Sever, 1982).

The uterine location of the developing conceptus appears to impact on foetal body weight and prenatal mortality (McLaren and Michie, 1959, 1960; Barr et al., 1970; Norman and Bruce, 1979a,b; Cornwall et al., 1984). Mice appear to exhibit a 'concave' profile, i.e. foetuses at the ovarian and cervical ends are heavier than those in the middle position (McLaren and Michie, 1959) while rats exhibit a 'convex' profile where the heavier foetuses are in the middle positions (Barr et al., 1969, 1970; Norman and Bruce, 1979a,b; Cornwall et al., 1984). Ward et al. (1977) reported a convex pattern for male rate foetuses, but observed that the weight of female foetuses was independent of uterine position. Runts in mice are more frequent at the extreme ovarian position (McLaren and Michie, 1960), while runts in rats are observed disproportionately at both ovarian and cervical ends (Barr et al., 1969). Embryonic resorptions in rats appear to be more frequent at both ovarian and cervical ends (Cornwall et al., 1984), or only at the cervical end (Barr et al., 1970). In rats, at least, the foetal weight and resorption patterns appear to be related, and indicate that the middle portions of both uterine horns provide the best environment for normal development. In the mouse, the highest incidence of foetal deaths or malformations occurred at uterine terminal positions, never in the middle positions, e.g. spontaneous cleft lip (Trasler, 1960), death from anoxia (Woollam and Miller, 1962), vitamin A (Woollam and Miller, 1961), or trypan blue (Beck, 1967). The mechanism for such differential response based on uterine location appears not to be haemodynamic since the rat and mouse exhibit opposite weight patterns with similar uterine vasculature (Cornwall et al., 1984). The structural arrangement, and therefore blood flow, of the uterine artery differs to the left and right uterine horns with some reports of differing foetal weights in the two horns (Wilson, 1965), or no difference in foetal weight reported between the two horns (Cornwall et al., 1984). These patterns appear to be species specific (Cornwall et al., 1984) and are relevant only to multifoetal pregnancies. They may be distorted by, or

Table 8.7. Historical control data on foetal body weight relative to litter size[a].

	Fischer 344 rat		
Litter size (live foetuses)	*Number of litters*	*Foetal weight per litter*[b]	*Significant difference*[c]
1– 2	7	4.84 ± 0.26	*v*. 11–12, 13–14
3– 4	7	4.59 ± 0.21	NS[e]
5– 6	13	4.57 ± 0.21	NS[e]
7– 8	26	4.45 ± 0.13	*v*. 11–12, 13–14
9–10	55	4.38 ± 0.13	*v*. 13–14
11–12	65	4.33 ± 0.17	*v*. 1–2, 7–8
13–14	16	4.25 ± 0.10	*v*. 1–2,7–8, 9–10
15–16	None	—	—
17–18	None	—	—
19–20	None	—	—
Total	189	4.40 ± 0.21	

	CD® rat		
Litter size (live foetuses)	*Number of litters*	*Foetal weight per litter*[b]	*Significant difference*[d]
1– 2	1	3.94	*v*. 3–4
3– 4	3	5.67 ± 0.62	*v*. 1–2, 15–16, 17–18
5– 6	2	5.24 ± 0.47	NS[e]
7– 8	None	—	—
9–10	1	5.10	NS[e]
11–12	13	5.03 ± 0.30	NS[e]
13–14	33	5.07 ± 0.38	NS[e]
15–16	28	4.90 ± 0.26	*v*. 3–4
17–18	7	4.72 ± 0.59	*v*. 3–4
19–20	1	4.50	NS[e]
Total	89	4.99 ± 0.40	

	New Zealand white rabbit		
Litter size (live foetuses)	*Number of litters*	*Foetal weight per litter*[b]	*Significant difference*[d]
1– 2	7	56.51 ± 3.38	*v*. 5–6, 7–8, 9–10, 11–12, 13–14
3– 4	4	52.50 ± 4.68	*v*. 1–2,7–8, 9–10, 11–12, 13–14
5– 6	15	46.00 ± 6.16	*v*. 1–2, 9–10, 11–12
7– 8	30	41.71 ± 6.18	*v*. 1–2, 3–4
9–10	42	39.93 ± 4.56	*v*. 1–2, 3–4, 5–6
11–12	13	39.31 ± 4.74	*v*. 1–2,3–4, 5–6
13–14	4	38.31 ± 5.36	*v*. 1–2, 3–4
15–16	None	—	—
17–18	None	—	—
19–20	None	—	—
Total	115	42.50 ± 6.90	

Table 8.7. Continued

[a] Data were collected from control litters from selected studies at Bushy Run Research Center; all control litters from each selected study with one or more live foetuses at scheduled sacrifice were included. Pregnant females were exposed to air (by inhalation), to carboxymethyl cellulose or corn oil (by gavage), on gestation day 6 through 15 (rats), or 6 through 18 (rabbits).
[b] Data are presented as grand mean ± standard deviation of litter means of the appropriate size, in grams. Rat foetuses were evaluated on gestational day 21, and rabbit foetuses on gestational day 29.
[c] Data were subjected to one-way analysis of variance (ANOVA, $p = 0{\cdot}000$), Levene's test for equal variances ($p = 0{\cdot}0025$) and separate variance t-test, with Bonferroni corrections for all pairwise comparisons. The criterion for significance was $p \leqslant 0{\cdot}05$ with correction.
[d] Data were subjected to one-way ANOVA ($p = 0{\cdot}0001$ for CD® rats and $p = 0{\cdot}0000$ for NZW rabbits), Levene's test for equal variances ($p = 0{\cdot}0688$ for CD® rats, $p = 0{\cdot}6942$ for NZW rabbits) and pooled variance t-test, with Bonferroni correction for all pairwise comparisons. The criterion for significance was $p \leqslant 0{\cdot}05$.
[e] NS = not significant in separate variance t-test (Fischer 344 rats) or in pooled variance t-test (CD® rats and NZW rabbits) with Bonferroni correction.

Table 8.8. Historical control data on foetal body weight by sex[a].

	Species and strain		
	Fischer 344 rat[b]	*CD® rat*[b]	*New Zealand white rabbit*[c]
Number of litters	189	89	89
Male weight/litter, g	4.50[d]	5.17	41.43[f]
Female weight/litter, g	4.24[e]	4.86	41.24
Difference, g	0.26	0.31	0.19
Female weight relative to male weight, %	94.22	94.00	99.54

[a] Data were pooled from control litters from selected studies at Bushy Run Research Center which were administered air (by inhalation), carboxymethyl cellulose or corn oil (by gavage); all control litters from each selected study with one or more live foetuses at scheduled sacrifice were included. Data are expressed as the grand mean of litter means for each sex, in grams.
[b] Timed-pregnant rat dams were treated on gestational days 6 though 15 and sacrificed on gestational day 21 (the day a dropped copulation plug was detected was designated gestational day 0).
[c] Timed-pregnant rabbit does were treated on gestational days 6 through 18 and sacrificed on gestational day 29 (the day of natural mating was designated gestational day 0). The number of rabbit litters used in this table differs from that used in *Table* 8.7 because rabbit foetuses in probe studies are weighed but not sexed in this laboratory, and therefore their data are not included in the evaluation of body weight by sex.
[d] N = 187, two litters contained only females.
[e] N = 188, one litter contained only males.
[f] N = 88, one litter contained only females.

interact with, exposure to a test agent, but they do indicate a differential susceptibility of certain conceptuses by virtue of their uterine position to reduced foetal weight, malformations and/or intrauterine death.

SUMMARY AND CONCLUSIONS

Developmental toxicity encompasses death, malformations, functional deficits and developmental delays in the conceptus. The developing conceptus is considered preferentially vulnerable to environmental insult relative to the adult, with qualitative and quantitative differences in vulnerability throughout its development from fertilization to sexual maturity. Governmental rules and guidelines have evolved to provide guidance and uniformity to the testing procedures for evaluating developmental and reproductive toxicity endpoints.

Important determinants and confounding factors of susceptibility include the genotype of the conceptus, i.e. genetic loci responsive to various environmental insults, and the repertoire of inducible and constitutive enzymes, cofactors, carriers, etc., available to manipulate a xenobiotic, including single gene and multifactorial interactions. Currently used laboratory animals differ in the type and frequency of spontaneous malformations and variations, which confound the extent of response and the detection of a response to insult. Evaluation of the maternal response to a test agent is critical for interpretation of developmental toxicity endpoints; this evaluation should include a thorough definition of maternal toxicokinetics to identify a number of parameters, e.g. blood levels of parent compound, identity and quantity of any metabolites, half-life, placental transfer and embryo/foetal levels of the test agent. In addition, organ function tests and histopathology of target organs should be performed, as well as the more typical relatively crude evaluations of body weights, weight change, organ weights, and food and water consumption. Maternal toxicity *per se* may cause the developmental toxicity observed, or it may be an independent response to the treatment. A beginning has been made in identifying those malformations and other developmental effects correlated with (but not necessarily caused by) maternal toxicity. More needs to be done to identify those responses in the conceptus due to maternal toxicity, and those due to the direct action of the test agent in each species and strain of animal evaluated. Further work must also be done to aid in the interpretation of findings, such as increased incidence of foetal variations, as to the implications for maternal or foetal toxicity versus teratogenicity. Publication of well-designed and well-performed developmental toxicity studies with so-called 'negative results', i.e. no teratogenicity or developmental toxicity in the presence of maternal toxicity, is strongly-encouraged.

Other confounding factors which impact on the response or detection of the response include the vehicle control chosen, litter size, foetal body weight, sex ratio, uterine position, and other factors yet unidentified.

Toxicity to the conceptus, including the spectrum of responses subsumed in this term, is a critical endpoint in reproductive and developmental toxicity testing and research in laboratory animals, in and of itself, for interpretation of other endpoints under test, for ascribing a mechanism of action of the agent, and for use in risk assessment for humans. It is dependent on maternal toxicity to varying degrees. It deserves closer examination and a more concerted effort by investigators to identify and evaluate aspects of its expression and confounding factors than it has been previously accorded.

ACKNOWLEDGEMENTS

Although all errors of omission or commission are the author's own, the author wishes to thank the following people: Dr Bryan Ballantyne for his perception and patience; Dr E. R. Homan, Dr E. H. Fowler and Dr D. E. McLain for their critical reading of the manuscript; Dr S. F. Preston, Dr C. J. Price and Dr C. A.

Kimmel for many fruitful discussions; Ms L. C. Fisher for her skill and enthusiasm in analysing historical control data; the author's staff at the University of Connecticut, the Chemical Industry Institute of Toxicology, the Research Triangle Institute, and Bushy Run Research Center for their expertise and support; and Ms R. K. Kephart for her skillful and patient typing of the manuscript.

REFERENCES

Aliverti V., Bonanomi L., Giavani E. et al., (1979). The extent of fetal ossification as an index of delayed development in teratogenic studies of the rat. *Teratology* **20**, 237–242.

Anderson D., Clode S. A., Stevenson B. I. et al. (1983) Genetic abnormalities in CD-a mice after dietary restriction. *Dev. Toxicol. Environ. Sci.* **11**, (*Dev. Sci. Pract. Toxicol.*), 541–544.

Ariyuki F., Higaki K. and Yasuda M. (1980). A study of fetal growth retardation in teratological tests: an examination of the relationship between body weight and ossification of coccygeal vertebrae in mouse and rat fetuses. *Teratology* **22**, 43–44.

Ariyuki F., Ishihara H., Higaki K. et al. (1982). A study of fetal growth retardation in teratological tests: relationship between body weight and ossification in rat fetuses. *Teratology* **26**, 263–267.

Balinsky B. I. (1975) *An Introduction to Embryology*, 4th ed. Philadelphia: Saunders.

Banerjee B. N. and Durloo R. S. (1973) Incidence of teratological anomalies in control Charles River CD strain rats. *Toxicology* **1**, 151–154.

Bankl H. (1977) *Congenital Malformations of the Heart and Great Vessels, Synopsis of Pathology, Embryology and Natural History. Part II.* Baltimore: Urban and Schwarzenberg.

Barr M. Jr., Jensh R. P. and Brent R. L. (1969) Fetal weight and intrauterine position in rats. *Teratology* **2**, 241–246.

Barr M. Jr., Jensh R. P. and Brent R. L. (1970) Prenatal growth in the albino rat: Effects of number, intrauterine position and resorptions. *Am. J. Anat.* **128**, 413–428.

Bear J. C. (1978) Spontaneous abortion, sex ratio, and facial cleft malformations. *Clin. Genet.* **13**, 1–7.

Beck S. L. (1967) Effects of position in the uterus of fetal mortality and on response to trypan blue. *J. Embryol. Exp. Morphol.* **17**, 607–624.

Brown K. S., Johnston M. C. and Murphy P. F. (1974) Isolated cleft palate in A/J mice after transitory exposure to drinking water deprivation and low humidity in pregnancy. *Teratology* **9**, 151–158.

Brown K. S., Johnston M. C. and Niswander J. D. (1972) Isolated cleft palate in mice after transportation during gestation. *Teratology* **5**, 119–124.

Bus J. S., White E. L., Tyl R. W. et al. (1979) Perinatal toxicity and metabolism of n-hexane in Fischer 344 rats after inhalation exposure during gestation. *Toxicol. Appl. Pharmacol.* **51**, 295–302.

Chapman R. R. and Roberts D. W. (1984) Humoral immune dysfunction as a result of prenatal exposure to diphenylhydantoin: Correlation with the occurrence of physical defects. *Teratology* **30**, 107–117.

Charles River Laboratories (1982) *Charles River Technical Bulletin* **1**, 4–5.

Chernoff N. and Kavlock R. J. (1980) A potential *in vivo* screen for the determination of teratogenic effects in mammals. *Teratology* **21**, 33–34A.

Chernoff N. and Kavlock R. J. (1982) An *in vivo* teratology screen using pregnant mice. *J. Toxicol. Environ. Health* **10**, 541–550.

Clark R. L., Robertson R. T., Minsker D. H. et al. Diflunisal-induced maternal anemia as a cause of teratogenicity in rabbits. *Teratology* **30**, 319–332.

Cole W. A. and Trasler D. G. (1980) Gene-teratogen interaction in insulin-induced mouse exencephaly. *Teratology* **22**, 125–139.

Cozens D. D. (1965) Abnormalities of the external form and of the skeleton in the New Zealand white rabbit. *Food. Cosmet. Toxicol.* **3**, 695–700.

Dagg C. P. (1967) Combined action of fluorouracil and two mutant genes on limb development in the mouse. *J. Exp. Zool.* **164**, 479–489.

DePass L. R. and Weaver E. V. (1982) Comparison of teratogenic effects of aspirin and hydroxyurea in the Fischer 344 and Wistar strains. *J. Toxicol. Environ. Health* **10**, 197–305.

Environmental Protection Agency (EPA) (1978) Environmental Protection Agency Pesticide Programs; Proposed Guidelines for Registering Pesticides in the US; Hazard Evaluation: Humans and Domestic Animals. Section F. Teratology and Reproduction Studies. *Fed. Reg.* **43**(163), 37347.

Environmental Protection Agency (EPA) (1979). Environmental Protection Agency proposed Health Effects Test Standards for Toxic Substances Control Act; Test Rules and Proposed Good Laboratory Practice Standards for Health Effects. Part IV. Subpart F—Teratogenic/Reproductive Health Effects. *Fed. Reg.* **44**(175), 44087–44092.

Environmental Protection Agency (EPA) (1983a) EPA Toxic Substances Control; Good Laboratory Practice Standards; Final Rule. Part III. *Fed. Reg.* **48**(230), 53922–53944.

Environmental Protection Agency (EPA) (1983b) Environmental Protection Agency Pesticide Programs; Good Laboratory Practice Standards; Final Rule. Part IV. *Fed. Reg.* **48**(230), 53946–53969.

Environmental Protection Agency (EPA)(1984a) Environmental Protection Agency, Federal Insecticide, Fungicide and Rodenticide Act (FIFRA); Good Laboratory Practice Standards; Effective Date. *Fed. Reg.* **49**(86), 18738–18739 (May 2, 1984).

Environmental Protection Agency (EPA)(1984b) *Guideline for the Health Assessment of Suspect Developmental Toxicants.* Draft Document from Office of Research and Development, EPA Washington DC, 29 pages (August 27, 1984).

Fabro S., Schull G. and Brown N. A. (1982) The relative teratogenic index and teratogenic potency: Proposed components of developmental toxicity risk assessment. *Teratogenisis Carcinog. Mutagen.* **2**, 61–76.

Filler R. (1982) The presence of metabolites in early embryos. *Teratology* **25**(2), 40A.

Fink B. R., Shepard T. H. and Blandau R. J. (1967) Teratogenic activity of nitrous oxide. *Nature* **214**, 146–148.

Food and Drug Administration (FDA) Advisory Committee of Protocols for Safety Evaluations (1970) Panel on reproduction report on reproduction studies in the safety evaluation of food additives and pesticide residues. *Toxicol. Appl. Pharmacol.* **16**, 264–296.

Food and Drug Administration (FDA) (1978) Good Laboratory Practice Regulations for Nonclinical Laboratory Studies. *Fed. Reg.*, **43**, 60013–60025.

Fritz H., Grauwiler J., Himmler H. et al. (1978) Collection of control data from teratological experiments in mice, rats and rabbits. *Arzneim-Forsch./Drug Res.* **28**, 1410–1413.

Gillette J. R. (1979) Chairman's introductory statement: Prenatal development of drug metabolism. In: Estabrook R. W. and Lindenlaut E. (ed.) *The Introduction of Drug Metabolism*, 501–506. Stuttgart and New York: F. K. Schattauer Verlag.

Goad P. T., Hill D. E., Slikker W. Jr. et al. (1984). The role of maternal diet in the developmental toxicology of ethanol. *Toxicol. Appl. Pharmacol.* **73**, 256–267.

Goldenthal E. I. (Chief, Drug Review Branch, Division of Toxicological Evaluation, Bureau of Scientific Standards and Evaluation). (Letter dated March 1, 1966) *Guidelines for Reproduction Studies for Safety Evaluation of Drugs for Human Use.*

Greenaway J. C., Bark D. H. and Juchau M. R. (1984) Embryotoxic effects of salicylates: Role of biotransformation. *Toxicol. App. Pharmacol.* **74**(1), 141–149.

Hamburgh M., Glezer I., Sabater J., et al. (1984) Evidence for repair in trypan blue-treated mouse egg cylinders: An electron microscopic study. *Teratology* **29**(3), 393–403.

Hardin B. D. (1987) Guest Editor. Evaluation of the Chernoff/Kavlock test for developmental toxicity. Proceedings of the Workshop on the Chernoff/Kavlock Short-Term in vivo Developmental Toxicity Test. *Teratogenesis, Carcinog. Mutagen.* **7**, 1–127.

Hemm R. D., Arslanoglou L. and Pollock J. J. (1977) Cleft palate following prenatal food restriction in mice: Association with elevated maternal corticosteroids. *Teratology* **15**, 243–248.

Hendrickx A. G., Prahalada S., Janos G. et al. (1983) Cardiac embryotoxicity studies on bendectin in macaques. *Teratology* **27**(2), 49A.

Inouye M. (1976) Differential staining of cartilage and bone in fetal mouse skeletal by alcian blue and alizarin red S. *Cong. Anom.* **16**, 171–173.

Interagency Regulatory Liaison Group (IRLG) (1980) Report on IRLG: Recent Accomplishments and 1980/81 Plans. *Fed. Reg.* **45**(18), 6276–6282.

James W. H. (1979) The sex ratio in anencephaly. *J. Med. Genet.* **16**, 129–133.

Janerich D. T. (1975) Female excess in anencephaly and spina bifida: Possible gestational influences. *Am. J. Epidemiol.* **101**, 70–76.

John J. A., Hayes W. C., Hanley T. R. et al. (1981) Behavioral and teratogenic potential of vitamin A in the Fischer 344 rat. *Teratology* **24**, 55A.

Johnson E. M. (1984) A prioritization and biological decision tree for developmental toxicity safety evaluations. *J. Am. Coll. Toxicol.* **3**(2), 141–147.
Johnson E. M. and Christian M. S. (1984) When is a teratology study not an evaluation of teratogenicity? *J. Am. Coll. Toxicol.* **3**(6), 431–434.
Johnson E. M. and Gabel B. E. G. (1983) An artificial embryo for detection of abnormal developmental biology. *Fund. Appl. Toxicol.* **3**, 243–249.
Juchau M. R. (1981) Enzymatic bioactivation and inactivation of chemical teratogens and transplacental carcinogens/mutagens. Juchau M. R. (ed.) *The Biochemical Basis of Chemical Teratogenesis*, Chapter 2, 63–84. New York: Elsevier/North-Holland.
Kalter H. (1954) The inheritance of susceptibility to the teratogenic action of cortisone in mice. *Genetics* **39**, 185–196.
Kalter H. (1965) Interplay of intrinsic and extrinsic factors. In: Wilson J. G. and Warkany J. (ed.) *Teratology Principles and Techniques*, Chapter 3, 57–80. Chicago. University of Chicago Press.
Kalter H. and Warkany J. (1983) Congenital malformations. *N. Engl. J. Med.* **308**, 424–431.
Kapron-Bras C. M. and Trasler D. G. (1984) Gene-teratogen interaction and its morphological basis in retinoic acid-induced mouse spina bifida. *Teratology* **30**, 143–150.
Kelsey F. O. (1982) Regulatory aspects of teratology: role of the Food and Drug Administration. *Teratology* **25**, 193–199.
Kenel M. F., Schardein J. L., Terry R. D. et al. (1984) Developmental variations as markers of maternal and embryotoxicity. *Teratology* **29**(2), 40–41A.
Khera K. S. (1981) Comman fetal aberrations and their teratologic significance: A review. *Fund. Appl. Toxicol.* **1**(1), 13–18.
Khera K. S. (1983) Materno-fetal toxicity—a possible cause of fetal malformations in the mouse. *Teratology* **27**(2), 56–57A.
Khera K. S. (1984) Maternal toxicity—a possible factor in fetal malformations in mice. *Teratology* **29**, 411–416.
Khera K. S. (1985) Maternal toxicity: A possible etiological factor in embryo-fetal deaths and fetal malformations of rodent-rabbit species. *Teratology* **31**, 129–153.
Kimmel C. A. and Kimmel C. L. (1986) Editors. Interagency Regulatory Liason Group Workshop on Reproductive Toxicity Risk Assessment. *Environ. Health Perspec.* **66**, 193–221.
Kimmel C. A., Price C. J., Sadler B. M. et al. (1985) Comparison of distilled water (DW) and corn oil (CO) vehicle controls from historical teratology study data. *The Toxicologist* **5**, 185.
Kimmel C. A. and Trammel C. (1981) A rapid procedure for routine double-staining of cartilage and bone in fetal and adult animals. *Stain Technol.* **56**(5), 271–273.
Kimmel C. A. and Wilson J. G. (1973) Skeletal deviations in rats: malformations or variations? *Teratology* **8**, 309–316.
Landauer W. (1960) Nicotine-induced malformations of chicken embryos and their bearing on the phenocopy problem. *J. Exp. Zool.* **143**, 107–122.
Lochry E. A., Hoberman A. M. and Christian M. S. (1984) Positive correlation of pup body weight with other commonly used developmental landmarks, *Teratology* **29**(2), 44A.
McLaren A. and Michie D. (1959) The spacing of implantations in the mouse uterus. *Mem. Soc. Endocrinol.* **6**, 65–74.
McLaren A. and Michie D. (1960) Congenital runts. In: Wolstenholme G. E. N. and O'Connor C. M. (ed). *Ciba Foundation Symposium on Congenital Malformations*, 178–194. Boston: Little Brown.
Miller K. K. (1977) Commercial dietary influences on the frequency of cortisone-induced cleft palate in C57BL/6J mice. *Teratology* **15**, 249–252.
Morgenroth III V. (Chairman, Testing Standards and Guidelines Work Group of the Interagency Regulatory Liaison Group (IRLG) (August 1979) *Draft IRLG Guidelines for Selected Acute Toxicity Tests*. 113–114.
Nau H., Merker H. J., Brendel K. et al. (1984) Disposition, embryotoxicity, and teratogenicity of valproic acid in the mouse as related to man. In Levy R. H., Pitlik W. H. and Eichelbaum M. (ed.) *Metabolism of Antiepileptic Drugs* (Proceedings of Workshop, 1982), 85–96. New York: Raven Press.
Nishimura M., Iizuka M., Iwaki S. et al. (1982) Repairability of drug-induced 'wavy ribs' in rat offspring. *Arzneimittelforsch/Drug Res.* **32**, 1518–1522.
Niswander J. D., Maclean C. J., Chung C. S. et al. (1972) Sex ratio and cleft lip with or without cleft palate. *Lancet* **ii**, 858–860.
Norman N. A. and Bruce N. W. (1979a) Fetal and placental weight relationships in the rat at days 13 and 17 of gestation. *J. Reprod. Fert.* **57**, 345–348.

Norman N. A. and Bruce N. W. (1979b) Fetal and placental weight relationships in the albino rat near term. *Teratology* **19**, 245–250.

Organization for Economic Cooperation and Development (OECD) (1981) *OECD Guidelines for Testing of Chemicals*, No. 414: Teratogenicity, Appendix Section 4—Health Effects.

Organization for Economic Cooperation and Development (OECD) (1983) *OECD Guidelines for Testing of Chemicals*, No. 415: One-Generation Reproduction Toxicity Study, 1–8; No. 416: Two-Generation Reproduction Toxicity Study, 1–8.

Palmer A. K. (1972) Sporadic malformations in laboratory animals and their influence in drug testing. In: Klingsberg M. A. et al., (ed.) *Drugs and Fetal Development. Adv. Biol. Med.* **27**, 45–60.

Palmer A. K. (1978) The design of subprimate animal studies. In: Wilson J. G. and Fraser F. C. (ed.) *Handbook of Teratology. Vol. 4*, 215–253. New York: Plenum.

Perraud J. (1976) Levels of spontaneous malformations in the CD rat and the CD-1 mouse. *Lab. Anim. Sci.* **26**, 293–300.

Price C. J., Tyl R. W., Marks T. A. et al. (1985) Teratologic and postnatal evaluation of aniline hydrochloride in the Fischer 344 rat. *Toxicol. Appl. Pharmacol.* **77**, 465–478.

Puro D. G. (1984) Use of a culture system to identify possible causes of abnormal retinal development. *Invest. Ophthalmol. Visual Sci.* **25**(6), 691–697.

Reel J. R., Lawton A. D., Wolkowski-Tyl R. et al. (1985) Evaluation of a new reproductive toxicology protocol using diethylstilbestrol (DES) as a positive control compound. *J. Am. Coll. Toxicol.* **4**(2), 147–162.

Rice J. M. (1976) Carcinogenesis: A late effect of irreversible toxic damage during development. *Environ. Health Persp.*, **18**, 133–139.

Rogers J. M. (1987) Comparison of maternal and fetal toxic dose responses in mammals. *Teratogenesis Carcinog. Mutagen.* **7**, 297–306.

Rogers S. C. and Morris M. (1973) Anencephalus: A changing sex ratio. *Br. J. Prev. Soc. Med.* **27**, 81–84.

Rosenzweig S. and Blaustein F. M. (1970) Cleft palate in A/J mice resulting from restraint and deprivation of food and water. *Teratology* **3**, 45–52.

Rugh R. (1968) Organogeny. In: *The Mouse Its Reproduction and Development*, Chapter 5, 208–216 (External Changes). Minneapolis: Burgess Publishing Company.

Salewski E. (1964) Färbemethode zum markoskopischen Nachweis von Implantations-Stellen am Uterus der Ratte. *Naunyn Schmiedebergs Arch Exp Pathol Pharmackol.* **247**, 367.

Saunders J. W. Jr (1966) Death in embryonic systems. *Science* **154**, 604–612.

Schuepbach P. M. and Schroeder H. E. (1984) Prenatal repair of experimentally induced clefts in the secondary palate of the rat. *Teratology* **30**, 131–142.

Schwetz B. A. and Tyl R. W. (1987) Consensus Workshop on the Evaluation of Maternal and Developmental Toxicity; Work Group III Report. Low dose extrapolation and other considerations for risk assessment - models and applications. *Teratogenesis Carcinog. Mutagen.* **7**, 321–327.

Scott W. J., Butcher R. L., Kindt C. W. et al. (1972) Greater sensitivity of female than male rat embryos to acetazolamide teratogenicity. *Teratology* **6**, 239–240.

Sever L. E. (1982) An epidemiologic study of neural tube defects in Los Angeles County. II. Etiologic factors in an area with low prevalence at birth. *Teratology* **25**, 323–334.

Slikker W. Jr, Bailey J. R., Newport G. D. et al. (1982b) Placental transfer and metabolism of 17-ethylnylestradiol-17β and estradiol-17β(E_2) in the rhesus monkey. *J. Pharmacol. Exp. Ther.* **233**, 483–489.

Slikker W. Jr, Hill D. E. and Young J. F. (1982a) Comparison of the transplacental pharmacokinetics of estradiol-17β and diethylstilbestrol in the sub-human primate. *J. Pharmacol. Exp. Ther.* **221**, 173–182.

Snellings W. M., Pringle J. L., Dorko J. D. et al. (1979) Teratology and reproduction studies with rats exposed to 10, 33 or 100 ppm of ethylene oxide (EO). *Toxicol. Appl. Pharmacol.* **48**, A84.

Spyker J. M. and Fernandes G. (1973) Impaired immune function in offspring for methylmercury treated mice. *Teratology* **7**, 28A.

Stadler J., Kessedjian M.-J. and Perraud J. (1983) Use of the New Zealand white rabbit in teratology: incidence of spontaneous and drug-induced malformations. *Food. Chem. Toxicol.* **21**(5), 631–636.

Staples R. E. (1974) Detection of visceral alterations in mammalian fetuses. *Teratology* **9**, A37.

Staples R. E. (with concurrence of J. G. Wilson) (1975) Definition of teratogenesis and teratogen. Chapter 4. In: Shepard T. H., Miller J. R. and Marois M. (ed.) *Methods for Detection of Environmental Agents that Produce Congenital Defects.* Proceedings of the Guadeloupe Meeting sponsored by the Institute de la Vie, North Holland Publishing Company, American Elsevier, 25–26.

Trasler D. G. (1960) Influence of uterine site on occurrence of spontaneous cleft lip in mice. *Science* **132**, 420–421.

Tyl R. W., Millicovsky G., Dodd D. E. et al. (1984) Teratologic evaluation of ethylene glycol monobutyl ether in Fischer 344 rats and New Zealand white rabbits following inhalation exposure. *Environ. Health Persp.* **57**, 47–68.

Ward W. F., Karp C. M. and Aceto H. Jr. (1977) Developmental effects of the uterine environment: dependence on fetal sex in rats. *J. Reprod. Fert.* **50**, 269–274.

Warshaw L. J. (1977) *Guidelines on Pregnancy and Work.* Washington DC: Government Printing Office.

Weil C. S. (1970) Selection of the valid number of sampling units and a consideration of their combination in toxicological studies involving reproduction, teratogenesis or carcinogenesis. *Food Cosmet. Toxicol.* **8**, 177–182.

Wilson J. G. (1965) Embryological considerations in teratology. In: Wilson J. G. and Warkany J. (ed.) *Teratology Principles and Techniques* 251–277. Chicago: The University of Chicago Press.

Wilson J. G. (1973) *Environment and Birth Defects.* New York: Academic Press.

Wilson J. G. (1979) The evolution of teratological testing. *Teratology* **20**(2), 205–211.

Winfield J. B. and Bennett D. (1971) Gene-teratogen interaction: potentiation of actinomycin D teratogenesis in the house mouse by the lethal gene Brachyury. *Teratology* **4**, 157–170.

Wolkowski R. M. (1974) Differential cadmium-induced embryotoxicity in two inbred mouse strains. 1. Analysis of inheritance of the response to cadmium and the presence of cadmium in fetus and placental tissues. *Teratology* **10**(3), 243–262.

Wolkowski-Tyl R. M. (1978) Strain and tissue differences in cadmium-binding protein in cadmium-treated mice. In: *Developmental Toxicology of Energy-Related Pollutants. DOE Symposium Series* **47**, 568–585.

Wolkowski-Tyl R. (1981) Reproductive and teratogenic effects: No more thalidomides? In: *The Pesticide Chemist and Modern Toxicology. ACS Symposium Series* **160**, 115–155.

Wolkowski-Tyl R., Phelps M. and Davis J. K. (1983a) Structural teratogenicity evaluation of methyl chloride in rats and mice after inhalation exposure. *Teratology* **27**, 181–195.

Wolkowski-Tyl R., Lawton A. D., Phelps M. et al. (1983b) Evaluation of heart and formations in B6C3F1 mouse fetuses induced by *in utero* exposure to methyl chloride. *Teratology* **27**, 197–206.

Wolkowski-Tyl R. and Preston S. F. (1979) The interaction of cadmium-binding protein (Cd-bp) and progesterone in cadmium-induced tissue and embryotoxicity. *Teratology* **20**(3), 341–351.

Woo D. C. and Hoar R. M. (1972) 'Apparent hydronephrosis' as a normal aspect of renal development in late gestation of rats: The effect of methyl salicylate. *Teratology* **6**, 191–196.

Woo D. C. and Hoar R. M (1979) Reproductive performance and spontaneous malformations in control Charles River CD rats: A joint study by MARTA. *Teratology* **19**, 54A.

Woo D. C. and Hoar R. M. (1982) Reproductive performance and spontaneous malformations in control New Zealand white rabbits: A joint study by MARTA. *Teratology* **25**(2), 82A.

Woollam D. H. M. and Miller J. W. (1961) Influence of uterine position on the response of the mouse embryo to the teratogenic effects of hypervitaminosis-A. *Nature* **190**, 184–185.

Woollam D. H. M. and Miller J. W. (1962) Influence of uterine position on the response of the mouse embryo to anoxia. *Nature* **194**, 990–991.

Yasuda M. and Maeda H. (1973) Significance of the lumbar rib as an index of teratogenicity. *Senten Ijo (Congenital Abnormality)* **13**, 25–29.

Zimmerman E. F. (1984) Neuropharmacologic teratogenesis and neurotransmitter regulation of palate development. *Am. J. Ment. Defic.* **88**(5), 548–558.

Chapter 9

The Role of Genetic Differences as a Determinant in Xenobiotic-Induced Developmental Toxicity

George H. Lambert

Developmental toxicology studies the effects of environmental agents on the developmental process. This chapter will first briefly present the scope and complexity of developmental toxicology. Then the role of genetics as a determinant in, and scientific probe of, developmental toxicology will be discussed, followed by an example of the application of a genetic probe, the inducibility of cytochrome P1-450 isozyme activity, in studying developmental toxicology. Detailed information on other aspects of developmental toxicology can be obtained from four recently published books (Kimmel and Monie, 1981; Juchau, 1981; Snell, 1982; Mattison, 1983).

THE COMPLEXITY OF DEVELOPMENTAL TOXICOLOGY

Developmental toxicology is an area of research which has been referred to as a Gordian knot (Ajl, 1982), a knot which is not yet untied but has begun to be unravelled. The intricacies of the knot are due to several factors, including the number of individual entities involved in the complex developmental process, the number and type of toxic effects (endpoints) that can alter the developmental process, and certain temporal features of development and developmental toxicology.

For development to occur, four specific entities—the mother, father, placenta and offspring—have to function separately and together in a genetically determined manner. Each individual entity has multiple complex biological functions to perform (*Table* 9.1) at specific times if normal development is to occur. In addition, these primary biological functions cannot occur unless a host of other organs function adequately.

The toxic endpoints seen in developmental toxicology are more diverse and complex than in any other field of toxicology, and include all those found in general toxicology such as cancer (transplacental), mutation, organ dysfunction and death (maternal or offspring). In addition, other toxic endpoints seen in the mother, father, placenta and offspring are unique to developmental toxicology (*Fig*. 9.1) and are often difficult to assess.

Table 9.1. Partial list of primary biological functions required for normal development.

Maternal:	*Paternal:*
oogenesis	spermatogenesis
ovulation	ejaculation
fertilization	fertilization
implantation	support of:
support of:	offspring
pregnancy	postnatal
placenta	
offspring:	
prenatal	
postnatal	
parturition	
Placental:	*Offspring:*
development	fertilization
transport	implantation
metabolism	placental development
endocrine function	support of:
support of:	pregnancy
pregnancy	placenta
offspring	organ:
parturition	
	development
	prenatal
	postnatal:
	physical
	functional

Temporal features of normal development and developmental toxicology create additional difficulties when determining the toxic potential of a xenobiotic. These include the length of the developmental process, the specific times during development when an organism is sensitive to a toxic xenobiotic (sensitive window), and the length of time before some toxic endpoints are apparent.

The developmental process can be considered to begin with the formation of the gametes and end with adulthood. In man, the length of this process spans two generations since the oocytes are formed in the mother when she is *in utero*. Exposure to a toxic xenobiotic can occur at anytime during development and persist throughout development, or can occur prior to development and result in a body burden of a xenobiotic in either parent at the beginning of development.

The sensitive window greatly complicates the study of a xenobiotic as a developmental toxin. The sensitive window is a specific period in development when a xenobiotic produces a specific toxic endpoint in a specific species, and the sensitive window is present usually only during a small portion of the developmental process. Sensitive windows are seen in transplacental carcinogenesis, abnormal organ maturation, placental and yolk sac dysfunction, and birth defects. The best recognized example of a sensitive window is the teratogenic window, and the best known teratogen with a well defined teratogenic window is thalidomide. In the human, the sensitive window of thalidomide is between days 27 and 40 of gestation (Lenz and Knapp, 1962; Mellin and Katzenstein, 1962; Shepard, 1980). This sensitive window of 14 days is less than 0·2% of the entire

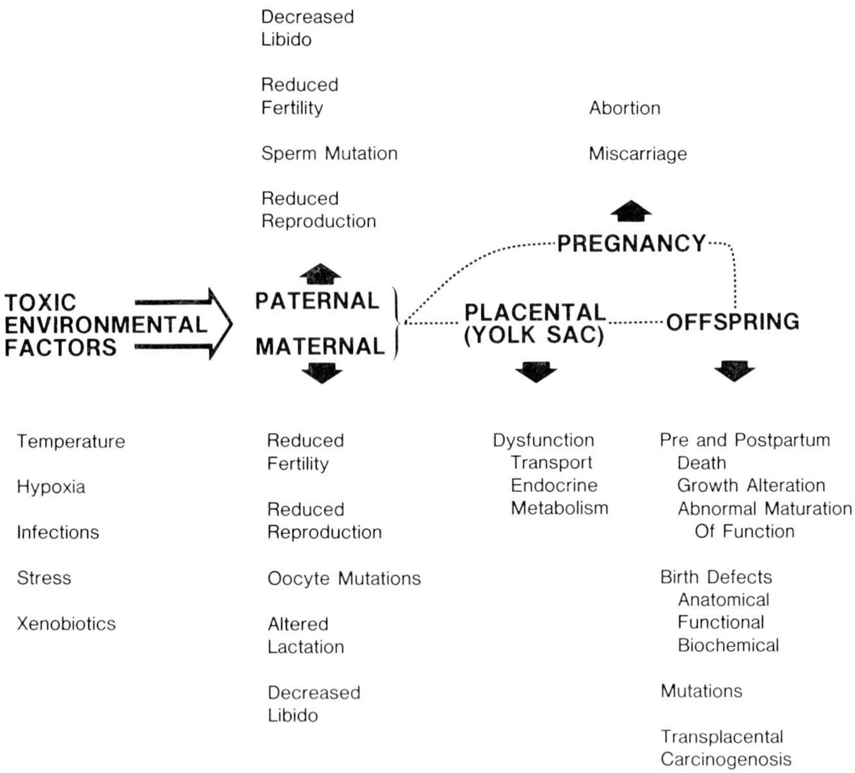

Fig. 9.1. Toxic endpoints in the developmental process.

40 to 50 year period of development in the human. At all times, thalidomide is a remarkable non-toxic xenobiotic.

Finally, certain toxic endpoints may not be apparent until the offspring is maturing into adulthood or later, even when the exposure has occurred in the perinatal period. An example of this is diethylstibesterol transplacentally-induced uterine cervical cancer occurring in the human female decades after the *in utero* exposure (Herbst et al., 1971). Another example of delayed manifestations of toxic endpoints is perinatal imprinting, where exposure to a xenobiotic in the perinatal period programmes a biochemical process or neurobehavioural activity to function differently than it would have otherwise functioned (Middaugh et al., 1975). An example of this is the perinatal exposure of the rodent offspring to methyl mercury which results in decreased hepatic enzyme function in the adult male (Robbins et al., 1977).

The above discussion demonstrates the complexity of developmental toxicology and the difficulty in determining if a xenobiotic has any toxic effect on the developmental process. The next portion of this chapter will discuss how genetics is a primary determinant of developmental toxicology and how the genetic-related differences in developmental toxicology can assist to unite this complex knot.

GENETICS

There is an ever increasing amount of data which demonstrate the dominant role genetics plays in developmental toxicology. In the animal model, species- and strain-specific differences of xenobiotic-induced toxic effects have been documented for many years. Most of the interspecies differences identified in animals have been derived from comparisons of the results from different studies using different species. However, the strain-specific differences in xenobiotic-induced toxic effects have been supported by data from different strains employed in the same experiment (*Table* 9.2). Intrastrain differences in the sensitivity to developmental toxins have been reported even in rodents of the same strain obtained from different suppliers (Nolen, 1969).

In the human, the data that support a dominant role of genetics in development toxicology are not as complete as the animal data. Thalidomide-induced birth defects demonstrate the interspecies differences in sensitivity to xenobiotics involving animals and man. As previously discussed, thalidomide taken by the human during a specific sensitive window causes phocomelia, an abnormality of limb development. However, in animal species thalidomide does not cause limb defects, and produces abnormalities only after multifold increases in the dose of

Table 9.2. Xenobiotics with strain-related differences in their induced developmental toxicities and the proposed genetic factors responsible for these differences.

Xenobiotic	*Species*	*Toxic endpoint(s)*	*Proposed Genetic difference (s)*	*References*
Ethanol	Mouse	IUGR[a] Birth defects Prenatal deaths	Maternal ethanol clearance rate	Cernoff 1980
Benzo[a]pyrene DMBA[b]	Mouse	IUGR[a] Prenatal deaths	Ah locus	Shum et al. 1979 Lambert and Nebert 1977
3-Methyl-cholanthrene TCDD[c]	Mouse	Birth defects Birth defects	Ah locus	Poland and Gover 1980
Corticosteroids	Mouse	Cleft palate	Amount of corticosteroid receptor H-2[a] locus	Levine et al. 1968 Goldman et al. 1977 Bonner and Tynan 1982
Cadmium	Hamsters	Testicular damage	109 C[d] uptake	Lucis and Lucis 1969
Insulin	Mouse	Birth defects	Delay in neuroectoderm cell division; delay in pattern of foetal turning; delay in neural tube closure	Cole and Trasler 1980
Phenytoin	Mouse	Birth defects	Maternal cardiovascular system's sensitivity to phenytoin H-2[a] locus	Watkinson and Millicovsky 1983 Goldman et al. 1983
Vitamin A	Mouse	Birth defects	Vitamin A carrier protein	Seller et al. 1983

[a] Intrauterine growth retardation.
[b] 7,12-dimethylbenz[a]anthracene.
[c] 2,3,7,8-tetrachlorodibenzo-p-dioxin.

thalidomide as compared to the human (Cahen, 1966). In no animal species was the sensitive window the same as was found in the human (Shepard, 1980).

Indirect data suggest intraspecies (interindividual) differences in the sensitivity to developmental toxins occur in the human as they do in animals. Many females are exposed during pregnancy to similar doses of developmental toxins, such as diphenylhydantoin or alcohol, but not all pregnancies or offspring are affected to a similar degree. This interpregnancy difference in xenobiotic-induced toxic effects may be due to alterations of the xenobiotic dose during pregnancy, to not being exposed to the xenobiotic during a sensitive window, or to different genotypes in the different sets of parents and offspring. The most convincing evidence that genetics can cause interindividual differences in the response to developmental toxins in the human is derived from studies of dizygotic twins. Dizygotic twins born to mothers who have taken alcohol (Christoffel and Salafsky, 1975), thalidomide (Mellin and Katzenstein, 1962; Schmidt and Salzano, 1980), or diphenylhydantoin (Loughnan, 1973) during pregnancy have been born with one twin having a different array of birth defects than the other twin. In at least one case when the mother had taken diphenylhydantoin (Loughnan, 1973), one twin was affected while the other twin was not affected. Therefore, the genotypes of the offspring and the parents appear to be important in developmental toxicology in humans as well as in animals. The importance of genetics in developmental toxicology is not surprising since two of the most pivotal parameters of developmental toxicology, (1) the normal developmental process and (2) the pharmacokinetics and pharmacodynamics of the xenobiotics, are under genetic control.

Normal Development

The entire developmental process is, as are all biological processes, under genetic control. As the result of genetic differences, there are many and diverse species- and strain-specific differences in the developmental process. These differences in development can be as distinct as different types of placenta or different degrees of maturity of the offspring at parturition; or as subtle as differences in timing of anatomical or functional organ development. The stage of embryonic development when the palate is closed, or the activity of maternal or embryonic hepatic enzyme functions during certain stages of gestation are examples of subtle differences. The timing of each step in development is important in and of itself, but also in relationship to the other components of development. Consider, for example, the time when the yolk sac (and not the placenta) is the primary organ of nutrition in relationship to organogenesis. If organogenesis occurs prior to the placenta becoming a functional organ, transport of a xenobiotic may be decreased and the toxic effect on the offspring decreases. On the other hand, if a xenobiotic affects yolk sac function, there would be a greater effect on these offspring than the offspring from a species where the placenta was the major organ of nutrition during organogenesis.

The factors listed in *Table* 9.1 are all under genetic control and have intra- and interspecies differences. It is these strain- and species-specific differences that are partially responsible for the genetic-related differences in developmental toxicology. Comparative placental morphology and function and offspring development of organ systems have been recently reviewed (Beck, 1981; Hoar and Monie, 1981).

As outlined previously, the normal developmental process requires four individual entities—the mother, father, offspring and placenta. Each of these entities has a different genotype, including the placenta which is made up of maternal cells and offspring's cells. The only time when the genotypes are similar is when an inbred strain of animal is studied. This genotypic mix not only complicates the study of developmental toxicology, but can be used to understand better the complexities of developmental toxicology.

Pharmacogenetics

The kinetics (absorption, distribution, metabolism and clearance) and dynamics (end-organ response) of xenobiotics are also under genetic control. Most of the pharmacogenetic studies have been conducted with drugs, but recently many studies have examined the pharmacogenetics of the kinetics and dynamics of environmental chemicals, including developmental toxins (Chernoff, 1980; Legraverend et al., 1984).

General toxicology studies have demonstrated with certain xenobiotics that species- and strain-specific differences in the toxicities of the xenobiotics were due to differences in the kinetics of the xenobiotic or end-organ response to the xenobiotic. A limited list of the genetically controlled factors that regulate the kinetics and dynamics of a xenobiotic during development in the mother, placenta and offspring are included in *Figs*. 9.2, 9.3 and 9.4. The interactions between the genetically controlled developmental process and the genetically regulated kinetics and dynamics of the xenobiotic are primarily responsible for the inter- and intraspecies differences in sensitivity to developmental toxins. For each developmental toxin, a different array of genetically controlled factors may be important in determining the type and incidence of toxic endpoints, and can

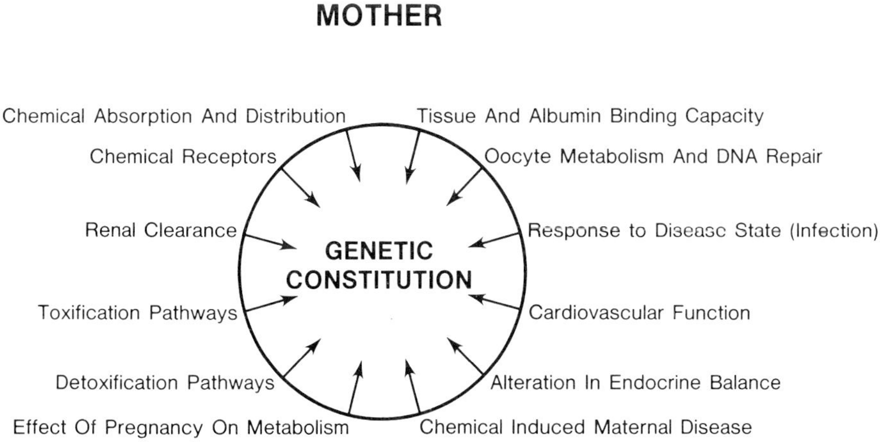

Fig. 9.2. Maternal factors which regulate the kinetics and dynamics of xenobiotics and are under genetic control.

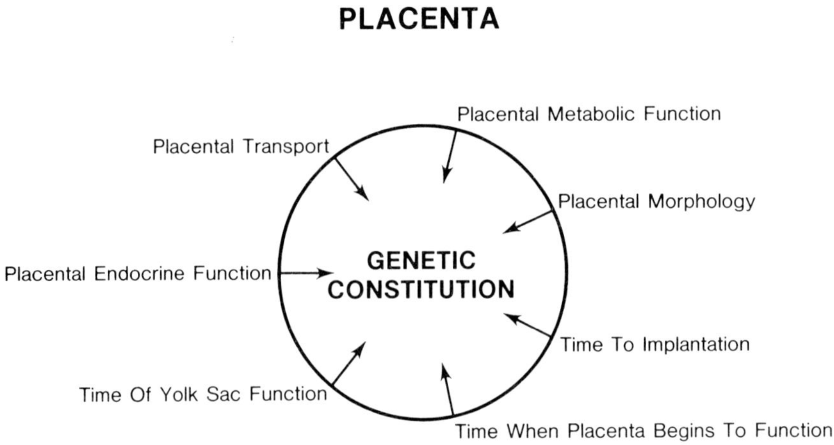

Fig. 9.3. Placental factors which regulate the kinetics and dynamics of xenobiotics and are under genetic control.

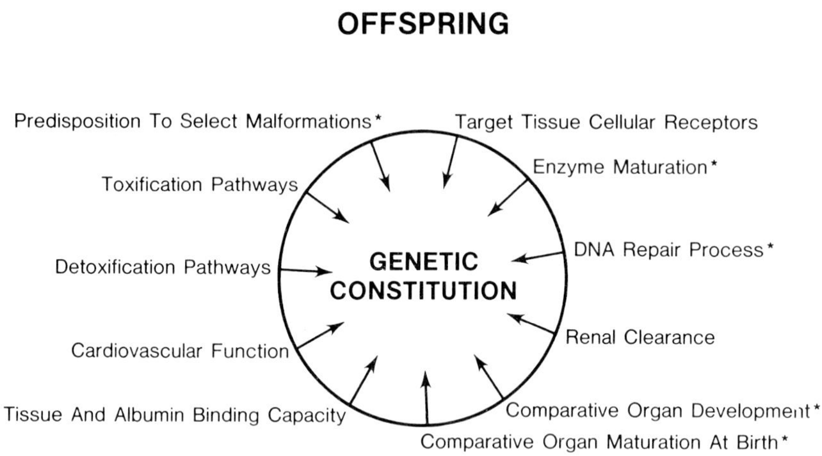

Fig. 9.4. Offspring's factors which regulate the kinetics and dynamics of a xenobiotic and are under genetic control. *Denotes genetically controlled factors of development that interact with the pharmacologic factors resulting in the strain - and species-specific differences seen in developmental toxicology.

explain some of the unique features of developmental toxicology such as the sensitive window.

As discussed previously, while thalidomide was a very potent human teratogen with a specific sensitive window during gestation, it was not nearly as potent a teratogen in any animal species and the sensitive window was not the same. The reason for this species-specific sensitivity to thalidomide has not been conclusively identified, but the increased sensitivity of man to thalidomide-induced limb anomalies may be due to the capacity of the human embryo to metabolize thalidomide to a toxic intermediate during limb bud formation (Gordon et al., 1981). In most other species, the development of drug metabolizing enzymes, such as cytochrome P-450 dependent mixed function monooxygenase (P-450) activity, reaches adult levels only after parturition (Neims et al., 1976). Another pharmacogenetic example is ethanol, which causes a species-specific array of toxic effects on the mother, father, placenta and offspring. Different inbred strains of mice have been studied and the species-specific ethanol-induced foetal toxicity closely correlated with the maternal clearance of ethanol (Chernoff, 1980). The strains of mice that had the highest rate of ethanol clearance were the strains which were least sensitive to ethanol-induced toxicity in the offspring.

Other xenobiotics have been reported to have strain-specific differences in the sensitivity to xenobiotic-induced toxicities. *Table* 9.2 lists several xenobiotics and the proposed genetically controlled features responsible for the strain-related differences in developmental toxicity. Although many other factors are involved in developmental toxicology, clearly the genotype of the mother, father and offspring are critical to the type and severity of developmental toxicity produced by a xenobiotic.

Genetics as a Probe of Developmental Toxicology

After a xenobiotic is identified which has a strain-specific difference in its toxic effect, this strain-specific difference can be exploited as a genetic probe to learn more about the developmental toxin and the genetic differences responsible for the observed differences. Classical breeding methods between the two strains can be employed to determine the mode of inheritance of the altered sensitivity to the xenobiotic, if the trait is controlled by one or more genetic loci, and if the inherited trait is closely linked to any other known loci.

Conversely, inbred strains of mice with known selective genetic differences in development, drug metabolism or organ function, etc. can be used to test a hypothesis regarding the mechanism of toxicity of a specific xenobiotic or class of xenobiotics. For example, as discussed in the next section, inbred strains of mice with and without the genetically controlled capacity to increase cytochrome P1-450 activity in response to polyaromatic hydrocarbons can be selected to test the hypothesis that this enzyme system is necessary to activate select xenobiotics to teratogens. If the results of the initial experiment using the two inbred strains of mice support the hypothesis, other genetic studies can be performed to test further the hypothesis. Classical breeding studies between the two inbred strains can determine if the proposed responsible trait and the altered sensitivity to a developmental toxin co-segregate. If they do not co-segregate, then the hypothesis is invalid.

The pharmacodynamics of a xenobiotic in different strains of mice has also been used to determine if a mechanism of action of toxin is the same in each strain. Biddle (1977, 1978) has suggested that by comparing specific dose-effect curves of a developmental toxin in different strains of mice one may determine if the mechanism of action of the developmental toxin is similar in both strains. For example, when comparing the effect of cortisone treatment on the formation of cleft palate in two strains of mice, parallel dose-response curves indicate a similar mechanism and non-parallel dose-effect curves suggest different mechanisms of action.

Toxicogenetics—Application

The discussion above demonstrates the major role of genetics in the developmental process and developmental toxicology, and how these genetic differences can be employed to understand better the developmental process and developmental toxicology. To illustrate these points, a brief review of previous studies exploiting the genetically controlled induction of the cytochrome P-450 dependent mixed function monooxygenase (P-450) isozymes will be presented.

The P-450 system is a family of isozymes responsible for the metabolism of many xenobiotics. Isozyme activity can be induced by certain xenobiotics, primarily polyaromatic hydrocarbons, in specific strains of animals. Strains of animals in which the P1-450 isozyme can be induced have a cytosolic receptor, the Ah receptor, which binds to polyaromatic hydrocarbons. In the nucleus, the Ah receptor–polyaromatic hydrocarbon complex activates a structural gene in an unknown fashion to cause an increase in P1-450 activity. The genetic locus controlling this response to polyaromatic hydrocarbons is the Ah locus (Nebert et al., 1982). The dominant allele which is 'responsive' to exposure to polyaromatic hydrocarbons is designated Ahb, while the recessive 'non-responsive' allele is Ahd. In strains of animals which have the Ahd allele, the receptor is either absent or it has a very low affinity for polyaromatic hydrocarbons, and P1-450 cannot be induced except by tetrachlorodibenzo-*p*-dioxin.

By using P1-450 induction capacity as a genetic probe, many researchers have studied xenobiotic-induced organ toxicity, cancer and mutations. The P1-450 was shown not only to be important in the metabolism and clearance of many xenobiotics, but P1-450 was capable of metabolizing many relatively non-toxic xenobiotics to toxic intermediates which were capable of causing organ damage (Potter et al., 1973), mutations (Felton et al., 1975) and cancer (Kouri, 1976).

It was hypothesized that some teratogens may also require metabolism by the P-450 system to toxic metabolites before they were foetotoxic. Therefore, the genetic probe of P1-450 induction was used to determine if P1-450 induction could play an important role in developmental toxicology (Lambert and Nebert, 1977). Two polyaromatic hydrocarbons, 7,12-dimethylbenz[*a*]anthracene or 3 methylcholanthrene, were administered to responsive strains (C57BL/6N, BALB/CAnN, ad C3H/HeN) and a non-responsive strain (AKR) of mice between day 5 and 13 of gestation. The responsive strains in comparison to the non-responsive strains had an increased incidence of xenobiotic-induced malformations and resorptions in the offspring.

To test further the hypothesis and to explore the interaction between the teratogen and genetics of the mother, father and offspring, backcross studies between responsive and non-responsive strains of mice were conducted (Shum and Nebert, 1979). The responsive strain, C57BL/6N, and the non-responsive strain, AKR, were mated and the (C57BL/6) (AKR)F1 generation backcrossed to the AKR adult male or female. The pregnant females were administered benzo[*a*]pyrene (BP) intraperitoneally on day 7, 10 or 12 of gestation. At the end of gestation, the mother was sacrificed and the offspring were weighed, examined for gross malformations and phenotyped for P1-450 inducibility by determining hepatic P1-450 dependent aryl hydrocarbon hydroxylase (AHH) activity. Some of the pregnant females were treated with generally labelled tritiated BP and the entire foetuses with the livers removed were monitored for protein and DNA bound radioactivity.

In the (AKR) × (C57BL/6) (AKR) mating the mother is non-responsive, and in the (C57BL/6) (AKR) × (AKR) the mother is responsive. In both matings, the expected phenotype of the offspring would be 50% responsive and 50% non-responsive mice. The results showed that when the mother was responsive, 50% of the offspring were non-responsive and 50% responsive. There was no difference between the responsive and non-responsive offspring in foetal losses, foetal weight, the incidence of malformations or the amount of radioactivity bound to foetal protein and DNA. However, when the mother was non-responsive, 62% of the offspring were non-responsive and 38% of the offspring were responsive. Therefore, the majority of the offspring that died *in utero* were responsive. The responsive offspring in comparison to the non-responsive offspring weighed less, had more malformations and had more radioactivity bound to foetal protein and DNA. This study confirmed the hypothesis and demonstrated that the genotypes of the mother and foetus (and therefore also the father) were important in determining BP-induced toxic effects on reproduction and the offspring. In the pregnancies with the non-responsive mother, the Ahb allele co-segregated with the increased sensitivity to xenobiotic-induced toxicity in the offspring.

In contrast to the above study, when BP is administered orally the non-responsive pregnant females had the higher rate of malformed offspring and reproductive losses (Legraverend et al., 1984). When maternal clearance and placental transport of orally administered radiolabelled BP were studied, the clearance rate of BP was higher in the responsive mother, and placental transport of BP was lower than in the non-responsive strain. Therefore, genetically controlled pharmacokinetics of the foetotoxin in the mother was a critical factor which appeared responsible for the intraspecies differences in reproductive and foetal toxicity.

A question of comparative development was raised suggesting that the mouse embryo did not have any P1-450 activity during organogenesis, and therefore the chemical could not have been metabolized to an active teratogen by the P1-450 system. To examine this question, explanted embryonic tissue from days 3·5, 5·5, 7·5, and 8·5 of gestation were cultured in a medium containing BP and supplemented with 5-bromodeoxyuridine to allow detection of sister chromatid exchange (Galloway et al., 1980). Five inbred, one outbred, and two recombinant inbred strains were studied. The results demonstrated an excellent correlation between increased sister chromatid exchange and the degree to which the strain of mouse was responsive to P1-450 induction. Other investigators (Filler and Lew, 1981) have monitored the formation of BP metabolites *in vitro*, and have shown that embryonic tissue can metabolize BP and the rate of metabolism can be increased in responsive strains of mice.

In the human, a recent study examined the correlation in smokers between placental P1-450 activity (BP metabolism) and birth defects (Manchester and Jacoby, 1984). Smoking during pregnancy had previously been shown to increase P1-450 activity in the human placenta (Nebert et al., 1969). Placental P1-450 activities were determined from pregnancies which resulted in normal and abnormal offspring. The mean P1-450 activity was four times higher in placentas from the normal than the abnormal offspring. Benzo[a]pyrene metabolism was detected in 97% of the placentas from normal offspring, but only 58% of placentas from abnormal offspring. The authors concluded that genetically controlled metabolism of select xenobiotics was an important determinant in embryotoxicity in the human.

The studies described above have increased the understanding of the genetic differences of polyaromatic hydrocarbon-induced developmental toxicities and some of the factors that can alter xenobiotic-induced developmental toxicities. Further studies exploiting the Ah locus as a genetic probe should provide more basic details of the mechanism of toxicity of BP and the normal developmental process. The toxic route of action of BP as a developmental toxin has not been definitely identified and may not be the metabolism of BP to a toxic metabolite. The toxic mechanism of action may be through a direct action of BP, the BP-Ah receptor binding, or the alteration of P-450 isozymes.

The BP may interact with chromosome 17 in the mouse. Chromosome 17 not only contains the locus which is responsible for P1-450 induction by the polyaromatic hydrocarbons (Legraverend et al., 1984), but also the H-2 locus and the T locus. The H-2a locus has been associated with increased sensitivity to xenobiotic-induced cleft palate (Bonner and Tynan, 1982; Goldman et al., 1983). The T locus is a complex region of the chromosome which is thought to have considerable control over embryonic development (Bennett 1975a,b). The Ah locus may be part of the T locus, or just closely linked to the T locus or the H-2 locus. Benzo[a]pyrene, as has been shown with other xenobiotics (Hamburgh et al., 1970; Lary et al., 1982), may directly or indirectly interact with the T locus causing malformations and resorptions in the offspring, or interact with the H-2 locus resulting in an increased incidence of birth defects. Future genetic studies in inbred strains of mice should be able to determine the relationships between these three important loci.

The toxic pathway may involve the Ah receptor binding to an aromatic hydrocarbon, and this temporal gene may then regulate another biochemical process, which is not P1-450, that results in alteration of cellular biochemistry and development (Poland and Grover, 1980). This may, in fact, be a possible mechanism of action since the Ah receptor has been shown to be important in epidermal keratinization (Knutson and Poland, 1980), epidermal growth factor (Ivanovic and Weinstein, 1982), and tumour promotion (Pitot et al., 1980).

The P-450 isozymes may themselves be involved in the toxic pathway and normal development in a yet to be discovered way. As discussed above, the Ah locus appears to control some basic cellular functions. In addition, a new isozyme of hepatic P-450, P-450-P, has been identified in pregnant female mice (Kotake and Lambert, unpublished data). P-450-P has only been found during pregnancy, and may be important in development. Alterations of P-450-P by BP could then alter development.

Future studies exploring the roles of chromosome 17, the Ah locus, and P-450 isozymes may not only identify the mechanism of action of BP as a developmental toxin, but also provide assistance in understanding developmental toxicology and normal development. The strain-specific genetically regulated Ah locus will be an invaluable aid in these future studies.

CONCLUDING REMARKS

The rapid increase in the number of chemicals synthesized and released into the environment continue to be a problem due to the difficulty in assessing their potential as biologic toxins. This is particularly true in developmental toxicology as discussed previously. The application of many different genetic probes may facilitate the assessment of these xenobiotics as developmental toxins. In addition, understanding the mechanism of action of developmental toxins and the specific genetic traits which make an individual or species sensitive to a developmental toxin will improve the capacity to identify specific individuals or species that are potentially at risk from a xenobiotic or class of xenobiotics. New sensitive methods have to be developed that are capable of efficient and non-invasive monitoring of the genetically controlled factors that are important in developmental toxicology. Methods such as the aminopyrine breath test, which is capable of non-invasively monitoring the P-450 system in animals (Kotake et al., 1982), including during pregnancy (Lambert et al., 1983), may help the investigator to understand further the role of specific traits throughout development.

In no species is the need for new methods so critical as the human. The extrapolation of developmental toxicology results between species, particularly from the rodents and rabbits usually employed in laboratory studies, is fraught with severe problems demonstrated in the research described above. It is by studying the human that we will be better able to understand the particular sensitivities of man. The development of new non-invasive *in vivo* or *in vitro* methods capable of measuring specific factors in the human, which have been shown to be important in determining a strain-related difference in animals, will facilitate research into the role of the genetically determined factors in human developmental toxicology (Adams et al., 1981; Shepard et al., 1983; Speilberg et al., 1983; Lambert et al., 1983; Seyler et al., 1984).

Developmental toxicology is the study of how environmental factors alter development from the gamete through adulthood. Since the developmental process and the kinetics and dynamics of xenobiotics are under genetic control, the effect of the environmental chemicals are different in different species. Genetic differences in sensitivity to developmental toxins are powerful tools which can help to unravel the Gordian knot of developmental toxicology, and ultimately improve our ability to predict potential toxicity in environmental chemicals.

REFERENCES

Adams J. and Buelke-Sam J. (1981) Behavioral assessment of the postnatal animal: testing and methods development. In: Kimmel C. A. and Buelke-Sam J. (ed.) *Developmental Toxicology*, 233–257. New York: Raven Press.

Ajl S. J. (1982) Birth defects research: 1980 and after. *Am. J. Med.* **72**, 119–126.

Beck F. (1981) Comparative placental morphology and function. In: Kimmel C. A. and Buelke-Sam J. (ed.) *Developmental Toxicology*, 35–54. New York: Raven Press.

Bennett D. (1975a) T-locus mutants suggestion for the control of early embryonic organization through cell surface components. In: Balles and Wild (ed.) *The Early Development of Mammals*, 207–218. Cambridge: Cambridge University Press.

Bennett D. (1975b) The T locus of the mouse. *Cell* **6**, 441–454.

Biddle F. G. (1977) 6-Aminonicotinamide-induced cleft palate in the mouse: the nature of the differences between A/J and C57BL/6J strains in frequency of response and its genetic basis. *Teratology* **16**, 301–312.

Biddle F. G. (1978) Use of dose-response relationships to discriminate between the mechanisms of cleft palate induction by different teratogens: an argument for discussion. *Teratology* **18**, 247–252.

Biddle F. G. (1981) The role of genetic studies in developmental toxicology. In: Kimmel C. A. and Buelke-Sam J. (ed.) *Developmental Toxicology*, 55–82. New York: Raven Press.

Bonner J. J. and Tynan M. L. (1982) Backcross test demonstrates the linkage of glucocorticoid-induced cleft palate susceptibility to H-2. *Teratology* **26**, 213–216.

Cahen R. (1966) Experimental and clinical chemoteratogenesis. *Adv. Pharmacol.* **4**, 263–349.

Chernoff G. F. (1980) The fetal alcohol syndrome in mice: maternal variables. *Teratology* **22**, 71–75.

Christoffel K. K. and Salafsky I. (1975) Fetal alcohol syndrome in dyzygotic twins. *J. Pediatr.* **87**, 963–967.

Cole W. A. and Trasler D. G. (1980) Gene-teratogen interaction in insulin-induced mouse exencephaly. *Teratology* **22**, 125–139.

Dagg C. P. (1963) The interaction of environmental stimuli and inherited susceptibility to congenital deformity. *Am. Zoologist* **3**, 223–233.

Felton J. and Nebert D. W. (1975) Mutations of certain activated carcinogens *in vitro* associates with genetically mediated increase in monooxygenase activity and cytochrome P1450. *J. Biol. Chem*, **250**, 6769–6778.

Filler R. and Lew K. J. (1981) Developmental onset of mixed-function oxidase activity in preimplantation mouse embryos. *Proc. Natl Acad. Sci. USA*, **78**, 6991–6995.

Fraser F. C. and Fainstat T. D. (1951) Production of congenital defects of mice treated with cortisone. *Pediatrics* **8**, 527–533.

Galloway S. M., Perry P. E., Meneses J. et al. (1980) Cultured mouse embryos metabolize benzo[*a*]pyrene during early gestation: Genetic differences detectable by sister chromatid exchange. *Proc. Natl Acad. Sci. USA* **77**, 3524–3528.

Goldman A. S. Katsumata M., Yaffe S. J. et al., (1977) Palatal cytosol cortisol-binding protein associated with cleft palate susceptibility and H-2 genotype. *Nature* **265**, 643–645.

Goldman A. S., Fishman C. L. and Baker M. K. (1983) Phenytoin teratogenicity in the primary and secondary mouse embryonic palate is influenced by the H-2 histocompatibility locus. *Proc. Soc. Exp. Biol. Med.* **173**, 82–86.

Gordon G. B., Spielberg S. P., Blake D. A. et al., (1981) Thalidomide teratogenesis: evidence for a toxic area oxide metabolite. *Proc. Natl Acad. Sci. USA* **78**, 2545–2548.

Hamburgh M., Herz R. and Landa G. (1970) The effects of trypan blue on expressivity of the brachyury gene 'T', in mice. *Teratology* **3**, 111–118.

Herbst A. L., Ulfelder H. and Poskanzer D. C. (1971) Adenocarcinoma of the vagina: association of maternal stilbesterol therapy with tumor appearance in young women. *N. Engl. J. Med.* **284**, 878–881.

Hoar R. M. and Monie I. W. (1981) Comparative development of specific organ systems. In: Kimmel C. A. and Buelke-Sam J. (ed.) *Developmental Toxicology*, 13–33. New York: Raven Press.

Ivanovic V. and Weinstein I. B. (1982) Benzo[*a*]pyrene and other inducers of cytochrome P1-450 inhibit binding of epidermal growth factor to cell surface receptors. *Carcinogenesis* **3**, 505–510.

Juchau M. R. (1981) *The Biochemical Basis of Chemical Teratogenesis*. New York: Elsevier/North-Holland.

Kimmel C. A. and Buelke-Sam J. (ed.) (1981) *Developmental Toxicology*. New York: Raven Press.

Knapp K., Lenz W. and Nowak E. (1962) Multiple congenital abnormalities. *Lancet* **2**, 725.

Knutson J. C. and Poland A. (1980) Keratinization of mouse teratoma cell line XB produced by 2,3,7,8-tetrachlorodibenzo-*p*-dioxin: An *in vitro* model of toxicity. *Cell* **22**, 27–36.

Kotake A. N., Schreider B. S. and Latts J. R. (1982) The *in vivo* measurements of expired 14C02 derived from the N-demethylation of aminopyrine as a reflection of *in vitro* hepatic cytochrome P-450 drug metabolism activity in the rat. *Drug Metab. Dispos.* **10**, 251–258.

Kouri R. E. (1976) Relationship between labels of aryl hydrocarbon hydroxylase activity and susceptibility to 3-methylcholanthrene and benzo[*a*]pyrene-induced cancers in inbred strains of mice. In: Freudenthal R. I. and Jones P. W. (ed.) *Polynuclear Aromatic Hydrocarbons, Metabolism and Carcinogenesis*, 139–169. New York: Raven Press.

Lambert G. H., Kotake A. N. and Schoeller D. A. (1983) The CO_2 breath test as monitors of the cytochrome P-450 dependent mixed function monooxygenase system. In: MacLeod S. M., Okey A. B. and Spielberg S. P. (ed.) *Developmental Pharmacology*, 119–145. New York:

Lambert G. H., Lietz H., Pang D. et al. (1983) Caffeine breath test in pregnancy. *Pediatr. Res.* **17**, 150A.

Lambert G. H. and Nebert D. W. (1977) Genetically mediated induction of drug metabolizing enzymes associated with congenital defects in the mouse. *Teratology* **16**, 147–153.

Legraverend C., Guenthner T. M. and Nebert D. W. (1984) Importance of the route of administration for genetic differences in benzo[a]pyrene-induced *in utero* toxicity and teratogenicity. *Teratology* **29**, 35–47.

Lenz W. and Knapp K. (1962) Thalidomide embryopathy. *Arch. Environ. Health* **5**, 100–105.

Levine A. I., Yaffe S. J. and Back N. (1968) Maternal-fetal distribution of radioactive cortisol and its correlation with teratogenic effect. *Proc. Soc. Exp. Biol. Med.* **129**, 86–88.

Loughnan P. M., Gold H. and Vance J. C. (1973) Phenytoin teratogenicity in man. *Lancet* **1**, 70–72.

Lucis O. J. and Lucis R. (1969) Distribution of cadmium 109 and zinc 65 in mice of inbred strains. *Arch. Environ. Health* **19**, 334–336.

Manchester D. and Jacoby E. (1984) Decreased placental monooxygenase activities associated with birth defects. *Teratology* **30**, 31–37.

Mattison D. R. (1983) *Reproductive Toxicology*. New York: Liss.

Mellin G. W. and Katzenstein M. (1962) The saga of thalidomide: neuropathy to embryopathy, with case reports of congenital anomalies. *N. Engl. J. Med.* **267**, 1238–1244.

Middaugh L. D., Santos C. A. III and Zemp J. W. (1975) Effects of phenobarbitol given to pregnant mice on behavior of mature offspring. *Dev. Psychobiol.* **8**, 305–313.

Nebert D. W., Negishi M., Long M. A. et al. (1982) The Ah locus, a family necessary for survival in a chemically adverse environment: comparison with the immune system. *Adv. Genet.* **21**, 1–52.

Nebert D. W., Winkler J. and Gelboin H. V. (1969) Aryl hydrocarbon hydroxylase activity in human placenta from cigarette smoking and nonsmoking women. *Cancer Res.* **29**, 1763–1769.

Neims A. H., Warner M., Loughnan P. M. et al. (1976) Developmental aspects of the hepatic cytochrome P-450 monooxygenase system. *Ann. Rev. Pharmacol.* **16**, 427–445.

Nolen G. A. (1969) Variations in teratogenic response to hypervitaminosis A in three strains of albino rat. *Food Cosmet. Toxicol.* **7**, 209–214.

Phelan M. C., Pellock J. M. and Nance W. E. (1982) Discordant expression of fetal hydantion syndrome in heteropaternal dizygotic twins. *N. Engl. J. Med.* **307**, 99–101.

Pitot H. C., Goldsworthy T., Campbell H. A. et al., (1980) Quantitative evaluation of the promotion by 2,3,7,8-tetrachlorodibenzo-*p*-dioxin of hepatocarcinogenesis from diethylnitrosamine. *Cancer Res.* **40**, 3616–3620.

Poland A. and Grover E. (1980) 2,3,7,8-tetrachlorodibenzo-*p*-dioxin: segregation of toxicity with the Ah locus. *Molec. Pharmacol.* **17**, 86–94.

Potter W. Z., Davis D. C., Mitchell J. R. et al. (1973) Acetaminophen-induced hepatic necrosis. III. cytochrome P-450 mediated covalent binding *in vitro*. *J. Pharmacol. Exper. Ther.* **187**, 203–210.

Robbins M. S., Hughes J. A., Sparber S. B. et al. (1977) Delayed teratogenic effect of methylmercury on hepatic cytochrome P-450-dependent monooxygenase systems of rats. *Life Sciences* **22**, 287–294.

Sang J. H. and McDonald J. M. (1954) Production of phenocopies in *Drosophila* using salts, particularly sodium metaborate. *J. Genet.* **52**, 392–412.

Schmidt M. and Salzano F. M. (1980) Dissimilar effects of thalidomide in dyzygotic twins. *Acta Genet. Med. Gemellol. (Roma)* **29**, 295–297.

Seller M. J., Perkins K. J. and Adinolfi M. (1983) Differential response of heterozygous curly-tail embryos to vitamin A teratogenesis depending on maternal genotype. *Teratology* **28**, 123–129.

Seyler D. E., East J. M., Condie L. W. et al. (1984) The use of *in vitro* methods for assessing reproductive toxicity. Dichlorophenols. *Toxicol. Lett.* **20**, 309–315.

Shepard T. H. (1980) *Catalog of Teratogenic Agents*, 3rd ed., 317–320. Baltimore: Johns Hopkins University Press.

Shepard T. H., Fantel A. G., Mirkes P. E. et al. (1983) In: MacLeod S. M., Okey A. B. and Speilberg S. S. (ed.) *Developmental Pharmacology*, 147–164. New York: Liss.

Shum S., Jensen N. M. and Nebert D. W. (1979) The murine Ah locus: *in utero* toxicity and teratogenesis associated with genetic differences in benzo[*a*]pyrene metabolism. *Teratology* **20**, 365–376.

Snell K. (1982) *Developmental Pharmacology*. New York: Praeger.

Spielberg, S. S. (1983) *In vitro* human pharmacogenetics of reactive drug metabolite detoxification. In: MacLeod S. M., Okey A. B. and Speilberg S. S. (ed.) *Developmental Pharmacology*. 107–118. New York: Liss.

Watkinson W. P. and Millicovsky G. (1983) Effect of phenytoin on maternal heart rate in A/J mice: possible role in teratogenesis. *Teratology* **28**, 1–8.

Chapter 10

A Survey of *in vitro* Teratology Tests

John A. Thomas and Yigal Greener

INTRODUCTION

Several *in vitro* methods for assessing embryonic development (or lack thereof) are intriguing procedures from a conceptual viewpoint because in many cases they promise to supplant presumed equivalent *in vivo* assays (Homberger and Goldberg, 1985). Perhaps the most prominent and contemporary example of this *in vitro* and *in vivo* relationship is the use of the Ames mutagenicity assay as an equivalency for a chronic two-year carcinogenesis assay. It has been demonstrated for a host of chemicals that extension of short-term testing results to long-term *in vivo* results seldom reveals any strict correlation. Again, and drawing upon experiences gained from cancer screening procedures, no single short-term mutagenesis assay will elucidate all carcinogens. Similarly, no short-term *in vitro* teratology test will consistently predict those chemicals/drugs that produce birth defects in either vertebrates or invertebrates.

The notion of evaluating agents for teratogenicity using anything other than a pregnant mammal has consistently been rejected by the biomedical and regulatory community. Certainly the maternal–placental–embryonic relationship bears no resemblance to any *in vitro* teratology assay system, regardless of whether such a system is a mammalian form (Schardein, 1985). To date, no *in vitro* teratology assay system has been devised that can even begin to approximate the anatomical and physiological relationship between maternal and embryonic organisms.

Wilson (1978) has posed the question as to why there should be concern with the development of an *in vitro* assay system if such a system cannot possibly provide a reasonable model of human pregnancy. In part, the answer lies with the ever increasing volume of distinct chemical identities and the seeming impossibility of completing even subhuman *in vivo* teratology tests. Reportedly, there are over four million distinct chemical identities, and an estimated 6000 or so new entries are being added each week. To assess properly each of these agents, even excluding combinations, becomes a task of staggering dimensions.

Several of the *in vitro* teratologic methodologies are certainly attractive from a conceptual standpoint, particularly if they might supplant an equivalent *in vivo* test. Ideally, the Ames mutagenicity assay would be much preferred over a chronic two-year carcinogenesis assay. Likewise, although on a lesser scale, a predictive short-term *in vitro* teratogen-type assay would be preferred to an *in vivo* full-term pregnancy and offspring protocol. Unfortunately, the extrapolation of short-term tests, regardless of whether *in vitro* or *in vivo*, has not proven consistent with full-term pregnancy teratology assays. Cost and convenience aside, such extrapolations from *in vitro* findings to those of *in vivo* systems have always been difficult to accept scientifically, particularly in the area of teratology.

Steele et al. (1983a) have examined the use of cultures of whole embryos as a screening test for teratogens. The culture system is amenable to continuous scrutiny of any effects of a chemical/drug on embryonic development. The system also allows for precise dosage monitoring as related to the stage of development at the time of exposure or injection. Using this short-term *in vitro* culture system, the action of a suspected teratogen can be evaluated by:

a. Adding the chemical/drug directly to the culture medium;
b. Adding the chemical/drug directly to the culture medium together with specific maternal metabolic components; and
c. Growing the embryos in serum taken from animals dosed with the chemical/drug.

Each of these three approaches can yield valuable information, yet none will provide a complete model of the so-called embryonal/placental/maternal unit as it occurs in the pregnant animal (Steele et al., 1983a).

Wilson (1978) has suggested a set of criteria that constitute highly desirable assay characteristics (*Table* 10.1). Such characteristics would include essential features and also non-essential, but desirable, features.

The need for a short-term test is evident, even if one considers only the cost- and labour-intensive methodologies of the *in vivo* assay. Unfortunately, the ideal system for *in vitro* testing does not yet exist. Lacking a single, simple screening assay, one might instead employ a battery or tier of *in vitro* assays under certain conditions.

Finally, a statistical structure-activity model has been used to predict the probable teratogenicity of chemicals (Enslein et al., 1983). Structure-activity models have also been employed to predict mutagenicity and carcinogenicity. According to Enslein (1983), such a teratogenic model can be compared to the rat acute oral LD_{50}. The teratogenesis model is based on responses, collected from existing biomedical literature, to about 400 chemicals. The mathematical equation used for this structure-activity model results in about an 8% false positive

Table 10.1. Characteristics of an ideal short-term *in vitro* teratogen assay.[a]

Essential features:
Employs biologic subjects available in large numbers
Possesses aspects of progressive development
Related to mechanism(s) of teratogenesis
Readily performed and reproducible
Desirable features:
Employs an intact organism
Renders few so-called false negatives
Universally reactant to chemicals/drugs

[a] Modified from Wilson (1978).

classification and about a 10% false negative. Approximately 25% of the compounds tested are classified neither as teratogens or non-teratogens. This statistical model could represent a short-term evaluation procedure, but is quite limited in its usefulness because it is based on only about 400 chemicals, an exceedingly small sample size given the total number of potential teratogens.

LIMITATIONS OF SHORT-TERM *IN VITRO* ASSAYS

Extrapolation of teratogenic findings from animals to man has been, and will continue to be, a perplexing problem. The use of *in vitro* systems compounds the dilemma. The fact that a substance exhibits detrimental effects in embryonic cells and tissues *in vitro* does not necessarily render it a teratogen *in vivo*.

Generally, the use of an *in vitro* screening test provides no information regarding placentation, and also excludes data regarding potential biochemical conversion to more toxic metabolites. The normal physiologic barriers to the transport of chemicals and/or drugs certainly differ between *in vitro* and *in vivo* tests. While certain *in vitro* test systems allow for precise dosing or concentrations, such information in itself precludes establishing so-called safe levels of the drug or chemical.

ADVANTAGES OF *IN VITRO* TESTING

Kochhar (1981) has described a number of advantages to certain *in vitro* testing methodologies (*Table* 10.2). More particularly, tissue culture methods can be employed for assessing aspects of teratogenicity. Many of the advantages enjoyed by *in vitro* tests for teratogenesis are also appropriate for mutagenicity and carcinogenicity testing.

Subsequent sections of the chapter will deal with specific advantages (or disadvantages) of a variety of *in vitro* tests, whether they involve organ explants or whole embryos obtained from mammalian and non-mammalian organisms.

MAMMALIAN EMBRYO

Over the past several years there has been a resurgence of interest in designing *in vitro* methods (systems) for the determination of the potential toxic effects of various chemicals on the developing mammalian embryo. These systems, utilizing either whole explanted mammalian embryos or embryonic cells, organs and tissues, are considered relevant to studies on teratogenesis as they offer a number of advantages (Kochhar, 1981; *Table* 10.2).

Yet, in spite of these advantages, the *in vitro* maintenance of mammalian embryo has the following limitations:

a. The period of observation provided does not exceed several hours or a few days;
b. The embryo undergoing advanced organogenesis and beginning to show a degree of functional maturation does not thrive under *in vitro* conditions, probably because of lack of maternal environment; and

Table 10.2. Advantages of *in vitro* testing.[a]

1. Embryonic cells and tissues are made accessible to direct observation.
2. The stage of development of the target organ or tissue at the time of exposure can be precisely determined.
3. Variability in tissue response is reduced or eliminated by direct control over the experimental conditions.
4. Replicate samples can be obtained from the same litter or even from the same embryo.
5. Control can easily be exercised over the duration of exposure of the target cells and tissues to the agent.
6. Maternal/placental metabolism of the drug is circumvented; hence, rather precise assessment of the active form of the chemical agent can be made.

[a] Modified from Kochhar (1981).

c. The *in vitro* system does not provide for teratogenic effects manifested during the postnatal period.

Nevertheless, a number of *in vitro* techniques employing the mammalian embryo have been used as teratology-monitoring or screening systems. These systems can be classified into three categories:

a. Direct exposure of the explanted embryo in culture to various chemicals and environmental conditions (e.g. temperature);
b. Exposure of the explanted embryo in culture to serum from treated animals (i.e. 'treated serum' system); and
c. Exposure of the mammalian embryo *in utero* and observation of the embryo response *in vitro* (i.e. '*in vivo*/*in vitro*' system).

Using the explanted (10-day-old) rat embryo culture system, Mirkes et al. (1981) demonstrated that phosphoramide mustard was the teratogenic metabolite of cyclophosphamide since the effects of the metabolite resembled those of the *in vivo* bioactivated cyclophosphamide. These effects were reductions in total embryo protein content, crown–rump length and number of somites, in addition to exencephaly, cleft lips/palate, skeletal defects and pattern of cell necrosis. In a more recent study, Mirkes et al. (1984) suggested that acrolein may play a role in cyclophosphamide teratogenesis, but only if it is generated at the 'teratogenic sites' within the embryo. Greenaway et al. (1982) showed that embryos cultured with cyclophosphamide were indistinguishable from embryos cultured in medium only, and thus concluded that the 10-day-old rat embryo was apparently deficient in enzymes necessary for the metabolic activation of cyclophosphamide. However, the *in vitro* exposure of the 10-day-old rat embryos to the teratogenic dosage of cyclophosphamide in the presence of a metabolic system produced molecular lesions necessary to elicit the teratogenic effects of the chemical seen *in vivo* (Mirkes et al., 1983). In addition to the effects of various chemicals, the explanted embryo system has been used to assess the teratogenic effects of hyperthermia (Cockroft and New, 1978). This procedure, which eliminated maternal effects, subjected the embryo directly to temperature increase, thus resulting in malformed and growth retarded embryos.

In order to quantitate the *in vitro* morphological development of rat embryos (aged 9.5–12.5 days—late presomite to 40-somite stage), Brown and Fabro (1981) proposed a morphological score that was to be directly proportional to the embryonic age, suggesting that such application can provide essential information on morphological development, facilitate the detection of abnormalities and organ-specific retardations, and allow a quantitative comparison of growth and development.

In addition to screening for the direct effects of drugs or their metabolites, the *in vitro* system can be utilized in investigating the mechanism(s) involved in drug teratogenicity/embryotoxicity using the 'treated serum' system. Steele et al. (1983b) showed that it was the direct action of two hypolipidaemic agents on the embryo itself, and not the hypolipidaemic serum, that was harmful to embryonic development. In another study, Klein et al. (1980) demonstrated the usefulness of rat embryo cultures to monitor serum teratogenic activity, using serum taken at intervals from rats treated with either cadmium or cyclophosphamide.

The *in vivo/in vitro* system has the advantage of *in utero* exposure; thus, a drug or chemical would be processed by the maternal placenta–embryo unit. Evaluation of the potential teratogenic agent is carried out using the explanted embryo cultured in serum obtained from untreated animals (Beaudoin and Fisher, 1981; Steele et al., (1983a). Although this system provides that the exposure of the pregnant animal to the chemical agent simulates the human exposure, it nevertheless has its limitations. Beaudoin and Fisher (1981) reported that teratogenic agents (i.e. thiadiazole, cadmium sulphate, 1,2-dibromo-2,2-dichloroethyl dimethyl phosphate, 2-(sec-butyl)-4,6-dinitrophenol, lead nitrate, trypan blue, polybrominated biphenyls and sodium arsenate) inhibited the subsequent rate of development of the embryos in culture. The pattern of malformations observed, however, bore little resemblance to that found in embryos allowed to continue development in the mother. Conversely, Steele et al. (1983a) suggested that the evaluation of embryos in culture (using the *in vivo/in vitro* method) can provide a good indication of the effects of the teratogenic agent (e.g. vitamin A) *in vivo*.

Tissue culture methods can provide sufficient information to compare the results with *in vivo* development. These methods are simple, reliable (Warner et al., (1983), and show resemblance to specific stages in organogenesis *in vivo* (New, 1978). However, it seems that although these methods provide a valuable additional screening procedure for new drugs and potential teratogens and can contribute to an understanding of developmental mechanisms and congenital malformations in mammals, they cannot, at present, replace the classic *in vivo* procedures used to screen chemicals for teratogenicity.

INVERTEBRATE EMBRYOS

Wilson (1978) has outlined the ideal teratogenic screening assay (*Table* 10.1). Such criteria, particularly as they relate to invertebrate embryos, include the availability of large numbers of organisms, and the ease with which such tests can be performed, and also the interpretation of the endpoints. A likely advantage, in the case of the invertebrate embryo, is that the test can evolve around an intact organism capable of absorbing, circulating, metabolizing and excreting the chemical or drug. Several species of invertebrate embryos above the protozoa possess all of the aforementioned criteria for *in vitro* screening. That *Drosophila*, sea urchins and sand dollars can be grown under laboratory conditions in large numbers renders these species particularly suitable for *in vitro* teratogenicity screening.

Bournias-Vardiabasis et al., (1984) have utilized an *in vitro* assay employing *Drosophila* embryonic cell cultures. The endpoint selected in assessing the teratogenic potential of a chemical or drug involves detection of interference with normal muscle and/or neurone differentiation. In evaluating or comparing the *Drosophila* test with teratogenicity data obtained in animals and humans, there appears to be a rather favourable correlation among several drugs (*Table* 10.3). It would appear that some strains of *Drosophila* are more sensitive than others with regard to detecting teratogenicity. Results of the *Drosophila* test included only a low percentage of false positives and false negatives.

Table 10.3. Comparison of the *Drosophila* assay with *in utero* development tests.[a]

Agent	*Drosophila assay*	*In utero assay*
Acetazolamide	–[b]	–
Actinomycin D	+[c]	+
Aspirin	+	+
Amphotericin	+	+
Caffeine	–	–
Dexamethasone	+	+
Phenytoin	+	+
Pentobarbital	+	+
Sulphonamides	–	–
Thalidomide	+	+

[a] Excerpted from Bournias-Vardiabasis (1983).
[b] Non-teratogenic.
[c] Teratogenic potential.

Embryos of the cricket *Acheta domesticus* (L.) have been shown by bioassay to develop gross morphological abnormalities after exposure to a variety of different chemicals (Walton, 1983). The major advantages of the *A. domesticus* embryo assay are that it is inexpensive and that it requires only a small investment for commercially available equipment.

Crickets are easily acquired and can be bred very readily so as to obtain sufficiently large numbers. The cricket embryo exhibits a critical period of teratogen sensitivity and has the ability to metabolize xenobiotics. Genetic marker strains are not available for *A. domesticus*, but this disadvantage can be overcome by using cricket species with different responses to the same teratogen for comparative studies.

The major disadvantage of the cricket embryo assay as a screen for chemical teratogens is that it currently remains an unvalidated system. Using the cricket embryo, several different polycyclic aromatic hydrocarbons, azaarenes, and certain primary aromatic amines were observed to be toxic, but not teratogenic. Of some 30 chemicals reported to be non-teratogenic to *A. domesticus*, only benzo[*a*]pyrene is reported to be teratogenic in other species (Walton, 1983).

Additional studies using the cricket embryo assay may establish its relative importance as a predictive teratogen screening method.

AQUATIC EMBRYOS

In the search for *in vitro* teratogenicity screening systems, aquatic (e.g. fish and amphibian) embryo-larval stages offer some ideal characteristics as animal models that satisfy the requirements for such systems. They are available in large numbers, the tests are easily performed and yield interpretable results, and they are capable of absorbing, circulating and excreting the agents under investigation. Using the amphibian and fish embryos system, Birge et al. (1983) exposed trout, narrow-mouth toads and catfish to inorganic mercury, boron or atrazine and observed malformations in the developing embryos. Embryos of amphibia have also been used as models for assessing the toxicity of organophosphorus compounds (Fulton and Chambers, 1985). Nakatsuji (1983) observed craniofacial malformations in the amphibian embryos *Xenopus laevis* following exposure to ethanol. The malformations were similar to those observed in the human foetal alcohol syndrome. It thus seems that fish and amphibian developmental stages can serve effectively as models for:

a. Studying mechanisms of the teratogenic effects of environmental xenobiotics; and
b. Screening environmental toxicants, including teratogens.

The fresh water coelenterate *Hydra attenuata* has been recently presented as a model for studying the teratogenic effects of xenobiotics (Johnson, 1980; Johnson and Gabel, 1982, 1983; Chun et al., 1983a,b,c). Adult hydra are readily dissociable into their component cells, which can then be packed into pellets of randomly reaggregated cells. These cells, i.e. artificial 'embryos', will begin to regenerate into multiple adult hydra. During this regeneration, 'embryos' will go through the developmental events similar to those seen in mammalian embryogenesis, i.e. changes in cell shape and size, selective cell death, spatial orientation with formation of junctions, formation of inert cellular matrix, cell migration and association into tissues (Johnson, 1980). Yet, despite these similarities, which provide excellent opportunity for direct observations of several aspects of embryogenesis in higher animals, this system has its limitations, as it represents only a very limited segment of the developmental process. Furthermore, the extent to which the system can simulate the teratogenic effects of xenobiotics on mammalian embryos remains to be established.

AVIAN EMBRYO

The chick embryo has been used widely for model systems in experimental embryology and teratology. This model, which is independent of maternal circulation, offers a number of advantages in the studies of teratogenesis (*Table* 10.4).

Recently, a number of techniques employing the chick embryo have been developed for the assessment of potential teratogens and their effects on embryonic development. These techniques can be classified into three categories:

a. Direct exposure of the explanted embryo in culture to various chemicals;
b. Dosing and monitoring the development of early chick embryo, i.e. age 1–3 days; and
c. Use of the chick embryo at a later stage of development, i.e. dosing during the early stage of development and monitoring during incubation and up to and beyond hatching.

Table 10.4. Advantages of using the chick embryo in studying teratogenesis.[a]

1. It can be practicably used in larger numbers than any mammal.
2. The self-contained nature of the embryonated egg permits instillation of exogenous materials with the assurance that these will not be diluted, metabolized, or otherwise affected by a maternal system.
3. Sampling of embryo blood and tissues is feasible during development.
4. Various tissues, e.g. nervous system, are at an advanced stage of development at hatching and thus a comparison between the early stage of embryonic development and the advanced stage with regard to morphology as well as quantitative analysis can be made.
5. The viability of embryos can be easily determined and closely followed.

[a] Modified from Greener and Kochen (1983).

The explanted chick embryo in culture media was used by Nadeau and Mun (1978) to study the mechanism(s) that lead to the formation of rumplessness in the chick embryo. They concluded that trypan blue acts directly, rather than indirectly, through interference with osmoregulatory mechanisms on organs and structures in the caudal region of the chick embryo, thus resulting in rumplessness. Employing the explanted chick embryo technique, Lee and Nagele (1979) showed that papaverine (6,7-diethoxy-1-veratrylisoquinoline hydrochloride) preferentially inhibited uplifting of neural folds (and hence closure of the neural tube) in the cultured chick embryo. This technique, used as a tool to study the mechanisms of neurolation, shed more light on the cause(s) of various congenital central nervous system defects.

Studying the early (1–3 days old) chick embryo presents a number of problems not encountered during subsequent development stages. The target is much smaller, positioning of the embryo is difficult, the embryo is invisible to candling (particularly prior to the onset of blood flow at about 48 hours), and it is possible to cause some embryo malformations (e.g. neural tube defects) when windowing eggs during the first day of incubation. Therefore, various procedures and techniques have been devised in order to circumvent these problems. Wyttenbach et al. (1981) and Kitos et al. (1981) devised a set of guidelines for locating and positioning the young embryo prior to intravitelline injection of the chemicals. Additionally, they described an instrument that makes it possible to inject small liquid volumes into the yolks of incubating eggs. Fisher and Schoenwolf (1983) showed that during the windowing procedure, filling the suprablastodermal air space with saline or albumin reduced the frequency of neural tube defects, thus allowing the administration of teratogens to young embryos by subblastodermic injection.

Using the early chick embryo model system, the effects of amphetamine and trypan blue on chick morphogenesis were studied (Kolesari and Kaplan, 1979; Grala and Kaplan, 1980a,b; Weaver et al., 1981). Swartz (1980) showed that the embryotoxic and teratogenic effects of busulphan were dependent on the age of the embryo and the duration of the exposure. Prenalterol, a cardiac β-adrenergic receptor blocker, which has been shown to be teratogenic in the rabbit, induced cardiovascular malformations when administered topically to 2·5 through 5·5-day-old chick embryos (Bruyere et al., 1983). Cameron et al. (1984) modified a technique wherein the mean ventricular blood pressure was measured in the 4-day-old chick embryo. Using dextroamphetamine, Cameron et al. (1983) proposed that elevation of embryonic blood pressure during a critical period of aortic arch and ventricular septal morphogenesis might be an aetiological factor in the genesis of their malformations. The early chick embryo was also used as a model system for determining the teratogenic potential of the food additive carrageenan (Monis and Rovasio, 1981).

While the explanted-culture and the early chick embryo model systems have been used for studies in experimental teratology, a large number of studies have been published in which the chick embryo at a later stage of development has been described. This model was used by Verrette et al. (1980) in the determination of the toxicity and teratogenicity of food additive chemicals. Kochen and Greener (1974, 1976, 1977a,b), Roy et al. (1974), Kochen et al. (1977), and Hirano and Kochen (1977a,b) studied the dose-effect and temporal relationship, as well as morphological effects, of lead on the developing chick embryo. Using the same model, Greener and Kochen (1983) studied the teratogenic effects of methyl mercury on the developing chick embryo. Various drugs and environmental teratogens and their effects on specific organ systems have been studied using the chick embryo model. Gilbert et al. (1980) suggested that practolol prevented isoproterenol-induced acute heart failure in the embryonic chick. Ishikawa et al. (1978) studied the morphogenic effects of theophylline on cardiac tissues. Kuhlmann et al. (1983) and Cameron et al. (1983) demonstrated the teratogenic effects of catecholamines and amphetamines, respectively, on the cardiovascular system. Bruyere et al. (1983) demonstrated the synergistic effects of methylxanthines and β-adrenomimetic agents on the morphology of the cardiac system. The chick embryo model was also used in the studies of steroids (Fisher and Sawyer, 1980; Peterka and Jelinek, 1983), environmental teratogens, such as 2,3,7,8-tetrachlorodibenzo-*p*-dioxin (Cheung et al., 1981), aliphatic and aromatic fractions of crude and fuel oil (Ellenton, 1982), trichloroethylene (Bross et al., 1983), insecticides (Eto et al., 1980; Misawa et al., 1981), chlorinated biphenyls (Brundstrom and Darnerud, 1983), irradiation (Schneider and Norton, 1980), carbon monoxide (Daughtrey et al., 1983), and mycotoxins (Gilani et al., 1978). As an alternative to the chick embryo, a number of investigators used other avian model systems for the studies of teratogenic effects of drugs (Meiniel, 1981—quail) and environmental hazardous chemicals (Hoffman, 1982—duck and quail).

The chick embryo is commonly used as a model system in pharmacological and toxicological research. Several ways of exposing the chick embryo to xenobiotics have been described. They include immersing the egg totally in the test solution, culturing the explanted embryo, cutting a window in the shell and either pipetting the agent onto extra-embryonic membranes overlying the embryo, injecting it into the extra-embryonic coelom directly beneath the embryo, or into the air chamber. Results obtained using such procedures indicate that the chick embryo test system is capable of demonstrating teratogenic potential of compounds because it is selective and generally does not respond non-specifically to agents introduced during development. Therefore, the chick embryo model system is useful for screening large numbers of compounds to identify those that should be subjected to more critical teratogenicity studies. However, it should not replace currently used teratology and reproduction tests in mammals where the drugs and other chemicals tested might involve exposure of pregnant women.

SUMMARY

Teratology testing in experimental animals will never resolve the issue of extrapolation of findings to the human. Furthermore, *in vitro* tests will never fully replace *in vivo* teratologic studies. However, properly conducted *in vitro* teratogenesis assays can provide a useful screen for both chemicals and drugs. Additionally, the *in vitro* teratology model system can aid significantly in elucidating certain aspects of the mechanism of toxic action of a particular chemical or drugs. The shortcomings in an *in vitro* teratogenesis assay are not unique in so far as the general use of any *in vitro* system.

REFERENCES

Beaudoin A. R. and Fisher D. L. (1981) An *in vivo/in vitro* evaluation of teratogenic action. *Teratology* **23**, 57–61.

Birge W. J., Black J. A., Westerman A. G. et al. (1983) Fish and amphibian embryos—a model system for evaluating teratogenicity. *Fund. Appl. Toxicol.* **3**, 237–242.

Bournias-Vardiabasis N., Teplitz R. L., Chernoff G. E. et al., (1983) Detection of teratogens in the *Drosphila* embryonic cell culture test: Assay 100 chemicals. *Teratology* **28**, 109–122.

Bross G., DiFranceisco D. and Desmond M. E. (1983) The effects of low dosages of trichloroethylene on chick development. *Toxicology* **28**, 283–284.

Brown N. A. and Fabro S. (1981) Quantitation of rat embryonic development *in vitro*: a morphological scoring system. *Teratology* **24**, 65–78.

Brundstrom B. and Darnerud P. O. (1983) Toxicity and distribution in chick embryo of 3,3′,4,4′ tetrachlorobiphenyl injected into the eggs. *Toxicology* **27**, 103–110.

Bruyere H. J. Jr., Fallon J. F. and Gilbert E. F. (1983) External malformations in chick embryos following concomitant administration of methylxanthines and β-adrenomimetic agents: 1. Gross pathologic features. *Teratology* **28**, 257–269.

Bruyere H. J. Jr., Matsuoka R., Carlsson E. et al. (1983) Cardiovascular malformations associated with administration of prenalterol to young chick embryos. *Teratology* **28**, 75–82.

Cameron R. A., Kolesari G. H. and Kallifleisch J. H. (1983) Pharmacology of dextroamphetamine-induced cardiovascular malformations in the chick embryo. *Teratology* **27**, 253–259.

Cameron R. H., Kolesari G. L. and Rajala G. M. (1984) Elevated blood pressure in the embryonic chick induced by a teratogenic dose of dextroamphetamine sulfate. *Teratology* **29**, 87–92.

Cheung M. O., Gilbert E. F. and Peterson R. E. (1981) Cardiovascular teratogenicity of 2,3,7,8-tetrachlorodibenzo-*p*-dioxin in the chick embryo. *Toxicol. Appl. Pharmacol.* **61**, 197–204.

Chun Y. H., Johnson E. M., Gabel B. E. G. et al. (1983a) Regeneration by dissociated hydra cells: a histologic study. *Teratology* **27**, 81–87.

Chun Y. H., Johnson E. M., Gabel B. E. G. et al. (1983b) Effects of vinblastine sulfate on the growth and histologic development of reaggregated hydra. *Teratology* **27**, 89–94.

Chun Y. H., Johnson E. M. and Gabel B. E. G. (1983c) Relationship of developmental stages to effects of vinblastine on artificial 'embryo' of hydra. *Teratology* **27**, 95–100.

Cockroft D. L. and New D. A. T. (1978) Abnormalities induced in cultured rat embryo by hyperthermia. *Teratology* **17**, 277–284.

Daughtrey W. C., Newby-Schmidt M. B. and Norton S. (1983) Forebrain damage in chick embryos exposed to carbon monoxide. *Teratology* **28**, 83–89.

Ellenton J. A. (1982) Teratogenic activity of aliphatic and aromatic fractions of Prudhoe Bay crude and fuel oil No. 2 in the chicken embryo. *Toxicol. Appl. Pharmacol.* **63**, 209–215.

Enslein K., Lander T. R. and Strange J. R. (1983) Teratogenesis—a statistical structure-activity model. *Teratogenesis Carcinog. Mutag.* **3**, 289–309.

Eto M., Seifert J., Engel J. L. and Casida J. E. (1980) Organophosphorus and methylcarbamate teratogens: structural requirements for inducing embryonic abnormalities in chickens and kymurenine formamidase inhibition in mouse liver. *Toxicol. Appl. Pharmacol.* **54**, 20–30.

Fisher M. and Schoenwolf G. C. (1983) The use of early chick embryos in experimental embryology and teratology: improvements in standard procedures. *Teratology* **27**, 65–72.

Fisher C. J. and Sawyer R. H. (1980) The effects of triamcinolone on the development of the bursa fabricius in chick embryos. *Teratology* **22**, 7–12.

Fulton M. H. and Chambers J. E. (1985) The toxic and teratogenic effects of selected organophosphorus compounds on the embryo of three species of amphians. *Toxicol. Lett.* **26**, 175–180.

Gilani S., Bancroft J. and Reily M. (1978) Teratogenicity of ochratoxin A in chick embryo. *Toxicol. Appl. Pharmacol.* **46**, 543–546.

Gilbert E. F., Bruyere H. J. Jr., Ishikawa S., Foulke L. M. and Heimann S. R. (1980) Role of decreased cardiac output in isoproterenol-induced cardiovascular teratogenesis in chick embryos. *Teratology* **21**, 299–307.

Grala G. M. and Kaplan S. (1980a) Abnormally elevated blood pressure in trypan blue-treated chick embryo during early morphogenesis. *Teratology* **21**, 247–251.

Grala G. M. and Kaplan S. (1980b) The formation of caudal hematomas in trypan blue-treated chick embryo as a function of morphological stage at treatment. *Teratology* **21**, 265–269.

Greenaway J. C., Fantel A. G., Shepard T. H. et al. (1982) The *in vitro* teratogenicity of cyclophosphamide in rat embryos. *Teratology* **25**, 335–343.

Greener Y. and Kochen J. A. (1983) Methyl mercury toxicity in the chick embryo. *Teratology* **28**, 23–28.

Hirano A. and Kochen J. A. (1977a) Experimental lead encephalopathy. Morphologic studies. Vol. III. In: Zimmerman H. M. (ed.) *Progress in Neuropathology*, 319–341. New York and London: Grune and Stratton.

Hirano A. and Kochen J. A. (1977b) Relationship of blood and brain lead levels to morphologic changes in lead-induced chick embryo encephalopathy. I. Morphological studies. In: Roizin L., Shiraki H. and Grcevic N. (ed.) *First International Symposium of Neurotoxicology*, 307–308. New York: Raven Press.

Hoffman D. J., Eastin W. C. Jr. and Gay M. L. (1982) Embryotoxic and biochemical effects of waste crankcase oil on birds' eggs. *Toxicol. Appl. Pharmacol.* **63**, 230–241.

Homberger F. E. and Goldberg A. N. (1985) *In Vitro Embryotoxicity and Teratogenicity*. Basel: Karger.

Ishikawa S., Gilbert E. F., Bruyere H. J. Jr et al. (1978) Aortic aneurism associated with cardiac defects in theophylline stimulated chick embryos. *Teratology* **18**, 23–30.

Johnson E. M. (1980) A subvertebrate system for rapid determination of potential teratogenic hazards. *J. Environ. Pathol. Toxicol.* **4**, 153–156.

Johnson E. M. and Gabel B. E. G. (1982) Application of the hydra assay for rapid detection of developmental hazards. *J. Am. Coll. Toxicol*, **1**, 57–71.

Johnson E. M. and Gabel B. E. G. (1983) An artificial 'embryo' for detection of abnormal developmental biology. *Fund. Appl. Toxicol.* **3**, 243–249.

Kitos P. A., Wyttenbach C. R., Olson K. et al. (1981) Precision delivery of small volumes of liquid to very young avian embryos. II. Description of the injection system. *Toxicol. Appl. Pharmacol.* **59**, 49–53.

Klein N. W., Vogler M. A., Chatat C. L. et al. (1980) The use of cultured rat embryo to evaluate the teratogenic activity of serum: cadmium and cyclophosphamide. *Teratology* **21**, 199–208.

Kochen J. A. and Greener Y. (1974) Lead toxicity and tissue levels in the embryo. *Pediatr. Res.* **8**, 358.

Kochen J. A. and Greener Y. (1976) Lead encephalopathy: a consequence of capillary dysfunction. *Pediatr. Res.* **10**, 449.

Kochen J. A. and Greener Y. (1977a). Brain lead levels in hemorrhagic lead encephalopathy. *Pediatr. Res.* **11**, 563.

Kochen J. A. and Greener Y. (1977b) Microvascular injury in chick embryo lead encephalopathy. *Bibl. Anat.* **15**, 199–201.

Kochen J. A., Greener Y. and Hirano A. (1977) Relationship of blood and brain lead levels to morphologic changes in lead-induced embryo encephalopathy. II. Biochemical studies. In: Roizin L., Shiraki H. and Grcevic N. (ed.) *Neurotoxicology*, 309–311. New York: Raven Press.

Kochhar D. M. (1981) Embryo explant and organ cultures in screening of chemicals for teratogenic effects. In: Kimmel C. A. and Buelke-Sam J. (ed.) *Developmental Toxicology*, 303–319. New York: Raven Press.

Kolesari G. L. and Kaplan S. (1979) Amphetamines reduce embryonic size and produce caudal hematomas during early chick morphogenesis. *Teratology* **20**, 403–412.

Kuhlmann R. S., Kolesari G. L. and Kallifleisch J. H. (1983) Reduction of catecholamine-induced cardiovascular malformations in the chick embryo with metoprolol. *Teratology* **28**, 9–14.

Lee H. and Nagele R. G. (1979) Neural tube closure defects caused by papaverine in explanted early chick embryo. *Teratology* **20**, 321–332.

Meiniel R. (1981) Neuromuscular blocking agents and axial teratogenesis in the avian embryo. Can axial morphogenetic disorders be explained by pharmacological action upon muscle tissue. *Teratology* **23**, 259–271.

Mirkes P. E., Fantel A. G., Greenaway J. C. et al. (1981) Teratogenicity of cyclophosphamide metabolites: phosphoramide mustard, acrolein, and 4-ketocyclophosphamide in rat embryos cultured *in vivo*. *Toxicol. Appl. Pharmacol.* **58**, 322–330.

Mirkes P. E., Greenaway J. C., Rogers J. G. et al. (1984) Role of acrolein in cyclophosphamide teratogenicity in rat embryo *in vitro*. *Toxicol. Appl. Pharmacol.* **72**, 281–291.

Mirkes P. E., Greenaway J. C. and Shepard T. H. (1983) A kinetic analysis of rat embryo response to cyclophosphamide exposure *in vitro*. *Teratology* **28**, 249–256.

Misawa M., Doull J., Kitos P. A. et al. (1981) Teratogenic effects of cholinergic insecticides in chick embryos. I. Diazinon treatment of acetylcholinesterase and choline acetyltransferase additives. *Toxicol. Appl. Pharmacol.* **57**, 20–29.

Monis B. and Rovasio R. A. (1981) Teratogenic effects of lambda-carrageenan on the chick embryo. *Teratology* **23**, 273–278.

Nadeau J. H. and Mun A. M. (1978) The induction of axial blisters in chick embryo by trypan blue. *Teratology* **17**, 341–352.

Nakatsuji N. (1983) Craniofacial malformation in *Xenopus laevis* tadpoles caused by the exposure of early embryo to ethanol. *Teratology* **28**, 299–305.

New D. A. T. (1978) Whole-embryo culture and the study of mammalian embryos during organogenesis. *Biol. Rev.* **53**, 81–82.

Peterka M. and Jelinek R. (1983) Origin of hydrocortisone-induced orofacial clefts in chick embryo. *Cleft Palat. J.* **20**, 35–46.

Roy S., Hirano A., Kochen J. A. and Zimmerman H. M. (1974) Ultrastructure of cerebral vessels in chick embryo lead intoxication. *Acta Neuropath.*, **30**, 287–294.

Schardein J. L. (1985) *Chemically Induced Birth Defects*. New York: Dekker.

Schneider B. F. and Norton S. (1980) Neuronal damage in chick and rat embryos following X-irradiation. *Teratology* **22**, 303–309.

Steele C. E., Transler D. G. and New D. A. T. (1983a) An *in vivo/in vitro* evaluation of the teratogenic action of excess vitamin A. *Teratology* **28**, 209–214.

Steele C. E., New D. A. T., Ashford A. et al. (1983b) Teratogenic action of hypolipidemic agents: an *in vitro* study with post implantation rat embryos. *Teratology* **28**, 229–236.

Swartz W. J. (1980) Response of early chick embryos to busulfan. *Teratology* **21**, 1–8.

Verrette M. J., Scott W. F., Reynaldo E. F. et al. (1980) Toxicity and teratogenicity of food additive chemicals in the developing chick embryo. *Toxicol. Appl. Pharmacol.* **56**, 265–273.

Walton B. T. (1983) Use of the cricket embryo (*Acheta domesticus*) as an invertebrate model. *Fund. Appl. Toxicol.* **3**, 233–236.

Warner C. W., Sadler T. W., Shockey J. et al. (1983) A comparison of the *in vivo* and *in vitro* response of mammalian embryos to a teratogenic insult. *Toxicology* **28**, 271–282.

Weaver T. E., Kaplan S. and Grala M. G. (1981) Vascular hypervolemia and hematoma formation in chick embryos treated with trypan blue. *Teratology* **23**, 403–409.

Wilson J. G. (1978) Review of *in vitro* systems with potential for use in teratogenicity screening. *J. Environ. Pathol. Toxicol.* **2**, 149–167.

Wyttenbach C. R., Collins B., Thompson S. et al. (1981) Precision delivery of small volumes of liquids to very young avian embryos. I. Locating and positioning the embryo *in ovo*. *Toxicol. Appl. Pharmacol.* **59**, 40–48.

Chapter 11

Carcinogenicity Tests in Animals: Some Pitfalls That Could Be Avoided

Paul Grasso

INTRODUCTION

Laboratory animals had been employed in the study of biological phenomena long before cancer research became an established branch of the biological sciences, and these early workers noticed that if animals are kept till the end of their life span, they developed a number of tumours, some of which caused their demise (IARC 1973, 1976, 1979, 1983). This striking similarity to the development of cancer in man, where the highest incidence occurs in the last decades of life, could not have escaped the attention of these early workers, and may have been an important factor in creating a climate of opinion for the use of animals in research on cancer. It was then perhaps quite natural to think of using these animals as surrogates for man when Percival Pott in the United Kingdom and Rehn in Germany drew attention to the development of cancer from occupational exposure to soot on the one hand and to products of the dye industry on the other (Pott 1775; Rehn 1985).

The early experience in the use of animals in cancer research gave some justification to the view that animals may be sufficiently sensitive to serve as efficient models for the identification of carcinogens. First Yamagiwa (1918) and then others showed conclusively that tar and soot produced skin tumours when painted on to the shaved dorsal skin of rabbits and mice, and that the tumours were of the same type as the scrotal tumours in chimney sweeps. Furthermore, the identification of carcinogenic chemicals in soot and coal tar was possible because of the sensitivity of laboratory animals, in particular mice and rabbits, to these chemicals (Cook, 1983).

Attempts to reproduce bladder cancer in laboratory rodents, however, did not meet with much success until Hueper (1938) employed the dog, a non-rodent species, several years after Rehn's observations. Conversely, early Japanese workers showed that glucose and common salt could be carcinogenic in animals if given by subcutaneous injection (Grasso and Goldberg, 1966).

This early work provided a warning that although animals may be useful in detecting chemicals which possess a carcinogenic potential for man, they may also give misleading results. And yet these early warnings were largely ignored. It became widely accepted that chemicals which were carcinogenic for animals must also be carcinogenic for man. In support of this attitude, many would point out that chemicals (drugs and industrial chemicals) and processes which are carcinogenic to humans are also carcinogenic to laboratory animals (IARC, 1979) and consequently there is no alternative way for looking at positive animal data.

It is difficult to disagree with this view and yet commonsense would suggest that cancer, like many other human diseases, is very probably a multifactorial disease so that a mere increase in the incidence of tumours in a carcinogenicity test is not necessarily an indication that these tumours have been induced by the test substance. Over the years, experience has shown that a number of endogenous and environmental factors can lead to an increased incidence of tumours in experimental animals, chiefly rats and mice, and it is important to search for these factors to establish the extent to which they may be responsible for the production of tumours before assuming a causal relationship between an increased tumour incidence and the administration of a test chemical.

Some of the important criteria for validating a carcinogenicity study will be mentioned in the first part of this chapter. The role played by diet, genetics, viruses and hormones in influencing the natural incidence of tumours will be outlined in the second part, and the last section will contain a brief account of pathological changes that could lead to tumour formation irrespective of the nature of the test substance administered.

EVALUATION OF RESULTS

The objective of a carcinogenicity study is to determine the ability of a substance to enhance tumours in animals. An important first step is to establish whether any difference in tumour incidence could have occurred by chance. There are a number of statistical methods that could be used to achieve this end, and the subject is treated in detail by Peto (IARC, 1978). But even if the difference is statistically significant, it may not be sufficient to establish a cause and effect relationship. For example, let us take a hypothetical result of a long-term test in rats in which more lymphomas are reported in a treated group in males compared with controls. Statistically the difference is significant at the middle dose but not significant at the higher or lower dose. In females there is only a significant increase in tumour incidence at the lowest dose. Clearly there is no dose-response relationship here and despite statistical significance, there is a strong possibility that these results are a chance occurrence.

Dose-response Relationships

Over the last three or four decades several experiments have shown that the larger the dose of a carcinogen, the greater the number of tumours induced. In this respect, carcinogens resemble most other toxic and pharmacologic substances which elicit a stronger response as the dose administered is increased. The basis of the dose-response relationship of carcinogens was established by Druckery in the late 1950s and has been amply confirmed in subsequent experiments (Druckery and Schmahl, 1962). In my view, this link between dose and response is one of the most important pieces of evidence linking causally the test compound with an increased incidence of tumours. The greater the number of dose-levels used (within reason) the better can such a link be established. In practice three dose-levels have been found to be adequate.

Data from dose-response relationships are sometimes employed to estimate the expected tumour incidence at dose-levels very much lower than those which could possibly be employed in conventional experiments. A number of mathematical models have been employed in such estimates (FDA, 1971; IARC, 1980) and the results obtained vary considerably. Despite these uncertainties—and the possibly greater ones in extrapolating from animals to man—such models are often employed in some quarters to estimate the likely risk to man.

Nature and Type of Tumours Induced

Malignant and Benign Tumours

In order to establish the carcinogenic property of a test compound, some of the tumours induced must be malignant. Although there is no general agreement with this view it would seem illogical to label a compound as a 'carcinogen' unless it has been shown to induce 'cancer', and the word 'cancer' is widely held to be a fatal disease brought about by malignant tumours.

This statement does not mean that benign tumours are to be ignored. Chemical carcinogens induce both benign and malignant tumours and many hold that benign tumours may progress to become malignant (Foulds, 1975). Others hold the view that benign tumours represent an 'endpoint' and do not progress further. At the moment it is doubtful whether this controversy could be resolved since the evidence for either point of view is inconclusive, but the fact that both types of tumours of the same histogenetic origin occur in animals treated with carcinogens indicates that benign tumours must be taken seriously into account. In the writer's view, however, benign tumours do not have the same significance as malignant tumours and could be looked upon with a lower level of concern. The scheme recently devised by Squires supports this view and attempts to give some numerical rating score to it (Squires, 1981).

Types of Tumours Induced

Over the years, experience has shown that tumours arising in some organs (e.g. subcutaneous tissue, mammary gland tissue) are less reliable as an index of carcinogenicity than other types irrespective of their benign or malignant nature. Tumours of this sort often have a high and variable natural incidence which can often be altered by clearly definable factors unconnected with the test substance, or else they can be determined by factors which are clearly connected with local pathological changes in the target organ.

DIET

The first experiments designed to explore the effect of diet on cancer development were conducted on mice. The early workers directed their attention to the effects of restricted calorie intake or of a high fat, protein or carbohydrate diet on the natural incidence of tumours. Restriction of calorie intake was found to inhibit the formation of many types of tumours particularly those of the mammary gland and of the liver. For example, Tannenbaum (1947) compared the mammary tumour incidence in DBA mice maintained on a normal or restricted diet. One group received 2·0 g only of basic ration daily (normal consumption about 3·0 g) and the other group received the same amount of the basic diet but supplemented with an additional 1 g of corn starch . The average body weight of the mice on a restricted diet was in the range of 19 to 21 g while the others attained a normal size (29–31 g body weight). By 100 weeks of age about half the mice on the corn-starch supplemented diet had developed spontaneous mammary cancer. None had occurred in the calorie restricted group. This striking difference cannot be attributed to early deaths or disease from undernutrition since the mice on a restricted diet were more active and had a better fur than the mice on the supplemented diet and lived as long as the ones on an unrestricted diet.

In another experiment (Tannenbaum, 1942) female mice of the C3H strain (another strain of a high mammary tumour incidence) were fed *ad libitum* for 2, 5 or 9 months and then transferred to a calorie-restricted diet. It was found that calorie restriction was as effective when commenced at 9 months as when commenced at 2 months suggesting that the main effect of calorie restriction occurs at the time the tumour begins to develop.

The incidence of hepatomata is reduced as dramatically as that of mammary carcinoma by restricting the diet. In a series of observations Tannenbaum and Silverstone (1949) found that the incidence of tumours, measured in probits, was a straight-line function of the logarithm of the caloric intake. The incidence of other commonly occurring spontaneous tumours in mice, such as pulmonary adenomata and leukaemia (Tannenbaum, 1942; Saxton, 1944) was also reduced by calorie restriction but not to the same extent as mammary gland tumours or hepatomata.

Recent investigations by Tucker (1979) and Conybeare (1980) have confirmed the findings of the early investigators. Tucker (1979) showed that Charles Rivers mice on a 20% restriction of diet developed fewer hepatic tumours than mice allowed to feed *ad libitum*. This effect was more marked in females than in males, presumably reflecting the higher incidence of tumours in this sex. A marked reduction in the incidence of tumours of the pituitary, lung and lymph nodes also occurred. A reduction in the incidence of the same tumours was also observed by Conybeare (1980) in another strain of mice. This author reported that the incidence of liver tumours in his strain of mice fell from 47% to 12% by reducing food intake to 75% of the usual amount (approximately 5 g of diet). A reduction of pulmonary and lymphoid tumours was also observed by this dietary restriction.

Calorie restriction has some effect on induced tumours as well. A reduction in the incidence of sarcomata, induced by the injection of polycyclic aromatic hydrocarbons and of skin carcinomata by painting these compounds on the skin of mice was observed (Rusch et al., 1945; Tannenbaum and Silverstone, 1949) in calorie-restricted mice.

Some studies have been conducted to examine the relationship of the major components of the diet to tumour incidence. In one of the early studies (Watson and Mallanby, 1930) it was found that feeding mice on a diet containing a high percentage (about 20–25%) of butterfat, caused a definite increase in the incidence of skin tumours from the topical application of coal tar. This led to other investigations on the role of a high fat diet on the incidence of spontaneous tumours. It was found that mice fed high fat diets (up to 16–20%) developed more mammary tumours than mice of the same strain concurrently fed on a low fat diet. Furthermore, the tumours in the animals fed a high fat diet appeared significantly earlier. The same enhancement of tumour incidence occurred in the liver when the fat content of the diet was raised from 2% to 20% (Silverstone and Tannenbaum, 1951). High fat diets did not influence the incidence of spontaneous lung adenoma or leukaemia (Tannenbaum, 1942).

It is not known for certain whether a change in the total protein content of the diet can affect the incidence of tumours but a change in some of the constituent proteins can do so. Thus, a distinct increase in the incidence of hepatomata was observed when the casein content of the diet (maintained isocalorically) was increased from 9% to 18%. A further increase of the casein content (up to 45%) did not materially increase the incidence of hepatomata. This result was observed in more than one strain of mice and occurred in both males and females. The increase in tumour incidence does not appear to be due to an increase in the protein content *per se*, since the addition of 9% gelatin to 9% casein in the diet did not affect the incidence of hepatomata. On the other hand, supplementing a 9% casein diet with small amounts of methionine and cystine augmented the hepatoma incidence to that observed in mice on an 18% casein diet (Tannenbaum, 1959). Although an increase in the protein content of the diet may increase the incidence of spontaneous tumours there is some indication that induction of chemically induced tumours of liver are affected in the opposite way by the protein content of the diet. Thus Silverstone (1948) found that a high protein diet reduced the incidence of hepatic tumours induced by *p*-dimethylaminoazobenzene. Chemically induced tumours in sites other than the liver do not appear to be affected by the protein content of the diet.

The diet of rats may also exert a profound influence on both naturally occurring and chemically induced tumours (Tucker, 1979), while the observations of Ross and Bras (1965) indicate that the total incidence of tumours in untreated rats was directly and exponentially related to calorie intake.

In rats, as in mice, total protein intake would appear to influence tumour development. Rats on a high protein diet had a higher incidence of malignant lymphomas than rats on a low protein diet. In addition, the total tumour incidence was higher in this group than in the group with a low protein intake (Ross and Bras, 1965). Furthermore, Ross and Bras (1971) found that restriction of both the calorie and the protein content of the diet in early life had the same effect as if the restriction was carried out throughout the life-span.

The fat content of the diet also influences tumour incidence in rats. Benson et al. (1956) showed that rats developed a higher incidence of spontaneous mammary adenocarcinoma when olive oil was added to the diet and Chan and Dao (1981) observed a higher incidence of naturally occurring mammary tumours in Sprague–Dawley rats on a semisynthetic diet containing 16% corn oil, compared to rats on a standard laboratory chow diet.

Both the protein and fat content of the diet of rats may influence the chemical induction of tumours in certain organs. A high fat diet enhances the mammary tumour incidence induced by DMBA (Carroll and Khor, 1975) in Sprague–Dawley rats, the hepatocellular carcinomas induced by *p*-dimethylaminoazobenzene in the liver of rats from various strains (Miller and Miller, 1953), colon cancers by 1,2-dimethylhydrazine (Reddy et al., 1976) and the pancreatic adenocarcinomas by azaserine (Roebuck, 1981). A high protein diet may also lead to an increased tumorigenic response in liver and intestine to chemical carcinogens. Thus, the response of the rat to the development of hepatocellular carcinomas from aflatoxin (Madhaven, 1968) and of colon carcinomas from 1,2-dimethylhydrazine are enhanced by a high protein diet (Reddy et al., 1976).

These studies indicate that diet exerts an important influence on the natural incidence of liver, mammary and lymphoid tumours in mice, and mammary gland tumours in the rat. The total calorie content of the diet appears to be the most important factor in this respect but the composition of the diet, in particular the high fat or protein content, may also be important.

VIRUSES

Although under experimental conditions a variety of viruses are known to produce tumours in a number of organs in mice (Gross, 1978; Friend, 1977), only two naturally occurring tumours are known to have a viral aetiology, lymphomas and mammary adenocarcinomas.

The mouse lymphoma virus was discovered by Gross in 1951 while investigating an outbreak of malignant lymphoma in a colony of mice (Gross, 1978). This virus has now been characterized both immunologically and in terms of its molecular structure (Friend, 1977). It is not the only virus that is responsible for this disease in the mouse (Lilly and Pincus, 1973). The results of investigations carried out over several years revealed that most mice carry one or more of these lymphoma viruses. Only a few strains (e.g. Balb/c) appear to be exempt (Lilly and Pincus, 1973). Since not all mice that are allowed to live out their life span succumb to this disease, it would appear that the virus may exist in an unexpressed form. The factors that determine its expression are not clearly understood. The genetic constitution of the animal clearly has a major role (Lilly and Pincus, 1973). Other factors which may also be important are the strength and frequency of infection by the virus, the virulence of the strain and the adequacy of the antigenic response. These factors determine the onset and outcome of virus infections in most mammalian organisms and one would expect them to operate as well in the mouse. These factors probably also account for the variability in incidence which has been reported in several publications. This variability is quite marked both among inbred and outbred strains of mice (Lilly and Pincus, 1973). The unexplained early appearance of this type of tumour in some studies could also be accounted for by the multifactorial nature of this disease and may reflect a particularly heavy infection or a particularly weak host resistance.

A similar explanation could be advanced to account for the variability of mammary tumour incidence in mice. It is now widely acknowledged that mammary tumour development is determined principally by the presence of the mammary tumour virus (MTV) which is present in most strains of mice that exhibit a high natural incidence of these tumours (Squartini, 1979), but genetic and hormonal factors also play important roles (Nandi and McGrath, 1973). It is probable that these factors, as well as immunological defense mechanisms, may vary considerably in the strength with which they operate in individual mice and may account for the wide intra- and interstrain variability in mammary tumour incidence (Sher, 1974).

By comparison with the mouse, there is little knowledge of the role played by viruses in determining the incidence of tumours in rats. There is some suspicion, however, that viruses may play some role in the development of the mononuclear cell leukaemia, discovered by Moloney (1969) in the Fischer rat, and the mammary gland tumours found in the Sprague–Dawley rat. Both of these tumours have a high natural incidence (approximately 25% of untreated rats). Despite the fact that the natural history of these tumours (i.e. a high and variable incidence in untreated rats, and an early appearance of a few tumours) is strongly reminiscent of that of the virus-induced tumours in the mouse, there is no cultural or immunological evidence that viruses are involved in the genesis of these tumours (Young and Hallowes, 1973; Swaen and Van Heerde, 1973).

GENETIC FACTORS

Genetic factors appear to dominate the production of pulmonary tumours in mice. In a series of investigations involving many strains it was shown that hybrids of high-tumour and low-tumour strains resulted in F_1 generations that resembled the high-tumour strain. The back-cross generations resembled the strain to which the F_1 mice were mated. This was interpreted to indicate that susceptibility to the development of pulmonary tumours was inherited in a dominant manner (Heston and Vlahakis, 1961; Falconer and Bloom, 1964). According to Bentvelzen and Szalay (1966), a single gene appears to exert a major effect on the resistance of C57BL mice to the development of pulmonary tumours. In contrast, other investigators have found that the difference in susceptibility between a strain with low incidence (C57BL) and a strain with high incidence (strain A) is controlled by more than one pair of genes.

The pulmonary tumour incidence in the progeny of high- or low-tumour strains follows the pattern of the parent generation so that the incidence appears to be reasonably stable (Shimkin and Stoner, 1973). This stability, however, does not exclude a substantial variation in incidence when small groups of mice are compared with one another. Such variations are very probably due to chance.

Genetic factors play a less dominant role in the production of mammary tumours than they do in pulmonary tumours in mice. Nevertheless, many workers consider that the role they play is an important one.

It has been known for several years (Murray, 1911) that female mice are most prone to the development of mammary tumours when this tumour had occurred in their immediate ancestors. The later development of inbred strains confirmed this observation and demonstrated that the tumour incidence in BALB/c mice (a high incidence strain) maintained free from the mammary tumour virus is reasonably stable, suggesting that there is a genetic basis for its development. Recent work suggests that mammary tumour incidence in mice is influenced by an interplay of factors which include the level of hormones involved in the development of mammary gland tumours (principally prolactin and oestrogens), the responsiveness of mammary tissue to these hormones, the susceptibility of mammary tissue to infection, and to tumour formation by MTV (Nandi and McGrath, 1973).

Although genetic factors have been known to play an important role in the development of pulmonary and mammary tumours in mice, it is only comparatively recently that an important role has been assigned to genetic factors in the production of lymphoreticular tumours in this species.

For several years, attention had been directed to the viruses which appeared to have an aetiological relationship with the occurrence of these malignant tumours. Recent work, however, suggests that the genetic constitution of the host plays an important part in determining whether the viruses establish themselves in the target tissue and whether they produce any tumours (Lilly and Pincus, 1973). The identity of these genes is not known for certain, but a study of mice infected by Friend virus suggests that at least three genes are involved, namely: Fv-1, which governs the likelihood that infection by leukaemia virus will be successful; Fv-2, which governs the capacity of cell transformation; and H-2, which determines the host response to the tumour antigens (Lilly and Pincus, 1973). It would appear that these genetic factors are more important than is generally thought in the development of lymphomas in mice. According to several workers, the lymphoma virus genome is present in an unexpressed form in virtually all strains of mice; its expression may be determined by the genetic constitution of the host (Huebner et al., 1968, 1970). It is not certain if there is any genetic involvement in susceptibility to experimental induction of leukaemias (Laws, 1952).

There is some indication that genetic factors may also influence the incidence of hepatic tumours in mice. The clearest evidence comes from the work of Heston (1963) who showed that a 'viable yellow' gene is responsible for the high incidence of hepatic tumours in some strains of C3H mice. It is not known, however, whether genetic factors of this type are found in other strains of mice which also have a high incidence of tumours (e.g. CF strain) but Heston's work would lead one to suspect that the high incidence of tumours in such strains of mice is probably genetically determined.

Few systematic studies have been conducted on the rat to explore the role of genetic factors in determining the natural incidence of tumours and none of these are on the same scale depth as those conducted on the mouse. It is probable, however, that such factors may operate in the production of tumours which have a high natural incidence; for example, the atypical mononuclear leukaemia in the F344 rat and the mammary tumours in the Sprague–Dawley rat.

HORMONES

The role of hormones in determining the natural tumour incidence in mice and rats is poorly understood but, nevertheless, there are indications that they may play a very important part. The high incidence of mammary gland tumours in female but not in male mice was regarded by early workers as a strong indication that hormonal influences play a major role in the development of these tumours (Bittner, 1957). Earlier, Lacassagne (1936) and others had shown in a series of experiments that oestrogenic hormones caused both proliferative and neoplastic lesions in the mammary tissue of male mice and these results were reproducible.

More recently it has been shown that prolactin appears to be implicated as well as oestrogens in the production of these tumours (Gardner, Pfeiffer and Trentin, 1959).

Although the investigations of Lacassagne (1936) and others have indicated that hormones can, on their own, induce malignant tumours of mammary gland tissue, Nandi and McGrath (1973) seem to favour the view that hormones, under natural conditions, act largely indirectly by aiding the mammary tumour virus to become established in the mammary gland tissue or by promoting the production of precancerous lesions which would then progress to frankly malignant tumours. Thus, there seems to be a clear co-carcinogenic effect between hormones and the mammary tumour virus.

Hormones do not appear to exert such a clear influence on tumour development in other tissues, but there is some evidence suggesting that they may play an important role. The striking sex difference which exists in the natural incidence of hepatic tumours in mice have led to suggestions that some hormonal factors may be involved (Grasso and Hardy, 1975). Some confirmation of this view was obtained when it was demonstrated that both castration and hypophysectomy reduced the natural incidence in male mice (Heston, 1963), but no further confirmation of this hypothesis has been forthcoming despite the many experiments that have been carried out to investigate this phenomenon.

There does not appear to be any hormonal influence in the production of lymphomas or lung adenomas in this species.

In the rat there are two tumours which appear to be dependent on hormone production: pituitary and mammary gland tumours. Some strains of rats, for example the Wistar, have a high incidence of pituitary tumours. In this species, the incidence in female rats may be as high as 47% (Kroes, 1980). The pituitary is known to be regulated from the hypothalamus and at least one hormone called prolacting inhibiting factor (PIF) is involved in this regulatory control (Frantz, 1978). As in other glands, a disturbance in this control mechanism may result first in hyperplasia, and then in tumour production. In fact Russfield (1967) suggested that spontaneous hypothalamic failure in the ageing rat may be the cause of most pituitary tumours. At first, the rat pituitary tumours were thought to be non-secretory, but by refinements in staining techniques it is now known that a substantial proportion of these tumours are functional. The principal hormones they secrete are prolactin and growth hormones (Berkvens et al., 1980).

Various authors have suggested a possible association between the occurrence of pituitary tumours and mammary tumours in the rat. A high incidence of pituitary tumours occurs in the Sprague–Dawley and Wistar rats and is thought partially to account for the high natural incidence of mammary tumours in these strains of rats (Russfield, 1967; Murakoa et al., 1977).

There is also some indication that an increased incidence of tumours in other tissues may be associated with pituitary tumours. For example, pituitary tumours in rats appear to precede the occurrence of islet cell tumours of the pancreas (Murakoa et al., 1977; Kroes et al., 1980). These pancreatic tumours are more common in Wistar and Sprague–Dawley rats which have a high incidence of pituitary adenomas (Gillman et al., 1953; Rosen et al., 1961; Berg, 1967).

A similar picture would appear to occur also in the mouse but because the incidence of pituitary adenomas is much less frequent than in the rat it is difficult to establish an association between the two (Russfield, 1967b).

Thus, there would appear to be a link between the development of pituitary tumours and tumours of the mammary glands and of the pancreatic islet cells. Recent work suggests that pituitary tumours may also be associated with other endocrine abnormalities such as phaeochromocytomas, thyroid tumours, and testicular and ovarian tumours, giving rise to the concept of multiple-endocrine neoplasia (Bardjis, 1960, 1963; Rosen et al., 1961; Rowlatt, 1967).

THE ROLE OF TISSUE DAMAGE AND HYPERPLASIA IN THE PRODUCTION OF TUMOURS

So far we have evaluated the role of diet, viruses, genetics and endogenous hormone imbalance in influencing the occurrence of naturally occurring tumours in animals and we shall see later the way in which these might act as confounding factors. Other confounding factors may arise from chronic tissue damage induced by the compound. Experience has shown that such damage and the consequent reactive process may lead to an increased incidence of tumours irrespective of chemical nature of the agent. Examples of tumours induced in several organs will be presented to substantiate this view.

Tissue Damage and Subcutaneous Sarcoma

Early work revealed that sarcomas which developed at the site of subcutaneous injections could be readily induced by a wide variety of polycyclic aromatic hydrocarbon carcinogens and other carcinogens. This site proved to be more sensitive than the skin in detecting the carcinogenic activity of test chemicals since tumours could be induced with much smaller quantities than the amounts applied topically to mouse or rabbit skin. Furthermore, administration by injection was found to have two further advantages: accurate control of dosage, and prevention of oxidation by atmospheric oxygen (Grasso and Golberg, 1966).

In the early 1950s Oppenheimer discovered that sarcomas developed around cellophane films which he had wrapped around the kidneys of rats to induce hypertension (Oppenheimer et al, 1933). This accidental discovery led to a re-appraisal of the validity of this tumour as an indication of carcinogenic activity when induced by implantation of solids or by injection. In the course of these investigations, a variety of solids including polymeric materials, gold, silver and glass were implanted subcutaneously and all produced sarcomas (Bischoff and Bryson, 1964). In these investigations, it was customary to implant relatively large pieces (about 2 cm square) of solid material in the subcutaneous tissue of rodents. When smaller pieces of 0·5 cm or less were implanted no tumours at all appeared even though several pieces were implanted together at the same site.

It was at first thought that the tumours arose as a consequence of the molecular interaction at the interface between the test material and the surrounding tissue. However, this could not explain the total absence of tumours when a large number of small pieces were implanted subcutaneously where the possibility of the same reaction occurring was the same or greater. Attention then turned towards the nature of the tissue reaction. It was found that a florid reactive lesion made up of fibroblasts and macrophoges occurred around the large implants whereas the small implants were surrounded by a thin capsule of connective tissue. It was further shown that if a large implant was allowed to remain in the subcutaneous tissue for at least four months, then its removal was not followed by the resolution of the tissue reaction. Instead this reaction persisted and led to the development of local sarcomas (Bischoff and Bryson, 1964; Grasso and Golberg, 1966).

Subcutaneous sarcoma was also induced by injecting hyperosmolar, surface active, acidic or alkaline solutions subcutaneously once or twice weekly for 12 months or more. When these substances were administered at a concentration compatible with the mammalian tissue osmolality, pH or surface tension then no sarcomas were observed.

Injection of hyperosmolar, acidic, alkaline or surface active solutions is known to produce severe tissue damage and repeated injection of solutions of this sort at the same site led first to granulamatous reaction and then to severe tissue fibrosis which resembled the thick connective tissue capsule that developed around the large solid implants mentioned in the previous paragraphs. When the solutions injected were isoosmolar with tissue fluids, at neutral pH and without surface activity, then little or no reaction was induced (Grasso and Golberg, 1966; Grasso et al., 1971).

There is another group of compounds which when injected subcutaneously resulted in extensive tissue fibrosis and sarcoma. These were substances which possessed a viscosity similar to that of an oil and which were not absorbed easily from the site of injection. Examples of such substances are vegetable and mineral oil and polymeric materials in suspension (Grasso and Golberg, 1966).

It would, thus, appear that although carcinogens can produce tumours when injected repeatedly subcutaneously, so can many substances which are commonly regarded as innocuous and these do so by causing excessive tissue fibrosis and maintain the connective tissue in an active state.

Epithelial Tissues, Tissue Hyperplasia and Cancer

The determining nature of hyperplasia in the development of cancer is not limited to connective tissues. Tumours develop also in epithelial tissues if a state of hyperplasia is first induced and then maintained for some considerable time. This is exemplified by experiments involving chronic damage to the urothelium and skin epithelium.

The implantation of small pellets of wax or cholesterol or glass beads is known to induce transitional carcinoma of the bladder in both rats and mice. The tumour incidence varied from 1·2 to 15%. Attempts were made to explain this tumorigenic response on residues of carcinogens on the surface of these foreign bodies but careful cleaning of the pellets did not alter the outcome: carcinomas still appeared (Ball et al., 1964; Roe, 1964). A study of the local pathological changes in the urothelium revealed that both hyperplasia and metaplasia developed shortly after the implant was placed surgically inside the bladder and that a correlation existed between the changes in the urothelium and the development of tumours. Further light on the development of carcinoma in the urinary bladder of rodents from an implanted foreign body was shed by Flaks et al., (1973) in an important experiment on mice. These authors noted that

4-ethylsulphonylnaphthalene-1-sulphonamide (ESNS) was a potent carcinogen to the mouse bladder and that it produced both hyperplasia and stones as well as tumours. The urine in the treated animals was alkaline and the stones were thought to be due to this change in urinary pH. When the urine was corrected by the administration of NH_4Cl in the drinking water neither calculi nor tumours developed in the urinary bladders of the treated animals. Acidification of the urine led also to an amelioration of the hyperplasia. Whereas urothelial reaction was severe when stones were present, it was observed to be very mild when the urinary pH was brought back to normal.

Hyperplasia in the skin of mice would appear also to be important in the evolution of tumours. Narat (1925) and Schmahl (1984) have produced squamous cell carcinoma by repeated painting of sodium hydroxide or hydrochloric acid on mouse skin.

These experiments leave little room for doubt that hyperplasia is involved in the production of tumours both in the connective and the epithelial tissues of mice.

Liver Tumours in Rodents

Apart from the connective tissue and epithelial tissues of the skin and bladder, the liver provides yet another example of cancer development following prolonged periods of hyperplasia.

Tumours of the liver are induced more frequently than tumours in any other organ of the rodent by chemical carcinogens (ECETOC, 1982). A large proportion of hepatocarcinogens in rodents are non-genotoxic and include most of the chlorinated hydrocarbon carcinogens and substances such as phenobarbitone (Schulte-Hermann, 1974), BHT (Olsen, 1983) and selenium (Wilbur, 1980).

Most, if not all, non-genotoxic hepatocarcinogens either produce hepatocellular necrosis or some type of subcellular change such as SER hypertrophy, peroxisome proliferation, or increased lysosomal activity (Schulte-Hermann, 1974; Cohen and Grasso, 1981; ECETOC, 1982). Hepatocellular necrosis stimulates a reparative process which involves active cell proliferation. Continued damage to the liver leads to a cycle of cell necrosis and regeneration. This type of regenerative hyperplasia has been shown to induce hepatocellular carcinoma if maintained for a significant portion of the animal's lifetime (Eschenbrenner and Miller, 1945).

The subcellular changes in the liver mentioned earlier are almost invariably associated with liver enlargement, a process which involves an initial phase of hyperplasia. If the liver is maintained in an enlarged state by the continued administration of the chemical a subsequent and gradual increase in ploidy levels occurs (Schulte-Hermann, 1974) by a process of endonuclear reduplication. This process is considered to be the counterpart of hyperplasia (Brodsky and Uryvaeva, 1977). The continued replication of DNA which endonuclear reduplication entails would appear to be as prone to lead to the development of transformed cells as the replication that takes place prior to cell division since the majority of compounds that cause liver enlargement also cause tumours (Schulte-Hermann, 1974; Cohen and Grasso, 1981).

Experimentally Induced Hormonal Imbalance and Neoplasia

In a previous section we have indicated that a naturally occurring hormonal imbalance can influence significantly tumour induction. In this section we will indicate that hormonal imbalance brought about by test chemicals can be directly responsible for the induction of malignant tumours.

Some early experiments gave an indication that such a mechanism might operate under experimental conditions. Carter et al. (1976) mentioned the production of granulosa cell tumours in pieces of an ovary implanted underneath the capsule of internal organs or in the anterior chamber of the eye after a bilateral ovariectomy, while Mostofi et al. (1976) mentioned that Leydig cell tumours are readily induced in infantile rat testes implanted in the spleen of castrated rats. Obviously the pituitary gonatrophic hormones must have been responsible for the production of the tumours on both occasions, presumably because of the high levels achieved in the absence of 'feed-back' from the ovarian and testicular hormones. Pituitary tumours can be induced by techniques which either reduce or greatly increase the levels of circulating hormones. For example, experimentally produced chronic thyroid deficiency or excessive oestrogen levels may lead to an increased incidence of pituitary tumours (Watari and Tsukagoshi, 1968; Furth et al., 1976). Overproduction of the pituitary hormones themselves may result in tumours of the 'target' organs. For example, excessive production of TSH, such as may occur from the administration of thiourea, produces thyroid adenomas and carcinomas (Purves and Greisbach 1947); an excess of prolactin, such as may occur after the administration of reserpine, produces an increased incidence of mammary tumours (Welsch and Nagasawa 1977); while an excess of growth hormone may produce pancreatic islet tumours (Quitkin et al., 1978). Hormonal imbalance may lead to tumour production in paracrine organs as well, for example omeprazole, a suppressor of gastric acid secretion, may lead to a great increase in gastrin which in turn leads to the formation of carcinoids (Harvey et al., 1985).

These examples indicate that cancer in rodents can be induced by an interference with the physiological control mechanism that regulates hormonal balance. In general terms this imbalance involves an overproduction of a particular hormone, which in turn leads to an increased functional activity of the receptive gland. An increase in the number of functional cells would normally accompany glandular overactivity, so that hyperplasia is a feature of the response of the overstimulated gland. Since hormonally induced tumours have a long latent period, this overstimulation must have been present for several months before tumours appeared.

CONCLUSION

There is ample experimental evidence that tumours can be induced in animals by the administration of chemicals. All compounds which produce tumours in man also produce tumours in experimental animals and there would appear to be little doubt that animals can serve as a useful screen for assessing the carcinogenic activity of chemicals.

It would be foolish, however, to accept a mere increase in tumour incidence in test over control as clearly indicative of carcinogenic action. For logistic reasons carcinogenicity studies have to be conducted on groups of a few animals and a variable tumorigenic response between such groups may occur quite by chance. This variability may be greatly increased if the tumour has a high natural incidence, and we have outlined some of the factors which may, and often do, contribute to a high natural incidence of tumours in rats and mice. Critical attention to these factors is essential if one is to arrive at a valid causal relationship between test chemical and cancer production.

Attention needs also to be directed to any tissue injury or profound hormonal imbalance produced by the chemical at the dose-levels employed in the carcinogenicity test. If the test chemical clearly produces recognizable tissue injury at the dose-levels tested then serious consideration should be given to chronic damage and repair as possible causal factors in tumour production. The same considerations apply if there is any evidence of hormonal imbalance.

In such circumstances, strategically planned experiments can often help to unravel the role played by any one or more than one of these factors in tumour production. It cannot be stressed too strongly that if a mammalian cell is called to undergo repeated cycles of mitosis over and above that which would normally occur in the life-time of untreated animals, that cell is at a much greater increased risk of developing into a cancer. It is a moot point whether environmental carcinogens are involved in this process (a dividing cell being more prone to damage by such an agent than a resting cell), or whether the cell suffers spontaneous genetic error. The real issue is that the transformation was not brought about directly by the test compound. The test compound merely played a 'permissive' role by causing tissue changes which allowed such a transformation to take place.

In attempting to assess risk to man two points become clear:

1. If the increased tumour incidence is clearly due to the operation of diet, endogenous hormonal imbalance, viral infection, or genetics, then clearly the experiment does not indicate hazard to man. If the evidence is not clear then further studies should be undertaken to learn more about the role they might have played in causing an increase in tumour incidence.
2. If the evidence clearly incriminates tissue damage as playing a key role in the production of tumours then some safety factor or factors could be employed to estimate risk for man. It must be clearly stated, however, that demonstration of tissue injury as a causative factor in tumour production does not mean that there is no risk for man since tissue damage may lead to cancer in man as well as it does in animals.

REFERENCES

Ball J. K. et al. (1964) The carcinogenic and co-carcinogenic effects of paraffin wax pellets and glass beads in the mouse bladder. *Br. J. Urol.* **36**, 225.

Bardijis C. C. (1960) Pluriglandular syndrome. I. Multiple endocrine adenomas in irradiated rats. *Oncologia* **13**, 441.

Benson J., Lev M. and Grand C. G. (1956) Enhancement of mammary fibroadenomas in the female rat by a high fat diet. *Cancer Res.* **16**, 135–137.

Bentvelzen P. A. J. and Szalay G. (1966) Some genetic aspects of differences in susceptibility to the development of lung tumours between inbred strains of mice. In: Severi L. (ed.) (1965) *Lung*

Tumours in Animals, Proceedings of the 3rd Quadrennial Conference on Cancer, 835. University of Perugia.

Berg B. N. (1967) In: Cotchin E. and Roe F. J. C. (ed.) *Pathology of Laboratory Rats and Mice*, 102, Oxford: Blackwell Scientific.

Bischoff F. and Bryson G. (1964) Carcinogenesis through solid state surfaces. In: Homburger F. (ed.) *Progress in Experimental Tumour Research*, 85. Basle: Karger.

Bittner J. J. (1957) Recent studies on the mouse mammary tumour agent CMTA. *Ann. NY Acad. Sci.* **68**, 636.

Boot L. M. (1969) *Induction by prolactin of mammary tumours in mice*. Amsterdam: North-Holland Publishing Co.

Brodsky W. Y. and Uryvaeva I. V. (1977) Cell ploidy: its relation to tissue growth and function. *Int. Rec. Cytol.* **50**, 275.

Carroll K. K. and Khor H. T. (1975) Dietary fat in relation to tumorigenesis. *Prog. Biochem. Pharmacol.* **10**, 303–353.

Carter R. L. and Ird E. A. (1976) Tumours of the ovary. In: Turusov V. S. (ed.) *Pathology of Tumours in Laboratory Animals, Vol. 1*. Lyon: IARC.

Chan P. C. and Dao T. L. (1981) Enhancement of mammary carcinogenesis by a high fat diet in Fischer, Long–Evans and Sprague–Dawley rats. *Cancer Res.*, **41**, 164–167.

Cohen A. J. and Grasso P. (1981) Review of the hepatic response to hypolipidaemic drugs in rodents and assessment of its toxicological significance to man. *Food Cosmet. Toxicol.* **19**, 585–605.

Conybeare G. (1980) Effect of quality and quantity of diet on survival and tumour incidence in outbred Swiss mice. *Food Cosmet. Toxicol.* **18**, 65.

Cook J. W., Hieger O., Kennaway E. L. et al., (1932) The production of cancer by pure hydrocarbons—Part I. *Proc. Roy. Soc. B.* **iii**, 455.

Druckrey H. and Schmahl D. (1962) Quantitative Analyse der experimentellen Krebserzegung. *Naturwissenschaften* **49**, 19.

ECETOC (1982). *Heptocarcinogenesis in Laboratory Rodents: Relevance for Man*. Brussels: ECETOC.

Esschenbrenner A. B. and Miller E. (1945). Induction of hepatomas in mice by repeated oral administration of chloroform, with observation on sex differences. *J. Natl Cancer Inst.* **5**, 251.

Falconer D. S. and Bloom J. L. (1964) Changes in susceptibility to urethane-induced lung tumours produced by selective breeding in mice. *Br. J. Cancer* **18**, 322.

Flaks A. et al. (1973) Effect of ammonium chloride on incidence of bladder tumours induced by 4-ethylsulphonylnapthalene-1-sulphonamide. *J. Natl Cancer Inst.* **51**, 2007.

Food and Drug Administration Committee on Protocols for Safety Evaluation (1971). Panel on carcinogenesis report on cancer testing in the safety of food additives and pesticides. *Toxicol. Appl. Pharmacol.* **20**, 419–430.

Foulds L. (1975a) Introduction. *Neoplastic Development, Vol. 2*, 6. London: Academic Press.

Foulds L. (1975b) *Neoplastic Development, Vol. 2*, 345. London: Academic Press.

Frantz A. G. (1978) Physiology in medicine. *N. Eng.. Med.* 298, 201–207.

Friend C. (1977) The coming of age of tumour virology. *Cancer Res.* **37**, 1255–1263.

Furth J. (1955) Experimental pituitary tumours. *Recent Prog. Horm. Res.* **ii**, 221.

Gardner W. U., Pfeiffer C. A. and Trentin J. J. (1959) Hormonal factors in experimental carcinogenesis. In: Homberger F. (ed.) *The Physiopathology of Cancer*, 2nd ed., 152. New York: Holber-Harper.

Gillman J., Gilbert C, and Spense I. (1953) Phaeochromocytoma in the rat. Pathogenesis and collateral reactions and its relation to comparable tumours in man. *Cancer* **6**, 494.

Grasso P., Gangolli S. D., Golberg L. et al. (1971) Physico-chemical and other factors determining local sarcoma production by food additives. *Food Cosmetic. Toxicol.* **9**, 463–478.

Grasso P. and Golberg L. (1966) Subcutaneous sarcoma as an index of carcinogenic potency. *Food Cosmet. Toxicol.* **4**, 297–320.

Grasso P. and Hardy J. (1975) Strain difference in natural incidence and response to carcinogens. In: Butler W. H. and Newberne P. M. (ed.) *Mouse Hepatic Neoplasia*. Amsterdam: Elsevier.

Gross L. (1978) Viral aetiology of cancer and leukaemia—a look into the past, present and future (GHA Clowes Memorial Lecture) *Cancer Res.* **38**, 485–493.

Harvey R. H., Bradshaw M. J., Davidson C. M. et al. (1985) Multifocal gastric carcinoid tumours, achlorhydria and hypergastrinaemia. *Lancet* April 27, 951–952.

Heston W. E. (1963) Complete inhibition of occurrence of spontaneous hepatomas in highly susceptible (C3H × YBR) F_1 male mice by hypophysectomy. *J. Natl Cancer Inst.* **31**, 467–474.

Heuper W. C., Wiley F. H. and Wolfe H. D. (1938) Experimental production of bladder tumours in dogs by the administration of beta-naphthylamine. *J. Ind. Hyg.* **20**, 146.

Heubner R. J. and Todaro G. J. (1969) Oncogenesis of RNA tumour viruses as determinants of cancer. *Proc. Natl Acad. Sci. (USA)* **64**, 1087.

Huebner R. J., Kelloff F. J. Sarma P. S. et al. (1970) Group-scientific antigen expression during embryogenesis of the genome of the C-type RNA tumour virus: implication for ontogenesis and oncogenesis. *Proc. Natl. Acad. Sci.* (USA) **67**, 366.

IARC (Turusov V. S. (ed. in chief)) *Pathology of Tumours in Laboratory Animals*: (1973, 1976) *Vol 1 Tumours of the Rat*; (1979) *Vol. 2 Tumours of the Mouse*; (1983) *Vol. 3 Tumours of the Hamster*. Lyon: IARC.

IARC (1979) Chemical and industrial processes associated with cancer in humans. *Monographs on the evaluation of the carcinogenic risk of chemicals to humans*. Lyon: IARC.

IARC (1980) Long-term and short term screening assays for carcinogens: a critical appraisal. *Monographs on the evaluation of the carcinogenic risk of chemicals to humans. Supplement 2.* Lyon: IARC.

Kroes R., Garbis-Berkvens J. M., deVries T. and van Nesselrooy J. H. J. (1986) Histopathological profile of a Wistar rat stock including a survey of the literature. (In press.)

Lacassagne A. (1936) A comparative study of the carcinogenic action of certain estrogenic hormones. *Am. J. Cancer* **28**, 735–740.

Law L. W. (1952) The flexed tail anaemia gene(s) and induced leukaemia in mice. *J. Natl Cancer Inst.* **12**, 1119.

Lilly F. and Pincus T. (1973) Genetic control of murine viral leukaemogenesis. *Adv. Cancer Res.* **17**, 231.

Madhavan T. V. and Gopalan C. (1968) The effect of dietary protein on carcinogenesis by aflatoxin. *Arch. Pathol.* **85**, 133–137.

Miller J. A. and Miller E. C. (1953) The carcinogenic aminoazodyes. *Adv. Cancer Res.* **1**, 339–396.

Moloney W. C., Boschetti A. E. and King V. P. (1969) Observation on leukaemia in Wistar Furth rats. *Cancer Res.* **29**, 938

Moon H. D., Koneff A. A., Li C. H. et al. (1956) Phaeochromocytomas of adrenals in male rats chronically injected with pituitary growth hormone. *Proc. Soc. Exp. Biol.* **93**, 74–77.

Mostofi F. K. and Bresler V. M. (1976) Tumours of the testis. In: Turusov V. S. (ed.) *Pathology of Tumours in Laboratory Animals: Vol. 1 Tumours of the Rat,* Part 2 (IARC Scientific Publication No. 5). Lyon: IARC.

Murakoa Y., Itoh M., Yamashita F. et al. (1977) Spontaneous tumours in aged SD–JCL rats. *Exper. Anim.* **26**, 13.

Murray J. A. (1911) Cancerous ancestry and the incidence of cancer in mice. *Scie. Rep. Invest. Imp Cancer Res. Fund* **4**, 114.

Nandi S. and McGrath C. M. (1973) Mammary neoplasia in mice. *Adv. Cancer Res.* **17**, 353.

Narat J. K. (1925) Experimental production of malignant growths by simple chemicals. *J. Cancer Res.* **9**, 135.

Olsen P., Bille N. and Meyer O. (1983) Hepatocellular neoplasms in rats induced by butylated hydroxytoluene. *Acta Pharmocol. Toxicol* **53**, 433–434.

Oppenheimer B. S., Oppenheimer E. T. and Stout A. P. (1953) Carcinogenic effect of imbedding various plastic films in rats and mice. *Surg. Forum* **4**, 672.

Pott P. (1775) *Chirurgical Observations*.

Purves H. D. and Griesbach W. E. (1947) Studies on experimental goitre, VIII. Thyroid tumours in rats treated with thiourea. *Br. J. Exp. Path.* **28**, 46–53.

Quitkin F., Rifkin A., Kane J. et al. (1978) Long-acting oral *vs* injectable antipsychotic drugs in schizophrenics. A one-year double-blind comparison in multiple episode schizophrenics. *Arch. Gen. Psych.* **35**, 889.

Reddy B. S., Narisawa T., Vukusich D. et al. (1976) Effects of quality and quantity of dietary fat and dimethyl hydrazine in colon carcinogenesis in rats. *Proc. Soc. Exp. Biol. Med.* **151**, 237–239.

Rehn L. (1895). Über Blasentamoren bei Fuchsinarbeitern. *Arch. Klin. Chir.* **50**, 588.

Roe F. J. C. (1964) An illustrated classification of the proliferative and neoplastic changes in mouse bladder epithelium in response to prolonged irritation. *Br. J. Urol.* **36**, 238.

Roebuck B. D., Yager J. D. and Longnecker D. S. (1981) Dietary modulation of azaserine induced pancreatic carcinogenesis in the rat. *Cancer Res.* **41**, 888–893.

Rosen V. J., Castanera T. J., Jones D. C. et al. (1961) Islet cell tumours of the pancreas in the irradiated and non-irradiated rat. *Lab. Invest.* **10**, 608.

Ross M. H. and Bras G. (1965) Tumour incidence patterns and nutrition in the rat. *J. Nut.* **87**, 245–260.

Rusch H. P., Johnson R. O. and Kline B. E. (1945) The relationship of caloric intake and of blood sugar sarcogenesis in mice. *Cancer Res.* **5**, 705–712.

Russfield A. B. (1967) Pathology of the endocrine glands, ovary and testis of rats and mice. In Cotchin E. and Roe F. J. C. (ed.) *Pathology of Laboratory Rats and Mice*, 391. Oxford: Blackwell Scientific.

Saxton J. A. Jn., Boon M. C. and Furth J. (1944) Observations on the inhibition and development of spontaneous leukaemia in mice by underfeeding. *Cancer Res* **4**, 401–409.

Schmahl D. (1984) Carcinogenic activity of KOH and NaOH by topical application to mice. In: Schmahl D. (ed.) *Maligne Tumoren—Entstehung Wachtsum Chemotherapie*, 290–291.

Schulte-Hermann R. C. (1974) Induction of liver growth by xenobiotic compounds and other stimuli. *Crit. Rev. Toxicol.* **13**, 97–158.

Sher A. P. (1974) Tumours in control mice—literature tabulation. *Toxicol. Appl. Pharm.* **30**, 337–359.

Shimkin M. B. and Stoner G. D. (1975) Lung tumours in mice: application to carcinogenesis bioassay. *Adv. Cancer Res.* **21**, 1.

Silverstone H. (1948) The levels of carcinogenic azo dyes in the livers of rats fed various diets containing *p*-dimethylaminozobenzene: relationship to the formation of hepatomas. *Cancer Res.* **8**, 301–308.

Silverstone H. and Tannenbaum A. (1951) The influence of dietary fat and riboflavine on the formation of spontaneous hepatomas in the mouse. *Cancer Res.* **11**, 200–203.

Squartini F. (1979) Tumours of the mammary gland. In Turusov V. S. (ed.) *Pathology of Tumours in Laboratory Animals*: *Vol. 2 Tumours of the Mouse* (IARC Scientific Publication No. 23.) Lyon: IARC

Squires R. A. (1981) Ranking animal carcinogens: a proposed regulatory approach. *Science* **214**, 877–880.

Swaen G. J. V. and Heerde Van P. (1973) Tumours of the haematopoietic system. In Turusov V. S. (ed.) *Pathology of Tumours in Laboratory Animals: Vol. 1 Tumours of the Rat* (IARC Scientific Publication No. 5.) Lyon: IARC.

Tannenbaum A. (1942a) The genesis and growth of tumours. II. Effect of caloric restriction *per se*. *Cancer Res.* **2**, 460.

Tannenbaum A. (1942b) The genesis and growth of tumours. III. Effects of a high fat diet. *Cancer Res.* **2**, 468–475.

Tannenbaum A. (1947) The role of nutrition in the origin and growth of tumours. In: *Approaches to Tumour Chemotherapy*, 96–127. Lancaster: Pa Science Press.

Tannenbaum A. (1959) Nutrition and cancer. In: Homburger F. (ed.) *Physiopathology of Cancer*, 517–565. New York: Hoebe-Harper.

Tannenbaum A. and Silverstone H. (1949) The influence of the degree of caloric restriction on the formation of skin tumours and hepatomas in mice. *Cancer Res.* **9**, 724–727.

Tucker M. J. (1979) The effect of long-term food restriction on tumours in rodents. *Int. J. Cancer* **23**, 803–807.

Watari N. and Tsukagoshi N. (1968) Electron-microscopic observations on the estrogen-induced pituitary tumours. In: *Gunma Symposium on Endocrinology, Vol. 6*, 297.

Watson A. E. and Mellanby E. (1930) Tar cancer in mice. II. The condition of the skin when modified by external treatment or diet, as a factor in influencing the cancerous reaction. *Br. Exper. Path.* **11**, 311.

Welsch C. W. and Nagasawa H. (1977) Prolactin and murine mammary tumourigenesis: a review. *Cancer Res.* **37**, 951–963.

Wilbur C. G. (1980) Toxicology of selenium—a review. *Clin. Toxicol.* **17**, 171–230.

Yamagiwa K. and Ichikawa K. (1918) Experimental study of the pathogenesis of carcinoma. *J. Cancer Res.* **3**, 1.

Yound G. and Hallowes R. C. (1973) Tumours of the mammary gland. In: Turusov V. S. (ed.) *Pathology of Tumours in Laboratory Animals: Vol. 1. Tumours of the Rat* (IARC Scientific Publication No. 5). Lyon: IARC.

Chapter 12

Experimental Approaches to the Design and Assessment of Antidotal Procedures

Timothy C. Marrs

The introduction into clinical practice of a new antidotal procedure for a poison is generally the culmination of a large amount of experimental work (*Fig.* 12.1). This may include some or all of the following processes:

1. Determination of toxic effects in experimental animals, together with the nature of the target organ.
2. Study of the absorption, distribution and excretion of the toxicant in several animals species together with its metabolism.
3. Identification of animal models in which the poisoning may be studied.
4. Identification of a promising antidotal procedure based on knowledge of the behaviour of the poison in the body.
5. Antidotal efficacy studies in experimental animals.
6. Studies on the toxicity of the proposed antidote.

At all points in the work, any information available from experience in human poisoning will be extremely valuable. Although such exposures will by their nature be uncontrolled, and important features, such as the dose of toxicant, unknown, they may provide considerable assistance in extrapolating animal data to man.

ACUTE TOXICITY OF THE TOXICANT

The LD_{50} test has attracted criticism (e.g. Brown, 1983; British Toxicology Society Working Party on Toxicity, 1984). Indeed it has been stated (Rumack and Peterson, 1980) that the LD_{50} and MLD, gained from animals, are of little clinical use in the management of poisoned patients. There are, however, instances in experimental clinical toxicology where a detailed estimate of lethality is required. Notably, some measure of toxicity is needed for the design and interpretation of experiments in which the efficacy of antidotal procedures is to be assessed. This use of the LD_{50} test is further discussed on page 296. Secondly, marked interspecies differences in acute toxicity, such as occur with ethylene glycol (Gessner et al., 1961; Patty, 1963), may be an indication that particular

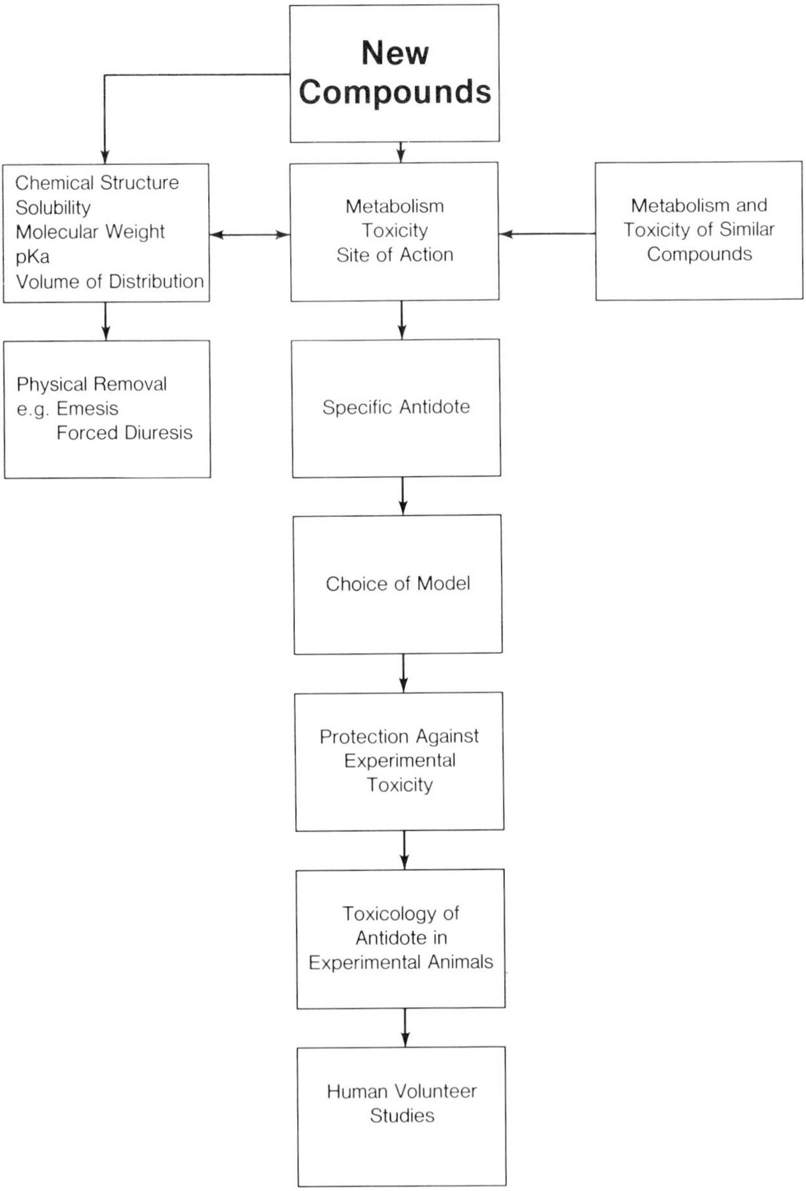

Fig. 12.1. Flow-diagram of approach to antidotal therapy for a new poison.

care will have to be taken with choice of animal model. Careful planning at this point is essential to ensure the validity of the work whilst keeping the number of animals used to a minimum.

The LD_{50} should be determined in more than one species using the route of administration by which the toxicant is usually taken. It should be in its usual physical state, and with substances such as drugs and pesticides, considerations of formulation are important. Because the slope of the log dose-probit mortality line may give some indication of the mode of action, that also should be recorded. Furthermore, the slope as well as the LD_{50} of a substance may be altered by antidotal treatment (Natoff and Reiff, 1970). In order to obtain the greatest possible amount of information, examination both of decedents and survivors should be undertaken at autopsy, since this may give some indication of organ-specific toxicity.

Additional single-dose toxicity studies may be necessary in special circumstances. Thus, if a delayed effect of the toxicant is sought, the animals may have to be retained for a longer period than is usual during LD_{50} tests. Compounds in which delayed toxicity is important include the organophosphate pesticides and nerve agents (Aldridge et al., 1969; Murphy, 1980) and carbon monoxide (Garland and Pearce, 1967). In these and in other cases where survival of sublethal doses of a poison give rise to crippling sequelae (e.g. blindness in methanol poisoning), it may be adjudged that treatment should be directed at ameliorating that effect, as well as preventing death. In such cases, acute studies should include the ED_{50} (effective dose in 50% of the animals) for the effect in question.

CHOICE OF ANIMAL MODEL

Further study of the behaviour of the toxicant brings one to the central problem in experimental clinical toxicology: the problem of the choice of animal model for the poisoning in humans. It must be borne in mind that during the development of antidotal procedures the model will have to serve for study of both the toxicant and the antidote, as well as their interactions *in vivo*. Before any antidote has been proposed, the only basis for the choice of experimental model is comparison of the effects of the poison in animals and in man. This means that at this stage a model cannot be chosen with certainty. Therefore, probably the best course is to study the response of several species to the toxicant, in the expectation that one or more of them will also resemble man in his response to the antidote.

Amongst the determinants of choice of animal model are differences or similarities in absorption, distribution and excretion of the toxicant together with its metabolism. Unfortunately it is also necessary to consider other factors, such as availability and cost of animals and animal husbandry. This is especially the case since use of the larger and more expensive animals, or unusual ones, will tend to limit the numbers that can be studied. Another consideration which may enter into the decision is the availability of information in the scientific literature on the handling of xenobiotics by particular species. It is necessary to make a judgement on the basis of all these factors, weighing carefully metabolic and toxicological considerations on the one hand, and factors such as expense and availability on the other.

Source of Interspecies Variation

Interspecies differences in response to toxicants may arise from dissimilarities in absorption, distribution, metabolism, excretion or receptor response. Because such differences may arise in so many ways, it is only possible to indicate some of the more important ones affecting toxicants and antidotes.

Interspecies Differences in Absorption, Distribution and Excretion

The most important factors to consider during absorption of the toxicant are those affecting the similarity of the experimental model to man in respect of the route of entry into the body by which poisoning usually takes place. In many cases this will be by mouth, in which case it is important to bear in mind that there are considerable anatomical differences between ruminants and other animals. Additionally, since small alterations in pH may profoundly affect ionization of weak electrolytes (Moffat, 1978), species differences in gastrointestinal pH will cause absorption differences. Where the poisoning normally occurs after percutaneous absorption, interspecies differences in rate of entry by that route will have to be considered. These have been reviewed by Calabrese (1983) who concluded that the pig and monkey most closely approximate to the human in skin absorption capability.

Included amongst substances in which significant interspecies differences exist in absorption after oral administration is pentobarbitone (Hume et al., 1968); this drug is significantly more slowly absorbed through the gastric mucosa of humans than that of dogs or rats. Several ways around this type of problem are possible. One is to give the poison parenterally either by slow intravenous infusion or intramuscularly, but this avoids any first pass effect. In small laboratory animals the intraperitoneal route may be used. A problem with using any route other than the oral one to study poisoning which takes place after ingestion is that it represents a departure from the clinical situation which the animal is supposed to model. It will certainly make the design of protection and therapy experiments more difficult, and careful attention will have to be paid to time relationships between giving the poison and administering the antidote.

Many antidotes are given intravenously in clinical practice, in which case it is logical to do the same in the animal model during therapy studies. No problem thus arises from different gastrointestinal absorptive capacities. In instances where the antidote is normally given by mouth, e.g. methionine for paracetamol poisoning (Vale et al., 1981), similar considerations of interspecies differences in absorptive capacity will have to borne in mind both with the antidote and the poison.

Another cause of interspecies differences in response to toxicants is the extent of plasma protein binding. Sturman and Smith (1967) investigated the effect of this on salicylate added to human plasma, and also plasma from a variety of animal species. The rhesus monkey, rabbit and guinea-pig resembled man in having a relatively high affinity for binding salicylate, whilst the baboon, horse, dog, rat, mouse, turkey and toad had a low binding capacity. With amphetamines, human blood has a relatively low plasma protein-binding capability; Baggot et al. (1972) determined the extent of plasma protein binding *in vitro* by equilibrium dialysis using radionucleide labelled-amphetamine at a concentration of 10^{-6} mol l^{-1}. Plasma from all the mammals they studied bound a greater proportion of the amphetamine than did human plasma. A large number of important toxicants are bound to a greater or lesser extent by plasma proteins, including cyanide (Christel et al., 1977) which is reported to be bound to plasma proteins in dogs to the extent of about 60%: morphine (Baggot and Davis, 1973) and many heavy metals are amongst other compounds found to be protein bound. Since methods are available for the determination of protein binding in human and animal plasma *in vitro*, and such methods are fairly straightforward, the procedure should be carried out as a preliminary to the choice of animal model. It should, of course, be remembered that as the blood concentration of the toxicant increases, the fraction of the drug unbound increases, so that plasma protein binding studies of compounds at low, or in the case of drugs, therapeutic concentrations are not reliable guides to the situation in overdose (Rosenburg et al., 1981). Protein binding studies should be designed accordingly.

Examples of antidotes showing a degree of plasma protein binding include the chelating agent D-penicillamine (Neugebauer, 1977) and the morphine antagonists naloxone and nalorphine (Misra et al., 1976). Reuning et al. (1977) investigated the plasma protein binding of another morphine antagonist, naltrexone, in six species including man, monkey and guinea-pig. The proportion of the drug bound to plasma protein varied from 20% to 26%.

With some poisons, biliary or urinary excretion (particularly the former) may be important processes which influence the choice of model, and there is evidence for interspecies differences in the biliary excretion of a number of foreign compounds. Abou-el-Makarem et al. (1967) classified animals into three groups; poor, good and intermediate excretors. Monkeys fall into the poor group, and Calabrese (1983) suggests that man may be similar. Biliary excretion of xenobiotics has been fully reviewed by Klaasen and Watkins (1984).

Interspecies Differences in Metabolism

Among the most frequent causes of differences in susceptibility of various species to toxicants are dissimilarities in intermediary metabolism. Because metabolic differences may also affect the response to antidotes, the subject is a complex one in so far as it affects the experimental treatment of poisoning. The variety of known interspecies differences is very great (Burns, 1970; Testa and Jenner, 1976; Calabrese, 1983), therefore only a few of the most important ones affecting toxicants and antidotes are discussed.

With respect to phase I reactions, several notable species differences have been reported. Dring et al. (1970) showed that 60% of a dose of ^{14}C-labelled amphetamine was excreted as *p*-hydroxyamphetamine by rats in 24 hours, whilst over the same period men excreted only 3% in that form: the largest fraction in man appearing in the urine was unchanged amphetamine. This difference in aromatic *p*-hydroxylation extends to a number of similar drugs (Williams et al., 1973). The oxidation of methanol is the subject of another important interspecies difference. The work of Tephly et al. (1964) suggests that a peroxidative system involving hepatic catalase plays an important role in methanol oxidation in rats, and that this system is not primarily responsible for oxidation of ethanol. In monkeys the toxicity of methanol is abolished by 4-methylpyrazole, an inhibitor of alcohol dehydrogenase, so the difference in toxicity between the monkey and the rat probably lies in the specificity of alcohol dehydrogenase (Clay et al., 1975). Because the acidosis found in methanol poisoning in humans can only be reproduced experimentally in primates, no other animals can satisfactorily be used as the experimental model for human methanol intoxication. Clay et al. (1975) showed that the metabolic dissimilarities extended to primates, the rhesus monkey only sometimes developing acidosis, whilst the pigtail macaque reliably did so. Another alcohol metabolized by alcohol dehydrogenase and giving rise to metabolic acidosis is ethylene glycol. Gessner et al. (1961) showed that cats form much more oxalic acid in response to a dose of ethylene glycol than rabbits and guinea-pigs, a fact which is paralleled by a lower lethal dose in the cat. Man appears to resemble the cat in susceptibility to ethylene glycol poisoning (Troisi, 1950; Gessner et al., 1961), rendering the use of small laboratory animals unsuitable as a model for man in this poisoning. In the metabolism of the important organophosphate group of compounds, several species differences in metabolism have been reported. Thus, hepatic demethylation of dimethylvinphos occurs to a greater extent in dogs than in rats, accounting for LD_{50}s of less than 200 mg kg^{-1} in rats, and greater than 2 g kg^{-1} in dogs (Crawford et al., 1976). Another species difference affecting organophosphate metabolism was demonstrated by Mendoza et al. (1977), who showed significantly different esterase activities toward three organophosphate compounds, malaoxon, fenitroxon and paroxon, in sera from a number of mammalian species.

Amongst important species differences in phase II reactions is the failure of cats to form glucuronides with a number of substances such as phenol (Capel et al., 1972). This defect, which is not a complete one, extends to morphine (Millburn, 1974) and to paracetamol (Savides et al., 1984). Caution should be exercised in extrapolating findings on the effects of aromatic substances from cats to humans.

Species differences in the metabolism of substances used as antidotes are perhaps less common, but include the opiate antagonist naltrexone (Reuning et al., 1975), where the ratios of α- and β-naltrexol appearing in the urine varies with species. With the cyanide antidote 4-dimethylaminophenol, substantial differences exist in the urinary excretion products in man, dog and rat (Eyer and Kiese, 1976; Eyer and Gaber, 1978; Eyer and Kampffmeyer, 1978; Jancso et al., 1981; Klimmek et al., 1983).

An unusual and interesting example of species difference in enzymic activity against a substance which can be both a poison and an antidote is responsible for differences in susceptibility to atropine. Esterase activity, capable of hydrolysing atropine, is found in rat and guinea-pig serum, but not usually in that of humans: interestingly, only a proportion of rabbits possess atropine esterase activity, an example of intraspecies variation (Szoradi et al., 1970; Weiner, 1980).

In their review of drug metabolism in non-human primates, Smith and Caldwell (1977) tabulated similarities and differences in metabolism of 23 drugs by rhesus monkeys, man and rats, and other non-primate species. Primates generally appeared to have a considerable advantage over other animals as metabolic models for man, but there were sufficient exceptions to render an uncritical use of primates unwise. If primates be used, it should be remembered that they are not metabolically homogeneous, and different species of primates, even closely related ones, may show metabolic dissimilarities: thus, as is discussed above, rhesus and pigtail macaques differ in their response to methanol (Clay et al., 1975).

The species most used in experimental toxicology are dogs, rabbits and rodents. Non-mammals have been used rarely because of major differences from man in structure, physiology and biochemistry. An important exception is the use of hens to detect delayed neurotoxicity caused by organophosphates (Aldridge et al., 1969; Murphy, 1980). In this unusual instance the 70-day-old hen is regarded as the only animal model completely suitable for demonstrating the effect.

Other Considerations in Choice of Model

In certain types of poisoning, factors other than those discussed above may enter into the choice of animal model. In complex behavioural studies, ability of the animal to perform the test may loom larger than considerations of toxicological similarity to man. In the study of poisons acting at pharmacological receptors, differences in their specificity, distribution and density must be considered. This factor may affect important toxicants such as the opiates (Buatti and Pasternak, 1981).

Choice of Model—Conclusions

Ultimately the choice is made by comparing data on the metabolism of toxicology of the poison with that obtained from humans. Comparison of urinary excretion products in man and laboratory animals is particularly helpful. The former may come from volunteer studies, or case reports of overdosage with drugs, or from accidental or other contaminations with pesticides and industrial chemicals. Manufacturers may possess relevant information.

TYPE OF THERAPY AND EXPERIMENTAL APPROACH

Although regimens available for the treatment of poisoning show a spectrum of specificity, it is frequently convenient to divide them into non-specific physicochemical methods, and more or less specific antidotes (Goldstein et al., 1979). Physicochemical methods prevent absorption from the gastrointestinal tract, or hasten the removal of toxicants from the body. They include gastric lavage, emesis and the administration of activated charcoal. The last method has achieved some popularity (Saxena and Kingston, 1982; Prescott, 1983), but has to be given fairly soon after poisoning if a successful outcome is to be achieved.

Measures that work by removal of poisons from the body include charcoal haemoperfusion (Volans et al., 1977; Raper et al., 1982), peritoneal dialysis and haemodialysis (Watanabe, 1977). The main factors determining the efficacy of the dialysis procedures are the molecular weight of the compound, its volume of distribution and extent of plasma protein binding.

The main method used to hasten excretion through the urinary tract is forced diuresis. In salicylate poisoning the pH of the urine is rendered alkaline by the infusion of sodium bicarbonate or citrate (forced alkaline diuresis). The rationale depends on two factors: one is highly non-specific, namely greater urine flow; the other, ion trapping, depends on the relationship between urinary pH and the pK_a of salicylate (3·2). Alkalinization of the urine increases ionization of the salicylate, and hence decreases renal tubular reabsorption (Hill, 1973). Forced alkaline diuresis has been used with a number of drugs with acid pK_as, whilst forced acid diuresis promotes the excretion of amphetamine, a drug with a pK_a of 9·8 (Anggard et al. 1973).

What specificity the physicochemical procedures possess depends more on the physical or chemical characteristics of the poison than in its metabolism or precise mode of action. Thus, they can be used when detailed information on the toxicant is not available, a state of affairs which often obtains with newly introduced compounds.

Specific Antidotes

Unlike the non-specific treatments for poisonings discussed above, the design and application of a specific antidotal procedure depends on a detailed substructure of information on the biochemical and toxicological mechanisms which underlie the poisoning. This information will include the identification of target organs and the nature of the toxicant's effects on these organs, as well as the absorption, distribution, excretion and metabolism of the poison. Furthermore, information from animal studies should be complemented by investigation of any human exposures. The physicochemical properties of the poison such as pK_a may be of interest as with non-specific therapies. Because the relative importance of these various factors depends to some extent on the mode of action of the proposed antidote, it is worthwhile briefly to consider the various processes which antidotal therapy may exploit.

A number of antidotes bind directly to the toxicant, including dicobalt edetate (Paulet, 1958) and hydroxocobalamin (Mushett et al., 1952), both of which have been used experimentally and clinically to combat cyanide poisoning. A form of treatment which is presently applicable to digoxin poisoning, but which may later become of more general utility, is the administration of Fab fragments (Smith et al., 1976; Lloyd and Smith, 1978). A similar procedure is the use of complete monoclonal antibodies; these are reported to confer some protective effect against the organophosphate nerve agent soman (GD) in experimental animals (Lenz et al., 1984). These direct binding antidotes present perhaps the least difficulty with choice of animal model. The reason for this is that the concentration of the reactant species and the stability of the product are the main factors determining antidotal efficacy. In certain cases, e.g. the heavy metal chelators, it is possible to study the reaction *in vitro*. Indeed, with this family of antidotes one is to some extent able to predict the efficacy of particular chelating agents against the various metals on the basis of theoretical considerations (Pearson, 1968). Moreover, the interaction between chelating agents and metals can be described quantitatively (Ringbom, 1963). In spite of these models, Aaseth (1983) states that animal experiments are essential for the evaluation of chelating agents, a conclusion also reached by Stradling et al. (1986) studying actinide poisoning with chelating agents. One of the reasons for this is the complexity of the *in vivo* situation, not only enhancement of excretion of the metal being important, but also its concentration in the critical organ. Moreover, stability constants for the metal chelator complex may sometimes be misleading. Thus, Catsch and Harmuth-Hoene (1975) found that penicillamine mobilized mercury better than diethylenetriamine pentacetate, whereas the corresponding stability constants would predict the reverse. These workers suggested that the effect might be due to the superior penetration of penicillamine into the intracellular space.

The action of oximes such as pralidoxime mesylate in organophosphate poisoning involves binding to the enzyme-inhibitor complex and rupturing of the enzyme-inhibitor bonds. In this way cholinesterases are reactivated. The process has been studied *in vitro* by many workers (e.g. Hobbiger et al., 1960; Hobbiger and Vojvodic, 1966). Recently van Helden et al. (1983) have proposed marmoset muscle as a suitable *in vitro* model for the study of organophosphate poisoning and its antidotes. However, the disadvantages of using *in vitro* models are likely to be similar to those found with chelating agents and metals, namely that the complicated situation in the whole animal cannot adequately be simulated *in vitro*. Much experimental work has been carried out on organophosphate poisoning in small laboratory animals, but there has been no agreement on which is the most suitable small animal for use as a model for the poisoning in humans. Inns and Leadbeater (1983) justify their use of guinea-pigs by stating that these animals are closer than others in their similarity to primates with respect to sensitivity to organophosphate poisoning. Other groups (e.g. Kepner and Wolthuis, 1978; Wolthuis and Vanwersh, 1984) have not been unanimous in their choice of that experimental model.

A related mechanism of antidotal action is the production of a therapeutic methaemoglobinaemia by compounds such as sodium nitrite and 4-dimethylaminophenol. The methaemoglobin is capable of binding both cyanides (Rose et al., 1946) and sulphides (Smith et al., 1976). In the case of cyanide, efficacy of treatment is partly determined by the equilibrium constant for the reaction between cyanide and methaemoglobin, $10^{7.9}$ for dogs according to Christel et al. (1977), $10^{8.06}$ for humans (Christel et al., 1977, from data of Anusiem et al., 1968). Assuming that methaemoglobin is the mediator of the therapeutic benefit of these compounds (and this has been doubted in the case of sodium nitrite by Way et al., 1984), the ability of the animal to produce a similar methaemoglobinaemic response to humans should be the first criterion on which choice of animal model is made. The major determinant of the degree and duration of methaemoglobinaemia after administration of compounds such as 4-dimethylaminophenol seems to be the erythrocyte NADH-linked methaemoglobin reductase activity, which varies quite substantially in different species (Kiese and Weis, 1944; Malz, 1962; Smith and Beutler, 1966; Robin and Harley, 1966; Stolk and Smith, 1966; Agar and Harley, 1972). This is reflected in marked interspecies differences in time-profiles of blood methaemoglobin after addition of 4-dimethylaminophenol to blood *in vitro* (Marrs et al., 1987). In general, small laboratory animals, especially mice, have high methaemoglobin reduction rates while man, the dog and the cat have similar and considerably lower ones. Information on the methaemoglobin reduction potentialities of the erythrocytes of non-human primates is extremely sparse. There is some evidence that cynomolgus monkeys are more similar to man than to rodents (Hawkins et al., 1981), while the marmoset may be intermediate between the high and low reductase group (Marrs et al., 1987). Because of the lack of information on primates, and in view of the inadvisability of extrapolating to man data obtained using aromatic compounds in cats, dogs appear to be the most satisfactory model for the study of 4-dimethylaminophenol in cyanide poisoning. Even dogs are reported to differ to some extent from humans in their response to 4-dimethylaminophenol independently of differences in methaemoglobin reductase activity (Bright and Marrs, 1982).

A further variant of the direct binding mechanism may occur where a foreign substance requires metabolic conversion before it is toxic, and it is the toxic product which is bound by the antidote. It has been suggested that this might be the mode of action of N-acetylcysteine in paracetamol poisoning, where the toxic metabolite is thought to be N-acetyl-*p*-benzoquinoneimine (Huggett and Blair, 1983; but see also Dawson et al., 1984). With an antidote acting in this fashion a suitable animal model for man would obviously be an animal metabolizing the compound by the same route.

Where antidotes act by hastening metabolism of a toxicant to a less toxic product, metabolic similarities between animal model and man are paramount. An example of this type of action would be the use of sodium thiosulphate as a substrate for the enzyme rhodenese (Mintel and Westley, 1966) in cyanide poisoning. However, reported interspecies differences in rhodenese activity (e.g. Sörbo, 1951) do not appear to have greatly influenced choice of model in investigation of the antidote. In actual fact, this omission may not be of any great consequence since it has been doubted whether, in acute cyanide poisoning, there is time for substantial transulphuration to occur (Drawbaugh and Marrs, in press).

A related action of an antidote on a metabolic pathway can be used where the foreign compound is not itself toxic, but is enzymatically converted, as is paracetamol, to a toxic metabolite. The antidote may block the conversion either by acting as an alternative substrate, or as a specific inhibitor of the enzyme responsible for the conversion. Both types of antidotal action can be used to block alcohol dehydrogenase, the enzyme responsible for oxidation of methanol and ethylene glycol as well as ethanol in man. Thus, in methanol intoxication, where the deleterious effects are thought to be due to formaldehyde and formic acid (Cooper and Kini, 1962), subjects may be beneficially treated with ethanol. Ethylene glycol poisoning can be similarly treated (Peterson et al., 1963; Wacker et al., 1965). The alternative approach, the administration of specific inhibitors, is exemplified by the use of pyrazole (van Stee et al., 1975) and 4-methylpyrazole (Clay and Murphy, 1977). Both these substances have been used in the experimental treatment of ethylene glycol poisoning in animals.

Antagonism of poison and antidote at receptors is usually highly specific, and it is exploited clinically in the use of opiate antagonists naloxone, nalorphine and levallorphine (Jefferys and Volans, 1983; Prescott, 1983). Clearly, similarity in distribution, specificity and density of receptors in man and the animal model is important, but information on this is often limited. In the case of the antidotal action of atropine in anticholinesterase poisoning (Taylor, 1980), and physostigmine in atropine poisoning (Rumack, 1973; Weiner, 1980), similar considerations apply. These are not cases of true receptor antagonism, but wherever poison or antidote act at specific receptors, distribution of them should be considered in choice of model.

A further type of poison antidote interaction is sometimes called functional antagonism. The therapy is directed primarily at an important clinical sign or pathological effect. Atropine, which opposes anticholinesterases by blocking the muscarinic receptors at which they cause acetylcholine to accumulate, might be included in this group. More typical examples would be provided by the use of benzodiazepines in soman poisoning (Lipp, 1973), and the action of etomidate, flunarizine or verapamil in cyanide poisoning (Ashton et al., 1981; Dubinsky et al., 1984). This type of antagonism is particularly difficult to model in animals because of differences in physiological, pathological and clinical responses in different species, including man.

Toxicity of Antidotes

A clear requirement of the antidote is that it does not give rise to toxic effects comparable with those produced by the poisoning, and this should be established early in the experimental programme. If there is any doubt about this, it is possible to include a 'treatment only' group in studies where experimental poisoning is to be treated.

Where an antidote is being evaluated against existing therapies, the acute toxicity of the antidote may be a major factor affecting the choice. With a number of competing antidotes, neither the efficacy nor the toxicity alone determine the choice. Rather it is the relationship between the effective doses and the LD_{50}s of the antidotes which should be the criterion on which a decision is reached. An example may be seen amongst chelating agents where Aposhian et al. (1981, 1983) compared the LD_{50}s of various dimercapto compounds with their ED_{50}s in mice. A therapeutic index was derived which suggested that mesodimercaptosuccinic acid was the most effective of the four chelating agents tested. A similar study in which the toxicity of a family of antidotes was compared was that of Lovett Evans (1964). He tabulated the lethal doses of cobalt acetate, dicobalt edetate, cobaltous chloride and cobalt histidine, and also evaluated their antidotal efficacy in experimental cyanide poisoning.

An antidote newly demonstrated to be effective has to be treated very much in the same way as any other new drug. The acute toxicity of the antidote is useful in fixing doses for experimental treatment studies, but it will also, accompanied by further toxicological data, by needed for drug licensing. Included in the more detailed toxicology required may be acute, subacute, chronic, reproductive and teratological studies, together with mutagenicity tests. An example of the type of work needed can be found in the thorough study on the toxicity of N-acetylcysteine by Johnston et al. (1983). The precise requirements for clinical trial certificates or equivalent and drug licensing vary from country to country, and can be obtained from appropriate government departments; they are discussed in such texts as Jones (1981) and Morton (1981).

A particular problem with some antidotes is unpredictable reactions of the type occasionally encountered with N-acetylcysteine (Vale and Wheeler, 1982) and dicobalt edetate (Tyrer, 1981). These can rarely be predicted from animal tests.

THE ASSESSMENT OF EFFICACY OF ANTIDOTES IN EXPERIMENTAL ANIMALS

The object of treatment of experimental poisoning in animals is to demonstrate that a therapy or prophylaxis, believed to be valuable on the basis of *in vitro* work or theoretical considerations, is in fact effective *in vivo*. It is a mandatory preliminary to the use of the antidote in clinical practice.

The major factors influencing the design of the experiment are those that influence the design of any biological experiment. There is also the need to follow as closely as possible the clinical situation in which the antidote will be used. The latter consideration must be balanced against the fact that a major advantage of animal experimentation over case reports of uses of the antidote in humans is that the dose of poison and the time relationship between poisoning and administration of antidote can be controlled. This advantage should never be sacrificed. Furthermore, all possible steps should be taken to eliminate bias, and the time of day of the experiment, diet, and age and sex of the animals should be standardized.

Protocols used for antidotal efficacy experiments have varied widely, the main sources of variation being species and numbers of animals, and whether controls were used. Differences have also occurred in dose and route of administration of the poison, dose and route of administration of the antidote and the outcome to be observed.

Types of Design

The most frequently used experimental designs are those in which the LD_{50} of the poison is measured with and without therapy or prophylaxis with the antidote to give a protection ratio*, and those in which the animals are given a multiple of the lethal dose, and survival in the treated group is compared with that in the controls (multiple lethal dose design). The protection ratio type of design has the advantage that the result can be expressed as a single figure, but the approach cannot be used if the supply of animals is limited. Doubtless for that reason the protection ratio design has most frequently been employed where small laboratory animals have been the experimental model. Heilbron and Tolagen (1965), Hobbiger and Vojvodic (1966), Fleisher et al. (1970), Berry and Davies (1970), Gordon et al. (1978), Kepner and Wolthuis (1978) and Inns and Leadbeater (1983) all used this type of design in the course of their studies on therapies and prophylaxes for organophosphate poisoning in small laboratory animals. Using a similar design and investigating the same poisoning, Natoff and Reiff (1970) pointed out the problems that arise if the log dose-probit mortality curves with and without the antidote deviate from parallelism (this is further discussed below). Other poisonings and their treatments have been investigated using protection ratios; thus R. P. Smith (1969) determined the LD_{50} of sodium sulphide and sodium cyanide in mice, with and without prior treatment with sodium cobaltinitrite. Schwartz et al. (1979) investigated the prophylactic effect of cyanide antidotes, including sodium pyruvate, using a protection ratio design. Other workers studying cyanide poisoning who have used this general type of experiment protocol have included Frankenberg (1980) who studied purified bovine rhodenese and Moore et al. (1986) who studied α-ketoglutarate. Both these groups of workers used mice. The protection ratio type of design has been used in a few instances in larger animals. Dirnhuber et al. (1979) studied the

* This has been variously called the potency ratio (Schwartz et al., 1979; Burrows and Way, 1979), dose reduction factor (Frankenberg, 1980), or protective ratio (Gordon et al., 1978). The protective index is an alternative (Boskovic, 1979) and equals the LD_{50} protection ratio minus one.

protection of rhesus monkeys and marmosets against soman poisoning by pyridostigmine, while Burrows and Way (1979) studied sodium nitrite, sodium thiosulphate and cobaltous chloride as therapies in cyanide-poisoned sheep. In the latter case, the experiment was not primarily directed towards the treatment of human cyanide poisoning.

The substitution of ED_{50} (effective dose in 50% of the animals) for LD_{50} has allowed workers to use the protection ratio design for experiments where the outcome observed is something other than death, for instance an effect on a behavioural test (D'Mello, 1983).

The multiple lethal dose design requires less animals: there has been a consequent tendency to use it where the larger and more expensive animals have had to be used as the experimental subjects. Thus, Weger and Szinicz (1981) gave supralethal doses of organophosphate nerve agents ($5\times$ or $10\times LD_{50}$) to beagle dogs and subsequently treated them with various oximes. They simply recorded the proportion surviving. Lörcher and Weger (1971), Klimmek et al. (1979) and Marrs et al. (1985) working on cyanide prophylaxis, all in dogs, used the same type of design. Some of these workers evaluated more than one antidote. Other examples are provided by van Stee et al. (1975) who studied the treatment of experimental ethylene glycol poisoning with pyrazole in rats and dogs, and by Pill et al. (1980) who used mice and rabbits in experimental sodium nitroprusside poisoning. An instance of the use of the multiple lethal dose design entirely in small laboratory rodents is Klemm's evaluation of various antidotes in physostigmine poisoning (Klemm, 1983).

The choice between these two types of experimental design is extremely difficult. The view is held by some that the log dose-probit mortality response is such a well established concept that a protection ratio design should always be adopted. Quite apart from the statistical and interpretative difficulties, discussed below, which may arise when the slopes of control and treated animals differ, it has to be faced that the species that can be used will be limited. Species differences in toxicology are so widespread that the use of a biochemically unsuitable animal model may be positively misleading, however well designed the study is in other respects.

Controls

Failure to use controls considerably diminishes the value of the experiment. In the protection ratio design, the main alternative to determination of the LD_{50} in animals not treated with the antidote is to use an LD_{50} from the scientific literature as denominator in the protection ratio. Such a figure would be most unreliable, whilst the use of an historical LD_{50} in a multiple lethal dose type of study would mean that there would be no certainty that a lethal dose had in fact been administered.

These problems arise because of the difficulty in comparing work done in different laboratories, using different preparations, administered under different conditions, to animals which may or may not be nominally of the same species or strain. If the protection ratio design be adopted, it is almost essential to perform an LD_{50} on untreated animals, whilst with multiple lethal dose studies, the toxicant should at least be administered to a number of control animals, the outcome being observed to ensure the chosen dose is in fact a lethal one.

Challenge

If the LD_{50} of the toxicant has been determined earlier in the experimental programme, this may be used as a guide to dosage. If no such guide is available, a pilot study may be necessary. In protection ratio studies, 4 or 5 doses, designed to bracket the putative LD_{50}, are usually used (Finney, 1971). A similar procedure is followed to determine the LD_{50} in treated animals, but uncertainty over the likely therapeutic benefit may necessitate further pilot studies.

In the multiple lethal dose design, a multiple of the LD_{50} is chosen against which it is expected that the antidote will give significant protection. If protection is found to be successful, the dose of toxicant may be increased; where protection is unsuccessful, the dose of poison may be reduced, the aim being to find the maximum dose of poison against which the antidote will protect.

In the experimental protocol, all aspects of dosing, including route and speed of administration, should be standardized. The toxicant should generally be given using the route by which it normally gains entry to the body; thus, gavage may be used for poisons usually taken orally. There are permissible exceptions: thus, it may be impracticable to poison by inhalation. Toxicants normally absorbed through the skin pose a problem because a completely satisfactory model for man does not exist (Calabrese, 1983), although as has been discussed above the pig and the monkey may be the least unsatisfactory animal models.

Certain poisons may pose special problems in that they are difficult to handle safely. This may be the case with highly toxic and volatile substances, with irritants, or even be caused by consideration of cost. In these cases it is tempting to use a substitute toxicant. Such a procedure, which is often adopted for perfectly valid reasons, can raise serious problems of interpretation. Examples of this abound, especially in inhalation toxicology. Thus, the arsenical lewisite is an unpleasant compound to handle. Consequently, it would be very convenient to use inorganic arsenic salts when evaluating arsenic antidotes intended for use against lewisite; however, there are major differences in toxicity between this compound and inorganic arsenic compounds such as sodium arsenite. These differences relate both to comparative molar lethality figures, and to organ specific toxicity and appear to be reflected in different tissue distribution of the arsenic after administration of the two compounds (Inns et al., 1986). This type of situation, which is paralleled by dissimilarities between salts of other heavy metals and corresponding organic forms, points towards caution in substituting one toxicant for another, however closely related chemically.

If there is any doubt about the stability of the toxicant, the material should be assayed before use. Some workers, e.g. Marrs et al. (1982), have even assayed the individual doses given to the animals; if it is already intended to measure blood levels of the toxicant during the study, this procedure may not greatly add to the complexity of the experiment.

Antidote

The antidote should be given in the formulation it is proposed to be used in clinical practice. The dose will depend on the toxicity and efficacy of the antidote, and pilot studies may be needed. A systematic approach where there is no guide to the efficacy of the antidote might be to give a high dose and, having shown efficacy, reduce it stepwise. Such a procedure was followed by Pill et al. (1980) studying two nitroprusside antidotes. Some workers (e.g. Mushett et al., 1952) have varied the dose of both antidote and poison. Unless very large numbers of animals are used, there studies may be difficult to interpret.

A difficult problem to solve is the time relationship of poison and antidote. In different studies the antidote has been variously administered before the poison, after the poison and, perhaps with a different object in mind, simultaneously with it (de Vries et al., 1984). Logically, when prophylaxis is being studied the antidote should be given before the poison, and when therapy is being studied it should be given afterwards. The use of prophylactic experimental designs to evaluate therapies has been criticized as giving rise to misleading results (Way et al., 1984), and it seems logical to treat after the poisoning if that is to be the procedure in clinical practice.

Unfortunately there has been no agreement on how to define the time relationship between poisoning and subsequent administration of the antidote, the two commonest procedures being to give it at a fixed time after poisoning, or at the onset of a particular clinical sign. The former approach was adopted by Kepner and Wolthuis who gave oximes 1·5 minutes after soman injection. A similar procedure was applied to the therapy of cyanide poisoning by Burrows and Way (1979) who have their antidote after a 5 minute interval, and by Klimmek et al. (1979) who administered their therapies one or four minutes after poisoning. The criticism of these procedures, if such a short time interval be used, is their implication that therapy will only be effective if given within a very few minutes of poisoning. In reality this is unlikely to be a sufficient time for a poisoned patient to receive help. An alternative approach is to delay treatment until the onset of poisoning. Thus, Lörcher and Weger (1971) injected 4-dimethylaminophenol at the onset of convulsions caused by administration of cyanide. Sanderson (1965) used a similar approach in a part of his study on an organophosphate, morphothion. The advantages of waiting until toxic signs occur are that there is no doubt that a toxic dose has been given, and that it may be more realistic than using a very short time interval after poisoning. The disadvantage is that it can only be used when a poison gives fairly clear-cut signs of the onset of intoxication. Furthermore, there is the possibility of introducing bias if exact criteria are not used as the cue for giving the antidote. A more realistic approach, not giving rise to the possibility of bias, might be to use a fixed time interval after administration of the poison, but a rather longer one than most workers have employed.

On occasion it is desirable to study the use of more than one antidote simultaneously, perhaps because the protection offered by each singly is insufficient. The simplest approach to this is to compare a poisoned but untreated group of animals with a group treated with all the antidotes. This procedure has the major disadvantage that there is no way of knowing which antidote has contributed to any successful outcome. A better approach is to use all possible combinations of the antidotes separately, a procedure which will give information on separate antidotal effects as well as interactions. Several studies have used this type of design, including Schwartz et al. (1979) who studied sodium pyruvate, nitrite and thiosulphate alone, and in combination in the treatment of experimental cyanide poisoning. A large number of studies of multiple therapies for anticholinesterase poisoning have been published, including those of Natoff and Reiff (1970), Fleisher et al. (1970), Gordon et al. (1978) and Klemm (1983). Most of these studies used a protection ratio type of design with various antidotal and pretreatment combinations.

Outcome

In most of the examples quoted above, the outcome of the experiment has been determined by death or survival of the experimental animals. A variant on this has been to use survival time; thus, Hopff et al. (1981) reported increased survival times in rats poisoned with organophosphate and treated with methyl-methane thiolsulphonate, while using a monoclonal antibody against soman; Lenz et al. (1984) also found increased times to death. In fact, it is always useful to record survival times, even when death or survival is the prime outcome being determined.

There are several reasons why an experimenter may want to study the effects of sublethal doses of a poison. He may be primarily interested in the prophylaxis or therapy of sublethal effects, or he may wish to reuse the animals, although the latter may not be scientifically sound. One example of a behavioural end point for an experiment has already been cited (D'Mello, 1983). In this study the ability of guinea-pigs to undertake a swim test after treatment with organophosphates or cyanides, with or without appropriate antidotal pretreatment, was used as the indicator of therapeutic benefit. A protection ratio type of design was adopted by substituting ED_{50} for the LD_{50}, the ED_{50} being defined as that dose which produced a significant decrement in swim test performance in 50% of the animals. A significant decrement was considered to exist when the time taken to undertake the swim test was greater than the mean swim time for control animals plus three standard deviations. A somewhat different protocol involving ED_{50} for behavioural effects was adopted by Palfai and Felleman (1982), investigating the effect of clonidine or propranolol on digitoxin toxicity in mice. Other examples of behavioural endpoints include McMillan et al. (1970) and Goldberg et al. (1974), who investigated opiates and their antagonists in pigeons.

Another type of endpoint that may be employed is a biochemical indicator. This is almost the norm in metal chelation studies, where the criterion studied has often been increased elimination of the metal, perhaps expressed as biological half life (e.g. Aaseth, 1976). However, the same worker (Aaseth, 1983) suggests that decreased concentration in the critical organ should be the prime criterion of successful treatment. The importance of this point is shown by the work of Aposhian et al. (1984). These workers showed that BAL (dimercaprol or British anti-lewisite), the drug of choice in arsenic poisoning, actually increased the concentration of that metal in the brain. In the case of an antidote that binds the poison the concept may be refined further; a poison bound to a specific antidote is usually, but not always, biologically inactive. Thus we can say that decreased concentration of biologically active toxicant in the critical organ should be the criterion of success. Unfortunately, biologically active toxicant is often difficult to measure, which brings us back to lethality as an endpoint. For this reason, in spite of the widespread use of metal excretion, some workers have performed lethality studies (e.g. Inns et al., 1986; Athar et al., 1987).

Another possibility where it is essential to measure the biological activity of a poison, independent of its amount, is to use a biochemical indicator of activity of the poison. De Vries et al. (1984) used plasma alanine and asparatate aminotransferases, as well as glutathione levels in liver homogenates and histological studies to evaluate the protection offered by simultaneous administration of acetylsalicylic acid against paracetamol-induced hepatotoxicity. In the case of nitroprusside poisoning, where the toxic metabolite is cyanide, Krapez et al. (1981) used the concentrations of that ion, and of thiocyanate as indicators of antidotal activity. In the case of methanol and ethylene glycol poisoning, both of which are characterized by a severe organic acidosis, blood pH can be used to evaluate the success of therapy. This course was pursued by Clay and Murphy (1977) investigating ethylene glycol poisoning and its treatment with 4-methylpyrazone. If a poison be a known inhibitor of an enzyme system, it is possible to use the enzyme as marker for the presence of the poison. Thus, Aposhian et al. (1983) used sodium arsenite inhibition of mouse kidney pyruvate dehydrogenase when evaluating DL and mesodimercaptosuccinic acid as chelating agents in arsenic poisoning. In the experimental treatment of lung fibrosis, lung hydroxyproline can be used as an indicator of collagen deposition. Thus, Kehrer and Witchi (1981) used hydroxyproline measurement as an adjunct to percentage survival when evaluating the effect of indomethacin, prednisolone and *cis*-4-hydroxyproline on butylated hydroxytoluene-induced pulmonary fibrosis. To assess another type of pulmonary injury, namely the oedema seen in response to thiourea, Fox et al. (1983) used as well as lung weights, lung-lavage albumin concentrations.

Statistics

The protection ratio type of study gives its results in the form of a single figure, the ratio LD_{50} treated to LD_{50} untreated. If the figure is significantly greater than one, therapeutic benefit has accrued. In the event of the two log dose-probit mortality curves being parallel, the isolated use of the protection ratio is fairly satisfactory (*Fig*. 12.2). It frequently happens that the two curves are not parallel, i.e the slopes for the treated animals and for the untreated ones are

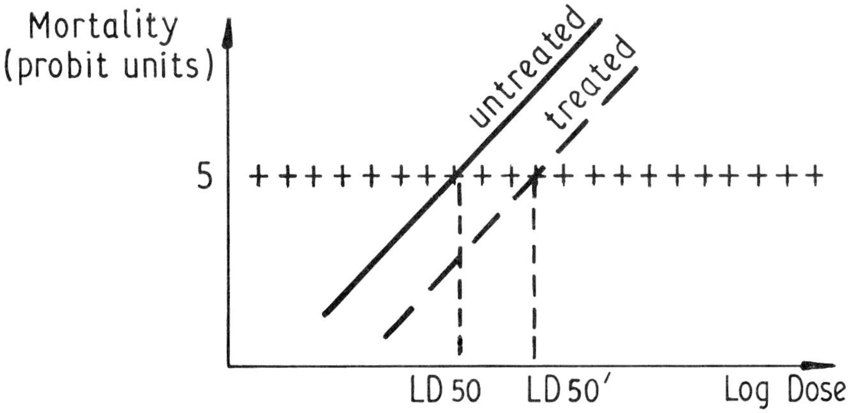

Fig. 12.2. Log dose-probit mortality lines with and without antidote. The slopes are the same in both cases so that the LD_{50}, LD_{90} and LD_{10} protection ratios are all equal.

different (Natoff and Reiff, 1970). In cases where the log dose-probit mortality curve is more shallow in the treated animals than in the untreated ones (e.g. Natoff and Reiff, 1970; Dirnhuber et al., 1979), the implication is that the treatment is less beneficial at low doses of toxicant (*Fig.* 12.3) and, if the lines cross, there is a therapeutic penalty (*Fig.* 12.4). Often in the therapy of poisoning, one is interested in the effect of supralethal doses: a shallower slope in treated animals implies that the LD_{50} protection ratio would underestimate the benefit. The reasons for deviation from parallelism are unclear; two possibilities might be that the treatment has its own intrinsic toxicity which is large enough to contribute towards mortality, or that the treatment alters the mechanism of death. The most common situation seems to be that shown in *Fig.* 12.3.

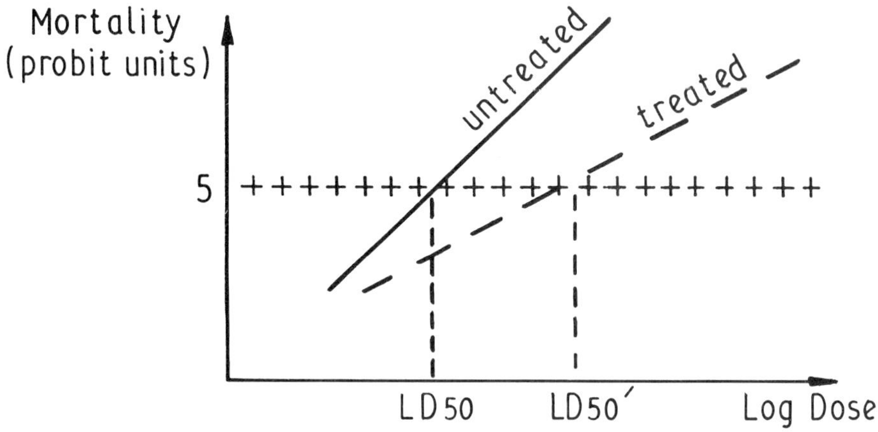

Fig. 12.3. Log dose-probit mortality lines with and without antidote. The slopes differ so that the LD_{10} protection ratio is less than, and the LD_{90} protection ratio is more than, the LD_{50} protection ratio.

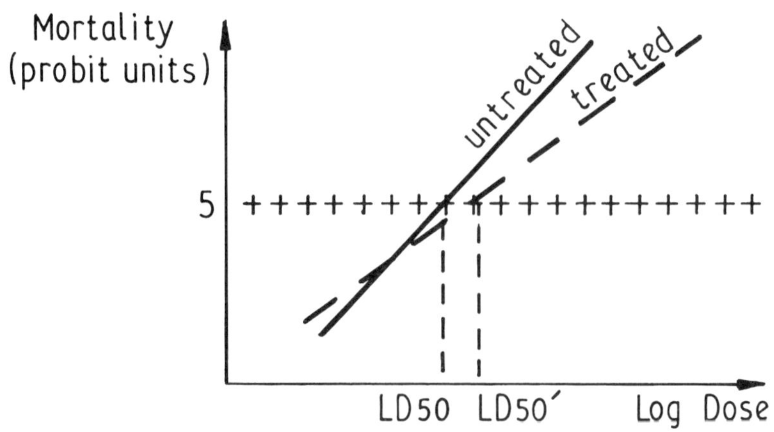

Fig. 12.4. Log dose-probit mortality lines with and without antidote. The slopes differ in such a way that the lines intersect implying an LD_{10} protection ratio of less than 1—a penalty.

Different log dose-probit mortality slopes give rise to problems in the presentation of data because the LD_{50} protection ratio no longer adequately describes the result of the study. Natoff and Reiff (1970) suggested that the reduction of an LD_{90} to an LD_{10} might provide a better indication of efficacy than the protection ratio, while it has been suggested (N. L. Cross, personal communication) that the percentage mortality in the treated animals, when given the dose that is the LD_{90} in the untreated animals, could be used. This measurement has the great advantage of giving a single figure which estimates the benefit accruing after treatment at a dose of toxicant well above the LD_{50}. Certainly if the LD_{50} protection ratio is to be retained, both slopes should be quoted in cases of non-parallelism, or alternatively LD_{10} and LD_{90} protection ratios in addition to the LD_{50} protection ratio.

If the multiple lethal dose design is to be used, the χ^2 or the Fisher exact tests can evaluate the significance of the difference in survival in the test and control groups. An important consideration is the use of large enough numbers to detect a difference between the survival rate in the two groups where such exists. The smaller the difference it is expedient to detect, the larger the sample needs to be. This problem has been considered by Freiman et al. (1978) in relation to clinical trials, but the same considerations apply to an efficacy study in experimental clinical toxicology.

Where outcomes other than death are considered, the methods of treating the data are as above, providing the outcome is an all or nothing event. If it is a measurement, e.g. enzyme activity, other statistical methods such as student's *t*-test should be used to compare control and test groups. In some cases (e.g. D'Mello, 1983), workers have converted what is essentially a continuously variable measurement into an all or nothing event by considering the results in test animals as being within or outside a normal range derived from control animals. Choice of appropriate statistical tests in these matters depends on considerations such as the normality of distribution of the data, and is fully discussed in texts on statistics in biological experimentation such as that of Bliss (1967) and Finney (1971).

CONCLUSION

It is clear that most workers have employed an *ad hoc* approach to the study of antidotal efficacy. It is obviously unreasonable to suggest that a standard model or protocol can be used for experiments of this type, but a more thoughtful approach might decrease the amount of animal experimentation necessary, while increasing the information acquired. It would also enable experimental antidotes to be brought into use more quickly, increasing the number of poisons which can be treated by specific therapy.

REFERENCES

Aaseth J. (1976) Mobilization of methyl mercury *in vivo* and *in vitro* using N-acetyl-DL-penicillamine and other complexing agents. *Acta Pharmacol. Toxicol.* **39**, 289–301.

Aaseth J. (1983) Recent advances in the therapy of metal poisonings with chelating agents. *Human Toxicol.* **2**, 257–272.

Abou-el-Makerem M. M., Millburn P., Smith R. L. et al. (1967) Biliary excretion of foreign compound. *Biochem. J.* **105**, 1289–1293.

Agar N. S. and Harley J. D. (1972) Erthrocytic methaemoglobin reductase of various mammalian species. *Experientia* **28**, 1248–1249.

Aldridge W. N., Barnes J. M. and Johnson M. K. (1969) Studies on delayed neurotoxicity produced by some organophosphorus compounds. *Ann. NY Acad. Sci.* **160**, 314–322.

Anggard E., Jonsson L-E., Hogmark A-L. et al. (1973) Amphetamine metabolism in amphetamine psychosis. *Clin. Pharm. Therap.* **14**, 870–879.

Anusiem A. C., Beetlestone J. G. and Irvine D. H. (1968) Reactivity differences between haemoglobins. Part VIII. *J. Chem. Soc. A.* 960–969.

Aposhian H. V., Carter D. E., Hoover T. D. et al. DMSA, DMPS and DMPA—as arsenic antidotes. *Fund. Appl. Toxicol.* **4**, S58–S70.

Aposhian H. V., Hsu C-A. and Hoover T. D. (1983) DL- and meso-dimercaptosuccinic acid: *in vitro* and *in vivo* studies with sodium arsenite. *Toxicol. Appl. Pharmacol.* **69**, 206–213.

Aposhian H. V., Tadlock C. H. and Moon T. E. (1981) Protection of mice against lethal effects of sodium arsenite—a qualitative comparison of a number of chelating agents. *Toxicol. Appl. Pharmacol.* **61**, 385–392.

Ashton D., van Reempts J. and Wauquier A. (1981) Behavioural, electroencephalographic and histological study of the protective effect of etomidate against histotoxic dysoxia produced by cyanide. *Arch. Int. Pharmacodyn. Ther.* **254**, 196–213.

Athar M., Misra N. and Srivastara R. C. (1987) Evaluation of chelating drugs on the toxicity, excretion and distribution of nickel in poisoned rats. *Fund. Appl. Tox.* **9**, 26–33.

Baggot J. D. and Davis L. E. (1973) Species differences in plasma protein binding of morphine and codeine. *Am. J. Vet. Res.* **34**, 571–574.

Baggot J. D., Davis L. E. and Neff C. A. (1972) Extent of plasma protein binding of amphetamine in different species. *Biochem. Pharmacol.* **21**, 1813–1816.

Berry W. K. and Davies D. R. (1970) The use of carbamates and atropine in the protection of animals against poisoning by 1,2,2-trimethylpropyl-methylphosphonofluoridate. *Biochem. Pharmacol.* **19**, 927–934.

Bliss C. I. (1967) *Statistics in Biology*. New York: McGraw-Hill.

Boskovic B. (1979) The influence of 2-/*o*-cresyl/4H-1:3:1-benzodioxaphosphorin-2-oxide (CBDP) on organophosphate poisoning and its therapy. *Arch. Toxicol.* **42**, 207–216.

Bright J. E. and Marrs T. C. (1982) A model for the induction of moderate levels of methaemoglobinaemia in man using 4-dimethylaminophenol. *Arch. Toxicol.* **50**, 57–64.

British Toxicology Society, Working Party on Toxicity (1984) Special Report. A new approach to the classification of substances and preparations on the basis of their acute toxicity. *Human Toxicol.* **3**, 85–92.

Brown V. K. H. (1983) Acute toxicity testing. In: Balls M., Riddell R. J. and Worden A. N. (ed.) *Animals and Alternatives in Toxicity Testing*, 1–16. London: Academic Press.

Buatti M. C. and Pasternak G. W. (1981) Multiple opiate receptors: phylogenetic differences. *Brain Res.* **218**, 400–405.

Burns J. J. (1970) Species differences in drug metabolism and toxicological implications. *Proc. Eur. Soc. Study Drug Tox.* **11**, 9–13.

Burrows G. E. and Way J. L. (1979) Cyanide intoxication in sheep: enhancement of efficacy of sodium nitrite, sodium thiosulfate and cobaltous chloride. *Am. J. Vet. Res.* **40**, 613–617.

Calabrese E. J. (1983) *Principles of Animal Extrapolation*. New York: Wiley.

Capel I. D., French M. R., Millburn P. et al. (1972) The fate of [^{14}C] phenol in various species. *Xenobiotica* **2**, 25–34.

Catsch A. and Harmuth-Hoene A-E. (1975) New developments in metal antidotal properties of chelating agents. *Biochem. Pharmacol.* **24**, 1557–1562.

Christel D., Eyer P., Hegemann M. et al. (1977) Pharmacokinetics of cyanide in poisoning of dogs, and the effect of 4-dimethylaminophenol or thiosulfate. *Arch. Toxicol.* **38**, 177–189.

Clay K. L. and Murphy R. C. (1977) On the metabolic acidosis of ethylene glycol intoxication. *Toxicol. Appl. Pharmacol.* **39**, 39–49.

Clay K. L., Murphy R. C. and Watkins W. D. (1975) Experimental methanol toxicity in the primate: analysis of metabolic acidosis. *Toxicol. Appl. Pharmacol.* **34**, 49–61.

Cooper J. R. and Kini M. M. (1962) Biochemical aspects of methanol poisoning. *Biochem. Pharmacol.* **11**, 405–416.

Crawford M. J., Hutson D. H. and King P. A. (1976) Metabolic demethylation of the insecticide dimethylvinphos in rats, in dogs and *in vitro*. *Xenobiotica* **6**, 745–762.

Dawson J. R., Norbeck K., Anundi I. et al. (1984) The effectiveness of N-acetylcysteine in isolated hepatocytes against the toxicity of paracetamol, acrolein and paraquat. *Arch. Toxicol.* **55**, 11–15.

de Vries J., de Jong J., Lock F. M. et al. (1984) Protection against paracetamol-induced hepatotoxicity by acetyl-salicyclic acid in rats. *Toxicology* **30**, 297–304.

Dirnhuber P., French M. C., Green D. M. et al. (1979) The protection of primates against soman poisoning by pretreatment with pyridostigmine. *J. Pharm. Pharmacol.* **31**, 295–299.

D'Mello D. G. (1983) Drug treatment for organophosphate and hydrocyanic acid poisoning in the guinea pig. *Proc. Int. Symposium on Protection Against Chemical Warfare Agents*, Stockholm, 6–9 June, 89–93.

Drawbaugh R. and Marrs T. C. (1987) Interspecies differences in rhodanese (thiosulfate sulfurtransferase, EC 2.8.1.1) in liver, kidney and plasma. *Comp. Biochem. Physiol.* **86B**, 307–310.

Dring L. G., Smith R. L. and Williams R. T. (1970) The metabolic rate of amphetamine in man and other species. *Biochem. J.* **116**, 425–435.

Dubinsky B., Sierchio J. N., Temple D. E. et al. (1984) Flunarizine and verapamil: effects on central nervous system and peripheral consequences of cytotoxic hypoxia in rats. *Life Sci.* **34**, 1299–1306.

Eyer P. and Gaber H. (1978) Biotransformation of 4-dimethylaminophenol in the dog. *Biochem. Pharmacol.* **27**, 2215–2221.

Eyer P. and Kampffmeyer H. G. (1978) Biotransformation of 4-amethylaminophenol in the isolated perfused rat liver and the rat. *Biochem. Pharmacol.* **27**, 2223–2228.

Eyer P. and Kiese M. (1976) Biotransformation of 4-dimethylaminophenol: reaction with glutathione and some properties of the reaction products. *Chem-Biol. Interact.* **14**, 165–178.

Finney D. J. (1971) *Probit Analysis*, 3rd ed. Cambridge: Cambridge University Press.

Fleisher J. H., Harris L. W., Miller G. R. et al. (1970) Antagonism of sarin poisoning in rats and guinea pigs by atropine, oximes and mecamylamine. *Toxicol. Appl. Pharmacol.* **16**, 40–47.

Fox R. B., Harda R. N., Tate R. M. et al. Prevention of thiourea-induced pulmonary edema by hydroxyl-radical scavengers. *J. Appl. Physiol.* **55**, 1456–1459.

Frankenberg L. (1980) Enzyme therapy in cyanide poisoning: effect of rhodenese and sulfur compounds. *Arch. Toxicol.* **45**, 315–323.

Freiman J. A., Chalmers T. C., Smith H. et al. (1983) The importance of beta, the type II error and sample size in the design and interpretation of randomized control trial. *N. Engl. J. Med.* **299**, 690–694.

Galinsky, R. E. and Levy, G. (1979). Effect on N-acetylcysteine on the pharmacokinetics of acetaminophen in rats. *Life Sci.* **25**, 693–700.

Garland H. and Pearce J. (1967) Neurological complications of carbon monoxide poisoning. *Q. J. Med.* **36**, 445–455.

Gessner P. K., Parke D. V. and Williams R. T. (1961) Studies in detoxication. *Biochem. J.* **79**, 482–489.

Goldberg S. R., Morse W. H. and Goldberg D. M. (1974) Naltrexone and naloxone agonist and antagonist effects in key-press responding of pigeons maintained under a multiple schedule of food preservation. *Pharmacologist* **16**, 226.

Goldstein A., Aronow L. and Kalman S. M. (1979) *Principles of Drug Action*, 357–436. New York: Wiley.

Gordon J. J., Leadbeater L. and Maidment M. P. (1978) The protection of animals against organophosphate poisoning by pretreatment with a carbamate. *Toxicol. Appl. Pharmacol.* **43**, 207–216.

Hawkins S. F., Gross W. A., Johnson R. P. et al. Comparison of the *in vivo* formation of methaemoglobin by 4-dimethylaminophenol and sodium nitrite in cynomolgous monkeys. *Fed. Proc.* **40**, 718.

Heilbron E. and Tolagen B. (1965) Toxogonin in sarin, soman and tabun poisoning. *Biochem. Pharmacol.* **14**, 73–77.

Hill J. B. (1973) Salicylate intoxication. *N. Engl. J. Med.* **288**, 1110–1113.

Hobbiger F., Pitman M. and Sadler P. W. (1960) Reactivation of phosphorylated acetocholinesterases by pyridinium aldoximes and related compounds. *Biochem. J.* **75**, 363–372.

Hobbiger F. and Vojvodic V. (1966) The reactivating and antidotal action of N,N′-trimethylbis(pyridinium-4-aldoxime)(TMB4) and N,N′-oxydimethylenebis(pyridinium-4-aldoxime) (toxogonin) with particular reference to their effect on phosphorylated acetylcholinesterase in the brain. *Biochem. Pharmacol.* **15**, 1677–1690.

Hopff W. H., Riggio G. and Warner P. G. (1981) Another approach to the treatment of organophosphate poisoning. *Pharmacology*. **37**, 671.

Huggett A. and Blair I. A. (1983) The mechanism of paracetamol-induced hepatotoxicity: implications for therapy. *Hum. Toxicol.* **2**, 399–405.

Hume A. S., Bush M. T., Remick J. and Douglas B. H. (1968) Comparison of gastric absorption of thiopental and pentobarbital in rat dog and man. *Arch. Int. Pharmacodyn.* **171**, 122–127.

Inns R. H., Bright J. E. and Marrs T. C. (1986) Comparative acute toxicity of sodium arsenite and dichloro(2-chlorovinyl) arsine. *Hum. Toxicol.* (In Press.)

Inns R. H. and Leadbeater L. (1983) The efficacy of bispyridinium derivatives in the treatment of organophosphonate poisoning in the guinea-pig. *J. Pharm. Pharmacol.* **35**, 427–433.

Jancso P., Szinicz L. and Eyer P. (1981) Biotransformation of 4-dimethylaminophenol in man. *Arch. Toxicol.* **47**, 39–45.

Jefferys D. B. and Volans G. N. (1983) An investigation of the role of the specific opioid antagonist naloxone in clinical toxicology. *Hum. Toxicol.* **2**, 227–231.

Johnston R. E., Hawkins H. C. and Weikel J. H. (1983) The toxicity of N-acetylcysteine in laboratory animals. *Semin. Oncol.* **10**, 17–24.

Jones G. (1981) Toxicity requirements of the UK and EEC. In: Gorrod J. W. (ed.) *Testing for Toxicity*, 1–10. London: Taylor and Francis.

Kehrer J. P. and Witchi H. (1981) The effect of indomethacin, prednisolone and *cis*-4-hydroxyproline on pulmonary fibrosis produced by butylated hydroxytoluene and oxygen. *Toxicology* **20**, 281 288.

Kepner L. A. and Wolthuis O. L. (1978) A comparison of the oximes HS-6 and HI-6 in the therapy of soman intoxication in rodents. *Eur. J. Pharmacol.* **48**, 377–382.

Kiese M. and Weis B. (1944) Die Reduction des Hämiglobins in den Erythrocyten verschiedener Tiere. *Naunyn Schmiedebergs Arch. Pharmacol.* **203**, 493–501.

Klaasen C. D. and Watkins J. B. (1984) Mechanisms of bile formation, hepatic uptake, and biliary excretion. *Pharmacol. Rev.* **36**, 1–67.

Klemm W. R. (1983) Efficacy and toxicity of drug combinations in treatment of physostigmine toxicosis. *Toxicology* **27**, 41–53.

Klimmek R., Krettek C., Szinicz L. et al. (1983) Effect and biotransformation of 4-dimethylaminophenol in man and dog. *Arch. Toxicol.* **53**, 275–288.

Klimmek R., Fladerer H. and Weger N. (1979). Circulation, respiration and blood homeostasis in cyanide-poisoned dogs after treatment with 4-dimethyl-aminophenol or cobalt compounds. *Arch. Toxicol.* **43**, 121–133.

Krapez J. R., Vesey C. J., Adams L. et al. (1984) Effects of cyanide antidotes used with sodium nitroprusside infusions: sodium thiosulphate and hydroxocobalamin given prophylactically to dogs. *Br. J. Anaesth.* **53**, 793–804.

Lenz D. E., Brimfield A. A., Hunter K. W. et al. (1984) Studies using a monoclonal antibody against soman. *Fund. Appl. Toxicol.* **4**, S156–S164.

Lignian H., Fontaine J. and Askenasi R. (1983) Naloxone and alcohol intoxication in the dog. *Hum. Toxicol.* **2**, 221–225

Lipp J. A. (1973) Effect of benzodiazepine derivatives on soman-induced seizure activity and convulsions in the monkey. *Arch. Int. Pharmacodyn.* **202**, 244–251.

Lloyd B. L. and Smith T. W. (1978) Contrasting rates of reversal of digoxin toxicity with digoxin-specific IgG and Fab fragments. *Circulation* **58**, 208–283.

Lörcher W. and Weger N. (1971) Optimal concentration of ferrihemoglobin for the treatment of cyanide poisoning. *Naunyn Schmiedebergs Arch. Pharmakol.* **270**, R88.

Lovett Evans C. (1964) Cobalt compounds as antidotes for hydrocyanic acid. *Br. J. Pharmacol.* **23**, 455–475.

McMillan D. E., Wolf P. S. and Carchman R. A. (1970) Antagonism of the behavioural effects of morphine and methadone by narcotic antagonists in the pigeon. *J. Pharmacol. Exp. Therap.* **175**, 443–458.

Malz E. (1962) Vergleichende Untersuchungen über die Methamoglobinreduktion in kernhaltigen and kernlosen Erythrozyten. *Folia Haematol.* (*Leipz.*) **78**, 510–515.

Marrs T. C., Bright J. E. and Swanston D. W. (1982) The effect of prior treatment with 4-dimethylaminophenol (DMAP) on animals experimentally poisoned with hydrogen cyanide. *Arch. Toxicol.* **51**, 247–253.

Marrs T. C., Bright. J. E. and Woodman A. C. (1987) Species differences in methaemoglobin production after addition of 4-dimethylaminophenol, a cyanide antidote to blood *in vitro*: a comparative study. *Comp. Biochem. Physiol.* **86B**, 141–148.

Marrs T. C., Swanston D. W. and Bright J. E. (1985) 4-Dimethylaminophenol and dicobalt edetate (Kelocyanor) in the treatment of experimental cyanide poisoning. *Hum. Toxicol.* **4**, 591–600.

Matsumoto S., Oka T., Akira E. J. et al. (1972) Comparative studies on the antagonism of naloxone and nalorphine to the morphine-induced respiratory depression in rabbits.

Mendoza C. E., Shields J. B. and Greenhalgh R. (1977) Activity of mammalian serum esterase towards malaoxon, ferritroxon and paraoxon. *Comp. Biochem. Physiol.* **566**, 189–191.

Millburn P. (1974) Factors affecting glucuronidation *in vivo*. *Biochem. Soc. Trans.* **2**, 1182–1186.

Mintel R. and Westley J. (1966) The rhodenese reaction. *J. Biol. Chem.* **241**, 3381–3385.

Misra A. L., Pontani R. B., Vadlamani N. L. and Mule S. J. (1976) Physiological disposition and biotransformation of [allyl-1′,3′-^{14}C] naloxone in the rat and some comparative observations on nalorphine. *J. Pharmacol. Exp. Therap.* **196**, 257–268.

Moffat A. C. (1978) Absorption of drugs In: Gorrod J. W. and Beckett A. H. (ed.) *Drug Metabolism in Man*, 1–23. London: Taylor and Francis.

Moore S. J., Norris J. C., Ho I. K. and Hume A. S. (1986) The efficacy of α-ketoglutaratic acid in the antagonism of cyanide intoxication. *Toxicol. Appl. Pharmacol.* **82**, 40–44.

Morton D. M. (1981) Requirements for the toxicological testing of drugs in the USA, Canada and Japan. In: Gorrod J. W. (ed.) *Testing for Toxicity*, 11–19. London: Taylor and Francis.

Murphy S. D. (1980) Pesticides. In: Doull J., Klaasen C. D. and Amdur M. O. (ed.) *Casarett and Doull's Toxicology, the Basic Science of Poisons*, 2nd edn. 357–408. New York: Macmillan.

Mushett C. W., Kelley K. L., Boxer G. E. and Rickards J. C. (1952) Antidotal efficacy of vitamin B_{12a} (hydroxo-cobalamin) in experimental cyanide poisoning. *Proc. Soc. Exp. Biol. Med.* **81**, 234–237.

Natoff I. L., and Reiff B. (1970) Quantitative studies of the effect of antagonists on the acute toxicity of organophosphates in rats. *Br. J. Pharm.* **40**, 124–134.

Neugebauer G. (1977) Einfluss hoher i.v. Dosen von D-Penicillamin auf toxische Herzglycosid-wirkungen am Meerschweinchen. *Arzneimittel Forsch.* **27**, 2073–2074.

Paddleford R. R. and Short C. E. (1973) An evaluation of naloxone as a narcotic antagonist in the dog. *Am. Vet. Med. Assoc.* **163**, 144–146.

Palfai T. and Felleman V. H. (1982) Effect of age, clonidine or propranolol on behavioral toxicity induced with digitoxin in mice. *Pharmacol. Biochem. Behavior* **17**, 399–404.

Patty F. A. (1963) *Industrial Hygiene and Toxicology Vol. 2*, 2nd ed., 1499. New York: Interscience Publishers.

Paulet G. (1958) Intoxication cyanhydrique et chélates de cobalt. *J. Physiol.* (*Paris*) **50**, 438–442.

Pearson R. G. (1968) Hard and soft acids and bases, HSAB. Part II. Underlying theories. *J. Chem. Educ.* **45**, 643–648.

Peterson D. I., Peterson J. E., Harding M. G. et al. (1963) Experimental treatment of ethylene glycol poisoning. *JAMA* **186**, 955–957.

Pill J., Engeser P., Höbel M. et al. (1980) Sodium nitroprusside (SNP): comparison of the antidotal effect of hydroxocobalamin and sodium thiosulfate in mice and rabbits. *Toxicol. Lett.* (*Suppl.*) **156**, P62.

Prescott L. F. (1983) New approaches in managing drug overdosage and poisoning. *Br. Med. J.* **287**, 274–276.

Raper S., Crome P., Vale J. A. et al. (1982) Experience with activated carbon-bead haemoperfusion columns in the treatment of severe drug intoxication. *Arch. Toxicol.* **49**, 303–310.

Reuning R. H., Malspeis L., Franks A. L. et al. (1977) Testing of drug delivery systems for use in the treatment of narcotic abuse. *Natl Inst. Drug Abuse Research Monograph* (US Government Printing Office 0-249-121) **141**, 43–45.

Ringbom A. (1963) *Complexation in Analytical Chemistry*. New York: Wiley Interscience.

Robin H. and Harley J. D. (1966) Factors influencing response to mammalian species to the methaemoglobin reduction test. *Aust. J. Exp. Biol. Med. Sci.* **44**, 519–526.

Rose C. L., Welles J. S., Fink R. D. et al (1947) The antidotal action of *p*-aminopropiophenone with or without sodium thiosulfate in cyanide poisoning. *J. Pharmacol. Exper. Therap.* **89**, 109–114.

Rosenburg J., Benowitz N. L. and Pond S. (1981) Pharmacokinetics of drug overdose. *Clin. Pharmacokin.* **6**, 161–192.

Rumack B. H. (1973) Anticholinergic poisoning treatment with physostigmine. *Pediatrics* **52**, 449–451.

Rumack B. H. and Peterson R. G. (1980). Clinical Toxicology. In: Doull J., Klaasen C. D. and Amdur M. O. (ed.) *Casarett and Doull's Toxicology, the Basic Science of Poisoning*, 2nd edn., 677–698. New York: Macmillan.

Sanderson D. M. (1965) Timing of therapy in experimental poisoning with organophosphorus compounds. Letter. *J. Pharm. Pharmacol.* **17**, 124–125.

Savides M. C., Oehme F. W., Nash S. L. et al. (1984) The toxicity and biotransformation of single doses of acetaminophen in dogs and cats. *Toxicol. Appl. Pharmacol.* **74**, 26–34.

Saxena K. and Kingston R. (1982) Acute poisoning. *Postgrad. Med. J.* **71**, 67–77.

Schwartz C., Morgan R. L., Way L. M. et al. (1979) Antagonism of cyanide intoxication with sodium pyruvate. *Toxicol. Appl. Pharmacol.* **50**, 437–441.

Smith J. E. and Beutler E. (1965) Methemoglobin formation and reduction in man and various animal species. *Am. J. Physiol.* **210**, 347–350.

Smith R. L. and Caldwell J. (1977) Drug metabolism in non-human primates. In: Parke D. V. and Smith R. L. (ed.) *Drug Metabolism—From Microbe to Man*, 331–358. London: Taylor and Francis.

Smith R. P. (1969) Cobalt salts: effects in cyanide and sulfide poisoning and on methemoglobinaemia. *Toxicol. Appl. Pharmacol.* **15**, 505–516.

Smith T. W., Haber E., Yeatman L. et al. (1976) Reversal of advanced digoxin intoxication with Fab fragments of digoxin specific antibodies. *N. Engl. J. Med.* **294**, 797–800.

Smith R. P., Kruszyna R. and Krusyna H. (1976) Management of acute sulfide poisoning. *Arch. Environ. Health.* **31**, 166–169.

Sörbo B. H. (1951) On the properties of rhodenese. *Acta Chem. Scand.* **5**, 724–234.

Stolk J. M. and Smith R. P. (1966) Species differences in methemoglobin reductase activity. *Biochem. Pharmacol.* **15**, 343–351.

Stradling, G. N., Stather J. W., Gray S. A. et al. (1986) Efficacies of LICAM (C) and DTPA for the recorporation of inhaled transportable forms of plutonium and Americium from the rat. *Human Toxicol.* **5**, 77–84.

Sturman J. A. and Smith M. J. H. (1967) The binding of salicylate to plasma protein in different species. *J. Pharm. Pharmacol.* **19**, 621–623.

Szoradi I., Szemere G., Magyarlaki A. et al (1970) Some observations concerning atropine esterase. *Acta Biol. Acad. Sci. Hungaricae* **21**, 293–297.

Taylor P. (1980) Anticholinesterase agents. In: Gilman A. G., Goodman L. S. and Gilman A. (ed.) *The Pharmacological Basis of Therapeutics*, 6th ed., 100–119. New York: Macmillan.

Tephly T. R., Parks R. E. and Mannering G. J. (1964) Methanol metabolism in the rat. *J. Pharmacol. Exper. Therap.* **143**, 292–300.

Testa B. and Jenner P. (1976) *Drug Metabolism: Chemical and Biochemical Aspects.* New York: Marcel Dekker, Inc.

Troisi F. M. (1950) Chronic intoxication by ethylene glycol vapour. *Br. J. Ind. Med.* **7**, 65–69.

Tyrer F. H. (1981) Treatment of cyanide poisoning. Letter. *J. Soc. Occup. Med.* **31**, 65–66.

Vale J. A., Meredith T. J. and Goulding R. (1981) Treatment of acetaminophen poisoning. *Arch. Intern. Med.* **141**, 394–396.

Vale J. A. and Wheeler D. C. (1982) Anaphalactoid reactions to acetylcysteine. *Lancet* **2**, 998.

van Helden H. P. M., van der Wiel H. J. and Wolthuis O. L. (1983) Therapy of organophosphate poisoning: the marmoset as a model for man. *Br. J. Pharmacol.* **78**, 579–589.

van Stee E. W., Harris A. M., Horton M. L. et al. (1975) The treatment of ethylene glycol toxicosis with pyrazole. *J. Pharmacol. Exper. Therap.* **192**, 251–259.

Volans G. N., Vale J. A., Crome P. et al. (1977) The role of charcoal haemoperfusion in the management of acute poisoning by drugs. In: Kennedy R. M., Courtney J. M., Gaylor J. D. S. and Gilchrist T. (ed.) *Artificial Organs*, 178–187. London: Macmillan.

Wacker E. C., Haynes H., Fisher W. et al. (1965) Treatment of ethylene glycol poisoning with ethyl alcohol. *JAMA* **194**, 1231–1233.

Watanabe A. S. (1977) Pharmacokinetic aspects of the dialysis of drugs. *Drug Intell. Clin. Pharm.* **11**, 407–416.

Way J. L., Sylvester D., Morgan R. L. et al. (1984) Recent perspectives in the toxicodynamic basis of cyanide antagonism. *Fund. Appl. Toxicol.* **4**, S231–S239.

Weger N. and Szinicz L. (1981) Therapeutic effects of new oximes, benactyzine and atropine in soman poisoning. Part I. Effects of various oximes in soman, sarin and VX poisoning in dogs. *Fund. Appl. Toxicol.* **1**, 161–163.

Weiner N. (1980) Atropine, scopalamine and related antimuscarinic drugs. In: Gilman A. G., Goodman L. S. and Gilman A. (ed.) *The Pharmacological Basis of Therapeutics*, 6th edn., 120–137. New York: Macmillan.

Williams R. J., Caldwell J. and Dring L. G. (1973) Comparative metabolism of some amphetamines in various species. In: Usden E. and Snyder S. H. (ed). *Frontiers in Catecholamine Research*, 927–932. New York: Pergamon.

Wolthuis O. L. and van Wersh R. A. P. (1984) Behavioral changes in the rat after low doses of cholinesterase inhibitors. *Fund. Appl. Toxicol.* **4**, S195–S208.

Chapter 13

The Interaction between Epidemiology and Animal Studies in Industrial Toxicology

H. Michael D. Utidjian

The question may be raised by some readers, especially those from the pure discipline of animal toxicology, as to what place a chapter on epidemiology has in a textbook on toxicology, even applied toxicology. At first glance the two disciplines seem to present more pointed contrasts than similarities. From the point of view of study design, epidemiology, essentially a study approach based upon opportunism, would appear to defy all the most cherished principles of animal toxicology. Thus, occupational epidemiology of necessity studies working populations of great genetic heterogeneity, of wide age distribution (at least within the 18 to 65 years industrial working age range), exposed intermittently to largely unknown concentrations of the toxicant of interest, by an ill-defined combination of routes (usually inhalation with a variable transdermal component), almost never in isolation, for outcomes or effects which are rarely determinable or even definable in the precise terms demanded of animal studies. Of the outcomes studied in occupational epidemiology, the 'underlying cause of death', usually taken from the death certificate, selected by conventional nosology from the various pathological entities inscribed thereon, rarely confirmed by autopsy or histopathology, is generally the best defined and most accurately ascertained. Moreover, the diet and other life-style variables in the free-living working population are not amenable to control, or even ascertainment, except in the broadest socioeconomic sense. Little wonder then that the inclusion of a small epidemiology unit in the industry-sponsored Chemical Industry Institute of Toxicology in North Carolina has been a hotly, sometimes acrimoniously debated topic, in meetings of the Scientific Advisory Panel of that institution. Happily, the modestly funded epidemiology unit has survived over the protests of a few toxicologic purists.

The answer to the question, or the justification of discussing epidemiology in a textbook of this scope, lies, of course, in the fact that epidemiology, with all its shortcomings from an experimental toxicological point of view, deals directly with the human as opposed to animal subjects. Moreover, it deals, in the occupational setting, with 'real life exposures' in the very mode of concern, for the regulation of which animal studies, by extrapolation, are ultimately designed to address. In this chapter an attempt will be made to review the ways in which epidemiology has historically interacted with experimental animal studies, sometimes in response to the findings of the latter, sometimes stimulating the initiation of animal studies for the first time, often in an alternating manner from one to the other.

EARLY INDUSTRIAL EPIDEMIOLOGY STUDIES

In recent years occupational epidemiology has been almost completely preoccupied with the issue of occupational cancer, and very largely through mortality studies in the historical perspective mode. Earlier in this century, however, before the spectre of occupational or industrial cancer had loomed so large, some occupational epidemiological morbidity studies, on a variety of industrial toxicants of importance, were published. These were often based on cross-sectional surveys of a work force, and were often not labelled or defined by their authors as 'epidemiological studies', though such they were. A good example of such a study is that published by Robert Kehoe and his colleagues (Kehoe et al., 1932) of health observations they performed on workers exposed to various levels of relatively pure and dust-free sulphur dioxide gas in the refrigeration industry, in which, at that time, liquified sulphur dioxide was commonly used as the refrigerant. Although several industrial morbidity studies have been published since, for example on oil refinery workers (Anderson, 1950), and on pulp and paper mills (Skalpe, 1964; Ferris et al., 1967), the Kehoe study was outstanding in that the exposure was to exceptionally pure sulphur dioxide virtually in isolation, a highly unusual circumstance in industry.

In the 1950s and 1960s a considerable amount of experimental work, mostly on the pathophysiological response and respiratory mechanics aspects of human exposures to sulphur dioxide, was undertaken (Amdur et al., 1953; Sim and Pattle, 1957; Frank et al., 1962, 1964; Nadel et al., 1965; Snell and Luchsinger, 1969; Burton et al., 1969; Melville, 1970). Sulphur dioxide represents, in fact, one of those less common situations where experimental studies on human volunteers, at least of short-term and acute exposures at low to moderate concentrations, have largely superseded animal studies. Sulphur dioxide has also attracted a great deal of attention from the Environmental Protection Agency as a significant constituent of community air pollution (as the original contaminant form of the sulphur oxides complex) and this has resulted in a series of community air pollution/health effects studies of an epidemiologic nature, for example the Community Health Environmental Surveillance System (CHESS). But by its very nature, 'air pollution epidemiology' has to address the combined effects of a particulate and irritant gas mixture of which sulphur dioxide is only one part, whose individual contribution has been quite probably exaggerated.

As to what interaction or cross-fertilization, if any, has taken place over the years between toxicological studies, whether in man or animals, and epidemiological studies, whether industrial or community-wide, it is difficult to say. Of the above cited authors, only Skalpe (1964) makes direct reference to human and animal experimental studies in the introduction to his epidemiological paper. The experimentalists all refer to preceding experimental work, never to epidemiological studies. However, it is difficult to imagine that there was no mutual influence between epidemiologic or clinical studies and the laboratory.

Another good example of early occupational epidemiological observation is the work of Neal and his co-workers of the US Public Health Service on the incidence of chronic mercurialism in the hatters' felt and felt hat making industries in New England (Neal et al., 1937, 1941). Although Neal's was pioneering work which has been followed by many other studies around the world (Smith and Moskovitz, 1948; Smith et al., 1949 (both US); Kesic and Haeusler, 1951 (Yugoslavia); Baldi et al., 1953 (Italy); McGill et al., 1964 (US); Ladd et al., 1966 (Philippines and Yugoslavia); West and Lim, 1968 (US); Trachtenberg, 1969 (USSR); Smith et al., 1970 (US), it was apparently on Neal's work, which was distinguished by excellent environmental data, that the occupational exposure standard of 0.1 mg Hg per cubic metre of air as an 8-hour time-weighted average which remained in effect for almost 30 years in the US was based (NIOSH, 1973).

There is a very extensive toxicological literature, both animal and human, on elemental and inorganic mercury and its compounds (Bidstrup, 1964; NIOSH, 1973). Toxicologist authors rarely make reference, let alone give credit, to epidemiological observations to justify or introduce their interest in a particular aspect of mercury toxicology—why should they? It has been known since the dawn of history that mercury is highly poisonous to man, at least in the form of its soluble salts such as 'corrosive sublimate', the evocative name given by medieval alchemists to mercuric chloride. (The toxic hazard of the vapour of the harmless looking elemental mercury or 'quicksilver' has not been fully appreciated until the post-World War II era, however.) The experimental toxicologist has therefore been largely concerned with studying the absorption, distribution and excretion of this insidiously poisonous metal, and the mechanisms of its peculiar toxicity to the central nervous system, and the kidneys in particular. The epidemiologist has in turn worked against a backdrop of historical knowledge, even folklore, of the human toxicity of mercury, including mass observations, which can be construed in an epidemiological manner. Only in that sense can it be said that the 'epidemiology of mercury' and its 'toxicology' have interacted.

THE ENVIRONMENTAL EPIDEMIOLOGY OF CANCER AND ITS INTERACTION WITH EXPERIMENTAL TOXICOLOGY

It is when we turn to the post-World War II era and the tremendous rise of concern over environmental, including industrial/occupational cancer, that the undoubted interaction between the very different investigatory disciplines of epidemiology and experimental toxicology, which is the theme of this chapter, begins to play a significant, if not always fully recognized, role. I prefer the more comprehensive term 'environmental' to 'industrial' or 'occupational' cancer epidemiology in this context to accommodate the most significant cancer increase of the last 30–40 years, the only one worthy of the term 'epidemic', namely lung cancer in cigarette smokers. Surely, not even the most zealous toxicologist would deny that epidemiology, and epidemiology alone, has indicted and incriminated the cigarette as a potent carcinogenic agent, or would claim that experimental animal toxicology could ever have done the job with the same definition. The epidemiologically established fact has, of course, stimulated a great deal of toxicological research into the proximal carcinogen, or carcinogens in the tobacco smoke, and a number of culprits have been found including polycyclic aromatic hydrocarbons, arsenic trioxide, nitrosamines, and radon daughters to name just a few. Skin cancers have been produced by the painting of tobacco tars on the skin of small animals, but due to the understandable difficulty of inducing laboratory animals to become the equivalent of 2-packs a day inhaler smokers (although I understand that zealous experimentalists have trained beagles and even miniature donkeys to 'smoke' through a suitable apparatus), the identification of specific carcinogenic agents in the tobacco smoke is very much 'after the fact' in terms of identifying the cigarette as Western man's most serious environmental carcinogen discovered to date.

The occupational cancer which produces the closest parallel to the cigarette-induced cancer situation, in that there still appears to be no unequivocal animal model, is that of arsenic, in the form of arsenic trioxide fume and, again, lung cancer. Arsenic has been a curiously elusive culprit as the cause of occupational cancer, longer and more often suspected than any other of being responsible for a variety of industrial cancers, now all attributed with some confidence to other causes, until arsenic trioxide was finally 'incriminated' of causing lung cancer in the 1970s (NIOSH, 1975a). Thus arsenic was erroneously suspected of being the cause of scrotal cancer in the smelters of arsenical copper in 1820, and was likewise suggested at one time as the carcinogenic agent in chimney soot in Pott's scrotal cancer of chimney sweeps, as the lung carcinogen in cobalt miners in Joachimstal (radon daughters are now considered responsible), as the carcinogen in the ethmoidal sinus and lung cancer experienced by workers in the carbonyl process of refining nickel in South Wales (now attributed to certain nickel ore dusts, such as the subsulphide) and, as already mentioned, as one of the potential carcinogens in cigarette smoke. At the same time, repeated attempts to induce cancer in small experimental animals by administration of arsenic in a variety of forms and by a variety of routes, have all failed (NIOSH, 1975a).

The first strongly suggestive evidence that occupational exposure to arsenic caused excesses of both lung and skin cancer came from a study, published as two adjacent papers, on a sodium arsenite sheep-dip factory in England, where exposures were to both the sodium arsenite salt and to the arsenic trioxide raw material (Hill and Faning, 1948; Perry et al., 1948). For some reason, the strong findings of this study were largely overlooked until two independent studies published in the United States in 1974 seemed to confirm the earlier British findings (Baetjer et al., 1974; Ott et al., 1974). These two latter studies reported moderate excesses of lymphopoietic cancer as well as lung cancer. In addition, there have been several studies of cancer mortality in non-ferrous smelter workers in the US who are exposed to varying degrees to arsenic trioxide in the fume from roasting and smelting of arseniferous ores, which have shown significant increases in lung cancer (Lee and Fraumeni, 1969; Rencher and Carter, 1971). One Japanese study (Kuratsune et al., 1974), while supportive of the findings of the preceding two US studies, is of methodological interest as it provides a rare example of a true retrospective or case-control study in an occupational setting. A remarkably high lung cancer mortality rate was observed among males in a particular town. The employment history of these lung cancer cases was compared with that of a control group of descendants who had died of other causes than lung, urinary bladder or skin cancer. A strong association was demonstrated between having died of lung cancer and having worked in the copper smelter.

If there has been interaction between epidemiology and experimental toxicology in the case of arsenic, it must all have been in the direction of human epidemiologic findings (or earlier suspicions, as already mentioned) suggesting to animal toxicologists that they might produce cancer in small animals with arsenic, but so far with no avail. Thus, those British pioneers of experimental cancer, Leitch and Kennaway, were already trying to induce cancer with arsenic as early as 1922 (Leitch and Kennaway, 1922; Leitch, 1923).

Hexavalent Chromium and Cancer—Which Chromates?

Another industrial metal, certain of whose compounds undoubtedly cause lung cancer with strikingly increased risk, in which epidemiological observation and later formal studies preceded and stimulated elucidatory animal toxicological work, is chromium. As far back as 1932 Lehmann in Germany published a paper with the quaintly old-fashioned title, which both asks a rhetorical question, and turned out subsequently to be quite prophetic: 'Is there a reason for special concern about the incidence of lung cancer in chromate workers....?' (Lehmann, 1932) To answer Lehmann's question, there is indeed a reason. To quote P. E. Enterline in a review article on chromate cancer epidemiology published 42 years later: 'Epidemiologic investigations of workers engaged in refining chromite ore show a remarkable excess in lung cancer....The magnitude of the excess in lung cancers has seldom been observed in human populations' (Enterline, 1974).

Further response to Lehmann's question is to be found in the considerable number of epidemiological studies which followed over the ensuing forty years in most of the countries with major chromate industries. The studies of Gross and Kolsch, (1943) (Germany), Machle and Gregorius (1948) (US), Baetjer (1950) (US), Mancuso and Hueper (1951) (US), Bidstrup and Case (1956) (UK), Taylor (1966) (US), Bittersohl (1972) (Germany), and Langard and Norseth (1975) (Norway) are a representative and chronological selection. Although all the foregoing studies showed excesses of lung cancer in their populations, the degree of excess varies considerably from one study to another, with the mean latent periods between onset of exposure to chromate and the development of lung cancer varying from 10·6 years (Mancuso and Hueper, 1951) to 14·5 years (Machle and Gregorius, 1948) to 21 years (Bidstrup and Case, 1956). These discrepancies led to much speculation as to the specific chromium compounds which might be the potent carcinogens, as the chemical processes and intermediates varied somewhat between certain plants, principally with respect to whether the chromate was leached from the roasted chromite ore as highly soluble sodium chromate or dichromate or as the more sparingly soluble calcium salts. These observations stimulated a great deal of animal toxicological experiments with the various chromium compounds encountered in the industry, including the basic chromite ore itself, administered by a variety of routes and techniques, but including, latterly, inhalation: Hueper (1958), Baetjer et al., (1959), Payne (1960), Nettesheim et al., (1961), Steffee and Baetjer (1965), Roe and Carter (1969), being but a representative selection. It is quite clear that this whole body of animal experimentation was originally and primarily instigated by the epidemiological observations already described in outline, another very clear cut example of interaction and mutual influence between the two investigatory disciplines. By a judicious combination of the evidence from both epidemiological and toxicological observations, it has been possible to identify a number of very sparingly soluble chromates, principally those of calcium and the other alkaline earth metals, but also lead and zinc chromates, as potent carcinogens, and to exonerate largely the highly soluble sodium and other alkali metal chromates (and dichromates and the corresponding ammonium salts) as carcinogens and also, by contrast, the highly insoluble compounds such as the sesquioxide and the unoxidized chromite ore itself, in which the chromium is in the trivalent form (NIOSH, 1975b).

Nickel and Cancer—Which Compounds?

A somewhat parallel situation evolved with respect to nickel industry carcinogenesis as has just been described historically for the chromate industry, in that an informal observation was initially made that there appeared to be an excessive incidence of lung cancer, and also of the much rarer cancer of the nasal cavities and paranasal sinuses, as far back as 1932 (Bridge, 1933), which was followed by a series of formal epidemiologic studies and other reports continuing through the late 1970s (Amor, 1938; Barnett, 1949; Morgan, 1958; Doll, 1958; Doll et al., 1970; Doll et al., 1977) which were remarkable for being all based upon the same plant, a nickel refinery at Clydach, South Wales. The excess cancer risk to the nasal and respiratory tracts was subsequently confirmed at a number of other plants in different countries, notably Canada (Sutherland, 1959, 1969), and Norway (Loken, 1959; Pedersen et al., 1973), a few cases additionally being reported from the USSR (Tatarskaya, 1965) and France (Bourasset and Galland, 1966). Speculation still continues as to what the specific carcinogenic agent or agents might be, although the field has narrowed down somewhat. Toxicology is once again being invoked in attempts to prove the carcinogenic potential of the various nickel compounds, and forms of metallic nickel itself, to which human, if not always strictly epidemiological, observations seem to point. As in the case of chromates research, it would appear that epidemiologic evidence has been the instigator, animal studies being conducted much more recently in an attempt to elucidate the situation. The first suggestion, by Amor in 1938, was that arsenic, present as an impurity in the sulphuric acid used to digest the nickel ores, was responsible for the excess respiratory cancer (Amor, 1938). Part of the reasoning was that a purer, arsenic-free source of acid was established in 1925, and it appeared that men first employed since that year had little or no excess risk of cancer. The next theory to prevail for some years was that nickel carbonyl, $Ni(CO)_4$, was responsible (Doll et al., 1977). This gaseous nickel compound is highly toxic on inhalation, causing life-threatening pulmonary oedema, and was at that time used only at Clydach as the intermediate in the Mond nickel-refining process. However, as cases of 'nickel cancer' started to appear at other plants and in other countries where nickel carbonyl is not employed at all, it became evident that if the carbonyl was the culprit at all, it could not be the sole one. Although under certain experimental conditions both metallic nickel and the carbonyl can cause cancer in animals (Sunderman, 1973), the epidemiological evidence points away from the nickel carbonyl process and rather to dust from the preliminary treatment of the ore, particularly dust formed during the roasting of impure nickel copper sulphide and nickel subsulphide to the oxides (Morgan, 1958; Doll, 1958; Sutherland, 1959; Pedersen et al., 1970; Doll et al., 1977). Some of the recent inhalation experiments on small animals have tended to confirm this circumstantial evidence against nickel subsulphide and oxide dusts (Kasprzak et al., 1973; Ottolenghi et al., 1975; Wehner et al., 1975).

The Beryllium Controversy

The still unresolved controversy over whether or not beryllium compounds are carcinogenic to man gives a further illustration of the considerable interplay possible between toxicology and epidemiology. Beryllium, an exotic and exceedingly toxic metal, has been known since the 1930s to cause a serious and life-threatening, though not strictly neoplastic, pulmonary granulomatous disease, clinically resembling Boeck's sarcoidosis, which was first given the name 'berylliosis' by Marradi-Fabroni in Italy, actually with reference to a similar lesion experimentally produced in guinea-pigs (Marradi-Fabroni, 1935). This led to a considerable proliferation of animal studies, as a result of which it was established that beryllium compounds could induce osteogenic sarcomas in rabbits and rats (Gardner and Heslington, 1946; Janes et al., 1954; Kelley et al., 1961). Also, in 1961 Schepers reported the induction of lung cancer in rats (Schepers, 1961). This observation spurred attempts by epidemiological mortality studies of beryllium workers to determine whether, in addition to the risk of berylliosis, such workers also experienced an increased risk of lung cancer (Mancuso, 1970). Such studies have been rendered very difficult as the primary metallurgy of this rare metal was originally confined to only two companies in the United States, and in recent years to one. A related series of studies of initially five plants, later confined to one, has been conducted by NIOSH and its predecessor agency, and were the subject of hearings held by the Occupational Safety and Health Administration (OSHA) in Washington in August–September 1977. The studies, which have never been published, were seriously flawed, and although the final one, based upon the smallest cohort, was claimed by its authors to show a small excess risk of lung cancer, this claim has not been widely accepted. NIOSH is apparently undertaking a fourth 'reworking and reanalysis' of the data (R. J. Waxweiler, personal communication, 1980). In the meantime, beryllium rightly remains on the list of 'suspect' or 'potential' human carcinogens on the basis of the animal data alone. In the Criteria Document of Beryllium (NIOSH, 1972), one of the first to be published, the following interesting statement appears under the provocative heading: 'Limitations of Experimental Toxicology'.'...An exact parallelism in the response of animals and man does not always exist. Animals respond toxicologically to beryllium with changes that are morphologically different from those observed in man....The epithelial proliferation and primary pulmonary cancer was induced in rats after long-term, daily repeated exposures to beryllium....and had not been reproduced in man even after long periods of time and high exposure levels....Hence, the carcinogenic exposure-effect relationship observed in animals does not correlate to man.' Once more, animal toxicology and (human) epidemiology are seen to interact, but in this case with apparent conflict.

Cadmium—Another Suspect Only

Before leaving the subject of the carcinogenic industrial metals, proven or merely suspect, one should briefly consider cadmium. This metal, the periodic neighbour and natural congener of zinc, is of very versatile toxicity in man and animals, and its carcinogenicity, if it exists, is probably of minor significance in industry relative to its profoundly damaging effects on the kidney and its probable life-long accumulation in that organ. The earlier epidemiological studies of cadmium workers addressed a variety of toxic effects, especially on the respiratory, renal, skeletal and haemopoietic systems, rather than the possibility of cancer (Hardy and Skinner, 1947; Princi, 1947; Friberg, 1950; Baader, 1951; Bonnell, 1955). The first indication that cadmium exposure might be associated with prostatic cancer was human and anecdotal/epidemiological (Potts, 1965; Kipling and Waterhouse, 1967; Lemen et al., 1976). These observations clearly preceded and no doubt largely inspired a series of animal studies for possible prostatic carcinogenesis, which appear, however, to have been entirely negative (Levy et al., 1973; Levy and Clack, 1975; Levy et al., 1975). Epidemiological studies will no doubt continue to be pursued where possible in this rather fragmented industry. However, as time goes by, exposures are likely to be so much reduced, in view of the general and cumulative toxicity of the metal, that the chances of demonstrating a carcinogenic effect by the relatively insensitive technique of epidemiology will become more remote.

Other metals and their compounds and industrial processes have been studied epidemiologically as well as toxicologically for evidence of carcinogenesis, including lead (negative so far), antimony (so close chemically and physically to arsenic as to be an obvious suspect and indicted), iron in the form of hematite (which ore is often associated with significant levels of radioactivity), not to mention the highly radioactive metals, especially radium (luminous dial-painters' osteogenic sarcoma of the mandible) and uranium (especially in the mining of the ores—radon-induced lung cancer).

Vinyl Chloride Cancer—A Humbling History

This gas, of great importance as the monomer in the enormous polyvinyl chloride (PVC) resin or polymer industry, presents a rich example of the interaction between toxicology and epidemiology, and a humbling reminder of the limitations of both disciplines in the timely detection of industrial carcinogenic risk when, in the former case, insufficiently long-term studies are performed and, in the latter, if the human tumour is of too great a rarity. For several decades, based upon acute animal exposure studies only, vinyl chloride was considered to be one of the least toxic of the halogenated hydrocarbons (Mastromatteo et al., 1960; Lester et al., 1963), and its use as an inhalation anaesthetic was even explored (Zenz, 1975). It was even used in the US as the propellant for certain domestic aerosol dispensers. Some capacity to cause liver and kidney injury in animals on repeated exposure had been reported in 1961 (Torkelson et al., 1961). The first focus of occupational hazard interest in vinyl chloride was in the area of a curious non-malignant lesion, acro-osteolysis, or resorption of the bone of the distal phalanges (believed to be secondary to an ischaemic bone necrosis) of the fingers in certain vinyl chloride polymerization workers (Harris and Adam, 1967; Wilson et al., 1967; Dinman et al., 1971; Dodson et al., 1971). This lesion, quite unique in the history of occupational pathology, appeared to be associated with a combination of high level exposures to the gas, and the heavy use of the fingers in the cleaning of caked PVC polymer from the interior of the reactor vessels. When this manual process was eliminated, the disease ceased to occur.

The author happened to be employed with a consulting firm in 1973 when it was approached by the then Manufacturing Chemists Association, on behalf of the majority of the vinyl chloride/PVC industry in the United States, and asked to perform, with some urgency, a multi-company mortality study on vinyl chloride producers and polymerizers in this country. When we asked for the underlying reason for such a study, which did not appear to be heralded by any human observations, we were told of then recent animal work by Viola and his co-workers in Italy who had reported tumours of the skin, lungs and bones of rats exposed to extremely high levels of vinyl chloride (30 000 ppm or 3% v/v) in studies originally attempting to reproduce acro-osteolysis in an animal model (Viola et al., 1971; Zenz, 1975).

This mortality study got underway by mid-1973, but before even any report of preliminary findings could be made, in August, 1974 (Tabershaw and Gaffey, 1974), the first finding of an excessive mortality from haemangiosarcoma in the liver among employees of one plant of the B. F. Goodrich Chemical Company in Louisville, Kentucky, manufacturing PVC resins, was reported by the plant physician, John Creech, in March of that year (Creech and Johnson, 1974). This striking observation was based initially upon only three cases, but so rare is this particular malignancy in the general population (only about 25 cases were being reported annually for the whole of the United States at that time (Falk et al., 1974a)), that it was immediately apparent that something was significantly amiss at this one plant. Further investigations at the same plant (Falk et al., 1974a) soon revealed the deaths of an additional four men from the same rare malignancy over the preceding few years.

However, the MCA sponsored study alone, although based upon the mortality experience of the employees of the majority of the vinyl chloride polymerizing industry of the US (i.e. over 10 000 workers in 37 plants), would have failed to reveal the association of VCM exposure with this exotic tumour. In the tables of Standardized Mortality Ratios (SMRs) in which the expected numbers of deaths from specific causes were conventionally derived from national mortality statistics, the five cases of haemangiosarcoma in the liver captured by this study were buried within the grouping: 'Malignant neoplasms, digestive organs and peritoneum. ICD Nos. 150–159', which overall showed a *deficit* relative to the expected number of deaths, with a group SMR of only 75%! Causes of death as rare as this are not broken out separately in the tables published annually by the National Center for Health Statistics. Moreover, if the primary malignancy associated with VCM exposure happened to be lung cancer, with the same *absolute* excess, five additional lung cancer deaths in this study would not have raised the SMR for lung cancer significantly above expectancy. Interestingly, the one cancer site which did show a significant excess in this study was that of the brain (primary), with an SMR of 215, based upon 12 observed cases (Equitable Environmental Health, Inc., 1978). Independently by this time Maltoni and Lefemine in Italy had demonstrated brain tumours induced by vinyl chloride exposures in rats (Maltoni and Lefemine, 1975).

During the subsequent furore among the regulatory agencies in Washington following this startling revelation from Louisville, Professor Maltoni attended the informal fact-finding hearings in the capital and revealed for the first time that he had demonstrated angiosarcoma in the liver and other tumours in rats exposed to much lower concentrations of VCM than those employed earlier by Viola, levels in fact well within the range obtaining in many workroom atmospheres in the polymerization plants within recent memory (Tabershaw, 1974).

Since the original observation at the Goodrich Plant in Louisville, Kentucky (Creech and Johnson, 1974), which attracted world wide attention, there have been many subsequent confirmatory studies of haemangiosarcomas in different countries, e.g. Frentzel-Beyme et al., (1978) in Germany, Saric et al., (1976) in Yugoslavia, and Monson et al., (1974) and Falk et al., (1974b) in the United States.

Also, attempts have been made to follow up the leads suggested by the original Tabershaw and Gaffey 1974 epidemiologic report by further animal studies e.g. Keplinger et al. (1975) and Maltoni and Lefemine (1974), and to confirm human risk of cancer at the additional sites of brain and lung (Waxweiler et al., 1976).

It was, however, really the informal observation of the original three fatalities to be noticed by a plant physician with 'epidemiological intuition' which led to the denouement of this significant new cause of occupational cancer, and which elicited the revelation of hitherto unpublished research by Maltoni in Italy (Maltoni, 1974; Tabershaw, 1974). Haemangiosarcoma in the liver, rare as it is, is not unique to vinyl chloride exposure. It is also known to be associated with the diagnostic use of 'Thorotrast', a contrast medium containing the radioactive element thorium in colloidal compound form, the use of which was not abandoned until the mid 1950s, and also, in all likelihood, with certain organic arsenical compounds. However, the revelation of this new occupational cancer, almost invariably fatal, in such a widespread industry, has brought the whole area of occupational cancer onto centre-stage of societal and political concern, a position which, ten years later, it is only beginning to share with occupational reproductive hazards (of infertility as well as teratogenesis) and, to a lesser extent, with occupational neurotoxicity.

Carcinogenesis Bioassays—Toxicology Takes the Lead

The vinyl chloride melodrama more or less coincided with a signal reversal of the relative roles of animal toxicology and (human) epidemiology, at least in the field of occupational cancer risk identification. With the coming of the carcinogenesis bioassay and the lifetime administration to large numbers of rats and other animals of often barely subtoxic doses of a wide variety of chemicals, established experimental carcinogens are now looking for epidemiological confirmation, often, though not exclusively, in the occupational or industrial sphere. In some respects, as one toxicologist informally put it to the author recently, by exposing large numbers of animals (e.g. the so-called 'mega-rat' studies) for periods approaching, if not equalling, the natural life-span of the animals, by using unexposed but otherwise identically maintained animals as controls, and then submitting the results to rigorous statistical analysis, the toxicologist is now virtually practising interventional 'epidemiology' on animals. If this view of modern toxicology, at least of the carcinogenesis bioassay, is accepted as more than a *jeu d'esprit*, then epidemiology can be said to have influenced experimental toxicology in a profound and philosophical sense, going far beyond the mere suggestion of worthwhile animal investigations.

Today we see animal studies of the carcinogenesis bioassay type instigating large-scale epidemiological studies into human cancer risk from occupational exposure to acrylonitrile, formaldehyde, ethylene oxide, and most recently and tentatively acrylamide, to mention only the salient examples.

Acrylonitrile

In the early years of the industrial use of acrylonitrile (AN) (in the production of synthetic rubber) the toxicity of the compound was more or less equated with that of inorganic cyanide ion, to which it is partially metabolized *in vivo*: Dudley and Neal (1942), Dudley et al., (1942), Wilson (1944), Wilson et al. (1948), Brieger et al. (1952). Later it came to be used also in the production of acrylic or PAN (polyacrylonitrile) fibre. In April 1977, the then Manufacturing Chemists Association reported interim results at the end of the first year of a life-long feeding water ingestion study in rats, and also of a parallel intermittent inhalation study, also in rats, more closely simulating occupational exposure. Both studies were being performed under multi-company sponsorship, at the laboratories of the Dow Chemical Company (NIOSH, 1977). In both series of animals an increased incidence of central nervous system tumours was reported. In the ingestion study, stomach papillomas and Zymbal gland carcinomas were seen. The inhalation study yielded an increased incidence of ear canal tumours and mammary masses (Quast et al., 1980a,b). In the same year a paper was published by the seemingly indefatigable Maltoni in Italy, reporting 'borderline oncogenic effects' in rats exposed to acrylonitrile by both inhalation and gavage (Maltoni et al., 1977). Still in the same year, the National Institute of Occupational Safety and Health received from the DuPont Company a preliminary report of an epidemiologic study of workers at their Camden, South Carolina, acrylic fibre plant, indicating an excessive incidence of cancer, both of the lung and the colon (NIOSH, 1977). In Current Intelligence Bulletin 18, on acrylonitrile, NIOSH quoted the DuPont investigators as stating that while they did not consider this study to provide definitive evidence of the carcinogenicity of acrylonitrile in man, the findings, when considered in the light of the recent animal tests, raise a serious suspicion that it may be a human carcinogen. A clear case of animal toxicologic evidence being seen as lending support to epidemiologic findings. The DuPont Camden plant epidemiology study, when finally published in 1980 (O'Berg, 1980), was found to have some problematic features. Innovatively the investigator had used a large DuPont employee population drawn from other chemical plants and not exposed to acrylonitrile, though doubtless exposed to other chemicals, to generate an expected incidence of the two cancers of interest, lung and colon, for comparison with the observed incidence at the acrylonitrile exposed workers at the Camden plant. It appeared, however, that for reasons unknown, the incidence of these two cancers in this larger 'control' DuPont population was lower than national rates in general, and the mortality rates for lung cancer in the county in which the Camden plant is located are significantly higher than the national average. This discrepancy and doubt as to the validity of the DuPont control population as an appropriate comparison group has led certain authorities to challenge the conclusions of the O'Berg study.

A further epidemiological study has been conducted at a different DuPont plant, in which 1083 male employees were identified as having potential exposure to acrylonitrile between 1944 and 1970, and who were followed through 1981 for mortality and through 1983 for cancer incidence (Chen et al., 1987). No statistically significant excesses were found for overall mortality or cancer incidence. Whilst an increased incidence of lung cancer was not found, they did report a statistically significant excess of cancer of the prostate, which was also noted in an update of the O'Berg study (O'Berg et al., 1985). It is clear, as has also been recommended in a report prepared for the National Cancer Institute (Syracuse Research Corporation, 1985), that further epidemiology studies are necessary to define the carcinogenic potential of acrylonitrile to humans.

Altogether nine additional epidemiological studies on vinyl chloride workers have been reported world-wide, of which four have been published. Of the total ten studies, six show no evidence of any carcinogenic risk, and four, including the O'Berg study, show suggestive evidence of carcinogenicity (EPA, 1983). All the studies to date have serious flaws, including paucity of numbers (O'Berg's cohort is by far the largest), confounding exposures to other carcinogens, paucity of environmental data, inadequacy of follow-up or tracing of cohort members, lack of information on cigarette smoking, and lack of convincing dose/duration-response relationship. An informal interest-group of acrylonitrile producing and/or using companies in the United States has approached the industrial field study section of the National Cancer Institute to conduct an industry-wide epidemiological study, thus maximizing the cohort size, to try to resolve this important issue—and possibly also to demonstrate an exposure level at which the risk of cancer, if such exists, is negligible.

Formaldehyde

Formaldehyde, a pungent, highly irritating and reactive gas, in industrial use longer than any of the other organic compounds discussed in this chapter, was recognized mainly as a respiratory irritant (Bohmer, 1934; Krans, 1935), and as both a primary irritant and sensitizer of the skin (Chajes, 1930).

Early epidemiological (morbidity) reports addressed the problem of dermatitis from direct contact with formalin or formaldehyde containing resins and glues (Schwartz, 1936; Schwartz et al., 1943; Markuson et al., 1943; Harris, 1953), or upper respiratory tract irritation by formaldehyde vapour (Zaeva et al., 1968; Shipkovitz, 1968; Yefremov, 1970). An early unsuccessful attempt to produce experimental cancer in mice by formaldehyde inhalation was reported in 1963 (Horton, 1963). Finally, in 1980 Swenberg and his colleagues, working at the Chemical Industry Institute of Toxicology in North Carolina, produced highly significant numbers of squamous cell carcinomas of the nasal turbinates of rats exposed intermittently for 18 months to only 15 ppm of formaldehyde by inhalation (Swenberg et al., 1980).

This definitive report has clearly triggered several epidemiological mortality studies, focusing on respiratory cancer (Wong, 1980; Marsh, 1982; Walrath and Fraumeni, 1983; Liebling et al., 1984). Only the last two have shown any suggestive evidence of carcinogenicity. So important an issue is the question of formaldehyde carcinogenicity with its widespread trace presence in buildings insulated with urea-formaldehyde foams, in garment making establishments using formaldehyde-based resins as permanent press agents, in iron and steel foundries using formaldehyde resins as core binders in the moulds, and in many branches of the chemical industry, that the Formaldehyde Institute, an American trade association, in 1982 sponsored a major industry-wide mortality study by the National Cancer Institute. This study is well under way at the time of writing.

Ethylene Oxide

Ethylene oxide, a highly reactive gas and the simplest epoxy compound, has been an important synthetic building block in the production of ethylene glycol and various glycol and 'crown' ethers since the 1930s. Even more important from the point of view of potential occupational exposures, however, is its widespread use as a sterilant in the food, drug and medical appliance industries, and for sterilizing instruments and dressings on site in hospitals. Until recently the main concern has been over its potency as a skin irritant (Taylor, 1977), and as a severe upper respiratory irritant (Thiess, 1963). Evidence of neurotoxicity in man (peripheral neuropathy) has also been reported (Gross et al., 1979). Well recognized as a potent experimental alkylating agent and mutagen in recent years (Wolman, 1979), it was inevitable that it would sooner or later be submitted to carcinogenesis bioassay. The definitive study was the two-year inhalation study in Fischer 344 rats, sponsored by a large group of industrial concerns and performed at the Bushy Run Research Center (BRRC), at that time administered by the Carnegie-Mellon University, supported by the Union Carbide Corporation (Snellings et al., 1981). Fischer 344 rats experienced an increased incidence of mononuclear cell leukemia and peritoneal mesotheliomas. Later, an increased incidence of primary brain neoplasms (gliomas) was also discovered (Sielken, 1983). A second inhalation study on rats, and also cynomolgus monkeys, was conducted by NIOSH and confirmed the enhancement of the rate of leukemia in the rats, but not in the monkeys (Lynch, 1982). A later report on this study also describes an increased incidence of central nervous system gliomas (Anonymous, 1982).

Three epidemiology (mortality) studies on ethylene oxide workers have now been reported. The one US study (Morgan et al., 1981) was negative. A Swedish study reported an excess of 'all malignant neoplasms', stomach cancer and leukemia, based, however, on extremely small numbers of cases (Hogstedt et al., 1979). A German study was reported as essentially negative (Thiess et al., 1981a).

The concern for human health hazards from ethylene oxide in two other areas has been heightened by reports of detection of increases in the rate of sister chromatid exchanges (SCEs) in cultured peripheral lymphocytes from ethylene oxide sterilizer operators (Garry et al., 1979; Abrahams, 1980; Thiess et al.,

1981b; Yager et al., 1983), and by one report of alleged increase in the spontaneous abortion rate in female hospital (sterilizer) workers in Finland (Hemminki et al., 1982).

In an attempt to resolve the carcinogenesis issue at least, NIOSH is undertaking, with the cooperation of US industry represented by the Health Industry Manufacturers Association (HIMA), a large-scale mortality study of a number of industrially based ethylene oxide sterilization facilities.

Acrylamide

Discovered in 1893, the major industrial uses of acrylamide had to await the commercial availability of acrylonitrile, from which it is made, in 1940 (Bikales and Kolodny, 1963). The major use of acrylamide monomer is in the production of gelatinous polymers which have widespread uses as flocculants in water and sewage treatment, and in paper-making (Bikales and Kolodny, 1963).

Until very recently the overwhelming toxicological concern over acrylamide monomer, a highly soluble crystalline solid of low vapour pressure, has been its profound and potent neurotoxicity in animals and man, by whatever route of absorption, including the unbroken skin (Hamblin, 1956). The compound causes primarily a peripheral neuropathy of the 'dying-back axonopathy' type in both sensory and motor nerves, but appearing to attack the sensory nerves first (Garland and Patterson, 1967; Takahashi et al., 1971). Extensive animal experimental work on the neurotoxic mechanism has been performed by Spencer and Schaumburg in this country, at the Albert Einstein Medical College Institute of Neurotoxicology (Spencer and Schaumburg, 1974).

Early in 1984, a jointly sponsored lifetime feeding studying of acrylamide in rats, intended as an investigation of long-term neurotoxicity as well as a carcinogenesis bioassay, under way at the toxicological laboratories of the Dow Chemical Company, began to show evidence of a carcinogenic effect involving the central nervous system and the gonads of animals of both sexes. The governmental regulatory agencies were promptly alerted, as were industrial customers and competitors. The reported study (Johnson et al., 1986) showed an increase in the incidence of several types of tumours in rats receiving the highest dose of acrylamide (2.0 mg/kg/day), with scrotal mesothelioma being the only tumour type increased at 0.5 mg/kg/day, and no tumour increase at 0.1 or 0.01 mg/kg/day. In a different study, Bull et al. (1984) showed acrylamide to be an initiator and to be active in the lung adenoma bioassay. The only epidemiology study published to date, as opposed to group clinical observations, is from the Dow Chemical Company who studied 371 employees assigned to acrylamide monomer or polymerization operations, and found no evidence for an association between exposure to acrylamide and overall mortality, total malignant neoplasms, or specific cancer types (Sobel et al., 1986). The same negative results have been established for a much larger international cohort of acrylamide workers employed by the American Cyanamid Company and its associates (Personal communication: J. J. Collins, 1987).

Until now, no epidemiological studies, as opposed to group clinical observations, have been undertaken on acrylamide. An historical perspective mortality study of acrylamide workers by one of the major companies in the industry is under active consideration at the time of writing.

SUMMARY

This chapter has been largely devoted to the application of occupational epidemiology, mostly in the mode of historical perspective mortality studies and their interaction with experimental toxicology. Epidemiology studies of this type lend themselves particularly well to cancer estimation because most occupational cancers, with the exception of those of the skin, have a high case fatality rate, so that mortality rates closely approximate incidence. Moreover, a death certificate, with all its shortcomings, represents a definite endpoint in which the certifying physician is strongly encouraged to arrive at a specific diagnosis or diagnoses. Also, cancer tends to be obtrusive as the single underlying cause of death for nosological selection.

As observed by Sir Richard Doll, most recognized occupational cancers have been discovered as a result of clinical intuition or epidemiological observation. However, most could have been avoided if modern toxicological techniques had been employed to test the substances used before men and women were exposed to them in the industrial environment (Doll, 1984).

Since the introduction of the costly carcinogenesis bioassay, which has for compelling economic reasons largely been employed on substances already in industrial use, epidemiology has started to lose its historic role as the initiating or 'hypothesis generating' study, and has become a secondary tool to follow and confirm, refute or quantify human carcinogenic effects—a 'hypothesis testing' and risk assessment role.

Therefore, we have seen that the two research disciplines of toxicology and epidemiology, apparently so different in approach, are in fact complementary, and both have a role to play. If carcinogenesis bioassay toxicology can be regarded as 'epidemiology on animals', by corollary, epidemiology could be seen as an opportunistic analysis of the results of inadvertent human experimentation in industry.

With the advent of computerized medical and industrial hygiene (environmental) surveillance systems in industry, it should be possible to pursue morbidity epidemiologic studies as opposed to exclusively mortality studies, and greatly extend the range of diseases for study beyond cancer to all chronic and debilitating diseases which may well have contributory occupational associations.

REFERENCES

Abrahams R. H. (1980) Recent studies with workers exposed to ethylene oxide. In: *HIMA Reports. The Safe Use of Ethylene Oxide*, Report No. 80-4, 27–38.

Amdur M. O., Melvin W. W. Jr. and Drinker P. (1953) Effects of inhalation of sulphur dioxide by man. *Lancet* **265**, 758–759.

Amor A. J. (1983) Growths of the respiratory tract. In: *Report of the VIII International Congress for Industrial Accidents and Occupational Diseases*, Frankfurt. **2**, 941–962.

Anderson A. (1950) Possible long-term effects of exposure to sulphur dioxide. *Br. J. Ind. Med.* **7**, 82–86.

Anonymous (1982). TSCA 8 (e) reports involving ethylene oxide. *Pesticide and Toxic Chemical News* **10**(41), 9.

Baader E. W. (1951) Chronic cadmium poisoning. *Dtsch. Med. Wochenschr.* (Germany) **76**, 484–487.

Baetjer A. M. (1950) Pulmonary carcinoma in chromate workers. I. A review of the literature and report of cases. *Arch. Ind. Hyg. Occup. Med.* **2**, 487–504.

Baetjer A. M., Levin M. L. and Lilienfeld A. (1974) *Analysis of mortality experience of Allied Chemical Plant—2000 Race St, Baltimore, MD.* Unpublished report submitted to the Allied Chemical Corporation (cited in NIOSH, 1975a (q.v). Morristown, NJ, 16 July.

Baetjer A. M., Lowney J. F., Steffee H. and Budacz V. (1959) Effect of chromium on incidence of lung tumors in mice and rats. *Arch. Ind. Health* **20**, 124–135.

Baldi G., Vigliani E. C. and Zurlo N. (1953) Chronic mercurialism in felt hat industries. *Med. Lav.* (Italy) **44**, 161–168.

Barnett G. P. (1949) Cancer of the nose and lung. In: *Annual Report of the Chief Inspector of Factories for the Year 1948*, 93. London: HMSO.

Bidstrup P. L. (1964) *Toxicity of mercury and its compounds.* New York: American Elsevier Publishing Company.

Bidstrup P. L. and Case R. A. M. (1956) Carcinoma of the lung in workmen in the bichromates-producing industry in Great Britain. *Br. J. Ind. Med.* **13**, 260–264.

Bikales N. M. and Kolodny E. R. (1963) Acrylamide. In: *Kirk-Othmer Encyclopedia of Chemical Technology*, Vol. 1, 2nd rev. edn., 274–284. New York: Interscience Publishers.

Bittersohl G. (November 1972) Health and the working environment—epidemiology of carcinomatosis in the chemical industry. *5th Merseburger Symposium* (Germany) 17–18.

Bohmer K. (1934) Formalin poisoning. *Dtsch. Z. Gesamte Gerichtl. Med.* (Germany) **23**, 7–18.

Bonnell J. A. (1955) Emphysema and proteinuria in men casting copper-cadmium alloys. *Br. J. Ind. Med.* **12**, 181–197.

Bourasset A. and Galland G. (1966) Carcinoma of the respiratory tract and exposure to nickel salts. *Arch. Mal. Prof. Med. Trav. Secur. Soc.* (France) **27**, 227–229.

Bridge J. C. (1933) 3—Health in Annual Report of the Chief Inspector of Factories for the Year 1932, 103–104. London: HMSO.

Brieger H., Rieders F. and Hodes W. A. (1952) Acrylonitrile: spectrophotometric determination, acute toxicity and mechanism of action. *Ind. Hyg. Occup. Med.* **6**, 128–140.

Bull R. J., Robinson M., Laurie R. D. et al. (1984) Carcinogenic effects of acrylamide in Sencar and A/J mice. *Cancer Res.* **44**, 107–111.

Burton G. G., Corn M., Gee J. B. L., Vasallo C. and Thomas A. P. (1969) Response of healthy men to inhaled low concentrations of gas-aerosol mixtures. *Arch. Environ. Health* **18**, 681–692.

Chajes B. (1930) Formaldehyde, formalin. In: International Labour Office, *Occupation and Health: Encyclopedia of Hygiene, Pathology and Social Welfare*, 806–810. Geneva: Noirclerc and Fenetrier.

Chen J. L., Walrath J., O'Berg M. T. et al. (1987) Cancer incidence and mortality among workers exposed to acrylonitrile. *Am. J. Ind. Med.* **11**, 157–163.

Creech J. L. and Johnson M. N. (1974) Angiosarcoma of liver in the manufacture of polyvinyl chloride. *J. Occup. Med.* **16**, 150–151.

Dinman B. D., Cook W. A., Whitehouse W. M. et al. (1971) Occupational acroosteolysis. I. An epidemiological study. *Arch. Environ. Health* **22**, 61–73.

Dodson V. N., Dinman B. D. and Whitehouse W. M. (1971) Occupational acroosteolysis. III. A clinical study. *Arch. Environ. Health* **22**, 83–91.

Doll R. (1958) Cancer of the lung and nose in nickel workers. *Br. J. Ind. Med.* **15**, 217–223.

Doll R. (1984) Epidemiologic discovery of occupational cancers. *Third Conference on Epidemiology in Occupational Health*, 28–30 (Singapore, September 1983). Abstracted in: *Scand. J. Work Environ. Health*, **10**, 121–138.

Doll R., Mathews J. D. and Morgan L. G. (1977) Cancer of the lung and nasal sinuses in nickel workers: a reassessment of the period of risk. *Br. J. Ind. Med.* **34**, 102–105.

Doll R., Morgan L. G. and Speizer F. E. (1970) Cancers of the lung and nasal sinuses in nickel workers. *Br. J. Cancer* **24**, 623–632.

Dudley H. C. and Neal P. A. (1942) Toxicology of acrylonitrile. I. A study of the acute toxicity. *J. Ind. Hyg. Toxicol.* **24**, 27–36.

Dudley, H. C., Sweeney, T. R. and Miller J. W. (1942) Toxicology of acrylonitrile (vinyl cyanide). II. Studies of effects of daily inhalation. *J. Ind. Hyg. Toxicol.*, **24**, 255–258.

Enterline P. E. (1974) Respiratory cancer among chromate workers. *J. Occup. Med.* **16**, 523–526.

EPA (1983) *Health Assessment Document for Acrylonitrile.* United States Environmental Protection Agency, Office of Health and Environmental Assessment, Washington DC, Section 13, p. 174.

Equitable Environmental Health, Inc. (1978) *Epidemiological Study of Vinyl Chloride Workers.* Unpublished report submitted to Manufacturing Chemists Association, Washington DC, August 1978.

Falk H., Creech J. L., Heath C. W. et al., (1974) Hepatic disease among workers at a vinyl chloride polymerization plant. *JAMA* **230**, 59–63.

Falk H., Heath C. W. Jr., Carter C. D. et al. (1974) Mortality among vinyl chloride workers. *Lancet* **2**, 784–785.

Ferris B. G. Jr., Burgess W. A. and Worcester J. (1967) Prevalence of chronic respiratory disease in a pulp mill and a paper mill in the United States. *Br. J. Ind. Med.* **24**, 26–37.

Fox A. J. and Collier P. R. (1977) Mortality experience of workers exposed to vinyl chloride monomer in the manufacture of polyvinyl chloride in Great Britain. *Br. J. Ind. Med.* **34**, 1–10.

Frank N. R., Amdur M. O. and Whittenberger J. L. (1964) A comparison of the acute effects of SO_2 administered alone or in combination with NaCl particles on the respiratory mechanics of healthy adults. *Int. J. Air Wat. Pollut.* **8**, 125–133.

Frank N. R., Amdur M. O., Worcester J. et al. (1962) Effects of acute controlled exposure to SO_2 on respiratory mechanics in healthy male adults. *J. Appl. Physiol.* **17**, 252–258.

Frentzel-Beyme R., Schmitz T. and Thiess A. M. (1978) Mortality study of VCM and PVC workers employed by BASF, Ludwigshafen/Rhein. *Arbeitsmedizin-Sozialmedizin-Praventivmedizin* (Stuttgart) **13/10**, 218–228.

Friberg L. (1950) *Health Hazards in the Manufacture of Alkaline Accumulators with Special Reference to Chronic Cadmium Poisoning—A Clinical and Experimental Study*. Stockholm: Ivar Haeggstroms Boktryckeri AB.

Gardner L. U. and Heslington H. F. (1946) Osteo-sarcoma from intravenous beryllium compounds in rabbits. *Fed. Proc.* **5**, 221.

Garland T. O. and Patterson M. W. H. (1967) Six cases of acrylamide poisoning. *Br. Med. J.* **4**, 134–138.

Garry V. F., Hozier F., Jacobs D. et al. (1979) Ethylene oxide: evidence of human chromosomal effects. *Environ. Mutagen.* **1**, 375–382.

Gross J. A., Haas M. L. and Swift T. R. (1979) Ethylene oxide neurotoxicity: report of four cases and review of the literature. *Neurology* **29**, 978–983.

Gross E. and Kolsch F. (1943) Lung cancer in the chromate dye industry. *Arch. Gewerbepathol. Gewerbehyg.* (Germany) **12**, 164–170.

Hamblin D. O. (1956) The toxicity of acrylamide—a preliminary report. *Hommage au Doyen René Fabre* (Paris), 195–199.

Hardy H. L. and Skinner J. B. (1947) The possibility of chronic cadmium poisoning. *J. Ind. Hyg. Toxicol.* **29**, 321–324.

Harris D. K. (1953) Health problems in the manufacture and use of plastics. *Br. J. Ind. Med.* **10**, 255–268.

Harris D. K. and Adam W. G. F. (1967) Acroosteolysis occurring in men engaged in the polymerization of vinyl chloride. *Br. Med. J.* **3**, 712–714.

Hemminki K., Mutanen P., Saloniemi I. et al. (1982) Spontaneous abortions in hospital staff engaged in sterilizing instruments with chemical agents. *Br. Med. J.* **285**, 1461–1463.

Hill A. B. and Faning E. L. (1948) Studies in the incidence of cancer in a factory handling inorganic compounds of arsenic. I. Mortality experience in the factory. *Br. J. Ind. Med.* **5**, 1–6.

Hogstedt C., Rohlen O., Berndtsson B. S. et al. (1979) A cohort study of mortality and cancer incidence in ethylene oxide production workers. *Br. J. Ind. Med.* **36**, 276–280.

Horton A. W., Tye R. and Stemmer K. L. (1963) Experimental carcinogenesis of the lung—inhalation of gaseous formaldehyde or an aerosol of coal tar by B3H mice. *J. Nat. Cancer Inst.* **30**, 31–40.

Hueper W. C. (1958) Experimental studies in metal cancerigenesis X. Cancerigenic effects of chromite ore roast deposited in muscle tissue and pleural cavity of rats. *Arch. Ind. Health* **18**, 284–291.

Janes J. M., Higgins G. M. and Herrick J. F. (1954) Beryllium-induced osteogenic sarcoma in rabbits. *J. Bone Joint Surg.* **36B**, 543–552.

Johnson K. A., Gorzinski S. J., Bodner K. et al. (1986) Chronic toxicity and oncogenicity study on acrylamide incorporated in the drinking water of Fischer 344 rats. *Toxicol. Appl. Pharmacol.* **85**, 154–168.

Kasprzak K. S., Marchow L. and Breborowicz J. (1973) Pathological reactions in rat lungs following intratracheal injection of nickel subsulfide and 3,4-benzpyrene. *Res. Commun. Chem. Pathol. Pharmacol.* **6**, 237–245.

Kehoe R. A., Machle W. F., Kitzmiller K. et al. (1932) On the effects of prolonged exposure to sulphur dioxide. *J. Ind. Hyg.* **14**, 159–731.

Kelley P. J., Janes J. M. and Peterson L. F. A. (1961) The effect of beryllium on bone. *J. Bone Joint Surg.* **43A**, 829–844.

Kerns W. D. (1980) *Long-term Inhalation Toxicity and Carcinogenicity Studies of Formaldehyde in Rats and Mice*. Presented at the Third CIIT Conference on Toxicology, Raleigh, North Carolina, 20–21 November.

Kesic B. and Haeusler V. (1951) Hematological investigation on workers exposed to mercury vapor. *Ind. Med. Surg.* **20**, 485–488.

Kipling M. D. and Waterhouse J. A. H. (1967) Cadmium and prostatic carcinoma. *Lancet* **1**, 730–731.

Krans E. W. (1935) Effects of fumes during the moulding of certain types of plastics. *Ind. Med. Surg.* **4**, 10–11.

Kuratsune M., Tokudome S., Shirakusa T. et al., (1974) Occupational lung cancer among copper smelters. *Int. J. Cancer* **13**, 552–558.

Kuschner M. and Laskin S. (1971) Experimental models in environmental carcinogenesis. *Am. J. Pathol.* **64**, 183–196.

Ladd A. C., Zuskin E., Valic F. et al. (1966) Absorption and excretion of mercury in miners. *J. Occup. Med.* **8**, 127–131.

Langard S. and Norseth T. (1975) A cohort study of bronchial carcinomas in workers producing chromate pigments. *Br. J. Ind. Med.* **32**, 62–65.

Laskin S., Capprello V., Isola D. et al. (1973) Chrome inhalation exposures with calcium chromate aerosols. *Am. Ind. Hyg. Assoc. J.* **164**.

Lee A. M. and Fraumeni J. F. Jr. (1969) Arsenic and respiratory cancer in man—an occupational study. *J. Natl Cancer Inst.* **42**, 1045–1052.

Lehmann K. B. (1932) Is there a reason for special concern about the incidence of lung cancer in chromate workers? With comments on lung cancer in general. *Zentralbl. Gewerbehyg.* (Germany) **9**, 168–170.

Leitch A. (1923) The experimental inquiry into the cause of cancer. *Br. Med. J.* **2**, 1–7.

Leitch A. and Kennaway E. L. (1922) Experimental production of cancer by arsenic. *Br. Med. J.* **2**, 1107–1108.

Lemen R. A., Lee J. S., Wagoner J. K. et al. (1976) Cancer mortality among cadmium production workers. *Ann. NY Acad. Sci.* **271**, 273–279.

Lester D., Greenberg L. A. and Adams W. R. (1963) Effects of single and repeated exposures of humans and rats to vinyl chloride. *Am. Ind. Hyg. J.* **24**, 265–275.

Levy L. S. and Clack C. (1975) Further studies on the effect of cadmium on the prostate gland. I. Absence of prostatic changes in rats given oral cadmium sulphate for two years. *Ann. Occup. Hyg.* **17**, 205–211.

Levy L. S., Clack D. and Roe F. J. C. (1975) Further studies of the effect of cadmium on the prostate gland. II. Absence of prostatic changes in mice give oral cadmium sulphate for eighteen months. *Ann. Occup. Hyg.* **17**, 213–220.

Levy L. S., Roe F. J. C., Malcolm D. et al. (1973) Absence of prostatic cancer changes in rats exposed to cadmium. *Ann. Occup. Hyg.* **16**, 111–118.

Liebling T., Rosenmann K. D., Pastides H. et al. (1984) Cancer mortality among workers exposed to formaldehyde. *Am. J. Ind. Med.* **5**, 423–428.

Lloyd J. W. (1975) Angiosarcoma of the liver in vinyl chloride/polyvinyl chloride workers. *J. Occup. Med.* **17**, 333–334.

Loken A. C. (1950) Lung cancer in nickel workers. *Tidsskr. Nor. Laegeforen* (Norway) **70**, 376–378.

Lynch D. W., Lewis T. R. and Moorman W. J. (1982) Chronic inhalation toxicity of ethylene oxide in rats and monkeys—a preliminary report. *The Toxicologist* **2**, 11.

Machle W. and Gregorius F. (1948) Cancer of the respiratory system in the United States chromate-producing industry. *Public Health Rep.* **63**, 1114–1127.

McGill C. M., Ladd A. C., Jacobs M. B. et al. (1964) Mercury exposure in a chlorine plant. *J. Occup. Med.* **6**, 335–344.

Maltoni C. (1974) *Preliminary report on the carcinogenicity bioassays of vinyl chloride*. US Dept. of Labor Informal Fact-Finding Hearing on Possible Hazards of Vinyl Chloride Manufacture and Use.

Maltoni C., Ciliberti A. and DiMaio V. (1977) Carcinogenicity bioassays on rats of acrylonitrile administered by inhalation and ingestion. *Med. Lav.* **68**, 401–411.

Maltoni C. and Lefemine G. (1975) Carcinogenicity bioassays of vinyl chloride: current results. *Ann. NY Acad. Sci.* **246**, 195–218.

Mancuso T. F. (1970) Relation of duration of employment and prior respiratory illness to respiratory cancer among beryllium workers. *Environ. Res.* **3**, 251–275.

Mancuso T. F. and Hueper W. C. (1951) Occupational cancer and other health hazards in a chromate plant: a medical appraisal. I. Lung cancers in chromate workers. *Ind. Med. Surg.* **20**, 358–363.

Markuson K. E., Mancuso T. F. and Soet J. S. (1943) Dermatitis due to the formaldehyde resins—prevention and methods of control. *Ind. Med.* **12**, 383–386.

Marsh G. M. (1982) Proportional mortality patterns among chemical plant workers exposed to formaldehyde. *Br. J. Ind. Med.* **39**, 313–322.

Mastromatteo E., Fisher A. M., Christie H. et al. (1960) Acute inhalation toxicity of vinyl chloride to laboratory animals. *Am. Ind. Hyg. J.* **21**, 394–398.

Melville G. N. (1970) Changes in specific airway conductance in health volunteers following nasal and oral inhalation of SO_2. *West Indian Med. J.* **19**, 231–235.

Monson R. R., Peters J. M. and Johnson M. N. (1974) Proportional mortality among vinyl-chloride workers. *Lancet* **2**, 397–398.

Morgan M. G. (1958) Some observations on the incidence of respiratory cancer in nickel workers. *Br. J. Ind. Med.* **15**, 224–234.

Morgan R. W., Claxton K. W., Divine B. J. et al. (1981) Mortality among ethylene oxide workers. *J. Occup. Med.* **23**, 767–770.

Nedel J. A., Salem H., Tamplin B. et al. (1965) Mechanism of bronchoconstriction during inhalation of sulfur dioxide. *J. Appl. Physiol.* **20**, 164–167.

Neal P. A., Flinn R. H., Edwards T. I., Reinhart W. H., Hough J. W., Dallavalle J. M., Goldman F. H., Armstrong D. W., Fray A. S., Coleman A. L. and Postman B. F. (1941) Mercurialism and its control in the felt hat industry. *Public Health Bulletin*, **263**. Federal Security Agency, US Public Health Service.

Neal P. A., Jones R. R., Bloomfield J. J. et al. (1937) Study of chronic mercurialism in the hatters' fur-cutting industry. *Public Health Bulletin*, **234**. Federal Security Agency, US Public Health Service.

Nettesheim P., Hanna M. G. Jr., Doherty D. G. et al. (1971) Effect of calcium chromate dust, influenza virus and 100 R whole-body X-radiation on lung tumor incidence in mice. *J. Natl. Cancer Inst.* **47**, 1129–1138.

Nicholson W. J., Hammond E. C., Seidman H. et al. (1975) Mortality experience of a cohort of vinyl chloride-polyvinyl chloride workers. *Ann. NY Acad. Sci.* **246**, 225–230.

NIOSH (1972) *Criteria for a recommended standard...occupational exposure to beryllium*. 18. US Dept. of Health, Education and Welfare, Health Services and Mental Health Administration, National Institute for Occupational Safety and Health.

NIOSH (1973) *Criteria for a recommended standard...exposure to inorganic mercury*, 72. US Dept. of Health, Safety and Welfare, Public Health Service, National Institute for Occupational Safety and Health.

NIOSH (1975a) *Criteria for a recommended standard...occupational exposure to inorganic arsenic —new criteria—1975*. US Dept. of Health, Education and Welfare, Public Health Service, Center for Disease Control, National Institute for Occupational Safety and Health.

NIOSH (1975b) *Criteria for a recommended standard...occupational exposure to chromium (VI)*, 133–153. US Dept. of Health, Education and Welfare, Public Health Service, National Institute for Occupational Safety and Health.

NIOSH (1977) Acrylonitrile. *Current Intelligence Bulletin*, **18**, 1 July 1977. US Dept. of Health, Education and Welfare, Public Health Service, Center for Disease Control, National Institute for Occupational Safety and Health.

O'Berg M. T. (1980) Epidemiologic study of workers exposed to acrylonitrile. *J. Occup. Med.* **22**. 245–252.

O'Berg M. T., Chen J. L., Burke C. A. et al. (1985) Epidemiologic study of workers exposed to acrulonitrile: An update. *J. Occup. Med.* **27**, 835–840.

Ott M. G., Holder B. B. and Gordon H. L. (1974) Respiratory cancer and occupational exposure to arsenicals. *Arch. Environ. Health* **29**, 250–255.

Ottolenghi A. D., Haseman J. K., Payne W. W. et al. (1975) Inhalation studies of nickel sulfide in pulmonary carcinogenesis of rats. *J. Natl. Cancer Inst.* **54**, 1165–1172.

Payne W. W. (1960) Production of cancers in mice and rats by chromium compounds. *Arch. Ind. Health* **21**, 530–535.

Pedersen E., Hogetveit A. C. and Anderson A. (1973) Cancer of the respiratory organs among workers at a nickel refinery in Norway. *Int. J. Cancer* **12**, 32–41.

Perry K., Bowler R. G., Buckell H. M. et al. (1948) Studies in the incidence of cancer in a factory handling inorganic compounds of arsenic. II. Clinical and environmental investigations. *Br. J. Ind. Med.* **5**, 6–15.

Potts C. L. (1965) Cadmium proteinuria—the health of battery workers exposed to cadmium oxide dust. *Ann. Occup. Hyg.* **8**, 55–61.

Princi F. (1947) A study of industrial exposures to cadmium. *J. Ind. Hyg. Toxicol.* **29**, 315–320.

Quast J. F., Wade C. E., Humiston C. G. et al. (1980) *A Two-Year Toxicity and Oncogenicity Study with Acrylonitrile Incorporated in the Drinking Water of Rats.* Prepared by the Toxicology Research Laboratory, Health and Environmental Sciences, Dow Chemical, USA, Midland, MI, for the Chemical Manufacturing Association, Washington DC. Available from: CMA, Washington DC.

Quast J. F., Schuetz D. J., Balmer M. F. et al. (1980) *A Two-Year Toxicity and Oncogenicity Study with Acrylonitrile Following Inhalation Exposure of Rats.* Prepared by the Toxicology Research Laboratory, Health and Environmental Sciences, Dow Chemical, USA, Midland, MI, for the Chemical Manufacturing Association, Washington DC. Available from: CMA, Washington DC.

Rencher A. C. and Carter M. W. (1971) Phase II. Mortality. *A Retrospective Epidemiological Study at Kennecott's Utah Smelter.* Unpublished report submitted to the Kennecott Copper Corporation, New York, NY, April. Cited in NIOSH, 1975a (q.v.)

Roe F. J. C. and Carter R. L. (1969) Chromium carcinogenesis—calcium chromate as a potent carcinogen for the subcutaneous tissues of the rat. *Br. J. Cancer* **23**, 172–176.

Saric M., Kulcar Z., Zorica M. et al. (1976) Malignant tumors of the liver and lungs in an area with PVC industry. *Environ. Health Persp.* **17**, 189–192.

Schepers G. W. G. (1961) Neoplasia experimentally induced by beryllium compounds. *Prog. Exp. Tumor Res.* **2**, 203–244.

Schwartz L. (1936) Dermatitis in the manufacture of synthetic resins and waxes in Skin Hazards in American Industry, Part II. *Public Health Bulletin*, **229**, 1–12. Treasury Dept., Public Health Service.

Schwartz L., Peck S. M. and Dunn J. E. (1943) Dermatitis from resin glue in war industries. *Public Health Rep.* **58**, 899–904.

Shipkovitz H. D. (1968) Formaldehyde vapor emissions in the permanent-press fabrics industry. Report No. TR-52. US Department of Health, Education and Welfare, Public, Health Service, Consumer Protection and Environmental Health Service, Environmental Control Administration, Cincinnati.

Sielken R. (1983) Primary neoplasms in the brains, dose-response models, risk assessment. *Ethylene oxide: BRRC two-year inhalation study in rats.* Supplemental submission to Occupational Safety and Health Administration, 17 August.

Sim V. M. and Pattle R. E. (1957) Effect of possible smog irritants on human subject. *JAMA.* **165**, 1908–1913.

Skalpe I. O. (1964) Long-term effects of sulphur dioxide exposure in pulp mills. *Br. J. Ind. Med.* **21**, 69–73.

Smith A. R., Goldwater L. J., Burke W. J. et al. (1949) Mercury exposure in the fur-felt hat industry. *Monthly Rev.* (NY State Dept. of Labor, Div. Ind. Hyg. Safety Standards) **28**, 17–24.

Smith A. R. and Moskovitz S. (1948) Urinary excretion of mercury. *Monthly Rev.* (NY State Dept. of Labor, Div. Ind. Hyg. Safety Standards) **27**, 45–47.

Smith R. G., Vorwald A. J., Patil L. S. et al. (1970) Effects of exposure to mercury in the manufacture of chlorine. *Am. Ind. Hyg. Assoc. J.* **31**, 687–700.

Snell R. E. and Luchsinger P. C. (1969) Effects of sulfur dioxide on expiratory flow rates and total respiratory resistance in normal human subjects. *Arch. Environ. Health* **18**, 693–698.

Snellings W. M., Weill C. S. and Maronpot R. R. (1981) Final report on ethylene oxide two-year inhalation study in rats. *Project Report No. 44-20.* Bushy Run Research Center, Pennsylvania.

Sobel W., Bond G. G., Parsons T. W. et al. (1986) Acrylamide cohort mortality study. *Br. J. Ind. Med.* **43**, 785–788.

Spencer P. S. and Schaumburg H. H. (1974) A review of acrylamide neurotoxicity. Part II. Experimental animal neurotoxicity and pathologic mechanisms. *Can. J. Neurol. Sci.* **1**, 152–169.

Steffee C. H. and Baetjer A. M. (1965) Histopathologic effects of chromate chemicals—report of studies in rabbits, guinea pigs, rats and mice. *Arch. Environ. Health* **11**, 66–75.

Sunderman F. W. Jr. (1973) The current status of nickel carcinogenesis. *Ann. Clin. Lab. Sci.* **3**, 156–180.

Sutherland R. B. (1959) *Summary of the Report on Respiratory Cancer Mortality, International Nickel Company of Canada, Ltd., Port Colborne Refinery,* 153. Ontario Dept. of Health, Toronto.

Sutherland R. B. (1969) *Mortality Among Sinter Workers, International Nickel Company of Canada, Ltd., Copper Cliff Smelter*, 22. Ontario Dept. of Health, Environmental Health Services Branch.

Swenberg J. A., Kerns W. D., Mitchell R. I. et al. (1980) Induction of squamous cell carcinomas of the rat nasal cavity by inhalation exposure to formaldehyde vapor. *Cancer Res.* **40**, 3398–3402.

Syracuse Research Corporation (1985) *Monograph on Human Exposure to Chemicals in the Workplace: Acrylonitrile*. Dated July, 1985. Prepared for the National Cancer Institute Betheda, MD. New York: Syracuse Research Corporation.

Tabershaw I. R. (ed.) (1974) Special communication: editor's note. *J. Occup. Med.* **16**, 151.

Tabershaw I. R. and Gaffey W. R. (1974) Mortality study of workers in the manufacture of vinyl chloride and its polymers. *J. Occup. Med.* **16**, 509–518.

Takahashi M., Ohara T. and Hashimoto K. (1971) Electro-physiological study of nerve injuries in workers handling acrylamide. *Int. Arch. Arbeitsmed.* **28**, 1–11.

Tatarskaya A. A. (1965) Occupational cancer of the upper respiratory passages in the nickel industry. *Gig. Tr. Prof. Zabol.* (Russia) **9**, 22–25.

Taylor F. H. (1966) The relationship of mortality and duration of employment as reflected by a cohort of chromate workers. *Am. J. Public Health* **56**, 218–229.

Taylor J. S. (1977) Dermatologic hazards from ethylene oxide. *Cutis* **19**, 189.

Thiess A. M. (1963) Observations concerning intoxication due to ethylene oxide exposure. *Arch. Toxicol.* **20**, 127.

Thiess A. M., Frentzel-Beyme R., Link R. et al. (1981a) Mortality study on employees exposed to alkylene oxides (ethylene oxide/propylene oxide) and their derivatives. *Proceedings, International Symposium on Prevention of Occupational Cancer*, Helsinki, Finland.

Thiess A. M., Schwegler H., Fleig I. et al. (1981b) Mutagenicity study of workers exposed to alkylene oxides (ethylene oxide/propylene oxide) and derivatives. *J. Occup. Med.* **23**, 343–347.

Torkelson T. R., Oyen F. and Rowe V. K. (1961) The toxicity of vinyl chloride as determined by repeated exposures of laboratory animals. *Am. Ind. Hyg. J.* **22**, 354–361.

Trachtenberg I. M. (1969) The chronic action of mercury on the organism, current aspects of the problem of micro-mercurialism and its prophylaxis. *Zdorov'ja* (Kiev).

Viola P. L., Biogotti A. and Caputo A. (1971) Oncogenic response of rat skin, lungs and bones to vinyl chloride. *Cancer Res.* **31**, 516–519.

Walrath J. and Fraumeni J. R. (1983) Mortality patterns among embalmers. *Int. J Cancer* **31**, 407–411.

Waxweiler R. J., Stringer W., Wagoner J. K., Jones J., Falk H. and Carter C. (1976) Neoplastic risk among workers exposed to vinyl chloride. *Ann. NY Acad. Sci.* **271**, 40–48.

Wehner A. P., Busch R. H., Olson R. J. and Craig D. K. (1975) Chronic inhalation of nickel oxide and cigarette smoke by hamsters. *Am. Ind. Hyg. Assoc. J.* **36**, 802–810.

West I. and Lim J. (1968) Mercury poisoning among workers in the California mercury mills—a preliminary report. *J. Occup. Med.* **10**, 697–701.

Wilson R. H. (1944) Health hazards encountered in the manufacture of synthetic rubber. *JAMA.* **124**, 701–703.

Wilson R. H., Hough G. V. and McCormick W. F. (1948) Medical problems encountered in the manufacture of American-made rubber. *Ind. Med.* **17**, 199–207.

Wilson R. H., McCormick W. E., Tatum C. F. et al. (1967) Occupational acroosteolysis. Report of 31 cases. *JAMA.* **201**,577–581.

Wolman S. R. (1979) Mutational consequences of exposure to ethylene oxide. *J. Environ. Pathol. Toxicol.* **2**, 1289–1303.

Wong O. (1980) An epidemiologic mortality study of a cohort of chemical workers potentially exposed to formaldehyde, with discussion of standardized mortality ratio and proportionate mortality ratio. *Formaldehyde Toxicity*, Third Chemical Industries Institute of Toxicology Conference on Toxicology, Raleigh, North Carolina, 21 November.

Yager J. W., Hines C. J. and Spear R. C. (1983) Exposure to ethylene oxide at work increases sister chromatid exchanges in human peripheral lymphocytes. *Science* **219**, 1221.

Yefremov G. G. (1970) The state of the upper respiratory tract in formaldehyde production employees. *Zh. Ushn. Nos. Gorl. Bolezn.* (Russia) **30**, 11–15.

Zaeva G. N., Ulanova I. P. and Dueva L. A. (1968) Materials for revision of the maximal permissible concentrations of formaldehyde in the inside atmosphere of industrial premises. *Gig. Tr. Prof. Zabol.* (Russia) **12**, 16–20.

Zenz C. (1975) *Occupational Medicine*, 805, 808. Chicago: Year Book Medical Publishers.

Chapter 14

Practical Assessment and Communication of Chemical Hazards in the Workplace

Tipton R. Tyler and Bryan Ballantyne

SCOPE

Toxicologists are called upon daily to assess the potential for adverse health effects from a wide variety of chemicals, and comment on the possible relevance of these to the likelihood of risk of injury to man under various conditions, some of which may not be too clearly defined. This activity has developed along with, and helped to shape, the science of toxicology itself, and is a major justification for expending human and economic resources on studying the potential adverse health effects that chemicals may cause to living organisms. The basic principles on which these assessments are made have been developed through years of practical experience, scientific investigation, and lessons from occupational and domestic accidents, and are being continually refined in parallel with the development of new tests, refinement of existing test systems, and greater appreciation of the mechanisms and determinants of toxicity. This chapter will discuss the basic principles which assist in reaching decisions concerning possible hazards that chemicals may pose in the workplace, and how these hazards may be communicated and avoided or minimized.

The general approach which is used in defining potential hazards, and making recommendations for the safe use of a specific material, consists essentially of the following sequence of steps:

1. A search for all available heath effects related information on the chemical and, where appropriate, for other chemicals which have close chemical structures. Information is required, for example, on physicochemical properties, *in vivo* and *in vitro* toxicology, epidemiology, known adverse occupational health effects and incidents, industrial hygiene, and current intended use patterns.
2. A detailed and impartial review of all relevant literature, placing emphasis on those studies which have been conducted by accepted and credible scientific standards, used relevant routes of exposure to the chemical, and, where toxicity has occurred, demonstrated dose-response relationships with regard to toxic effects. Such studies may cover a wide range of possible endpoints or be specific for a given target organ or tissue effect.
3. Interpretation of the credible and relevant literature, and a definition of the

toxicity of the material, in the light of the current knowledge of mechanisms of toxicity, biological variability, dose-response considerations, influence of environmental variants, and the possible multiple endpoints of a toxic response.

4. Conclusions regarding the potential adverse health effects of the chemical to man under specified conditions (i.e. hazard evaluation), and recommendations regarding the safe handling and acceptable exposure to the chemical under these conditions. Additionally, advice should be given on the immediate and long-term management of overexposure situations.
5. Communication of the toxicology review, hazard evaluation, recommended protective and precautionary measures, and medical management of overexposure in a manner which is capable of unambiguous interpretation by the particular audience for which a communication is intended.

In practice, and with many chemicals and mixtures, this process of hazard evaluation has often to be carried out with a minimum of available information on which to reach conclusions and base recommendations, and requires an extensive experience in subjective interpretation and professional judgement. Previous experience in laboratory toxicology, and a sound knowledge of animal and human biology, are essential prerequisites for those who undertake this work in a serious, professional and analytical scientific manner. A considerable effort is currently being devoted toward refining the decision-making process through the use of so-called quantitative risk assessment (Congressional Research Service, 1983; Ruckelshaus, 1985). However, these approaches are significantly limited by a lack of knowledge with regard to extrapolation of responses in various animal species to man, they do not take into account the biological variability in response, they do not allow for the small number of animals that may be technically and ethically incorporated into experimental design, and often ignore different mechanisms of toxicity. At the present time, and unfortunately in most cases, too little is known about any one mechanism of toxicity on which to base an appropriate mathematical model for a specific toxic response. Therefore, this quantitative approach also involves subjective decisions and judgemental conclusions which may ignore basic principles of biology. In most instances, chemicals for which an evaluation of hazard is required on a daily basis lack the extensive database which is ideally required to employ this type of mathematical manipulation. There are suggestions to incorporate consideration of mechanistic approaches, pharmacokinetics, and metabolism across different species, together with assessments of maximum tolerated doses into a process of qualitative and quantitative 'Biological Risk Assessment' (Clayson, 1987).

Decisions and recommendations regarding health effects of industrial chemicals are required for specific activities including compiling consumer product safety information, the setting of appropriate workplace exposure standards, and regulatory and legal considerations. In addition to formally published scientific reviews, information on the toxicity and potential hazards from exposure to industrial chemicals may be communicated in a variety of ways; these include customer letters, health effects statements in product information bulletins, material safety data sheets, and labels. The amount of detail and method of presentation may vary significantly between these different modes of communication.

Customers letters may be in response to technical inquiries from users, or potential users, or may be a rapid means of allowing customers to be made aware of new or important confirmatory information on potential adverse health effects and the conditions of their development. Product information bulletins may contain a health effect section which presents a short review of the toxicity and potential health hazards of the material(s) described in the bulletin. The review needs to be understood by a wide technical audience in order that they may clearly understand any limitations on the use and handling of the material(s) imposed by safety considerations.

Material safety data sheets provide a means to communicate potential health hazards, their management, and protective and precautionary measures to prevent their occurrence. This information is given in a condensed but detailed manner, giving all information which may have any relevance to human health hazards. The audience is mainly those who handle the material, either customer or workforce. In order to allow the most complete and understandable presentation of information, the arrangement and content of the material safety data sheet is generally along the following lines:

1. *Identification*. This includes chemical and product names, chemical family, formula, molecular weight, synonyms, CAS number and name.
2. *Physical data*. All relevant physical properties, e.g. boiling or melting point, specific gravity, solubility, vapour pressure, etc.
3. *Ingredients*. The composition of mixtures, or contaminants or additives in specific materials. The relative proportions of substances, their workplace exposure guidelines, and a brief statement on hazards each presents.
4. *Fire and explosion hazard data*. This will include flash point, flammable limits, extinguishing media, special firefighting procedures, and unusual fire and explosion hazards.
5. *Health hazard data*. The following are subsections for presentation of relevant information:

    a. Listing of known exposure guidelines, e.g. OSHA, ACGIH and industry-derived.
    b. Effects of single overexposure by swallowing, skin absorption, inhalation, skin and eye contact.
    c. Effects of repeated overexposure, by routes of exposure known or likely to produce these effects.
    d. Other effects of exposure not covered adequately by the above; this may be a convenient place to discuss, for example, immune-mediated hypersensitivity or teratogenicity.
    e. Significant laboratory data with possible relevance to human health hazard evaluation. This is a convenient section to present concise statements on *in vivo* or *in vitro* toxicology studies, the relevance of which to human health is unknown, or for which there is currently no evidence to implicate the findings as likely to occur in humans but nevertheless of possible toxicological relevance.
    f. Exacerbation of any co-existing diseases by exposure to the chemical.

g. Emergency first-aid procedures for the initial and later management of cases of poisoning by swallowing, skin and eye contact, or inhalation.
h. Notes to physician of a medical nature concerning special aspects of toxicity, complications, and management of poisoning.
i. Carcinogenic assessment by IARC, also OSHA or the National Toxicology Program list of carcinogens. Also, when materials shown to be carcinogenic by credible studies are not given the above authoritative lists, then the vendor may include this information as part of his own evaluation.

6. *Reactivity data*. Includes information on stability, incompatibility, hazardous polymerization, and hazardous combustion or decomposition products, each with advice on how to avoid dangerous conditions.
7. *Spill or leak procedures*. How to manage and how to dispose.
8. *Special protection information*. Includes information based on hazard evaluation (toxic, chemical and physical), on needs for respiratory protective equipment, ventilation, gloves, eye protection, and any other protective measures considered necessary.
9. *Special precautions*. Includes precautions necessary during handling, storage and other conceivable needs.
10. *Emergency telephone number*. For urgent advice on health hazards and their management, and environmental problems.

Overexposure in the context of the material safety data sheet, may be defined as exposure situations resulting in adverse health effects if the precautionary measures recommended with respect to exposure guidelines, spill or leak procedures, special protection or special precautions, are not obeyed. Clearly the above format allows for detailed and integrated presentation of potential adverse health effects, how to avoid them, or how to manage poisoning.

Labels should give a clear brief statement on hazards from handling materials, what precautions are necessary, and the immediate management of poisoning. Hazards which are appropriate for labelling include those which are life threatening, those producing irreversible or serious reversible effects which are detrimental to health, or reversible pharmacological effects which impair the normal or defensive reactions to the immediate environment (e.g. peripheral sensory irritation or narcosis). In some cases, it may be appropriate to warn of probable routes of exposure, e.g. harmful by inhalation or absorption through the skin. When a well defined target organ or tissue, or clear predominant effect, is known it may be possible to include this even under the more restrictive allowance of words possible with label size. These would include, for example, inflammation or corrosion, sensitization (skin and/or respiratory tract), neurotoxicity, reproductive toxicity (specified), teratogenic effects, carcinogenicity and pharmacological effects such as drowsiness or manifestations of peripheral sensory irritation.

The following discussion will concentrate on approaches used in the interpretation of data from animal studies, and consider how information from such studies can be used to address the practical needs of hazard evaluation and safety recommendations.

TERMINOLOGY

Precision in communication relies on a clear understanding of the definitions of technical and scientific terms in the context of their intended use. It is therefore appropriate to discuss the way in which terminology is used in toxicology as it relates to exposure conditions and effects produced. The following brief section reviews some essential general terms which have been discussed more fully by Ballantyne (1984a).

The type of toxicity produced, and the probability of its occurring, is often a function of the number of exposures (among a variety of other determinants). It is necessary to differentiate between acute (single) exposures and repeated exposures. The latter category covers a wide time span and, although somewhat artificial, it is convenient to refer to repeated exposure conditions as short-term repeated (i.e. not more than 5% of the life span), subchronic (5 to 15% of the life span), and chronic exposure conditions (the entire life span or a greater portion of it).

In describing toxicity and discussing hazard, it is clearly of importance to refer to the duration of any induced effects. Broadly, they may be spoken of as temporary (reversible or transient) or permanent (or persistent). Either may be produced as a result of acute or repeated exposure conditions. For example, transient effects may occur under the following differing conditions:

1. Peripheral sensory irritant effects may decline or disappear during exposure as a result of neurophysiological adaptive processes, or shortly following exposure due to decline in irritant molecule concentration at the sensory receptors in peripheral nerves of skin or mucosae.
2. Recovery from an acute central neuropharmacological effect, such as narcosis, following cessation of exposure due to diminished levels of the causative agent at the neural receptors.
3. Attenuation of an acute or repeated exposure biochemical and/or morphological injury due to adaptive enzyme formation in detoxification pathways.
4. The presence of biological repair mechanisms following acute or repeated exposure toxicity. This may occur at a cellular level, such as phagocytosis, or at a molecular level, for example DNA excision repair.
5. Reversion to normal processes of growth and differentiation, such as may occur in the regression of squamous metaplasia in epithelia following cessation of recurrent exposure to irritant materials.

Likewise, permanent effects may occur from acute or repeated exposure. Differing examples include blindness due to severe corneal injury following a single topical contamination of the eye with a corrosive material, kidney injury from massive acute overexposure to ethylene glycol, progressive liver fibrosis from frequent repeated peroral ethanol intoxication, and malignant neoplasia from repeated exposure to carcinogens. Although the majority of chemical carcinogens appear to require chronic exposure conditions, in a very few instances malignant neoplasia may occur as a delayed effect following an acute exposure e.g. certain polycyclic aromatic hydrocarbons can cause tumour development in three or four months following a single subcutaneous injection (Suss et al., 1983).

A convenient descriptive term for the development of certain effects as a result of repeated exposure conditions is cumulative toxicity; this involves progressive injury of a specific type produced by the summation of incremental injury resulting from successive exposures. Typical examples are progressive inflammation, epithelial thickening, and squamous metaplasia resulting from repeated exposure to irritant materials (Sellakumar et al., 1985; Miller et al., 1985) and peripheral neuropathy associated with repeated exposure to methyl *n*-butyl ketone (O'Donoghue, 1985).

A particularly important descriptive phrase, in its implications for hazard evaluation, is latent toxicity. This implies there is a period which is free from signs of toxicity following, usually, an acute overexposure to a chemical. Clearly, if there is a delay to onset of toxicity following exposure then this should be strongly emphasized in evaluations and recommendations in order that advice may be given to keep a subject overexposed to the chemical under observation for the latent period to ensure that any delayed toxicity that might be exhibited is recognized and appropriately treated at the earliest possible time. Examples of latent toxicity include delayed-onset pulmonary oedema following overexposure to phosgene (NIOSH, 1976), pulmonary fibrosis resulting from intoxication by the bipyridilium herbicide paraquat (Fletcher, 1974), and peripheral neuropathy from some anticholinesterase organophosphates (Davis and Richardson, 1980).

Finally, it is scientifically necessary and practical to differentiate those manifestations of toxicity where a material initially comes into contact with a surface membrane (local effects) from those occurring at sites remote from the site of contact after absorption into the organism (systemic effects).

CONSIDERATIONS IN THE DESIGN AND CONDUCT OF TOXICOLOGY STUDIES

Toxicology studies should allow, within the constraints of the time period studied, a quantitative determination of the potential for a chemical to produce local and systemic adverse effects, and an opportunity to define various factors which may influence the nature, severity and possible reversibility of effects. For the purpose of hazard evaluation, the identification of the nature of adverse effects which might occur to individuals exposed to a chemical, and determinants of these effects, is of utmost importance. Thus, particular consideration must be given to the following in both the design and interpretation of toxicology studies:

1. The route of exposure to the chemical, and variability in toxicity between different routes of exposure.
2. The clinical signs of toxicity which occur as a result of exposure, and the factors influencing their development.
3. A determination of the nature of structural and functional injury to tissues and organs by means of appropriate monitoring procedures.
4. The dosages at which effects occur, particularly an evaluation of whether there is clear dose-response relationship and a determination of doses producing no effects, threshold effects and definitive toxicity.

The above points are obviously of importance in any toxicological study; however, the relative emphasis may differ when the primary objective is not specific to hazard evaluation. For example, if a study is intended to examine mechanisms of toxicity, a route of administration may be selected which is not appropriate to hazard evaluation, but delivers the test material to the intended target organ under investigation. If on the other hand, the intended objective is to determine whether a structure-activity relationship exists between a series of chemicals, then the observation of general clinical condition may be of lesser importance than a specific effect of interest, and the relative potency at a particular dosage level for that effect.

For hazard evaluation purposes, there should be emphasis upon the exposure situations which exist under the practical conditions of use of the material under examination. However, exposure conditions may differ greatly between chemicals used in pharmaceutical preparations, chemicals used as food additives, chemicals used in cosmetics and fragrances, or industrial chemicals used as intermediates in industrial applications; specific guidelines may have to be developed for each particular case. The most important factors that need to be considered in hazard evaluation for an industrial chemical include physical and chemical properties, use patterns (including conceivable misuse), characteristics of the workplace, source(s) of exposure, duration, frequency and magnitude of exposure, route(s) of exposure, physical nature of the exposure conditions, population exposed, and variability of exposure conditions.

Consideration must also be given to the types of tests needed and the order in which they are to be conducted. For example, the design of repeated exposure toxicity studies is often guided by effects observed in single or shorter-term repeated studies, and the exposure conditions under which effects occurred. Therefore, initial studies in a toxicology testing programme are generally concerned with single (acute) exposure toxicity and primary irritancy. These tests have a long history of use, and yield information which, in most cases, generally provides a reasonably firm basis for predicting effects which are likely to occur in humans following a single overexposure. In this respect, acute toxicity information is extremely useful, frequently predictive, and is extremely valuable regarding the development of advice on necessary protective and precautionary measures, first-aid and medical considerations in the event of accidental single overexposures, and in developing easily understood advice for product safety guidance. In addition, more data are becoming available at very early stages in testing programmes concerning the mutagenic potential of chemicals. This information, in contrast with acute data, is more difficult to evaluate with respect to potential hazard because the endpoints are less well defined with respect to definitive toxicity, *in vitro* dose levels are not readily extrapolable to practical exposure settings, and the implications of chemically induced genetic damage in man have not been rigorously demonstrated.

In determining the testing needs for a particular material used in specific operations, it is important to take note of the possible influence of the use pattern on toxicity. For example, Agarwal et al. (1986) found that the aryl-hydrocarbon-hydroxylase-inducing activity of cutting oil was significantly enhanced after its industrial use, and this could be correlated with the formation of new and biologically active polycyclic aromatic hydrocarbons. They also demonstrated that the preferential removal of polycyclic aromatic hydrocarbons from used cutting oil considerably reduced the ability to induce skin and liver aryl hydrocarbon hydroxylase activity.

Development of Testing Programs

Toxicology testing programmes generally start with the single exposure *in vivo* or *in vitro* studies and progress to evaluating the effects of long-term repeated exposures and studies, with special endpoints, such as teratology and reproductive effects, being conducted as the end-use exposure pattern and the emerging toxicology profile dictate. Quite often, repeated exposure studies progress in sequence from short-term repeated studies (7 to 28 days in duration) to subchronic studies (around 90 exposure days) and thence to chronic studies involving exposure for a major portion of the life span of the animals. Special studies may be conducted in parallel or in sequence to these; they include effects of embryo/foetal development, effects on the reproductive capacity of animals, immune-mediated toxicity, neurological and behavioural toxicity, mechanisms of toxicity, metabolism, and pharmacokinetic studies. The design of repeated exposure studies should include provisions for the identification of multiple endpoints in different tissues and organs, including haematotoxicity, neurological and behavioural toxicity, and immunotoxicity. Additional tests may be required to evaluate potential genotoxic activity in the intact animal.

Study Design Considerations for Hazard Evaluation

The toxic potential of a chemical should be determined by several routes of administration, particularly if the effects result from acute exposure, are systemic in nature, or are modulated to a significant extent by metabolism, and this in turn may have a large influence on the perceived hazard of a chemical to man (Pepelko and Withey, 1985). For example, only direct local primary effects of a specific chemical of low percutaneous penetrability may be encountered upon skin contact, while systemic injury could occur after ingestion or inhalation of the same material.

Repeated peroral studies are conducted by various procedures, including administering the test material in food or water, using peroral gastric intubation, or (as in the case of studies in dogs) by placing the material in gelatin capsules and giving these by mouth. Repeated skin contact studies have been conducted either by placing the material directly on the dorsum in a position where it is difficult for it to be removed by licking or grooming activity, or by covering the area of application with an occlusive dressing. Acute and repeated percutaneous studies are generally conducted by the occlusive method. Inhalation studies are most conveniently conducted for 6 hours a day, 5 days a week, which presumably patterns the usual work-week in the occupational setting. However, a number of studies have been conducted using exposure times of 24 hours a day, 7 days a week, in order to evaluate the hazard from the chemical by continued exposure in ambient air.

A variety of animal species have been used in toxicity studies. However, for the vast majority of industrial chemicals, the range of animal species used have been reasonably limited; thus, rats and mice have been more commonly used in studies when materials are administered orally, by inhalation, and parenterally. Rabbits are more frequently used in cutaneous studies and in eye irritancy testing. Hamsters and non-rodent species, most commonly dogs, have also been used in repeated dosing studies. A large body of historical background information exists on the above animal models which usually allows a reasonably reliable interpretation of results.

Information from toxicology studies is necessary to develop hazard management programmes. These programmes should be designed such that recommendations can be developed for procedures to allow the safe handling of materials, preparation of reliable hazard warning statements and, if possible, to supply information which can assist first-aid and medical personnel in giving appropriate treatment in the event of overexposures. Overexposure is used to indicate those exposure conditions, acute or repeated, which may result in the development of signs and symptoms of irritancy or toxicity, or result in the production of potentially adverse health effects which are detected by routine or special clinical screening procedures. In addition, information of the type obtained from toxicology studies is required in order to establish credible workplace exposure standards, allowable concentrations for food additives, permissible concentrations in drinking water supplies, dose regimes for widely used therapeutic agents, and ambient air quality standards for potential pollutants. Toxicity data may also find a use in quantitating possible risk of adverse effects in exposed populations. Finally, the results from toxicity testing programmes may influence plant design, modify plans for applications and markets in which the material might be used, or contribute to the design and formulation of hazardous products in order to reduce the risk of accidental or purposeful misuse.

There are, unfortunately, few chemicals for which a totally adequate amount of information exists to accomplish the above goals. Indeed, for many chemicals little more than the acute toxicity and primary irritancy data are available. It is against this background that the day-to-day decisions of the hazards of various products must often be made.

APPLICATION OF TOXICOLOGY INFORMATION TO HAZARD EVALUATION

General Considerations on the Interpretation of Toxicology Information

Toxicology is concerned with defining the potential for a material to produce adverse health effects. Hazard evaluation is a procedure to determine if any of these known adverse effects will be exhibited under specific conditions of use. Thus, toxicology is but one of the many considerations in the hazard evaluation process. The following are some of the other important factors that need to be taken into account in defining whether a given workplace situation will be hazardous with respect to exposure to a chemical:

— Physicochemical properties of the material.
— Use pattern of the material.
— Characteristics of the workplace where the material is handled.
— Source of exposure, both normal and possible accidental.
— Control measures in place to regulate exposure.

— Magnitude, duration and frequency of exposure, with respect to normal and possible accidental situations.
— Route of exposure.
— Physical nature of exposure conditions (e.g. solid, liquid, gas, vapour aerosol, etc.).
— Variability in exposure conditions.
— Population exposed (e.g. number, sex, age, distribution, etc.).
— Any experience and information on exposed human populations.

Detailed review of the types of information listed above should allow exposure conditions to be precisely defined, and thus the likelihood of any known toxicity being exhibited under these conditions. The review and interpretation of toxicology information is a professional matter, requiring a knowledge of normal and pathological biology, together with practical experience in both the laboratory conduct of toxicology studies and the practice of applied toxicology. The review of toxicology studies should be on a case-by-case basis with particular, though not exclusive, attention being paid to the following:

a. It should be established that the laboratory reporting the study has the necessary scientific credibility, capabilities, experience and expertise in the area being investigated.
b. The objectives of the study should be precisely stated, and it should be confirmed that the overall design of the study satisfies the objectives.
c. The work should be presented in a clear and unambiguous way, with all necessary detail to allow the reviewer to undertake his or her own assessment and conclusions about the study.
d. It should be confirmed that there are adequate quality control procedures, and whether good laboratory practices and procedures have been followed.
e. The material(s) tested should be specified, including stability over the test period, and the nature and relative proportions of any impurities present.
f. It should be confirmed that the methods employed for exposing and monitoring the study are appropriate and sufficiently specific and sensitive for the endpoint(s) to be determined.
g. The study should be designed to allow a determination of the significance of results and permit hazard assessment processes. For example, the number of control and test animals should be sufficient in number to allow the detection of biological variability in response to exposure, and to permit statistical analysis. There should be sufficient dose-response information to allow decisions on causal relationships and the magnitude of doses which produce effects and those not producing effects.
h. It should be possible to determine whether any injury produced is a direct result of toxicity or a secondary effect. A primary toxic effect is one produced as a result of the direct adverse effect of a chemical, or a metabolite, on a target organ or tissue. Secondary effects are those occurring as a consequence of disturbed function in a primary target organ or tissue. For example, primary lung injury produced by inhaled severe irritants may result in hypoxaemia and secondary hypoxic injury in other organs, including the liver and kidney. In addition to confirming causal relationship between exposure and development of injury, the study should

be carefully assessed to determine if the available information is sufficient to allow any conclusion as to whether the effect(s) are caused by parent material or metabolite.

i. Extreme caution is needed to determine if numerical data have been correctly assessed. Thus, although a difference between the control group and a test group may reach statistical significance, this is not necessarily an implication that the difference is of important biological consequence. Conversely, some changes or trends, while not of statistical significance, may be of biological relevance. The quantitative information should be screened against a background of the study as a whole, the normal biological variability, quantitative changes which imply pathological processes, and the magnitude of any change relevant to what is known to constitute an adverse effect.

The above considerations indicate a need for careful design of toxicological studies, taking into account all those factors which are inherent in the defined objectives of the study. The relevance and credibility of a study can be no better than its study design and conduct allow. Ideally, the available toxicology information on a material should allow the following to be determined as part of the hazard evaluation procedure:

a. The nature of adverse effects produced.
b. The relevance of the conditions under which the toxicology studies were conducted to the practical in-use situation under consideration.
c. The average response, range of responses, presence of a hypersensitive group, and an indication of minimal or no-effects conditions.
d. Identification of factors likely to modify the toxic response.
e. Effects of gross overexposure.
f. Effects of repeated overexposure.
g. Recognition of adverse effects.
h. Assistance in the definition of allowable and non-allowable exposure conditions.
i. Assistance in the definition of monitoring requirements.
j. Guidance on the need for personal and collective protection measures.
k. Guidance on first-aid, antidotal, and medical support needs.
l. Relevance of toxicity to coincidental disease.
m. Definition of 'at risk' individuals e.g. pregnant and fertile females from teratogens and general reproductive toxic chemicals, males from chemicals causing testicular toxicity, and genetically susceptible individuals.

To illustrate the care needed in the interpretation of toxicity studies, some simple examples are given below of factors that need attention with respect to the determination of hazards from materials following peroral or inhalation exposure. With new materials, and indeed with many existing materials, information on acute peroral intoxication is not available, fortunately, from cases of human poisoning. Therefore, potential adverse effects and hazards from swallowing these materials has to be derived from animal toxicology studies. Interpretation of and extrapolation from such studies require detailed consideration with respect to the experimental conditions in order to avoid underestimating potential adverse human health effects and their management (Ballantyne,

1986a). Examples of some factors which may influence the results of acute peroral toxicity studies, and which can lead to possible misinterpretation with respect to potential health hazards, are as presented below:

1. *Feeding*. Acute peroral lethal toxicity may be influenced by whether animals have or have not been fed immediately before dosing. LD_{50} values for two materials are as follows for rats:

Epoxidized soybean oil:	Fasted	=	64.0 g/kg
	Unfasted	=	19.0 g/kg
Polypropylene glycol 425:	Fasted	=	0.81 g/kg
	Unfasted	=	4.00 g/kg

2. *Concentrations of test material*. Both lethal and sublethal toxicity may be influenced by the degree of dilution of the solution used for dosing. For example, undiluted diethylamine has an acute peroral LD_{50} in the rat of < 0.25 mg/kg, whereas the LD_{50} for a 10% solution in water is 1.41 ml/kg (95% confidence limits 1.03–1.95 ml/kg). The high acute peroral toxicity of the undiluted material is probably mainly due to a markedly irritant and ulcerogenic action on the gastrointestinal tract with consequent haemorrhage and hypovolaemic shock. In contrast, with the 10% dilution the systemic toxicity of the absorbed material is probably a more important determinant. Thus, the clinical management of the differing situations caused by dilution may require different approaches. A contrasting situation is seen with glutaraldehyde, also a primary irritant material, in which there is a reciprocal relation between acute peroral toxicity and the degree of dilution (*Table* 14.1). Thus, in contrast with the alkylamines, acute lethal peroral toxicity increases with dilution (in the concentration range 1 to 50% w/w), when expressed as absolute amounts of glutaraldehyde dosed. However, the relative hazard decreases with dilution in that the total volume of aqueous glutaraldehyde required to achieve a lethal dose increases with increasing dilution (Ballantyne et al., 1985). In this case, systemic toxicity may be of greater significance than local irritant effects on the gastrointestinal tract.

   In some cases dilution has little influence on acute lethal peroral toxicity. For example, with tetramethylhexanediamine (TMHDA), a highly irritant material, acute peroral LD_{50} values have been determined to be as shown in

Table 14.1. Acute peroral LD_{50} values in the rat for differing concentrations of glutaraldehyde (GA) in water.

Concentration of GA (% w/w)	LD_{50} (95% confidence limits)	
	As gavage solution (ml/kg)	*As contained GA (mg/kg)*
50	1·30 (0·87– 1·94)	733 (491–1094)
25	1·87 (1·26– 2·76)	497 (335– 734)
10	1·62 (1·01– 2·62)	168 (105– 273)
5	3·25 (2·40– 4·39)	165 (122– 223)
1	12·30 (9·13–16·70)	123 (92– 168)

Table 14.2 for undiluted TMHDA and a 5% aqueous solution. In this case it would appear that acute lethal toxicity due to corrosive effects with undiluted TMDHA approximates that for systemic toxicity from the diluted material.

Table 14.2. Acute peroral lethal toxicity of tetramethylhexanediamine (TMHDA) given to rats by gavage as either undiluted material or a 5% aqueous dilution.

Concentration	LD_{50} *as THMDA (95% confidence limits) in ml/kg*	
	Males	*Females*
Undiluted	0.42 (0.24–0.75)	0.30 (0.12–0.74)
5% aqueous	0.59 (0.51–0.70)	0.60 (0.39–0.90)

Examples of the above type highlight the need to interpret acute peroral toxicity data in terms of the concentration(s) of material tested. Information obtained from undiluted material may be quantitatively and functionally inappropriate for the diluted material, and thus statements of hazard evaluation and the magnitude and nature of poisoning may be required to be determined for differing concentrations, if these are used in practice. When dilution influences toxicity, the findings may give an indication of the biohandling of the material and possible different modes of toxicity. Statements on the acute peroral toxicity of a material may require to be qualified by the conditions of the study with respect to the concentration(s) of material tested. A potentially practical area of concern relating to the influence of dilution on peroral toxicity is a recommendation to give patients water to drink since this may enhance systemic toxicity. When the material is both systemically toxic and a local gastrointestinal irritant, then the relative disadvantages of giving water to drink must be considered on a case-by-case basis.

3. *Influence of solvent*. In some cases, and because of the nature of the material to be tested, it may be necessary to dissolve or suspend the material in an appropriate liquid vehicle. This may be required, for example, if the material to be tested is a solid, of high viscosity, or suspected to be of extremely high toxicity. In some cases a solvent may facilitate absorption (e.g. surfactants, dimethylsulphoxide) and hence enhance toxicity, and in other cases there may be a retardation of absorption, particularly if partition favours the diluent (e.g. oils with liphophilic materials). In yet other cases it may be suspected that the diluent or vehicle is itself responsible for the major fraction of the established toxicity of the material tested, and thus the toxicology studies *per se* could give a spurious estimate for the intrinsic acute peroral toxicity of the primary test material. To determine if this is in fact the case, it is necessary to make comparisons between the LD_{50} values for the material as tested with that for the material tested expressed as both contained primary test material and as contained solvent, and relate these values to the known (or determined) LD_{50} for the solvent alone. An example is shown in *Table* 14.3 for an epoxy resin formulation dissolved in 1-methyl-2-pyrrolidone (MPD). When the dose-mortality data is expressed solely as

contained epoxy compound, the acute peroral LD_{50} value of just below 1 g/kg suggests a moderate acute lethal toxicity for the resin given by gavage. However, when the LD_{50} of the material tested is expressed as contained MPD, the LD_{50} of around 3 ml/kg is close to that for the acute peroral LD_{50} of a separately tested sample of MPD alone. Thus, the acute toxicity of the tested solution (resin + MPD) can be attributed almost solely to the MPD content, indicating that the epoxy resin itself is of low acute peroral lethal toxicity. In such cases, the smaller the amount of dissolved primary test material, the greater will be the apparent toxicity when the dose mortality data for the total test solution is expressed in terms of contained primary test material.

Table 14.3. Acute peroral lethal toxicity to rats of an epoxy resin formulated material in 1-methyl-2-pyrolidone (MPD) and for MPD alone.

LD_{50} value calculated	*LD_{50}(95% confidence limits)*	
	Males	*Females*
Resin content (g/kg)	0·93 (0·03–1·14)	0·84 (0·03–1·11)
MPD in formulation (ml/kg)	3·00 (2·03–4·42)	2·70 (2·04–3·57)
MPD alone (ml/kg)	3·73 (2·52–5·52)	3·35 (2·86–3·92)

4. *Presence of known human toxicants.* It is of the utmost importance to be aware of the detailed composition of formulations before attempting to interpret acute peroral toxicity data in laboratory animals in terms of likely hazards to humans. For example, methanol and ethylene glycol are known to be of moderately high acute toxicity by swallowing in humans, but dose-mortality data in rats gives spuriously low estimates for the acute peroral lethal toxicity to humans. Thus, rat peroral LD_{50} values for 50% aqueous solutions are 12·9 (11·4–14·6) ml/kg for methanol, and 8·54 (7·31–9·99) ml/kg for ethylene glycol. Thus, formulations containing even high concentrations of these materials will be apparently of low acute peroral toxicity in rats, when the other constituents are also of low acute toxicity. For example, an amine alkyl silane ester, dissolved in methanol (50% content), was determined to have, in the rat, an acute peroral LD_{50} of 14·9 (10·3–21·6) ml/kg, suggesting a low order of toxicity. Without a knowledge that the formulation contains a high proportion of methanol, a serious misjudgement of the potential acute human toxicity could be made.
5. *Times to signs and death.* The time to onset of signs of toxicity and to death are of value in determining the magnitude of potential hazards and the urgency for management. For example, with two materials of similar acute peroral LD_{50} and slopes of dose-mortality regression lines, that having the more rapid time of onset of signs and of death should be reported as having the greatest acute peroral lethal hazard. An example is shown in *Table* 14.4 of two materials having a similar order of acute peroral LD_{50} values in the rat: on the basis of times to death, 2,4-pentanedione (mortalities in hours) should be regarded as being more lethally toxic and presenting a greater overall hazard than 2,2′-bis(4′-aminophenoxybenzyl)propane (mortalities in days).

Table 14.4. Acute peroral lethal toxicity to rats of two materials with differing times to death 2,2′-bis(4′-aminophenoxyphenyl) propane (BAPP) and 2,4-pentanedione (2,4-PD).

Material	*Sex*	LD$_{50}$ (95% confidence limits) (*g/kg*)	*Times to death* (*range*) (*range*)
BAPP	M	0·41 (0·25–0·66)	3–14 days
BAPP	F	0·31 (0·22–0·42)	3–14 days
2,4-PD	M	0·76 (0·64–0·89)	2–24 hours
2,4-PD	F	0·58 (0·50–0·68)	2–5 hours

6. *Irritant potential and acute peroral toxicity*. The majority of acute peroral toxicity studies are conducted by gavage, and thus local irritant effects on the oropharynx and oesophagus are not studied as such. This is important information to know for a variety of reasons, including (a) irritation of the mouth may give a warning of exposure, (b) the potential for upper alimentary inflammatory or corrosive lesions and complications thereof need to be mentioned in health effects literature, and (c) severe irritant effects on the alimentary tract may mask systemic toxicity, with the latter only being evident when dilute solutions are swallowed. When assessing the possible role of acute inflammatory effects on peroral toxicity, it is of considerable value to examine the results from acute skin and eye irritancy studies; the eye irritancy studies are particularly valuable to assess the inflammatory effects of irritants on mucosal surfaces. It is of the utmost importance to examine all information, and two examples are compared based on the information given in *Table* 14.5. The results for dimethylethanolamine (DMEA) indicate it to be of moderate acute peroral and percutaneous toxicity, and a severe skin and eye irritant. It is, therefore, expected that the material will cause

Table 14.5. Acute toxicity and primary irritancy of N,N-dimethylethanolamine (DMEA) and diethylene glycol monohexyl ether (DEGMHE).

Test	*Substance*	*Species (sex)*	*Results*
Peroral LD$_{50}$ (95% CL)[a]	DMEA[b]	Rat (M)	1.75 (1.15–2.03) ml/kg
	DEGMHE[c]	Rat (M)	4.02 (3.09–7.84) ml/kg
Percutaneous LD$_{50}$ (95% CL)[a]	DMEA[c]	Rabbit (M)	1.87 (1.26–2.76) ml/kg
(24-hour occlusion)	DEGMHE[c]	Rabbit (M)	2.14 (1.45–3.17) ml/kg
Skin irritation	DMEA	Rabbit (F)	Severe erythema, oedema and necrosis
(4-hour occlusion)	DEGMHE	Rabbit (F)	Mild erythema and oedema
Eye irritation	DMEA	Rabbit (F)	0.005 ml induced severe conjunctivitis and corneal injury
	DEGMHE	Rabbit (F)	0.1 ml caused moderate conjunctivitis and corneal injury

[a]95% Confidence limits.
[b]Tested as 20% in water (results as DMEA).
[c]Tested as undiluted DMEA.

marked irritation and possibly ulceration of the mouth, pharynx and oesophagus, and possibly haemorrhagic ulceration of the stomach with the undiluted material. The signs and symptoms which might therefore follow the swallowing of undiluted DMEA, and for which product safety warnings would be required, include pain or discomfort, with possible ulceration of the mouth and throat; discomfort or pain in the chest and/or abdomen; nausea, vomiting (possibly haematemesis), diarrhoea, thirst, drowsiness, dizziness, and loss of consciousness. Complications might include oesophageal perforation and mediastinitis, gastric perforation with peritonitis, hypovolaemic shock, and disseminated intravascular coagulation syndrome. A severe aspiration hazard exists, and it would be inappropriate to induce emesis. The percutaneous toxicity study indicates a potential for systemic toxicity with DMEA (albeit by another route) which may be masked perorally by the irritant effects. Therefore, in the absence of studies with diluted material it may be contraindicated to give water, other than to wash out the mouth. With diethylene glycol monohexyl ether (DEGMHE), on the other hand, systemic toxicity appears to be a more significant factor as indicated by a comparison of the acute peroral and percutaneous toxicities, and the lesser degrees of cutaneous and ocular irritancies. Thus, irritation of the mouth and throat may occur from DEGMHE, but the severe ulcerogenic effects which would occur with DMEA is unlikely. However, the eye irritation information suggests that pulmonary mucosal injury could occur from aspiration of undiluted material, and induction of emesis would be contraindicated for the undiluted material. Dilution by swallowing of water would probably be appropriate.

It is clear from the above considerations that an assessment of the potential for acute peroral adverse health effects requires that detailed attention be paid to all single exposure information and to the conditions under which the tests were conducted. Particular, though not exclusive, attention needs to be given to the following:

1. The LD_{50} values, although used in some mandatory classification schemes, give a minimum of information by themselves, and could be misleading if not considered along with the range of doses over which deaths occur, minimum lethal dose, slope of dose-mortality regression line, and whether the data follows a normal distribution or implies the existence for a hypersensitive group.
2. A detailed knowledge of the acute peroral sublethal toxicity can aid in defining what signs and symptoms are likely to occur, and how they may give an indication of the onset, progression and nature of poisoning. For example, irritation of the gastrointestinal tract may lead to nausea, vomiting, diarrhoea and abdominal discomfort; or decreased motor activity, slowed reactions to environmental stimuli and coma, indicate a generalized progressive depression of central nervous system function. As noted above, the time to onset of signs of toxicity and death are valuable in defining relative hazards and priorities for management of poisoning. Also, latency to onset of toxicity may be a determinant of cumulative toxicity by closely spaced repeated exposures.
3. Necropsy findings, although usually non-specific may give some indications

of general pathology or occasionally may suggest a target organ for toxicity. The value of routine histological examination of carefully selected tissues in acute toxicology studies has been undervalued and not appreciated by some.
4. Attention needs to be paid to the condition of the conduct of the study. Particularly important factors to consider are nutrition, the use of diluents or solvents, the precise chemical composition of formulations, and evidence for concentration of the test material influencing toxicity.
5. Results from other single-exposure studies of particular importance are potential for systematic toxicity as revealed by acute percutaneous or inhalation toxicity studies, and primary irritancy studies by application to the skin and eye. These may help clarify the acute peroral and systemic hazards.

The above brief considerations on interpretation of acute peroral toxicity studies can generally be applied to other single-exposure studies. However, route-specific considerations may apply, and a few examples of these are considered below for inhalation. A detailed review of the conduct and interpretation of toxicology studies by the inhalation route of exposure has been presented elsewhere (Ballantyne, 1981), and the following represent only some of the factors to be considered in assessing the significance and relevance of such studies.

1. When atmospheric concentrations of a material are quoted, do they represent measured concentrations (analytically or gravimetrically) or nominal concentrations based on metering rates? Is there good agreement between analytical and nominal concentrations? If the A/N ratio is significantly below unity what is the reason, since this may assist in defining generation and distribution properties of the material?
2. Detailed attention should be paid to the conditions of generation of the material. The following are specific examples of where such information is of value.
    a. The method of generation may be static, in which the material is placed directly into the exposure chamber, or dynamic by passing air over or through the material and then into the exposure chamber. There may be significant differences between the result from studies conducted by the two methods with materials containing small amounts of highly volatile and highly toxic materials. With static methods of generation, the volatile material may accumulate and reach toxic concentrations, whereas with dynamic methods the atmospheric concentration of toxic impurities will be a function of their concentration in the test material and their vapour pressure. Thus, the effects from highly toxic volatile contaminants may be exhibited in static generation methods but not necessarily if generation is dynamic. Chemical analysis of the sample and measurement of major components and contaminants in the atmosphere is highly desirable.
    b. Chamber humidity must be known in order to determine the possible contribution of mucosal dessication in an irritant response. Also, some materials may hydrolyze in a moist atmosphere to produce more, and sometimes less, toxic products.

c. Temperature of generation and exposure are needed. In most cases the statements on inhalation toxicity can only apply for ambient temperature, and the problems posed by high temperature or combustion products is an entirely different consideration.

3. When studies are conducted with fibres or particulates, their average size and distribution of sizes is required to be known in order to determine if they can be inhaled, or the fraction which is capable of being inhaled.
4. Most long-term repeated exposure studies are conducted by exposures to given relatively constant concentrations of the test material in the atmosphere for specific periods each day. However, for some situations additional studies may be required to assist in more precisely defining potentially hazardous conditions. Thus, Toft et al. (1982) studied bone marrow toxicity from benzene and found that, for example, 24 hours of exposure to 95 ppm (2280 ppm h) or 96 hours of exposure to 21 ppm (2016 ppm h) produced severe toxicity, while exposure to benzene vapour at 95 ppm for 2 hour/day, 5 days per week for 2 weeks (1900 ppm h) gave almost no effects. Also, at concentrations above an effective dose, intermittent exposure to a specific total dose was more effective the longer the duration e.g. 50 ppm for 8 hours/day (4000 ppm h). Differential effects on toxicity may result from variable exposure conditions. Thus, Appelman et al., (1986) found that with acetaldehyde, peak exposures up to 3000 ppm superimposed on 500 ppm caused irritation, excitation, and reduced body weight gain. No such effects occurred after interrupted or non-interrupted exposure to 500 ppm acetaldehyde without peak loads. Non-interrupted exposure to 500 ppm, however, produced a reduced phagocytic index of pulmonary macrophages and degeneration of nasal olfactory epithelium. With interruption of exposures or interruption plus peak exposures, there was enhancement of the effect on pulmonary macrophages, but no influence on the nasal olfactory pathology. As a further example, David et al. (1981) studied the relationship between exposure time and concentration of carbon tetrachloride vapour in rats, and found that the severity of liver lesions was influenced more by the atmospheric carbon tetrachloride concentration than by the total amount of carbon tetrachloride inhaled. Also, Wilmer et al. (1987), using histopathology and cell proliferation in the nasal mucosa as a monitor, also found for formaldehyde that the vapour concentration rather than the total dose determined the severity of the cytotoxic effects.
5. Inhalation toxicity information may be required to be examined for possible relevance to those individuals with established lung disease, as well as for those with normal lung function. For example, is an inhaled material likely to accelerate or precipitate a coexisting disease? Also does an existing lung pathology influence particle disposition in the respiratory tract, e.g. changes in airways diameter or geometry can influence dispositional mechanisms for particulates.

One area of concern in the extrapolation of inhalation toxicity data is the use of the inhalation exposure dose concept. The amount of airborne material to which the whole animal is exposed is a function of both the concentration (c) of the material in the atmosphere and the time of exposure (t); the product of these two (ct) is referred to as the inhalation exposure dosage. It is important to realize that this is the dose to which the animal is exposed, and not the dose inhaled or absorbed; there may be significant and variable differences between the exposure and absorbed inhalation doses. In order to extrapolate acute data outside the concentration time constraints of the experiments, some individuals and organizations assume Haber's rule, which states that for a given response (usually death) the product of concentration and time is constant (Haber, 1924). This is crudely used by some, for example, to re-evaluate an LC_{50} for a timed 4-hour exposure to a 1-hour LC_{50}. While within restricted ranges, it may be constant for some materials, this is not the case for many and could lead to grossly misleading extrapolations. For example, with hydrogen cyanide vapour, as the exposure concentration needed to produce a 50% morbidity (LC_{50}) is reduced, the time required to produce 50% mortality increases. However, up to an hour, as the time increases so does the (*ct*); the (*ct*) for 50% mortality of rats exposed for 1 minute to HCN vapour is 1129 mg min m^{-3}, but for a 1-hour exposure the $L(ct)_{50}$ increases to 9441 mg min m^{-3} (Ballantyne, 1983). The gross departure from Haber's rule with HCN vapour is due to its endogenous detoxification; thus, with high concentration-short duration exposure the detoxification mechanisms are swamped and lethal body concentrations build up rapidly, but with lower concentration-longer duration exposure significant proportions of the absorbed cyanide can be detoxified and lethal body loads take longer to develop. Derge et al., (1986) have re-evaluated raw data from acute lethal inhalation toxicology studies with several volatile industrial compounds and found that the product of *c* and *t* is not always a good parameter for predicting a mortality response.

Single-Exposure Studies

Data obtained from single-exposure studies are absolutely essential in order to define the potential acute handling hazards of chemical substances. Often these studies are conducted by the peroral, cutaneous and inhalation routes of exposure, and in some instances by parenteral injection. Studies designed to determine the dose which would be most likely expected to cause death in one half of the animals under the conditions to which the chemical is administered (LD_{50}) have come under criticism (Zbinden and Flury-Roversi 1981; Advisory Committee Report to the Home Office, 1979). The major criticisms levelled against single-exposure acute toxicity testing for the purposes of defining the LD_{50} values include a lack of predictability of lethal doses in humans, and human neonates and infants in particular, variability of LD_{50} according to test conditions, and the unnecessary use of animals for producing a number which is of minimal significance with regard to assessing hazard to humans. However, as has been noted by some investigators (Zbinden and Flury-Roversi, 1981; Gad et al., 1984; ECETOC, 1985), lethality is only one of a number of endpoints which can be obtained from a well designed single-exposure study. With regard to the utility of these tests from the standpoint of hazard evaluation, other and possibly more important endpoints include:

a. Clinical signs of toxicity, and their times to onset and duration.
b. Reversibility of toxic effects.

c. Sex-specific effects of toxicity.
d. Highest dosage without toxic effects and/or mortality.
e. Lowest dosage to produce toxic effects and/or mortality.
f. Range of doses over which signs and mortalities occur, and slope of dose-effects regression line.
g. Times to death, and relationship to doses.
h. Possible target organs demonstrating sensitivity to the toxic agent.

These endpoints and their dose-response relationships allow a reasonable assessment of acute hazard, and form a basis for developing warnings on product safety information statements. For example, a typical label statement for general use which could be developed for a minimally irritant material producing only transient central nervous system depression after a single peroral dose, and a single short-term inhalation exposure to the vapour generated at ambient temperature, might include:

WARNING! Harmful if inhaled or swallowed. May cause dizziness, faintness, drowsiness, incoordination of movements, blurred vision, and unconsciousness.

In contrast, a material such as a cholinesterase inhibitor, which causes prompt onset of signs of toxicity and at higher dosages a short time to death, would require a more detailed and emphatic warning statement, typical of which might be:

DANGER! Harmful if swallowed or if absorbed through the skin. May cause dizziness, headache, nausea and vomiting, diarrhoea, weakness, anxiety, tremors, salivation, lachrymation, visual disturbances, difficulty with breathing, convulsions, coma and death.

Additionally, if the material is an organophosphate anticholesterase, it may be necessary to draw attention to delayed peripheral neurotoxicity if this is indicated by laboratory studies or human experience. Examples of toxic processes and other potentially adverse health effects which can often be identified from single exposure studies include peripheral sensory irritant responses (excessive grooming, chromodacryorrhoea, blepharospasm, perinasal wetness, diarrhoea and rapid breathing), neurotoxic and neuropharmacologic effects (as determined by locomotory disturbances, behaviour and reaction to environmental stimuli), inflammatory effects (e.g. keratitis and conjunctivitis), and haemolysis (as detected by dark or discoloured urine in the dropping pans or in the bladder at necropsy). The information gained by careful observation of signs and necropsy findings can, therefore, be of great value in assessing the potential adverse health effects and thus potential hazards of a material, and in developing appropriate non-technical language for warning statements. In addition, the LD_{50} value does place the acute lethal toxicity of a chemical in perspective with regard to a large body of information available on other chemicals widely used in commerce, providing close attention is paid to 95% confidence limits and slope of regression line (Ballantyne, 1984a).

Information derived from carefully designed single-exposure toxicity studies is important in preparing guidance on what will constitute appropriate precautionary and protective measures, and often on treatment of overexposure situations. Many materials which demonstrate an appreciable order of toxicity by the peroral or parenteral routes may also be of slight to moderate toxicity when applied under occluded conditions to clipped skin. Also, some materials have been shown to be more acutely toxic by skin absorption than by peroral administration, or of equal toxicity by either of these routes of administration. This may reflect species differences, or the influence of differences in pharmacokinetics and biotransformation. In these instances, suggested precautionary measures and treatment requirements need to be tailored to the order of toxicity demonstrated in the specific tests. Thus, materials which have a percutaneous LD_{50} of 2 g/kg body weight or less, or that kill animals at dosages of 1 g/kg or less, require warning statements such as 'Harmful amounts may be absorbed through the skin', and advise for the use of protective clothing (including gloves) when handling the material, and washing clothing before re-use. This general statement is equally applicable whether the cause of death can or, more usually, cannot readily be ascertained from the available data. Other considerations are the need for washing of contaminated skin, and when medical advice is required.

The single dose LD_{50} values of chemicals are commonly used by regulatory agencies for classifying and controlling the use of chemicals, and defining the manner in which they may be legally transported and handled. Typical of such schemes is that used by the United States Department of Transportation (DOT) for categorizing materials for purposes of transportation under the restrictions applicable to Class B poisons (DOT, 1976). The conditions under which the single-exposure studies are to be conducted for purposes of classification are precisely specified, and include: the animal species, the number of animals to be used and the length of the observation time after the doses are administered. Under the DOT definitions, chemicals having LD_{50} values of 50 mg/kg body weight or less by the oral route in the rat, 200 mg/kg or less by the percutaneous route in the rabbit, or an LC_{50} of 2 mg/litre or less of vapour, mist or dust in the rat, would be regarded as Class B Poisons, and thus require special packaging and warning provisions for shipping in interstate commerce.

Recent interest in very short-term exposure to vapours of highly toxic chemicals has evolved as a result of accidents such as the discharge of methyl isocyanate into the atmosphere in Bhopal, India (Heylin, 1985). A number of procedures have been introduced in an attempt to identify these highly toxic chemicals. The DOT, for example, has developed a 'Poison-Inhalation Hazard Classification' which is based upon recommendations of the United Nations Committee of Experts on the Transportation of Dangerous Goods (DOT, 1985). The definition of a Poison-Inhalation Hazard is based on both the numerical value of the 1-hour LC_{50} in rats, and the ability of the material to produce vapour concentrations which would pose a hazard to human life. On these bases, the definition of a DOT Poison-Inhalation Hazard is:

> Any liquid material, other than a liquefied compressed gas, having a saturated vapour concentration equal to or greater than ten times its LC_{50} (vapour) value if the LC_{50} value is 1000 ppm or less.

It is the intention of the DOT not only to consider the toxicity of a chemical in assessing the hazard to humans, but also to consider, albeit in perhaps a somewhat simplistic manner, the probability that an event could occur in which the known toxicity could pose a real risk to human life and health. This latter question is addressed in the definition by including a consideration of the potential saturated vapour concentration.

The practical management and control of risks from a material which has been demonstrated to produce acutely toxic effects both in animals and in man can be conveniently illustrated by examining various measures which have been taken to reduce the possibility of exposure to potentially harmful amounts of the herbicide paraquat (Crome, 1986). This chemical has been responsible for a large number of deaths in children and adults, which have occurred as a result of accidental or intentional ingestion, or through gross misuse of the product (Fletcher, 1974). There is every indication that when used in the prescribed manner, paraquat presents no unacceptable health hazard (Howard, 1980). However, paraquat has been shown to cause severe liver, kidney and lung damage after a single large peroral dose. Death is usually delayed, and results from severe pulmonary insufficiency caused by interestitial pneumonitis and interalveolar fibrosis (Bismuth et al., 1982; Onyeama and Oehme, 1984; Seidenfeld et al., 1985) as a result of free radical injury to pulmonary alveolar macrophages (Wang and Stephens, 1986). In advanced cases, current antidotes are probably of marginal benefit. Therefore, the most successful strategy to reduce morbidity and mortality, by reducing hazard, has been to develop measures to prevent ingestion or subsequent absorption. One approach was the use of alerting agents. This included the addition of a blue dye to lessen the misidentification of the paraquat formulation in the event it were poured into a beverage or similar container. The colour blue was considered to be the least likely to be confused with a soft drink. A second alerting measure consisted of the addition of a stenching agent to discourage accidental or intentional consumption. Both alkyl pyridines and alkyl carboxylic acids have been used for this purpose. An attempt was also made to add a thixotropic material such that the formulated product consisted of a gel and could not be poured until vigorously shaken. This measure proved to be technically unworkable for the intended use of the product in the field, and could not be successfully incorporated into the risk management programme. The above example illustrates an important concept in development of 'warning' protective measures. Thus, successful consideration can be given to methods which reduce hazard yet do not interfere with intended use. Using a different principle many paraquat formulations now contain an emetic which has been shown to assist in reducing the absorbed dose, and increase the chances of survival in the event of ingestion (Denduyts-Whitehead et al., 1985). This covers those situations where warning measures may have been accidentally or deliberately avoided.

Primary Irritancy Studies

As with acute exposure toxicity studies, primary irritancy testing is an essential part of the initial programme to assess the handling hazards of a chemical. Reasonably predictive animal models exist for assessing the primary irritant properties of chemicals to both the skin and eyes of humans (Ballantyne and Swanston, 1977; McCreesh and Steinberg, 1983). Again, these testing procedures, and particularly those addressing eye irritancy, have come under attack by the animal rights activists. Although there is great pressure to develop, and use, *in vitro* model systems for the development of primary irritant hazard evaluation data, results obtained in some of these tests may be misleading because they do not possess the anatomical and pharmacokinetic elements found in the intact animal and these elements may significantly influence irritant responses. In particular, a key component of the rabbit ocular study is a determination of the differential response in the various tissues and completeness of the healing process.

Because of the emotive issues raised by eye irritancy testing in laboratory animals, methods have been suggested for simplifying the techniques, reducing numbers of animals, and limiting suffering (Seigfried, 1986). The use of enucleated eyes and various *in vitro* preparations have been proposed as alternatives for preliminary screening of materials for eye irritating potential (Borenfreund and Borrero, 1984), although the results may require confirmation by *in vivo* studies. Non-invasive methods have been described for the objective confirmation, *in vivo*, of eye irritating potential at applied doses less than those causing subjective indications of macroscopic eye injury (Ballantyne, 1986b).

Classification of materials as eye irritants on the basis of analogy with primary cutaneous irritation test results can be misleading. Thus, some materials which are not irritant by standard occlusive skin testing may be moderate eye irritants, and other materials shown to be moderate skin irritants may not be eye irritants by standard test procedures. The discrepancy in the latter case is often due to the difference in contact time with tissue between occluded cutaneous tests and the introduction of material onto the cornea or into the inferior conjunctival sac. In some cases the discrepancy may be due to the slow hydrolytic production of irritant species during the period of occlusion. Williams (1984) found that of 60 materials found to be severe cutaneous irritants or corrosives, only 39 were severe eye irritants and 15 were mild or non-irritant. Gad et al. (1986) found that severe skin irritation correlated with severe eye irritation in 66 of 72 cases, but skin irritation results failed to predict severe eye irritation in 6 of 72 cases.

With both skin and eye irritancy testing, it is important to obtain clinical evaluations over a period of time to determine if healing will occur. Different perceptions of hazard must be conveyed in cases where a splash in the eye might produce simple conjunctivitis compared with one producing permanent corneal injury. Typical warnings for product safety purposes would be as given below. For a severe eye irritant the following would be appropriate:

> DANGER! Causes severe eye burns! Blindness or major and incapacitating residual injury is likely in spite of prompt treatment! Wear eye protection when handling this material! If accidentally splashed in the eyes, promptly flush the eyes with water and continue washing for at least 15 minutes. Urgently seek the attention of a physician, preferably an ophthalmologist.

In comparison, a material that produces only conjunctival inflammation, but where there is rapid and complete healing of that injury, might have the following type of product safety warning:

> WARNING! Causes eye irritation. Wear eye protection when handling this material in a manner which might result in splashes. If accidentally splashed in the eyes, promptly flush eyes with water and continue washing for at least 15 minutes. Seek the attention of a physician.

The visual endpoints of primary irritancy studies for both eye and skin are well defined, and schemes have been developed to assign numerical values to the various effects for hazard evaluation purposes. The most frequently used schemes are those of Draize (1959), or modifications thereof. For skin studies, the lesions graded include erythema, eschar formation, oedema and necrosis. For eyes, independent grades are determined with regard to the cornea (the presence of opacity and the area affected by opacity), the iris and the conjunctiva. Often the values obtained by the Draize scheme are condensed into an integer value hazard warning; the National Paint and Coatings Association's HMIS ratings being typical of these procedures (NPCA, 1985). It should be pointed out, however, that arbitrary use of these schemes for hazard evaluation can be misleading, and may result in conclusions which could misrepresent the actual hazard of a material (Ballantyne and Swanston, 1977). This is particularly true, for example, in a few cases where experience in the workplace has established that humans may be more sensitive to the irritating properties of a chemical than laboratory animals on which the rating scale is based. In assessing irritant potential, it is necessary to examine information from all animal tests. For example, some low molecular weight oxirane/methyloxirane polymers produce minimal to slight irritant responses when tested on the clipped skin of rabbits by standard 4-hour occlusive procedures. However, in 24-hour occluded percutaneous toxicity studies a slightly more marked response which was obtained (Union Carbide, unpublished data). In some practical applications, the nature of the operation of equipment results in these materials coming into contact with skin for prolonged periods of time without the opportunity for washing them off. Under these circumstances, a large number of operators have experienced erythema, itching and a burning sensation of the skin of the hands and lower arms. This response is consistent with the response seen in the laboratory animals if one takes all the information into consideration, including the local effects in the percutaneous study. As a result of this human experience, the use of these materials and the precautionary measures used in handling them in this type of operation required re-evaluation.

Primary irritancy studies are used by regulatory agencies for the purpose of conveying hazard warning statements and prescribing appropriate packaging and handling procedures. Furthermore, the DOT also uses a protocol for classifying chemicals as corrosive materials. Thus, a material will be considered corrosive if it produces irreversible tissue injury (ulceration and/or necrosis) in 2 of 6 rabbits to which it is applied under prescribed conditions (Code of Federal Regulations (CFR), 1984). Materials which are classified as corrosive must be packaged in a prescribed manner and carry the specific warning statement 'DOT Corrosive'.

Peripheral Sensory Irritation

Many materials, with varying degrees of specificity and potency, are capable of producing peripheral sensory effects. That is to say, they interact with sensory receptors of peripheral nerves in skin and mucosae producing local sensation with associated reflexes, e.g. contamination of the eye produces local pain or discomfort together with excess lachrymation and blepharospasm. Effects such as these are clearly warning and protective; in the case of the eye, discomfort is warning, and lachrymation with blepharospasm protects the eye from further access of irritant material. However, from an occupational viewpoint, such effects may present a hazard by interfering with the ability of a person to see clearly, and thus predisposing that person to accidents (Ballantyne, 1984b). Thus, a knowledge of the peripheral sensory irritant effects of a material can be of considerable assistance in defining safe working conditions, in particular knowing what concentration is the threshold for sensory irritation. The latter consideration is of value in decisions on what constitute appropriate exposure guidelines for the workplace.

Careful observation of animals during the conduct of acute and repeated exposure inhalation toxicology studies gives a qualitative, and sometimes semi-quantitative, indication of the potential of an airborne material to produce sensory irritant effects. These may be exhibited, for example, as blepharospasm, periocular and perinasal moisture, and alteration in the pattern of breathing. A variety of methods are available to study more specifically peripheral sensory irritation. A few examples are:

a. Examination of laboratory animals for blepharospasm as a function of the concentration of material to which the eye is exposed (Ballantyne, 1984b).
b. Neurophysiological measurement of supraorbital nerve activity as a function of the concentration of material coming into contact with the cornea (Green and Tregear, 1964).
c. Measurement of the depression of respiratory rate by plethysmography (Alarie, 1981a).

Of all the laboratory methods used to investigate peripheral sensory irritation, that of plethysmography has received the most attention, and there now exists a large volume of information on the effects of a wide variety of chemicals tested in this way. In addition to its value for quantitatively determining sensory irritant response, the method has been extended to allow a comparison of the concentration of airborne material producing sensory irritation and that concentration resulting in early lung injury, and hence giving valuable information on the protective value of the subjective sensory irritant response (Alarie, 1981b; Matijak-Schaper et al., 1983).

Data for peripheral sensory irritation conditions may be obtained in the workplace by correlating subjective assessments of irritant sensation in workers with industrial hygiene measurements of the concentration of irritant material in the atmosphere. A more precise estimate may be obtained for specific materials by exposing human volunteer subjects to known atmospheric concentrations of test material. In this manner, a dose-response relationship, threshold value, and no-effect concentration may be derived (Ballantyne and Swanston, 1973, 1974). These mathematically derived precise values, however, should be viewed in the perspective of the modulating effects of various factors influencing sensory irritant responses, and the continually changing conditions in the workplace. Factors that may quantitatively influence peripheral sensory irritant responses include temperature, humidity, personality, motivation, distraction, tolerance and, for aerosols and dust, particle size (Ballantyne, 1983b). Clearly, controlled observations on human volunteer subjects should only be undertaken if there is adequate toxicological information to ensure that the procedure can be carried out with no risk to the subjects.

When communicating information about the peripheral sensory irritant effects of a material, it is of importance to differentiate mechanistically and functionally these neurophysiologically mediated effects, and their signs and symptoms, from those resulting from an inflammatory response to a primary skin, eye or respiratory tract irritant.

Repeated Exposure Studies

Although of the utmost importance for evaluating hazard by continued recurrent contact, repeated exposure information exists for considerably fewer industrial chemicals than does data from acute toxicity and primary irritancy studies. This is partly due to economic considerations. In many instances, and in particular for older studies, the information that does exist may lack sufficiently specific detail for rigorous evaluation with regard to hazard evaluation. However, even within these limitations, and when they are the only data available, they may be helpful in preparing warning statements and for recommendation of precautionary measures in the workplace. When information from well conducted studies is available, it provides valuable information that can be used not only for repeated exposure hazard evaluation, but can assist in setting appropriate exposure standards for the workplace and provide guidance in designing medical surveillance programmes. Protocols for repeated exposure studies should at least include general observations on the animals and a record of their behaviour; non-specific indices of toxicity (weight gain, water and food consumption, mortality); quantitative measures of toxicity, including haematology, serum chemistry and urinanalysis; organ weight data; and gross and microscopic observations for evaluating morphological tissue injury. A particularly important consideration in this type of study is the identification of any target organs and tissues which are most sensitive to toxic injury by the chemical. In addition, and for the purpose of hazard evaluation and risk assessment, it is imperative that dose-response relationships for toxic effects are established, and a 'no-observable-effect level' (NOEL) defined. The slope of the dose-response curve is critical to the establishment of appropriate safety factors. These safety factors are then applied to the NOEL for the most sensitive adverse effect caused by the chemical. The principles pointed out by Ballantyne (1984b) for establishing different levels of the margin of safety based upon the slope of the dose-response curve for respiratory irritants are also valid for other end points of toxicity, including target organ toxicity. Thus, for effects which elicit steep slopes, a small change in concentration could result in toxicity affecting a large portion of the exposed population, and therefore these chemicals require large safety factors. On the other hand, materials having shallow slopes would not produce the same impact with small increases in exposure concentrations; however these materials may present problems with the sensitive population represented at the left-hand side of the dose-response curve.

If a study is long, and particularly if it is in the chronic exposure category, it is useful to know the approximate time of appearance and subsequent progression of induced toxicity. For this reason it is valuable to include animals in the main exposure group that are to be sacrificed at various times during the exposure period. These interim sacrifice animals are examined and investigated in the same manner as those allowed to survive the total exposure period. Also, it is of practical value, particularly for the occupational health physician, to know if any induced toxicity is reversible. For this reason, it is often useful to have additional animals for exposure, but which are kept for several weeks after the end of the exposure period. These recovery group animals are examined and investigated in the same manner as those exposed animals which are sacrificed at the end of the exposure period. In this way, postexposure regression, progression or stasis of any induced structural and/or functional injury can be assessed.

Except for tumorigenesis, most types of repeated exposure toxicity will be detected by subchronic studies. Chronic exposure studies are conducted for the following reasons:

a. If there is a need to investigate the oncogenic potential of a chemical.
b. If it is necessary to determine a no-effect and a threshold level of toxicity for lifetime exposure.
c. If there is a reason to suspect that certain types of toxicity may only be exhibited under chronic exposure conditions.

Thus, chronic exposure studies are frequently designed to allow for combined observations for oncogenesis and non-neoplastic tissue injury. It is of considerable value to have interim sacrifices at 12 and 18 months to allow a determination of the onset and progression of tissue injury.

Although repeated exposure studies in animals generally supply the information needed for determining the nature of potential adverse health effects which might be encountered in workers who have continuous day-to-day contact with the chemical, the quantitative predictive value of these tests is often not as good as that for acute toxicity and primary irritancy. Since only a relatively few animals can technically and economically be used in most toxicity studies, the lowest incidence of an adverse effect which can be reliably detected is limited, particularly if the background (historical) incidence of the effect is high. When a larger exposed human population which has potential for exposure is considered, a low incidence of an adverse effect could result in a significant number of individuals being affected. For instance, an incidence of an adverse effect in the range of 0·1–1% or lower (1 animal in 1000 or 100) could be of major concern from a public health standpoint, and indicate a totally unacceptable risk in an application where several million people might be exposed. In order to minimize the possibility of missing a toxic effect which might occur infrequently, larger dosages are used than would be expected to be present in the environment, under the assumption that this will increase the chance for a toxic effect to occur, and also decrease the time to onset of that toxic effect (Gillette, 1984).

The interpretation of repeated exposure studies can be complicated by differences that are not related to treatment, but which may develop in groups of animals isolated from one another. Kjellstrand and Holmquist (1984), for example, kept several control groups of rats isolated in separate exposure chambers. After 30 days of exposure to filtered air, several endpoints were measured including body weight, organ weights and plasma esterase activity. The number of statistically significant differences in these indices between the respective control groups was greater than would be predicted by chance alone. These investigators attributed their findings to the slight differences in the environment caused by spatial location and/or intrinsic differences that develop within an isolated group, perhaps due to infections or unknown causes. They concluded that when testing for adverse effects of chemicals, such differences may be mistaken for treatment-related effects, and such conclusions would, in fact, be unwarranted. However, a clear dose-response relationship should indicate if effects are toxicologically significant.

Additional problems can be introduced into the interpretation of repeated exposure studies due to the sheer number of endpoints which are measured in order to ensure any organ or tissue effect is detected. The power of the statistical tests commonly used are often capable of assigning significance for very small numerical differences between treated and control groups. In addition, when multiple statistical tests are conducted, the opportunity for false positive results increases. It then becomes important to ensure that appropriate statistical tests have been applied, and also to determine which of the statistically significant effects observed in animals also have toxicological relevance. Zbinden (1979) has pointed out that many, if not most, changes that are observed and measured cannot be considered as relevant. In consideration of this fact, he has advocated that basic research on the mechanisms of toxicity be conducted, and results used in practical evaluation of hazard to man.

Differences in the toxicological manner by which various animal species respond to some chemicals, the way in which they absorb, distribute and excrete specific chemicals, and physiological differences which have an impact in the manifestation of a toxic response to a chemical, may also tend to weaken the predictability of repeated exposure test results as compared to those from acute toxicity and primary irritancy testing. However, well conducted short-term repeated studies, subchronic studies and chronic studies can supply a good deal of useful and relevant information regarding potential hazard to man in spite of the numerous shortcomings of the type discussed above, providing the information is carefully and critically examined. In particular, target organ toxicity is often identified, and the dose-response for injury defined (Heywood, 1983). The strength of evidence for toxicity is greatly enhanced if non-specific observations can be refined by more specific methods. For example, an increase in organ weight may be due to adaptive change (e.g. hypertrophy and adaptive enzyme formation), hyperplasia, metaplasia or neoplasia. Clearly the implications for each of these various responses is different and a knowledge of the cause of organ weight increase is of considerable functional importance. Thus, careful design and interpretation of experimental indices provides evidence for the nature of toxic injury at the cellular level, and the basis for impaired function. This type of information provides a valid and rational basis for developing strategies for managing the hazards which may occur from long-term repeated exposures to man, and for developing appropriate warning statements and precautionary and warning advice. As an example, several repeated exposure studies in animals and human cases have been able to delineate the neurotoxic effects of methyl *n*-butyl ketone. Recognition of this hazard has led to the removal of the solvent from the working environment and replacement with other less toxic solvents (O'Donoghue, 1985). The adverse effects produced in animals by ethylene glycol monomethyl ether on the blood forming tissues, testes and the central nervous system (Nagano et al., 1979; Hanley et al., 1984), coupled with results obtained in developmental toxicity studies in animals, have led to the withdrawal of this chemical from consumer products, and for strong warning statements to be placed on industrial labels and in product safety literature. The following is a typical example of a label warning for ethylene glycol monomethyl ether:

> WARNING!
> Harmful if inhaled, swallowed, or absorbed through skin. May cause damage to bone marrow resulting in anaemia. May cause damage to male reproductive organs leading to partial or total sterility. May produce tremors, speech difficulties, confusion, and unconsciousness. Has produced birth defects and embryofoetal toxicity in studies with laboratory animals.

Where there is appropriate evidence, statements are developed for specific types of target organ toxicity. For instance, ethylene glycol, which will cause kidney damage after either a single exposure or repeated exposures (Rowe and Wolf, 1982), might carry the following general warning statement with regard to its nephrotoxicity:

> DANGER! May be fatal if swallowed. Severe kidney damage follows the swallowing of large volumes of ethylene glycol or repeated ingestion of smaller volumes. This may result in abdominal discomfort or pain, malaise, pain in the loin, poor urine output, and kidney failure.

By careful observation of signs in animal toxicology studies, and particularly if appropriate monitoring for structural and functional injury is undertaken, information can be obtained which is of value to the occupational health and emergency room physician. The most valuable advice that can be given includes specific organ or tissue toxicity, any latency, the reversibility of induced lesions, and the most appropriate first-aid and antidotal measures. Clearly, this advice will be enhanced by the experience gained from human cases of intoxication. In cases where there is, unfortunately, experience with poisoning in humans it may be possible to be highly specific. The advice can also be enhanced by studies designed to study specifically the effects of antidotal procedures. This is discussed in detail by Marrs in Chapter 12. For materials where there is reasonably extensive and credible documentation, it is possible to provide reliable summarized advice. For example, with ethylene glycol the following brief statements can be made as 'Notes to Physician':

> The principal toxic effects of ethylene glycol, when swallowed, are kidney damage and metabolic acidosis. Ethanol is antidotal, and its early administration may block the formation of nephrotoxic metabolites of ethylene glycol in the liver. Ethanol should be given intravenously, as a 5% solution in sodium bicarbonate, at a rate of about 10 ml ethanol per hour. A desired therapeutic level of ethanol in blood is 100 mg/dl. Haemodialysis may be required. Pulmonary oedema with hypoxaemia has been described in a number of patients following poisoning with ethylene glycol. The mechanism of production has not been elucidated, but it appears to be non-cardiogenic in origin in several cases. Respiratory support with mechanical ventilation and positive end-respiratory pressure may be required.

At the other extreme, toxicology information may be so limited that the only definitive finding may be mortality or primary irritancy. In such cases, the only possible, and pathetically inadequate, advice that may be given with respect to treatment is:

> No known antidote. Treatment should be directed at the control of symptoms and the clinical condition of the patient.

Most advice falls between these two extremes. However, on the basis of toxicology studies it should be possible, at least, to give the following advice on first-aid and medical management:

a. The relative urgency with which treatment is required.
b. The order of magnitude of acute poisoning.
c. Guidance on the treatment of poisoning by swallowing, with particular reference to the need or otherwise of swallowing water, and whether emesis should be induced. With highly toxic or irritant materials, the maximum possible guidance should be given to the physician, e.g. anticipated complications, and any special treatment regimes such as the use of activated charcoal, cathartics, particular medicinal therapy or antidotes.
d. General guidance on the first-aid management of skin and eye contamination, and procedures necessary if material is inhaled.

Current regulatory activity in the United States, particularly in relation to the test rule provisions of the Toxic Substances Control Act, focuses on data collection with the objective of defining potential hazards of chemicals for which there is significant or substantial human exposure, or which may present an unreasonable risk of injury to health or the environment. Attempts are currently underway to formalize the process of assessing the risks of potential carcinogens, developmentally toxic substances and mutagens (Environmental Protection Agency, 1984a,b,c). These methods stress a mathematical extrapolation approach. There is little formal help available at the moment, however, for directing actions necessary to reduce the risks of adverse health effects once the hazards of a chemical have been defined.

Other Special Toxicology Studies

Although the previous sections have emphasized primary irritation, and acute and repeated exposure studies as sources of information on which to define hazards and their communication, many other special studies and specific potential adverse health effects exist which may require to be considered in detail. Some of these may present information indicating a new and specific health hazard from exposure, and others may allow a more precise definition of the condition under which toxicology may be exhibited. Some of the major specialized areas which may be investigated include the following:

1. *Immune-mediated hypersensitivity.* Industrial chemicals may produce hypersensitivity reactions by skin contact causing allergic contact dermatitis, or by inhalation resulting in occupational asthma. Methods are well established in laboratory animals for investigating skin sensitizing potential, and are developing in the area of assessing potential for respiratory sensitization. Case reports and experience with exposed humans are a major

source of information on sensitizing potential. Clearly, sensitizing reactions may represent a significant adverse health effect which may seriously limit allowable exposure of the worker.

2. *Reproductive and developmental toxicity.* Depending on the nature of the chemical, and its known or suspect toxicity, it may be appropriate to investigate its potential to cause abnormalities in reproductive function and to produce malfunctions in the foetus. Although teratogenic effects on the one hand may be an indication for specifically controlling exposure with respect to the pregnant or fertile woman, testicular toxicity on the other hand may be a valid reason for the reverse sex discrimination in workplace exposure.
3. *Metabolism and pharmacokinetics.* The potential for systemic toxicity may be highly dependent on the distribution, body burden and residence time of the parent material and/or its metabolites. Therefore, studies on the metabolism and pharmacokinetics of the parent material may yield valuable information on mechanisms of toxicity, target organ or tissues, relationship of environmental exposure dose to target organs dose, and the design of further studies to elucidate the toxicity of the material. Metabolic studies should yield information on the biotransformation of the material, the sites at which this occurs and the mechanism of biotransformation. Pharmacokinetic studies should quantitatively measure the rate of uptake, the absorbed dose, the distribution, residence, and the rate of elimination of parent material and metabolites. Such studies should allow a determination of the relationship between environmental exposure conditions, absorbed dose, and how these influence storage and elimination of parent material and metabolites and target organ doses.
4. *Genotoxicity.* Methods are available to screen for mutagenic and clastogenic potential *in vitro*, and confirm that these occur *in vivo*. A positive genotoxic result is not a directly useable endpoint *per se*, but may assist in defining a potential for adverse health effects or screening for potential toxicity. Thus, materials which show clear mutagenic activity may be suspect of being chemical carcinogens, and appropriate further studies may be required. Clastogenic materials may be suspect of reproductive toxicity.

PERMISSIBLE EXPOSURE STANDARDS

Any series of well conducted *in vivo* toxicology studies, particularly if examined along with human occupational health data from workplace experience, should allow a definition of what is expected to be a permissible level of exposure to the chemical, i.e. the exposure conditions for the majority of an exposed population which will not result in the exhibition of the known toxicity, sensory irritancy or incapacitating pharmacological effects associated with the material, under the specific time conditions for which the permissible conditions are defined. Differing values are necessary for differing purposes. In general, values are required either for repeated daily exposure conditions or for single short-term exposure emergency purposes. For short-term purposes, the most relevant information is that concerning acute injury, peripheral sensory irritation and pharmacological effects such as narcosis. The general workplace permissible exposure standards require, in addition to acutely mediated effects, a consideration of cumulative toxicity, carcinogenicity, and other specific aspects of repeated exposure toxicity.

General Workplace Atmosphere Standards

Most consideration has been given to general workplace standards. The guidelines are defined in various ways, but in general have as their objective the protection of individuals from the adverse effects of a chemical under particular time conditions of use, when rigorously adhered to. Perhaps one of the most widely recognized list of guidelines for airborne chemicals is that of the American Conference of Governmental Industrial Hygienists (ACGIH) for threshold limit values (TLVs). These values have been adopted by many organizations over the world. The TLV® is defined as the 'time-weighted average concentration for a normal 8-hour workday, and a 40-hour workweek, to which nearly all workers may be repeatedly exposed, day after day, without adverse effect' (ACGIH, 1986). The historical development of the TLV compilation has been reviewed by Paull (1984). This review adds valuable insight into concepts which guide the selection of specific values published for each of the chemicals on the ACGIH TLV list.

The efforts of the ACGIH were incorporated into the exposure standards adopted by the US government in the Occupational Safety and Health Act, which is administered by the Occupational Safety and Health Administration (OSHA). The list of Permissible Exposure Standards (PELs) published in this Act was adopted from the 1968 ACGIH TLV list. Unfortunately, the Act was so constructed that the published values could be changed only by Act of Congress or by formal rule-making procedures. Thus, while many significant changes have been made in the ACGIH TLV list, only a few changes have been transmitted to the OSHA PEL list. This is clearly an administratively, scientifically and ethically unacceptable position for ensuring occupational safety.

The actual TLV values are promulgated after careful consideration of all relevant data by various working committees of the ACGIH. Documentation for the guidelines, along with the basis on which specific exposure limits are proposed, are published (ACGIH, 1983). Smyth (1962) concluded that TLVs developed for specific materials could be categorized into groups providing protection against one or more of nine different adverse effects: acute systemic toxicity, asphyxiation, narcosis, chronic toxicity, fume fever, cancer, allergic sensitization, and eye pigmentation. More recently, a review identified 28 different effects on which TLVs were based, either in full or in part (Anger, 1984). Of these categories, sensory irritation played a role in determining the TLV values of approximately 73% of the 588 chemicals listed in the 1982 edition of the TLV booklet. Other notable categories included target tissue effects, nervous system effects and acute toxicity. Carcinogenicity entered into the considerations of TLVs for 59 chemicals, while teratogenic and mutagenic activity was a consideration in setting TLVs for 6 materials.

An early critique of the methods used to establish TLVs indicated that a majority of these values were established predominantly on the basis of studies conducted in laboratory animals (Smyth, 1959). Although over the years additional human experience has been gained with a large proportion of commodity chemicals, the primary basis for selecting values which are believed to provide minimal risk of adverse health effects to man still appear to be data obtained from studies in laboratory animals.

The general procedures by which exposure guidelines are established have been reasonably well standardized, based upon sound scientific and toxicological principles. However, often using the same information, a number of different standards have been established for the same chemical by different organizations and national regulatory commissions. A tabulation of these different standards has been compiled (ILO, 1980). Included in this latter monograph are brief descriptions of the procedures by which different countries develop standards, and in some instances, a brief description of the criteria used in the decision-making process. A particular contrast was noted between the criteria used by the ACGIH, where allowance is made for reversible clinical effects of chemicals, and the USSR, where no biological changes or functional decrements are permitted when setting a maximum allowable concentration (MAC).

In addition to considerations of criteria for establishing specific average exposure guidelines (e.g. average exposure over a 40-hour week), qualifications of the average value may be required to ensure that certain 'safe' upper limits are not exceeded. Thus, in addition to the establishment of TLV values, the ACGIH has adopted short-term exposure levels (STEL) for many chemicals. These STEL values are defined as 'a 15 minute time-weighted average exposure which should not be exceeded at any time during a work day, even if the 8-hour time-weighted average is within the TLV. Exposures at the STEL should not be longer than 15 minutes and should not be repeated more than 4 times per day. There should be at least 60 minutes between successive exposures at the STEL. An averaging period other than 15 minutes may be recommended when this is warranted by observed biological effects' (ACGIH, 1986). The ACGIH has also defined 'ceiling values' as air concentrations of a material which should not be exceeded even instantaneously during any part of the working exposure. Some attempts have also been made to develop dual workplace exposure standards which would be applied differentially to populations which clearly have different susceptibilities to the adverse effects of a chemical. This approach is particularly appropriate, for example, to teratogens or reproductively toxic materials. In this case, one standard might be developed for the most sensitive effect exclusive of developmental toxicity and be applied to all workers other than women of childbearing potential, and a second more stringent standard be developed for protection of the latter group. In Belgium, for instance, pregnant and nursing women cannot be exposed to certain chemicals; these include lead, mercury, carbon disulphide, arsenic compounds, benzene, aromatic amines, derivatives of aromatic hydrocarbons and carbon tetrachloride (ILO, 1980). Similar considerations might be applied to males for materials known to produce testicular toxicity. It has been the authors' experience that proposals for dual standards in the United States, particularly as applied to reproductive and developmental toxicity, have been far from successful. This reluctance to adopt dual standards results more from social, emancipating, union, business and political reasons, than from scientific and medical appropriateness.

Short-Term Emergency Standards

Several recent incidents, including chemical releases into the general environment, have accelerated the development of short-term air standards for highly toxic or irritant materials. Such standards would address exposure concentrations that could be tolerated for a short period of time without fatal or seriously injurious effects, or without incapacitating effects that would prevent escape from the contaminated atmosphere. These values are needed to formulate emergency response plans, and would be intended for incorporation into models which can be used to initiate response and evacuation actions within the plant and local community in the event of a major accidental spill or release of a toxic substance. All too often, however, the engineers developing these models are more interested in obtaining a number (any number!), to incorporate into their model, and give little thought to the appropriateness or scientific validity relating to the real health hazards of the material. This approach is exemplified, for example, in an EPA Guidance Document for Chemical Emergency Preparedness (EPA, 1985a). In this document it is suggested that an emergency exposure concentration (in g/m^3) may be determined from an oral LD_{50} value (in mg/kg) by multiplying the LD_{50} value by 0.1. There is no scientific, biological or mathematical justification for this simplistic approach to a serious safety consideration, and the toxicology community should regard these pseudoscientific approaches as abhorrent, and strongly object to such improper suggestions.

A compilation of values termed ‘immediately dangerous to life and health’ (IDLH) has been published in the NIOSH/OSHA *Pocket Guide to Chemical Hazards* (Department of Health and Human Services, 1985). These values are defined as the maximum concentrations from which one could escape in 30 minutes without any escape-impairing symptoms, or any irreversible health effects. They were defined for the purposes of respirator selection. The documentation for these values, and criteria by which they have been established, is not readily available.

The Toxicology Committee of the American Industrial Hygiene Association attempted to establish ‘emergency exposure limits’ (EEL) for a number of materials (Frawley, 1964). In recommending these limits, they considered six specific factors:

1. Exposure at the EEL will be by accident.
2. Normally, prevailing values of airborne contamination will be below the TLV.
3. Exposures will occur only once; further exposure will be prevented.
4. The levels are not designed to protect against idiosyncratic effects, sensitized individuals, or individuals predisposed to disease.
5. Exposed individuals will be under medical surveillance.
6. Effects which could lead to secondary injury (impairment of vision, judgement and coordination) must be considered in applying these values.

Values are presented for time periods of exposure ranging from 5 to 60 minutes. The documentation for a few of these materials is based predominantly on sensory irritation and respiratory effects. Thus, in considering levels for nitrogen dioxide, attention was given to short-term exposure levels which produced pulmonary oedema, death and chronic lung lesions in rats. Unfortunately, a compilation of EEL values is not readily available for use in emergency preparedness planning.

The authors believe the following are appropriate considerations in developing short-term emergency standards, which we will refer to as 'emergency response guidelines' (ERG). The use of an ERG is to trigger the use of protective equipment and/or evacuation of workforce personnel or those living in the immediate environment of a chemical facility. On this basis values should be assigned to avoid serious and permanent chemical injury and/or pharmacological incapacitating effects by single short-term exposure to airborne material. On this basis, an ERG may be defined as 'the maximum airborne concentration of a material that can be tolerated, as a single short exposure of specified duration, without the production of irreversible toxic injury and/or incapacitating pharmacological effects.' Values require to be cited as concentrations for a specific time period, the duration of which may depend on the precise local conditions. However, in most instances a time period between 30 and 60 minutes should be sufficient to allow appropriate protective and evasive actions, providing a well prepared action plan has been drawn up alongside, or as a consequence of, the development of an ERG. The use of inhalation exposure dosage units (*ct*) should be avoided because of the problems associated with extrapolation of inhalation exposure dosage values. ERG values require to be developed on a case-by-case basis, but the determinants for assignment will include: (*a*) toxicity (acute and short-term repeated) which may include local and/or systemic effects, structural and/or functional injury, and immediate or delayed effects; (*b*) major pharmacological effects, and will include peripheral sensory irritation of the eye and respiratory tract, and central nervous system depression; (*c*) certain special considerations may exist with a few materials, e.g. teratogenicity.

Biological Exposure Monitoring

In the context of this review, biological exposure monitoring is taken to mean the analysis of exhaled breath, body fluids and cells or tissues (including hair and nails) from workers to detect materials, or biological effects, which can be used to assess the exposure dosage of individuals to a chemical and give a warning level for overexposure. When a biological effect is assessed, this is usually a clearly definable toxic or toxic-related endpoint, or a specifically related biochemical feature; this definition, therefore, excludes the procedures carried out in routine occupational health monitoring procedures. Perhaps the most acceptable definitions of procedures related to monitoring of exposed individuals are those agreed upon by a CEC/NIOSH/OSHA meeting in 1980 (Berlin et al., 1984), as follows:

Biological monitoring—The measurement and assessment of workplace agents or their metabolites either in tissues, secretions, excreta, or any combination of these, to evaluate exposure and health risk compared to an appropriate referenced.

Health surveillance —The periodic medico-physiological examination of exposed workers with the objective of protecting and preventing occupational related diseases.

This definition of biological monitoring relates specifically to measurement of chemicals and does not include induced biological effects (such as enzyme inhibition, genotoxic endpoints, biological reactivity, etc.) directly attributable to exposure, but whose direct health impairing implications may be uncertain. Thus, an additional definition to cover these aspects has been proposed by Zielhuis and Henderson (1986), as follows:

Biological effect monitoring—The measurement and assessment of early biological effects, of which the relationship to health impairment has not been established, in exposed workers to evaluate exposure and/or health risks compared to an appropriate reference.

Since a biological endpoint or concentration of parent material or metabolite is being measured in biological fluids or tissues the particular parameter being monitored will give an indication of dosage for all routes of exposure through which the material in question can be absorbed. A few specific examples of the type of biological and biological-effect parameters are given in *Table* 14.6.

TLVs, and other proposed exposure guidelines, are meant to define what are safe working conditions for environmental exposures to airborne materials for the majority of the workforce. On the other hand, biological exposure monitoring is concerned with obtaining an estimate of the absorbed dose of a particular harmful exposure, and within the constraints of the methodology and the current knowledge give an early indication of when the absorbed dose reaches a level which is the threshold for reversible toxicity for an individual worker. As noted above, biological monitoring gives an index of the total dosage for individuals by all routes of exposure. With some materials, contribution to the absorbed dose by percutaneous absorption may be substantial, and in such cases there could be a discrepancy between the biological monitor and the recommended atmospheric exposure standard. In such situations, the biological indicator may be a more reliable and appropriate index for safe exposure conditions. The role of percutaneous absorption as a factor in biological monitoring has been reviewed by Thomas (1986).

In applying the methods of biological monitoring, particular attention should be paid to the development of reliable specific methods for sampling and analysis, determination of the variability in response for a given population, influence of exogenous factors and variables, and the assignment of a threshold or warning index above which hazardous overexposure is likely to occur. Genetically determined variation in metabolism may have a significant influence on biological monitoring procedures and their interpretation. Those who are likely to be hypersusceptible to xenobiotics because of genetic variability in specific biochemical features may require to be identified. Dewan et al. (1986) studying male workers engaged in the manufacture of benzidine hydrochloride found a substantial absorption of benzidine over an 8 hour workshift, and a significant

Table 14.6. Examples of biological and biological effects monitoring procedures currently in use in the workplace.

Effect or body fluid	*Example*	*Workplace agent*
Chemical monitoring:		
Exhaled air	Parent molecule	Ethanol, benzene, styrene, toluene
Urine	Parent material	Lead, acetone, methanol, pentachlorophenol
	Metabolite (parent exposure)	Phenol (benzene), Mandelic acid (methylbenzene, styrene)
Blood/plasma	Parent material	Dinitro-o-cresol, halothane, lindane
	Metabolite (parent exposure)	Trichloroethanol (trichloroethylene) Hippuric acid (toluene)
Biological effect:		
Enzyme inhibition	Erythrocyte acetylcholinesterase,	Organophosphates
	Blood δ-aminolaevulinic acid synthetase	Lead
Biochemical (non-enzymic)	Urinary β_2-microglobulin	Cadmium
	Urinary acetyl glucosaminidase	Nephrotoxins
Biochemical derivative	Carboxyhaemoglobin	Carbon monoxide
	Haemoglobin alkylation	Ethylene oxide
Genotoxic	Mutagenic activity (body fluids)	Ethylene oxide Cytotoxic drugs
	Clastogenic activity (lymphocytes)	Epoxides
	Increased sister chromatid exchange (lymphocytes)	Ethylene oxide

negative correlation between the rate of sulphamethazine acetylation and the urinary excretion of free benzidine. These data on benzidine excretion, therefore, need to be viewed in terms of the observation that slow acetylators may be more susceptible to arylamine-induced cancer than fast acetylators (Cartwright et al., 1982).

Additional factors to be considered in establishing permissible biological exposure limits, and in interpreting the data from such measurements, include the influence of physical activity, environmental conditions (e.g. temperature, diet, water consumption, changes in metabolism induced by the presence of another chemical, and methodology). These considerations indicate that the timing of specimen collection may have a significant influence on the results observed in a biological monitoring programme (ACGIH, 1984). The sources of error and variation in chemical biological monitoring have been reviewed by Aitio and Jarrisalo (1985) with respect to physiological environmental conditions and specimen collection and storage. Methods for biological monitoring of various specific materials are to be found in Aitio et al., 1984; Alessio et al., 1983; Lauwerys, 1983; WHO, 1985.

When there is exposure to mixtures of chemicals the enhancement of metabolic pathways by one chemical may influence the metabolism of another, and hence the concentration measured or effects detected. This enhancement is often reflected in changes in microsomal enzyme activity, which is principally related to the smooth endoplasmic reticulum of hepatocytes, and may result in modified metabolic activation and/or detoxification of the xenobiotic. Non-invasive methods are available for assessment of microsomal enzyme activity (Dossing, 1984), and may be useful in certain situations where there is exposure to mixtures.

ACGIH (1986) have used 'biological exposure indices' (BEIs) as values which represent warning levels of biological response to the material or its metabolites. Workers are not expected to suffer any ill effects so long as the described measurements of the determinant are maintained within the limits of the recommended BEI. Measurements outside these limits do not necessarily indicate a disease process. However, if deviant values persist, the advice of a physician should be sought. In the 1986–1987 ACGIH list, BEIs have been adopted for 6 materials, there is a 'notice of intent' to establish for 10, and a further 9 substances are under study. However, as currently discussed in the 1986–1987 booklet of threshold limit values and biological exposure indices, the BEI is not too clearly defined.

Testing of urine for mutagens and blood cells for chromosomal aberrations, increased sister chromatid exchanges and micronuclei has been proposed as possible useful screens for exposure to potential genotoxic and carcinogenic materials (direct or metabolically activated) in the occupational environment. Due to the influence of a variety of extraneous factors, including personal habits, the results from such studies and proposals for their use require careful consideration. Sequential observations should reduce the chance of irrelevant findings. It has been suggested that incorporation of biological monitoring methods into conventional epidemiological studies should increase the power to detect carcinogenic materials earlier, and at lower concentrations, as well as to estimate more accurately the magnitude of human risk (Vainio, 1985). A considerable literature is now accumulating on the rationale for urine screening, methodology and approaches for increasing specificity, and results on exposure to specific materials. Reviews and good sources of bibliography can be found by Ahlborg et al. 1985; Brewen, 1982; Lambert et al., 1982; Vainio, 1985.

Margins of Safety

Quite often, the process of setting exposure guidelines, recommending maximum tolerated daily intake, or merely giving advice concerning the safety of a particular chemical in a given application, comes down to the determination of an acceptable 'margin of safety' between the dosages which are known to be the threshold for causing adverse effects in animals or man and those estimated to represent non-harmful doses. As previously mentioned, much current activity in this direction deals with mathematical extrapolation and quantitative risk assessment. However, and to a large extent, individuals who find themselves involved in giving advice on a daily basis deal in terms of subjectively assessed margins of safety.

There is still considerable scientific and administrative controversy over which method, quantitative risk assessment or application of appropriate safety factors is more appropriate in developing realistic safety recommendations (Goldstein, 1983; Stockinger, 1987). Quantitative risk assessment, *per se*, does not result in decisions of what exposure levels are safe, and what levels are not safe. Generally, however, there are 'implied' or 'implicit' cut-off levels, any concentration above which would be deemed not to be safe. Thus, it might be considered that any concentration of chemical producing an annual excess of one case of cancer in 10^6 individuals exposed, presents unacceptable risk. Margins of safety, on the other hand, are applied directly to some exposure level which has been shown, in animals or in humans, to cause minimal or no observable adverse effects. The margin of safety that is used in this type of judgemental decision is affected by a number of variables. Traditionally, various factors of 10 have been applied to the NOEL to determine average daily intakes. The history of this logarithmatic approach has been extensively reviewed (Dourson and Stara, 1983; Gaylor, 1983). Generally, factors of 10 are applied for each of the following variables: intraspecies differences, variability within the human population, and relative degree of seriousness of the biological effect. Smyth (1959) pointed out the subjective nature of safety factors employed in establishing TLV values. At the time of that publication, the safety factors appeared to range from 0·2 to 10. Dourson and Stara (1983) have presented data which they contend support the value of 10 as an uncertainty factor for animal to animal variation, intraspecies adjustments, chronic toxicity, and in extrapolating from the information on lowest observable effect levels and NOELs. The consideration for intraspecies adjustment was based upon the variability of the dose-response for acute lethality of 490 chemicals in animals. Data supporting an intraspecies adjustment factor of 10 was based upon an analysis of metabolic body weight of different animal species. Analysis of NOELs and lowest observable exposure levels in subchronic and chronic studies resulted in evidence which would support another uncertainty factor of 10. The overall approach of Dourson and Stara (1983) was empirical in nature and did not take into consideration mechanisms of toxicity of individual chemicals.

Zielhuis and van der Kreek (1979) have proposed that safety factors between 3 and 10 should allow an acceptable level of safety for occupational settings. The magnitude of the safety factor used depends on the type of experimental data available. Thus, for animal studies, the length of exposure, the number of animals exposed, the number of animal species for which data exists, the number of treatment levels, the dose-response curve, and the seriousness of the toxic effect should all be taken into consideration. In addition, these factors should be applied to NOEL. Their proposal did not take into consideration carcinogenicity or developmental toxicity. Calabrese (1985) reviewed the intraindividual variation of a large number of enzymatic and biochemical responses in humans, and in many cases found variation in excess of 10-fold. He concluded that additional studies need to be conducted to establish firmer bases for regulatory approaches. As mentioned previously, Ballantyne (1984) has suggested that the slope of the dose-response curve for a specific effect should be used to guide decisions on the magnitude of the safety factor required.

It would seem reasonable to conclude that the less information that is available on a specific material, the more conservative (err on the side of safety) the selection of a margin of safety should be. This does not appear to be the case, and in fact exactly the reverse is the usual as demonstrated by the following. In reviewing the history of changes in TLVs, Smyth (1959) commented that, at that time, the TLVs for 45 substances were based in part on repeated inhalation or feeding studies in animals. Of these 45 materials, the TLVs for 15 were later revised. In all but one case, the changes involved reduction of the value first proposed. Smyth noted that: 'A single isolated observation of possible injury can result in reducing a threshold level, while it requires unusual opportunity, tenacity and motivation which would justify an increase in a threshold limit.' This situation does not appear to have changed appreciably in the intervening years. Of the 25 materials listed for notice of intended change in the 1985–86 ACGIH *Threshold Limit Handbook*, six were included to lower the existing TLV value, eight were included as new entries, six were included to propose the existing TLVs as ceiling levels, and one was included to add a carcinogen notation. Also included in this list was a proposal to increase the STEL value of carbon dioxide, to drop the carcinogen notation from a second material, amitrole, and to drop the ceiling notation from the TLV for 2-nitropropane. In the latter case, it was also proposed that the TLV be reduced from 25 ppm to 10 ppm. Thus, there remains a trend to take a more conservative stance with regard to exposure, as more information on materials becomes available.

Toxicology is concerned with defining the potential to cause injury, and toxicology study guidelines generally support the position that the highest exposure level included in a study should produce signs of toxicity, or be the highest practical exposure level attainable (EPA, 1985b; OECD, 1981). This requirement is needed in order to define the toxic response and identify organs and tissues susceptible to the chemical. These factors then play a major role in hazard evaluation, and in developing appropriate warning and precautionary statements, giving meaningful medical advice in the event of overexposure, and possibly giving guidance in developing medical surveillance programmes. The toxic response, and the dosage levels which produce the response, must be dealt with in an honest and rational manner in order to protect individuals from potential adverse effects of chemicals, but there may also be a need to give due consideration to possible economic impacts of decisions based on potential health risks. Health risks of chemicals may need to be balanced against health risks resulting from possible management options, which could lead to changes in work situations or actual loss of employment. The majority of provisions taken to reduce the likelihood of ill-health caused by exposure to chemicals in the workplace do not lead to plant or unit closure. However, in the event that loss of employment results from action taken to reduce health risks from potential exposure to a chemical, this loss of employment in and of itself has been shown to have adverse effects on health (Grayson, 1985). Thus, a balance must be found between the potential health effects caused by exposure to a chemical and the potential health effects which might be caused from the economic impact of actions taken to reduce exposure. It is therefore mandatory that exposure guidelines be based on strong scientific arguments which can be supported by relevant and credible information available concerning the toxic effects of the chemical.

SPECIAL CONSIDERATIONS

Most of the discussion in this essay has been limited to exposure to single chemical substances, and with the worker who forms part of a normal population. However, in most industrial situations, exposures are to more than one material. Also, there are requirements for special considerations for particular segments of the working population who could, for diverse reasons, be at greater risk than the majority of the workforce. The sensitive or susceptible members of the population are represented at the left-hand side of the dose-response curve for the adverse effects. In some cases this is due to a well defined biochemical and functional deficiency which increases sensitivity to the chemical. In such cases, the dose-response relationship for a population may show a biphasic plot with the susceptible individuals shown as a discrete subpopulation on the left-hand side of the distribution curve. In other cases, and particularly those at the left-hand side of a normally distributed dose-response curve, the cause for increased susceptibility to a given chemical may not be known. Other members of the workforce may be at increased risk because of sex or age-related physiological status, such as pregnancy, or because of coexisting disease, or certain potentially harmful personal habits which may increase susceptibility to toxic materials. Some of these factors requiring special considerations in the workplace are described briefly below.

Mixtures

Exposures to mixtures in the occupational environment may involve prior, coincidental or successive exposure to a multiplicity of chemicals, and the conditions of exposure may lead to significant alterations in toxicity from one or several of the chemicals by other constituents in the mixture. Thus, an evaluation of hazard from multiple chemical exposure can be a much more demanding procedure than evaluation of hazards from exposure to single chemicals, and is currently a much less satisfactory procedure. In addition to the factors necessary for evaluation of single exposure hazards, discussed above, it is also necessary to take into account factors such as chemical and/or physical interactions of the individual components; the effects that one chemical may have on the absorption, metabolism, or pharmacokinetic characteristics of another; and the possible interactions between parent compound and metabolites (Ballantyne, 1985). For simple mixtures the resultant toxicity may be an independent expression of those of the constituents; additive or antagonistic effects may occur, or there may be potentiation or synergism. In assessing the toxicity of mixtures, the following need to be considered with particular reference to assessing hazards (Ballantyne, 1985):

1. Possible physical and chemical interactions in the mixture, which may result in the formation of new compounds or groupings, or influence the bioavailability of materials in the mixture.
2. Time relationships of the exposure to the various components of the mixture.
3. Route and conditions of exposure.
4. Physical and physiological factors affecting absorption.
5. Mutual influences of absorbed materials and metabolites on biotransformation, pharmacokinetic characteristics, and target organ doses of toxic species.

6. Relative affinities at the target sites.
7. Potential for independent additive and interactive processes between the various chemical species.

Mixtures may be complex and contain unreacted parent materials, major reaction and degradation products, together with contaminants and trace additives. It is important to remember that small quantities may have equal, and sometimes greater, significance in respect of a potential for adverse health effects. Thus, serious consideration needs to be given to the possibility of harm from, for example, small quantities of monomer residuals in polymeric materials, e.g. ethylene oxide, propylene oxide and formaldehyde. The contribution to toxicity by trace materials is well exhibited, for example, from the presence of trialkyl phosphorothionate or phosphorothionate impurities in organophosphate anticholinesterases (Hollingshaus et al., 1981), and the presence in chlorophenols of 2,3,7,8-tetrachlorodibenzodioxin (Kimbrough et al., 1984).

On the skin, the systemic toxicity of a material may be enhanced by various materials which facilitate percutaneous absorption; this may include the presence of a surface-active material having a carrier function, the presence of an irritant which produces erythema resulting in increased local dermal blood flow, and changes in the ionization or solubility characteristics due to the influence of other materials present. Increasing the viscosity of a material may enhance local or systemic toxicity due to persistence of material on the skin.

By inhalation there may be a variety of differing factors to be considered. For example, inhalation exposure dosages of chemicals may be modified by the presence of irritants or low concentrations of HCN in the mixture which can modify the rate and depth of respiration. Particles in the air may absorb other, and toxic, materials, and if inhaled and retained in the lung increase the burden of the toxic material. Some materials may produce anosmia and hence remove the olfactory warning for other inhaled materials. The toxicity of vapour atmospheres generated from liquid mixtures will depend on the generation and atmospheric conditions. For example, in a static atmosphere the vapour concentration of the most volatile material will tend to be increased relative to that of other components of the mixture. It is therefore possible that in stagnant air conditions there may accumulate a hazardous concentration of a highly toxic material which is present in only a minor proportion in a liquid mixture. On the other hand, when there is free airflow, the vapour components of the atmosphere will be closer to their relative concentrations in the liquid mixture from which they are derived, and thus in these circumstances total masses of the particular constituents will be a major consideration. Thus, the degree of ventilation of an area may significantly influence the toxicity of an atmosphere resulting from vaporization of liquid mixtures.

Endogenous determinants of the toxicity resulting from exposure to a mixture may be extremely complex. Thus, toxicity may be modified by prior or simultaneous enhancement, or suppression, of metabolic activation or detoxification pathways, and the potential for toxicity will depend on the equilibrium state, although this may continually change. Modulation of toxicity may also result from modification of pharmacokinetic characteristics, variation in distribution of absorbed materials and their metabolites, increasing or decreasing elimination of the toxic species, and competition for binding sites or receptors.

The ultimate determinant of toxicity resulting from exposure to multiple chemicals depends on the relative and absolute concentrations of toxic species at the target sites, and their functional interrelationships and interactions. Detailed reviews on the toxicology and hazard evaluation of mixtures have been presented by National Research Council, (1980); World Health Organization, (1981); Murphy, (1983); Ballantyne (1985).

Genetically Susceptible Subpopulations

Several genetically determined biochemical variants are believed to cause individuals so affected to be more susceptible to xenobiotics than those with normal biochemical features. Such a phenomenon may show itself as a subpopulation in a biphasic frequency distribution in dose-response relationships for the toxicity to a chemical. For example, individuals with hereditary methaemoglobinaemia may develop marked methaemoglobin formation at exposure doses of nitrites or aromatic nitrophenols which only produce minor methaemoglobin concentrations in the majority of the population.

Glucose-6-phosphate dehydrogenase deficiency of the A^- variant is a sex-linked heritable state affecting approximately 14% of black males and 2% of black females in the United States of America (Calabrese et al., 1967). It has been suggested that individuals with G-6-PD deficient erythrocytes may be at risk from haemolytic effects of oxidant agents due to the inability of the erythrocyte to generate sufficient NADPH and maintain an adequate concentration of reduced glutathione, and hence there is resultant oxidant damage and haemolysis (Calabrese et al., 1982). However, Amoruso et al. (1986) studied the effects of oxidant gases on human G-6-PD deficient erythrocytes and in strains of mouse cells with differing G-6-PD activities. From the data derived, they estimated that for any haemolytic effect to occur exposure to toxic concentrations of oxidants would be required. They concluded that there is no basis to preclude employees with the A^- variant of G-6-PD deficiency from a workplace where they would be exposed to oxidant gases.

As mentioned previously, acetylator status may play a significant role in N-acetylation of arylamine compounds such as 2-naphthylamine, 4-aminobiphenyl and benzidine. Slow acetylators may be more susceptible to arylamine-induced cancer (Cartwright et al., 1982), and have a significantly greater urinary excretion of free arylamine (Dervan et al., 1986).

Other genetically determined factors that have been suggested as possible causes of increased susceptibility to chemicals in the workplace include serum α_1-antitrypsin deficiency (emphysema), aryl hydrocarbon hydroxylase deficiency (lung cancer), pseudocholinesterase variants (anticholinesterase toxicity), and thallasaemia (lead toxicity). Clearly there is a need for detailed laboratory and occupational clinical studies to confirm that, indeed, there is a significantly increased susceptibility in those affected. The ethical issues involved in testing for genetically induced differential susceptibility to occupational hazards has been reviewed by Lappé (1983).

Coexisting Disease

Workers with various general medical disorders may be at a greater risk from exposure to certain chemicals than those not so afflicted. For example, workers with cardiovascular disease may be at increased risk from carbon monoxide or carbon monoxide-generating materials such as methylene chloride, or from methaemoglobin generators, since both may compromise oxygen supply to the myocardium. Inhaled irritants may aggravate chronic progressive pulmonary disease. In the Hazards Communications Act of the US Occupational Safety and Health Administration, provisions have been made to draw attention to this special aspect of hazard evaluation in a requirement that material safety data sheets should provide a section to discuss medical conditions that may be aggravated by exposure to the material being reviewed.

The interactions between chemical exposure and coexisting pathology may be complex, and it may not be possible to allow for this in assigning (special) workplace exposure guidelines. Pre-employment medical examinations and frequent medical surveillance programmes may assist in avoiding the placement of individuals into situations where the chemicals to which they would be exposed could exacerbate an existing general medical condition. Clearly, the success of such programmes relies on an informed discussion between occupational health physicians and applied toxicologists.

Immune-Mediated Hypersensitivity Reactions

Those who become immunologically sensitized to certain materials may exhibit signs and symptons on challenge at very low concentrations, and often at levels considerably lower than those causing other adverse effects in non-sensitized individuals. This can be distressing, and occasionally life threatening, if it involves an immune-mediated hypersensitivity by airborne materials causing occupational asthma, as for example from formaldehyde or toluene di-isocyanate. In these cases, the workplace exposure standard needs to be set to prevent the induction of the immune response. These data can be derived with varying degrees of accuracy by careful analysis of workplace data when there is both good industrial hygiene monitoring data along with detailed medical surveillance programmes for respiratory disease. Screening of individuals for atopy and bronchial hyper-reactivity may assist in preventing the placement of potentially susceptible workers into areas where respiratory sensitizers may be present. However, in certain occupations it may be almost impossible to protect against sensitization, e.g. agricultural workers and the development of intrinsic allergic alveolitis.

Personal Habits

There are a variety of personal habits, including diet and the taking of medicinal products, which may influence a response to a toxic chemical in the workplace. Two areas that have received particular attention in this respect are the smoking of cigarettes and the consumption of alcoholic beverages.

General reasons for prohibition of smoking in the workplace include the problems associated with the ill-mannered passive contamination of non-smokers and predisposition to physical accidents because of the sensory irritant effects of smoke. Also, there are a variety of situations which may lead to an increase in the burden of chemical exposure by the smoker. The simplest situation is an increased uptake of chemical because of cigarettes becoming contaminated (NIOSH, 1979). In some circumstances, there are clear indications of significantly enhanced toxicity due to working in specific circumstances; the synergistic relationships between asbestos (Hammond and Selifoff, 1973) or radon (Archer et al., 1972) and smoking are well established. The intense heating of airborne chemicals when drawn through a lighted cigarette may result in combustion products being formed which are severely deleterious to health. Examples include polymer fume fever from polytetrafluoroethylene (Williams et al., 1976) and phosgene from dichloromethane.

Due to the significantly increased carboxyhaemoglobin concentrations in smokers, they will be at increased risk from workplace carbon monoxide and carbon monoxide-generating materials, compared with non-smokers. Indeed the carboxyhaemoglobin concentrations of smokers may be above that permitted by the ACGIH TWA-TLV or BEI for carbon monoxide. Other examples of materials produced by cigarette combustion, and which may add to the exposure burden of the workplace, include hydrogen cyanide, hydrogen sulphide, acrolein, phenol and polycyclic aromatic hydrocarbons.

Heavy alcohol consumption may lead to chronic progressive liver injury and fibrosis, and increase sensitivity to hepatotoxic substances, or impair hepatic detoxification pathways.

The question of controlling personal habits, such as smoking, clearly is a ready-made pitch for US First Amendment activists. It is rather disappointing, but perhaps not unexpected, that the rights of those who do not wish to have the results of unnatural and disease producing procedures enforced upon them should receive secondary considerations. However, in the workplace, protection against increased hazard and litigation, as well as the rights of those who prefer not to be passively contaminated, should receive equal or greater concern.

REFERENCES

Advisory Committee on the Administration of Cruelty to Animal Act 1876 (1979). *Report on the LD_{50} test*, 1–31. London: Home Office.

AGGIH (1983). *Documentation of the Threshold Limit Values*, 4th edn. Cincinnati, Ohio: American Conference of Governmental Industrial Hygienists, Inc.

ACGIH (1986). *Threshold Limit Values for Chemical Substances and Physical Agents in the Work Environment and Biological Exposure Indices with Intended Changes for 1986–87*. Cincinnati, Ohio: American Conference of Governmental Industrial Hygienists, Inc.

Agarwal R., Gupta K. P., Kumar S. et al. (1986) Assessment of some tumorigenic risks associated with fresh and used cutting oil. *Indian J. Exp. Biol.* **24**, 508–510.

Ahlborg G. Jr., Bergstrom G., Hogstedt C. et al. (1985) Urinary screening for potentially genotoxic exposures in a chemical industry. *Br. J. Ind. Med.* **42**, 691–699.

Aito A. and Jarvisalo J. (1985) Biological monitoring of occupational exposure to toxic chemicals. Collection, processing, and storage of specimens. *Ann. Clin. Lab. Sci.* **15**, 121–139.

Aito A., Jarvisalo J., Kilunun M. et al. (1984) *Int. Arch. Occup. Environ. Health* **54**, 241–249.

Alarie Y. (1981a) Bioassay for evaluating the potency of airborne irritants and predicting acceptable levels of exposure in man. *Food Cosmet. Toxicol.* **19**, 623–626.

Alarie Y. (1981b) Toxicological evaluation of airborne chemical irritants and allergens using respiratory reflex reactions. In: Leong B. K. J. (ed.) *Proceedings of the Inhalation Toxicology and Technology Symposium*, 207–231. Ann Arbor, Michigan.

Alessio L., Berlin A., Rot R. et al. (1983) *Industrial Health and Safety*. Human Biological

Monitoring of Industrial Chemical Series. Luxemburg: Commission of the European Communities.

Amoruso M. A., Ryer J., Easton D. et al. (1986) Estimation of risk of glucose 6-phosphate dehydrogenase-deficient red cells to ozone and nitrogen dioxide. *J. Occup. Med.* **28**, 473–479.

Anger W. K. (1984) Neurobehavioral testing of chemicals: impact on recommended standards. *Neurobehav. Toxicol. Teratol.* **6**, 147–153.

Appelman L. M., Woutersen R. A., Feron V. J. et al. (1986) Effect of variable versus fixed exposure levels on the toxicity of acetaldehyde in rats. *J. Appl. Toxicol.* **6**, 331–336.

Archer V. E., Waggner J. K. and Lurdin F. E. Jr. (1972) Uranium mining and cigarette smoking effects on man. *J. Occup. Med.* **15**, 204–211.

Ballantyne B. (1981) Toxic effects of inhaled materials. In: Ballantyne B. and Schwabe P. H. (eds) *Respiratory Protection: Principles and Applications*, 93–134. London: Chapman and Hall.

Ballantyne B. (1983) The influence of exposure route and species on the acute lethal toxicity and tissue concentrations of cyanide. In: Hayes A. W., Schnell R. C. and Miya T. S. (eds) *Developments in the Science and Practice of Toxicology*, 583–586. Amsterdam: Elsevier.

Ballantyne B. (1984a) Toxicology. In: Grayson M. and Eckroth D. (ed.) *Encyclopedia of Chemical Technology*, 3rd edn., Supplemental Volume, 874–924. New York: John Wiley and Sons.

Ballantyne B. (1984b) Peripheral sensory irritation as a factor in defining workplace exposure guidelines. In: Oxford R. R., Cowell J. W., Jamieson G. G. et al. (ed.) *Occupational Health in the Chemical Industry*, 119–149. Calgary: Medichem.

Ballantyne B. (1985) Evaluation of hazards from mixtures of chemicals in the occupational environment. *J. Occup. Med.* **27**, 85–94.

Ballantyne B. (1986a) Interpretation and extrapolation of acute peroral toxicity studies. *Vet. Hum. Toxicol.* **28**, 472.

Ballantyne B. (1986b) Applanation tonometry and corneal pachometry for the prediction of primary eye irritating potential. *The Pharmacologist* **28**, 173.

Ballantyne B., Garman R. H., Greenspan B. J. and Myers R. C. (1985) Acute toxicity and irritancy of glutaraldehyde. *Toxicologist* **5**, 204.

Ballantyne B. and Swanston D. W. (1973) The irritant potential of dilute solutions of orthochlorobenzylidene malononitrile (CS). *Acta Pharmacol. Toxicol.* **32**, 266–277.

Ballantyne B. and Swanston D. W. (1974) The irritant effects of dilute solutions of dibenzoxazepine (CR) on the eye and tongue. *Acta. Pharmacol. Toxicol.* **35**, 412–423.

Ballantyne B. and Swanston D. W. (1977) The scope and limitations of acute eye irritation tests. In: Ballantyne B. (ed.) *Current Approaches in Toxicology*, 139–157. Bristol, UK: John Wright and Sons, Ltd.

Berge W. F. ten, Zwart A. and Appelman L. M. (1986) Concentration-time mortality response relationships of irritant and systemically acting vapours and gases. *J. Hazard. Mat.* **13**, 301–309.

Berlin A., Yodaiken R. E. and Henman B. A. (1984) *Assessment of Toxic Agents in the Workplace. Roles of Ambient and Biological Monitoring*. Boston, The Hague, Dordrecht, Lancaster: Nijhoff.

Bismuth C., Garnier R., Dally S. et al. (1982) Prognosis and treatment of paraquat poisoning: a review of 28 cases. *J. Toxicol., Clin. Toxicol.* **19**, 461–474.

Borenfreund E. and Boriero O. (1986) *In vitro* cytotoxicity assays. Potential alternatives to the Draize ocular allergy test. *Cell. Biol. Toxicol.* **1**, 55–65.

Brewen J. G. (1982) Chromosome aberrations in mammals as genetic parameters in determining mutagenic potential and assessing genetic risk. In: Bora R. C., Douglas G. R. and Nestman E. R. (ed.) *Chemical Mutagenesis, Human Population Monitoring and Genetic Risk Assessment*, 261–274. Amsterdam: Elsevier Biomedical Press.

Calabrese E. J. (1985) Uncertainty factors and intraindividual variation. *Regulatory Toxicol. Pharmacol.* **5**, 190 196.

Calabrese E. J., Kojola N. H. and Garnow B. W. (1977) A possible cause of hemolytic anemia in glucose-6-phosphate dehydrogenase deficient individuals. *J. Toxicol. Environ. Health* **2**, 709–712.

Calabrese E. J., Moore G. S. and Williams P. (1982) The effect of methyl oleate ozonide, a possible ozone intermediate, on normal and G-6-PD deficient erythrocytes. *Bull. Eviron. Contam. Toxicol.* **29**, 498–504.

Cartwright R. A., Rogers H. J., Barham-Had D. et al. (1982) Role of N-acetyltransferase phenotype in bladder carcinogenesis: a pharmacogenetic epidemiological approach to bladder cancer. *Lancet* **11**, 842–846.

Clayson D. B. (1987) The need for biological risk assessment in reaching decisions about carcinogens. *Mutat. Res.* **185**, 243–269.

Code of Federal Regulations (1984) Title 49, part 173.240 and part 173.1300. Congressional Research

Service (1983) *A Review of Risk Assessment Methodologies*, 1–78. Washington DC: US Government Printing Office.
Crome P. (1986) Paraquat poisoning 1986. *Lancet* **i**, 333–334.
David A., Frantik E., Holuša R. et al. (1981) Role of time and concentration on carbon tetrachloride toxicity in rats. *Int. Arch. Occup. Environ. Health* **48**, 49–60.
Davis C. S. and Richardson R. J. (1980) Organophosphourus compounds. In: Spencer P. S. and Schaumburg H. H. (ed.) *Experimental and Clinical Neurotoxicology*, 527–544. Baltimore: Williams and Wilkins.
Denduyts-Whitehead A., Hart T. B. and Volans G. N. (1985) Effects of the addition of an emetic to paraquat formulations on acute poisoning in man. *Clin. Toxicol.* **23**, 422–423.
Department of Health and Human Services (1985) *NIOSH/OSHA Pocket Guide to Chemical Hazards*, DHEW (NIOSH) Publication No. 78-210. Washington DC: US Government Printing Office.
Department of Transportation (1976) *Department of Transportation Regulations for Shippers—Poisonous Materials, Etiologic Agents, and Radioactive Materials Definitions and Preparation.* 49 CFR 173.
Department of Transportation (1985) *Packaging and Placarding Requirements for Liquids Toxic by Inhalation.* 49 CFR, parts 172 and 173.
Dewan A., Jani J. P., Shah K. S. et al. (1986) Urinary excretion of benzidine in relation to the acetylator status of occupationally exposed subjects. *Human Toxicol.* **5**, 95–97.
Dossing M. (1984) Noninvasive assessment of microsomal enzyme activity in occupational medicine: present study of knowledge and future prospects. *Int. Arch. Occup. Environ. Health* **53**, 205–218.
Dourson M. L. and Stara J. F. (1983) Regulatory history and experimental support of uncertainty (safety) factors. *Regulatory Toxicol. Pharmacol.* **3**, 224–238.
Draize J. H. (1959) Dermal toxicity. In: *Appraisal of the Safety of Chemicals in Foods, Drugs and Cosmetics Division of Pharmacology, Food and Drug Administration*, 46–59. Austin, Texas: Texas State Department of Health.
Environmental Protection Agency (1984a) Proposed guidelines for carcinogen risk assessment; request for comments. *Fed. Reg.* **49**(227), 46294–46301.
Environmental Protection Agency (1984b) Proposed guidelines for mutagenicity risk assessment; request for comments. *Fed. Reg.* **49**(227), 46314–46321.
Environmental Protection Agency (1984c) Proposed guidelines for the health assessment of suspect developmental toxicants and request for comments. *Fed. Reg.* **49**(227), 46324–46331.
Environmental Protection Agency (1985a) *Chemical Emergency Preparedness Program-Interim Guidance.* Revision 1, PD5. Washington DC: Environmental Protection Agency.
Environmental Protection Agency (1985b) Toxic substances control act test guidelines; final rules. *Fed. Reg.* **50**(188), 39397–39471.
ECETOC (1985). *Acute Toxicity Tests, LD_{50} (LC_{50}) Determinations and Alternatives*, Monograph No. 6, 6. Brussels: European Chemical Industry Ecology and Toxicology Centre.
Fletcher K. (1984) Paraquat poisoning. In: Ballantyne B. (ed.) *Forensic Toxicology*, 86–98. Bristol: John Wright and Sons.
Frawley J. P. (1964) Emergency exposure limits. *Ind. Hyg. J.* Nov.–Dec., 578–584.
Gad S. C., Smith A. C., Cramp A. L., Gavigan F. A. and Derelanko M. J. (1984) Innovative designs and practices for acute systemic toxicity studies. *Drug Chem. Toxicol.* **7**, 423–434.
Gad S. C., Walsh R. D. and Dunn B. J. (1986) Correlation of ocular and dermal irritancy of industrial chemicals. *J. Toxicol., Cut. and Ocular Toxicol.* **5**, 195–213.
Gaylor D. W. (1983) The use of safety factors for controlling risk. *J. Toxicol. Environ. Health* **11**, 329–336.
Gillette J. R. (1984) Solvable and unsolvable problems in extrapolating toxicology data between animal species and strains. In: Mitchell J. and Horning M. G. (ed.) *Drug Metabolism and Drug Toxicity*, 237–260. New York: Raven Press.
Goldstein B. D. (1983) Toxic substances in the atmospheric environment—a critical review. *J. Air Pollut. Contr. Assoc.* **33**, 454–467.
Grayson J. P. (1985) The closure of a factory and its impact on health. *Int. J. Health Services* **15**, 69–93.
Green D. M. and Tregear R. T. (1984) The action of sensory irritants on the cat's cornea. *J. Physiol. (Lond)* **175**, 37–38.
Habet F. (1924) *Fünf Vortäge aus den Jahren 1920–1923.* Berlin: Springer-Verlag.
Hammond E. C. and Selikoff J. J. (1973) Relation of cigarette smoking to risk of death of asbestos

associated disease among insulation workers in the United States. In Bogorski P., Gilson J. C., Timbrell V., Wagner J. C. and Davis W. (ed.) *Biological Effects of Asbestos* (Scientific Publication No. 8) 312–317. Lyon, France: IARC.

Hanley T. R., Yano B. L., Nitschke K. D. et al. (1984) Comparison of the teratogenic potential of inhaled ethylene glycol monomethyl ether in rats, mice, and rabbits. *Toxicol. Appl. Pharmacol.* **75**, 409–422.

Heylin M. (1985) Bhopal report. *Chem. Eng. News* **63**, 14–65.

Heywood R. (1983) Target organ toxicity II. *Toxicol. Lett.* **18**, 83–88.

Hollingshaus J. G., Armstrong D. and Tora R. F. (1981) Delayed toxicity and delayed neurotoxicity of phosphorothionate and phosphorodithioate esters. *J. Toxicol. Environ. Health.* **8**, 619–627.

Howard J. K. (1980) Paraquat: a review of worker exposure in normal usage. *J. Soc. Occup. Med.* **30**, 6–11.

ILO (1980) *Occupational Exposure Limits for Airborne Toxic Substances*, Occupational Safety and Health Series No. 37, 2nd edn. Geneva: International Labour Office.

Kimbrough R. D., Falk H., Stehr P. et al. (1984) Health implications of 2,3,7,8-tetrachlorodibenzodioxin (TCDD) contamination of residential soil. *J. Toxicol. Environ. Health.* **14**, 47–93.

Kjellstrand P. and Holmquist B. (1984) Pitfalls in the interpretation of long-term inhalation experiments. *Toxicol. Lett.* **21**, 213–218.

Lambert B., Lindblad A., Holmberg K. et al. (1982) Use of sister chromatid exchange to monitor human populations for exposure to toxicologically harmful agents. In: Wolff S. (ed.) *Sister Chromatid Exchange*, 149–182. New York: John Wiley and Sons.

Lappé M. (1983) Ethical issues in testing for differential sensitivity to occupational hazards. *J. Occup. Med.* **25**, 797–808.

Lauwerys R. R. (1983) *Industrial Chemical Exposure: Guidelines for Biological Monitoring*. Davis, California: Biomedical Publications.

Matijak-Schaper M., Wong K-L. and Alarie Y. (1983) A method to rapidly evaluate the acute pulmonary effects of aerosols in unanesthetized guinea pigs. *Toxicol. Appl. Pharmacol.* **69**, 451–480.

Miller R. R. Young J. T., Kociba R. J. et al (1985) Chronic toxicity and oncogenicity bioassay of inhaled ethyl acrylate in Fischer 344 rats and B6C3F1 mice. *Drug Chem. Toxicol.* **8**, 1–42.

McCreesh A. H. and Steinberg M. (1983) Skin irritation testing in animals. In: Marzulli F. N. and Maibach H. I. (ed.) Dermatotoxicology, 147–166. New York: McGraw-Hill.

Murphy S. D. (1983) General principles in the assessment of toxicity of chemical mixtures. *Environ. Health Persp.* **48**, 141–144.

Nagano K., Nakayama E., Koyano M. et al (1979) Testicular atrophy of mice induced by ethylene glycol mono alkyl ethers. *Jap. J. Ind. Health* **21**, 29–35.

National Research Council (1980) *Principles of Toxicology Interactions Associated with Multiple Chemical Exposures*. Washington DC: National Academy of Sciences.

NIOSH (1976) *Occupational Exposure to Phosgene*, Publication No. 76-137. Washington DC: US Department of Health, Education and Welfare, National Institute for Occupational Safety and Health, Center for Disease Control.

NIOSH (1979) *Adverse health effects of smoking and the occupational environment*, Current Intelligence Bulletin No. 31, DHEW (NIOSH) Publication No. 79-122. Cincinnati: National Institute for Occupational Safety and Health.

NPCA (1985) *Hazardous Materials Identification System Revised—Implementation Manual*, 52. Chicago: Labelmaster, National Paint and Coatings Association.

O'Donoghue J. L. (1985) Alkanes, alcohols, ketones, and ethylene oxide. In: O'Donoghue J. L. (ed) *Neurotoxicity of Industrial and Commercial Chemicals. Vol. II*, 61–97. Boca Raton, Florida: CRC Press, Inc.

Onyeama H. P. and Oehme F. W. (1984) A literature review of paraquat toxicity. *Vet. Human. Toxicol.* **26**, 494–502.

OECD (1981) *OECD Guidelines for Testing*. Paris: Organization for Economic Cooperation and Development.

Paull J. M. (1984) The origin and basis of threshold limit values. *Am. J. Ind. Med.* **5**, 227–238.

Pepelko W. E. and Withey J. R. (1985) Methods for route-to-route extrapolation of dose. In: Stara J. F. and Erdreich L. S. (ed.) *Advances in Health Risk Assessment for Systemic Toxicants and Chemical Mixtures*, 153–175. Princeton: Princeton Scientific Publishing Co.

Rowe V. K. and Wolf M. A. (1982) Glycols. In: Clayton G. D. and Clayton F. E. (ed.) *Patty's Industrial Hygiene and Toxicology. Vol. IIC*, 3rd edn. 3817–3832. New York: Wiley-Interscience.

Ruckelshaus W. D. (1985) Risk, science and democracy. *Issues Sci. Technol.* **1**, 19–38.
Scaife M. C. (1985) The rabbit eye irritancy test—are these *in vitro* alternatives? *ATLA* **12**, 157–162.
Seidenfeld J. J., Sobonya R. E. and Toyoshima J. M. (1985) Recovery from paraquat pneumonitis. *Br. J. Ind. Med.* **42**, 178–183.
Seifried H. E. (1986) Eye irritancy testing: historical perspectives and future directions. *J. Toxicol. Cut. Ocular Toxicol.* **5**, 89–114.
Sellakumar A. R., Synder C. A., Solomon J. J. and Albert R. E. (1985) Carcinogenicity of formaldehyde and hydrogen chloride in rats. *Toxicol. Appl. Pharmacol.* **81**, 401–406.
Smyth H. F. Jr. (1959) The toxicological basis of threshold limit values: 1. Experience with threshold limit values based on animal data. *Am. Ind. Hyg. Assoc. J.* **20**, 341–345.
Smyth H. F. Jr. (1962) A toxicologist's view of threshold limits. *Am. Ind. Hyg. Assoc. J.* **23**, 37–44.
Stokinger H. E. (1987) Statistical versus illusory statistical approaches to the estimation of risk from environmental chemicals. *Dangerous Properties and Industrial Materials Report* **7**, 2–8.
Suss R., Kinzel V. and Scribner J. D. (1973) *Cancer—Experiment and Concepts*, 16. New York: Springer-Verlag.
Thomas A. A. (1986) Skin absorption: a potential contributing factor to the BEI. *Appl. Industr. Hyg.* **1**, 87–90.
Toft K., Olofsson T., Tunek A. et al. (1982) Toxic effects on mouse bone marrow caused by inhalation of benzene. *Arch. Toxicol.* **51**, 295–302.
Vainio H. (1985) Current trends in the biological monitoring of exposure to carcinogens. *Schand. J. Work Environ. Health* **11**, 1–6.
WHO (1980) *Recommended Health Based Limits in Occupational Exposure to Heavy Metals*, Technical Report Series No. 647. Geneva: World Health Organization.
WHO (1981) *Health Effects of Combined Exposure in the Workplace*. Technical Report Series No. 662. Geneva: World Health Organization.
Williams N., Atkinson G. W. and Patcheky A. S. (1974) Polymer-fume fever: not so benign. *J. Occup. Med.* **16**, 519–522.
Williams S. J. (1984) Prediction of ocular irritancy potential from dermal irritation test results. *Food Chem. Toxicol.* **22**, 157–161.
Wilmer J. W. G. M., Woutersen L. M., Appleman L. M. et al. (1987) Subacute (4-week) inhalation toxicity study of formaldehyde in male rats: 8-hour intermittent versus 8-hour continuous exposures. *J. Appl. Toxicol.* **7**, 15–16.
Wong R. C. and Stevens J. B. (1986) Bipyridylium herbicide toxicity *in vitro*: comparative study of the cytotoxicity of paraquat and diquat toward the pulmonary alveolar macrophage. *J. Toxicol. Environ. Health* **18**, 393–407.
Zbinden G. (1979) Application of basic concepts to research in toxicology. *Pharmacol. Reviews* **30**, 605–616.
Zbinden G. and Flury-Roversi M. (1981) Significance of the LD_{50}-test for the toxicological evaluation of chemical substances. *Arch. Toxicol.* **47**, 77–99.
Zielhuis R. L. and Henderson P. Th. (1986) Definitions of monitoring activities and their relevance for the practice of occupational health. *Int. Arch. Occup. Environ. Health* **57**, 249–257.
Zielhuis R. L. and van der Kreek F. W. (1979) The use of a safety factor in setting health based permissible levels for occupational exposure. *Int. Arch. Occup. Environ. Health.* **42**, 192–201.

Index